Handbook of Veterinary Microbiology and Disease

Handbook of Veterinary Microbiology and Disease

Edited by Emily Jackson

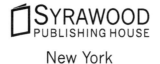

New York

Published by Syrawood Publishing House,
750 Third Avenue, 9th Floor,
New York, NY 10017, USA
www.syrawoodpublishinghouse.com

Handbook of Veterinary Microbiology and Disease
Edited by Emily Jackson

International Standard Book Number: 978-1-64740-442-0 (Hardback)

Cataloging-in-publication Data

Handbook of veterinary microbiology and disease / edited by Emily Jackson.
    p. cm.
Includes bibliographical references and index.
ISBN 978-1-64740-442-0
1. Veterinary microbiology. 2. Animals--Diseases. 3. Communicable diseases in animals.
4. Veterinary medicine. I. Jackson, Emily.
SF780.2 .H36 2023
636.089 690 41--dc23

TABLE OF CONTENTS

PREFACE

Veterinary microbiology is a field of microbiology that is concerned with bacterial and viral diseases of vertebrate animals, which are domesticated for providing food supply, companionship, or other useful products. These diseases have significance in veterinary medicine, as they have the capability for inducing illnesses in livestock and domesticated animals and causing economic loss. Furthermore, they are a significant threat towards animal welfare and health. Veterinary microbiology is involved in the study of the underlying mechanisms of virulence in pathogens, antimicrobial resistance and epidemiology of pathogens. Infectious diseases within this field are detected primarily through two methods, by confirming the traces of microorganisms or by detecting the presence of antibodies generated against the organism. Some of the different techniques used for the detection of diseases in animals are nucleic acid amplification, cytology, antigen assays, bacteriological culture, microarrays and fecal examination. This book explores all the important aspects of veterinary microbiology and disease. The readers would gain knowledge that would broaden their perspective in this area of veterinary science.

After months of intensive research and writing, this book is the end result of all who devoted their time and efforts in the initiation and progress of this book. It will surely be a source of reference in enhancing the required knowledge of the new developments in the area. During the course of developing this book, certain measures such as accuracy, authenticity and research focused analytical studies were given preference in order to produce a comprehensive book in the area of study.

This book would not have been possible without the efforts of the authors and the publisher. I extend my sincere thanks to them. Secondly, I express my gratitude to my family and well-wishers. And most importantly, I thank my students for constantly expressing their willingness and curiosity in enhancing their knowledge in the field, which encourages me to take up further research projects for the advancement of the area.

Editor

Usefulness of the Ranking Technique in the Microscopic Agglutination Test (MAT) to Predict the Most Likely Infecting Serogroup of *Leptospira*

Israel Barbosa Guedes, Gisele Oliveira de Souza, Juliana Fernandes de Paula Castro,
Matheus Burilli Cavalini, Antônio Francisco de Souza Filho and Marcos Bryan Heinemann*

*Departamento de Medicina Veterinária Preventiva e Saúde Animal, Faculdade de Medicina Veterinária e Zootecnia,
Universidade de São Paulo, São Paulo, Brazil*

Correspondence:
Marcos Bryan Heinemann
marcosbryan@usp.br

The microscopic agglutination test (MAT) used for the serological diagnosis of leptospirosis, as a robust and inexpensive method, is still the reality in many laboratories worldwide. Both the performance and the interpretation of the MAT vary from region to region, making standardization difficult. The prediction of the probable infecting serogroup using this test is indispensable for elucidating the epidemiology of the disease; however, in veterinary medicine, many studies consider any reaction detected with a titer of 100, which may ultimately overestimate some serogroups. Thus, the aim of this study was to evaluate the usefulness of the ranking technique for predicting the probable infecting serogroup identified by the MAT, eliminating cross reactions with other serogroups. *Leptospira* strains (12 samples) were inoculated in hamsters, and after 30 days, serology was performed by the MAT for these animals to confirm the infecting serogroup. Using the ranking technique, the probable infectious serogroup found with the MAT was the same as that in which the strains of inoculated leptospires belonged; additionally, the technique can be applied in epidemiological studies involving herds.

Keywords: leptospirosis, serology, MAT, diagnostic, epidemiology

INTRODUCTION

Leptospirosis is an emerging disease that affects various species of mammals, including humans. The disease is caused by pathogenic bacteria of the genus *Leptospira*, which encompass several serogroups that comprise a variety of serovars (1, 2). The great importance in knowing the predominant *Leptospira* serogroups circulating in a population is the contribution to elucidating the epidemiological chain of the disease, which influences the adoption of effective control measures (3).

The microscopic agglutination test (MAT) is considered a reference in the serological diagnosis of leptospirosis, mainly for epidemiological studies, as it is able to test for several serovars that represent different serogroups at once. The principle of the technique is based on the antigen-antibody reaction and detects both IgM and IgG classes of antibodies. The MAT is carried out in two stages. First is screening, in which only the reactive sera in the initial dilution (commonly

1:100) are considered positive and subjected to a second step for titration; in this case; the serum is diluted consecutively in a two-fold ratio and analyzed until the dilution where the serum stops reacting (between 50 and 100% leptospires free under dark field microscopy). In interpreting the results, many laboratories end up determining the positive limit of the test with a titer of 100 (1, 4).

Using the ranking technique, initially named the most likely serotype, only the reaction for a single serogroup with the highest titer is considered per animal, while other reactions with lower titers for other serogroups are disregarded, as well as samples in which a tie occurs for two or more serogroups with predominant titers (5). A general scheme for how the ranking technique can be used in MAT for a herd is shown in **Figure 1**. This technique can be very useful for epidemiological studies, as it seems to reduce paradoxical reactions, being used both for herds (5–8) and for humans (9); however, the ability of this technique to identify the presumptive infecting serogroup, namely, the most likely, has not been examined. Thus, the aim of this study was to evaluate the usefulness of the ranking technique for predicting the most likely infecting serogroup with the MAT carried out with serum from experimentally infected hamsters.

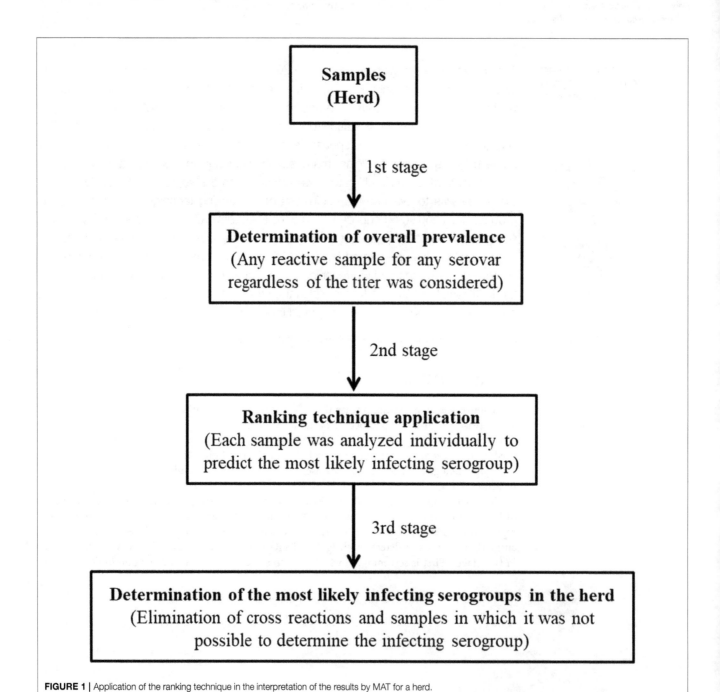

FIGURE 1 | Application of the ranking technique in the interpretation of the results by MAT for a herd.

TABLE 1 | Strains of leptospires used in this study (10).

Strain	Species	Serogroup
M02/20-52	*L. borgpetersenii*	Sejroe
M02/20-121	*L. borgpetersenii*	Sejroe
M02/20-144	*L. kirschneri*	Autumnalis
M02/20-126	*L. kirschneri*	Grippotyphosa
M02/20-111	*L. kirschneri*	Icterohaemorrhagiae
M02/20-03	*L. santarosai*	Autumnalis
M02/20-18	*L. santarosai*	Tarassovi
M02/20-114	*L. santarosai*	Not determined
M02/20-115	*L. santarosai*	Autumnalis
M02/20-46	*L. noguchii*	Panama
M02/20-155	*L. interrogans*	Canicola
M02/20-136	*L. interrogans*	Icterohaemorrhagiae

MATERIALS AND METHODS

This study was carried out from August to October 2020 and approved by the Ethics Committee on Animal Use of the School of Veterinary Medicine and Animal Science (Universidade de São Paulo) – CEUA/FMVZ no. 5724220920. Twelve strains of *Leptospira*, isolated from cattle raised in the Brazilian Amazon (**Table 1**), were grown in the EMJH medium (Ellinghausen-McCullough-Johnson-Harris) until they reached a concentration of ∼2×10^8 leptospires/mL. These samples were chosen because they were isolated from cattle, and most of the laboratory routine tested by us is focused on this species, further considering that it is a species in which cross reactions in serology are observed. In addition, since bovine leptospirosis is a herd disease, the diagnosis of this disease must always be performed at the herd level.

Before inoculation of the strains in hamsters (*Mesocricetus auratus*), blood was collected from the animals and subjected to serology using the MAT according to Faine et al. (1) to verify the absence of anti-*Leptospira* spp. antibodies. Then, 0.5 mL of each strain was inoculated intraperitoneally into hamsters weighing between 60 and 100 g for a total of 24 adult animals (2 animals per strain).

The animals were kept under observation for a period of 30 days or until the manifestation of clinical signs of leptospirosis (bristly hair, prostration, photophobia, jaundice, and weight loss), and the presence of these symptoms was the determining factor for carrying out euthanasia, thus avoiding natural death and prolonged stress. In this way, the hamsters were anesthetized, and blood collection was carried out through cardiac puncture. Immediately after, euthanasia and necropsy of the animals were performed, and fragments of the kidneys (1 × 1 cm) were obtained and macerated in sterile Sorensen buffered saline (1:10) and observed directly under dark field microscopy for detection of leptospires. Thus, tissue colonization and renal carriage were confirmed.

The serum samples from the animals were subjected to the MAT by applying a panel with 24 serovars of *Leptospira* spp.

used in the routine serological diagnosis of leptospirosis by the laboratory (**Supplementary Material 1**); moreover, the serum was also tested against the respective strain with which the animal was inoculated (challenge strains). The results were tabulated and analyzed using the ranking technique, considering only the predominant titers found in the MAT for each serum sample, and in this way, stipulating which serogroup was the most likely that infected the animal, discarding the cross reactions with the antigens of the standard MAT panel.

RESULTS

All animals used in this study, before the inoculation of the *Leptospira* strains, were negative in the MAT, ensuring that after the inoculation, the detected antibodies were obtained only due to the immune response against the inoculated strains. Furthermore, leptospires were detected in the kidneys of all post inoculation animals, demonstrating the ability of the strains to colonize renal tissue and consequently make the animal a carrier. No clinical signs suggestive of leptospirosis or macroscopic lesions on the organs of the animals were observed.

Regarding serology, the ranking technique did not alter the execution of the MAT in any way; it was only applied in the interpretations of MAT results, which were grouped into cases (**Table 2**). These cases represented possible situations that are commonly observed in the performance of serological studies. It is important to emphasize that the highest titers (800–6,400) were detected against the inoculated strains themselves (challenge strains), meaning there was an immune response from the animals, and any reaction to another serogroup other than that which the inoculated strain belonged was considered a cross reaction.

DISCUSSION

Despite in the literature there are no reports of evaluate the effectiveness of the ranking technique in a controlled way, when the infectious serogroup is known (experimental inoculation), this technique were used in MAT serology for random herds of cattle, buffaloes, sheep, horses and other species (5–8).

First, it is worth noting that the ranking technique, when used, does not negate any sample that was reactive for at least one antigen of the MAT panel, regardless of the titer found, and if there was a tie between antigens from different serogroups, the sample remains positive for leptospirosis and can be considered for calculating the general prevalence of the disease within a herd; however, it is not possible to predict the most likely infecting serogroup for this sample, so it is disregarded only to stipulate the serogroups prevalent in a herd (5–8).

In case 1, the predominant serogroup was the only serogroup detected in the MAT, and no cross reactions were detected since the only serogroups found were the same serogroups to which the challenge strains belonged.

In case 2, reactions were found for more than one antigen, but the antigens belonged to the same serogroup, and even though there was a tie between two antigens with the highest titer

TABLE 2 | Results obtained by serology performed with the serum of animals inoculated with *Leptospira* spp.

Case	Strain	Serogroup strain	Serology (MAT)		Serogroup (ranking technique)
			Challenge strain titer	Serovar/serogroup titer	
1	M02/20-126	Grippotyphosa	126: 800	**Grip/Grip: 400***	Grippotyphosa
	M02/20-46	Panama	46: 1600	**Pan/Pan: 800***	Panama
	M02/20-18	Tarassovi	18: 800	**Tara/Tara: 400***	Tarassovi
2	M02/20-52	Sejroe	52: 800	Gua/Sej: 100	Sejroe
				Hard/Sej: 400*	
				Hbov/Sej: 400*	
	M02/20-121	Sejroe	121: 800	Gua/Sej: 100	Sejroe
				Hard/Sej: 400*	
				Hbov/Sej: 400*	
	M02/20-136	Icterohaemorrhagiae	136: 1600	**Cope/Ict: 800***	Icterohaemorrhagiae
				Ict/Ict: 200	
3	M02/20-03	Autumnalis	03: 3200	**But/Aut: 1600***	Autumnalis
				Cyn/Cyn: 200	
	M02/20-155	Canicola	155: 3200	**Can/Can:800***	Canicola
				Pan/Pan:400	
	M02/20-144	Autumnalis	144: 6400	**But/Aut: 800***	Autumnalis
				Grip/Grip: 400	
	M02/20-111	Icterohaemorrhagiae	111: 1600	**Cop/Ict: 400***	Icterohaemorrhagiae
				Can/Can:100	
	M02/20-115	Autumnalis	115: 3.200	**Aut/Aut: 1600***	Autumnalis
				Brat/Brat:200	
				Pom/Pom: 100	
4	M02/20-114	Not determined	114: 800	Negative	Not determined

Grip, Grippotyphosa; Pan, Panama; Tara, Tarassovi; Gua, Guaricura; Sej, Sejroe; Hard, Hardjo-Prajitno; Hbov, Hardjo-Bovis; Cope, Copenhageni; Ict, Icterohaemorrhagiae; But, Butembo; Aut, Autumnalis; Cyn, Cynopteri; Can, Canicola; Brat, Bratislava; Pom, Pomona.
*Highest titer found and considered the most likely.

(Hard/Hbov), both are in the Sejroe serogroup; in this situation, the predominant serogroup was Sejroe. This phenomenon happens due to the cross reaction that normally occurs between serovars that belong to the same serogroup (1, 2).

In case 3, the animals were reactive for more than a single serogroup, and there was a variation in the titers, with the predominant titer attributed to the most likely serogroup, and the other reactions for the other serogroups disregarded. In addition, the most likely serogroup indicated by the ranking technique was compatible with the serogroup of the *Leptospira* strains inoculated in the respective animal. This seems to be the greatest utility of the ranking technique applied in the MAT for a herd because, if case 3 represented a herd, we would have identified the serogroups Autumnalis, Cynopteri, Canicola, Panama, Grippotyphosa, Icterohaemorrhagiae, Bratislava and Pomona, when in fact the real serogroups circulating in the herd would be Autumnalis, Canicola and Icterohaemorrhagiae; the other serogroups would be overestimated. In this case it is also common occurs a tie for two or more serogroups with predominant titers in a same sample, which would result in the disregard of this sample for the definition of the prevalent serogroups within the herd, however it would continue to be considered reactive for leptospirosis. This situation was not observed in this study.

During the organization and serological classification of leptospires, some serovars that belonged to a serogroup were removed and grouped into other serogroups due to serological affinity, such as what happened with the serovar Butembo, which previously belonged to the serogroup Cynopteri and was later added to the serogroup Autumnalis, remaining today in this serogroup (11). This indicates that antigens from different serogroups can be serologically related, which does not exclude the possibility of cross reaction between them.

Cross reactions between different serogroups usually occur in the MAT during acute cases of the disease since there is an increase in the production of IgM, a circumstance that makes it difficult to interpret the test (1, 12). Nevertheless, in this study, the serology of the animals was performed 30 days after inoculation, when the disease was in the chronic phase (13), and cross reactions were also found. This situation is frequently observed in epidemiological studies, wherein random sampling, it is not possible to establish which phase of the disease the animal is in (5–8).

The identification of acute cases occurs mainly in the presence of clinical signs of the disease (1); however, clinical signs may not be so easily detected, as occurs in cattle infected with strains adapted to them, such as those belonging to the Sejroe serogroup, which silently compromises the reproductive system of these animals (14). Further, different *Leptospira* strains (non-Sejroe) recovered from bovines without observation of clinical signs demonstrates the adaptability that these bacteria may have in the host (15).

We found it interesting to include a *Leptospira* strain in which the serogroup had not been determined, which was represented in case 4, and as a result, the animals were not reactive in the MAT and thus considered negative for leptospirosis; nonetheless, the animals were reactive for the strain that was inoculated and showed renal colonization. Apparently, strain M02/20-114 belongs to a serogroup that is not represented in the MAT panel that was used, which reinforces the importance of adapting the panel of antigens utilized in the MAT, inserting locally isolated strains to increase the sensitivity of the test (2, 7). It should be emphasized that, in cattle, leptospires can be recovered from the urine of negative animals in serology (16), which would be important for an efficient diagnosis the association with other techniques such as PCR, for example.

In conclusion, MAT is a traditional test and are provides a richness of information, therefore its replacement may be difficult to happen. The ranking technique is another way of interpreting the results obtained by MAT, in order to refine the data reducing the occurrence of cross reactions between the serogroups. Thus, we demonstrate how this technique can be useful in the MAT for predicting the most likely infecting serogroup of *Leptospira* and can be applied, especially in epidemiological studies involving herds.

ETHICS STATEMENT

The animal study was reviewed and approved by CEUA FMVZ 5724220920.

AUTHOR CONTRIBUTIONS

IG, GS, JC, MC, and AS performed the all laboratory tests. IG and MH performed the interpretation of the results. IG wrote the manuscript. MH accurately reviewed the manuscript. All authors contributed to the article and approved the submitted version.

ACKNOWLEDGMENTS

MH thanked CNPq (Conselho Nacional de Desenvolvimento Científico e Tecnológico) the fellowship. IG and JC thanked CAPES (Coordenação de Aperfeiçoamento de Pessoal de Nível Superior) for the scholarship.

REFERENCES

1. Faine S, Adler B, Bolin C, Perolat P. *Leptospira and Leptospirosis.* 2nd ed. Melbourne: Medisci. (1999). 272p.
2. Levett PN. Leptospirosis. *Clin Microbiol Rev.* (2001) 13:296–326. doi: 10.1128/CMR.14.2.296-326.2001
3. Assenga JA, Matemba LE, Muller SK, Mhampi GG, Kazwala RR. Predominant leptospiral serogroups circulating among humans, livestock and wildlife in Katavi-Rukwa ecosystem, Tanzania. *PLoS Negl Trop Dis.* (2015) 9:e0003607. doi: 10.1371/journal.pntd.0003607
4. World Health Organization (WHO). *Human Leptospirosis: Guidance for Diagnosis, Surveillance and Control.* Geneva: World Health Organization (2003).
5. Vasconcellos SA, Barbarini Junior O, Umehara O, Morais ZM, Cortez A, Pinheiro SR, et al. Leptospirose bovina. Níveis de ocorrência e sorotipos predominantes em rebanhos dos Estados de Minas Gerais, São Paulo, Rio de Janeiro, Paraná, Rio Grande do Sul e Mato Grosso do Sul, no período de janeiro a abril de 1996. *Arq Inst Biol.* (1997) 64:7–15.
6. Favero ACM, Pineiro SR, Vasconcellos SA, Morais ZM, Ferreira F, Ferreira Neto JS. Most frequent serovar of Leptospires in serological tests of buffaloes, sheeps, goats, horses, swines and dogs from several Brazilian states. *Cienc Rural.* (2002) 32:613–9. doi: 10.1590/S0103-84782002000400011
7. Sarmento AMC, Azevedo SS, Morais ZM, Souza GO, Oliveira FCS, Gonçalves AP, et al. Use of *Leptospira* spp. strains isolated in Brazil in the microscopic agglutination test applied to diagnosis of leptospirosis in cattle herds in eight Brazilian states. *Pesq Vet Bras.* (2012) 32:601–6. doi: 10.1590/S0100-736X2012000700003
8. Guedes IB, Souza GO, Oliveira LAR, Castro JFP, Souza-Filho AF, Maia, et al. Prevalence of *Leptospira* serogroups in buffaloes from the Brazilian Amazon. *Vet Med Sci.* (2020) 6:433–40. doi: 10.1002/vms3.271
9. Levett PN. Usefulness of serologic analysis as a predictor of the infecting serovar in patients with severe leptospirosis. *Clin Infect Dis.* (2003) 36:447–52. doi: 10.1086/346208
10. Guedes IB, Souza GO, Rocha KS, Cavalini MB, Damasceno Neto MS, Castro JFP, et al. *Leptospira* strains isolated from cattle in the Amazon region, Brazil, evidence of a variety of species and serogroups with a high frequency of the Sejroe serogroup. *Comp Immunol Microbiol Infect Dis.* (2021) 74:e101579. doi: 10.1016/j.cimid.2020.101579
11. Dikken H, Kmety E. Chapter VIII serological typing methods of leptospires. *Methods Microbiol.* (1978) 11:259–307. doi: 10.1016/S0580-9517(08)70493-8
12. Haake DA, Levett PN. Leptospirosis in humans. *Curr Top Mirobiol Immunol.* (2015) 387:65–97. doi: 10.1007/978-3-662-45059-8_5
13. Zuerner RL, Alt DP, Palmer MV. Development of chronic and acute golden Syrian hamster infection models with *Leptospira borgpetersenii* serovar Hardjo. *Vet Pathol.* (2012) 49:403–11. doi: 10.1177/0300985811409252
14. Loureiro AP, Lilenbaum W. Genital bovine leptospirosis: a new look for an old disease. *Theriogenology.* (2020) 141:41–7. doi: 10.1016/j.theriogenology.2019.09.011
15. Pinto PS, Pestana C, Medeiros MA, Lilenbaum W. Plurality of *Leptospira* strains on slaughtered animals suggest a broader concept of adaptability of leptospires to cattle. *Acta Trop.* (2017) 172:156–9. doi: 10.1016/j.actatropica.2017.04.032
16. Libonati H, Pinto PS, Lilenbaum W. Seronegativity of bovines face to their own recovered leptospiral isolates. *Microb Pathog.* (2017) 108:101–3. doi: 10.1016/j.micpath.2017.05.001

2

Detection of *Anaplasma Phagocytophilum* in Horses with Suspected Tick-Borne Disease in Northeastern United States by Metagenomic Sequencing

*Murugan Subbiah[1†], Nagaraja Thirumalapura[1], David Thompson[1], Suresh V. Kuchipudi[2,3], Bhushan Jayarao[2,3] and Deepanker Tewari[1]**

[1] Pennsylvania Veterinary Laboratory, Harrisburg, PA, United States, [2] Animal Diagnostic Laboratory, Pennsylvania State University, University Park, PA, United States, [3] Center for Infectious Disease Dynamics, Pennsylvania State University, University Park, PA, United States

*Correspondence:
Deepanker Tewari
dtewari@pa.gov

Metagenomic sequencing of clinical diagnostic specimens has a potential for unbiased detection of infectious agents, diagnosis of polymicrobial infections and discovery of emerging pathogens. Herein, next generation sequencing (NGS)-based metagenomic approach was used to investigate the cause of illness in a subset of horses recruited for a tick-borne disease surveillance study during 2017–2019. Blood samples collected from 10 horses with suspected tick-borne infection and five apparently healthy horses were subjected to metagenomic analysis. Total genomic DNA extracted from the blood samples were enriched for microbial DNA and subjected to shotgun next generation sequencing using Nextera DNA Flex library preparation kit and V2 chemistry sequencing kit on the Illumina MiSeq sequencing platform. Overall, 0.4–0.6 million reads per sample were analyzed using Kraken metagenomic sequence classification program. The taxonomic classification of the reads indicated that bacterial genomes were overrepresented (0.5 to 1%) among the total microbial reads. Most of the bacterial reads (~91%) belonged to phyla Firmicutes, Proteobacteria, Bacteroidetes, Actinobacteria, Cyanobacteria and Tenericutes in both groups. Importantly, 10–42.5% of Alphaproteobacterial reads in 5 of 10 animals with suspected tick-borne infection were identified as *Anaplasma phagocytophilum*. Of the 5 animals positive for *A. phagocytophilum* sequence reads, four animals tested *A. phagocytophilum* positive by PCR. Two animals with suspected tick-borne infection and *A. phagocytophilum* positive by PCR were found negative for any tick-borne microbial reads by metagenomic analysis. The present study demonstrates the usefulness of the NGS-based metagenomic analysis approach for the detection of blood-borne microbes.

Keywords: tick-borne disease, anaplasma, next- generation sequencing, metagenoimcs, blood, microbiome, horse

INTRODUCTION

Tick-borne pathogens pose a growing threat to both animals and public health because ticks often harbor multiple known and unknown pathogens and geographic range of ticks is expanding in recent decades (1). Ticks are known to transmit bacteria, viruses and protozoal pathogens, and tick-borne pathogens account for much of vector-borne diseases in temperate regions of North America, Europe and Asia (2). Important tick-borne diseases of horses include Lyme disease, equine granulocytic anaplasmosis, Tick-borne Encephalitis Virus (TBEV) and equine Piroplasmosis (3–6). While Lyme disease and equine granulocytic anaplasmosis are frequently reported in horses in the United States, TBEV and equine piroplasmosis are considered non-endemic (3–6).

Diagnosis of tick-borne diseases can be challenging due to non-specific clinical signs and transmission of multiple pathogens by ticks (7). Diagnosis is commonly based on history of tick bite, clinical suspicion, serology, and detection of antigen or pathogen nucleic acid. Although serology is a primary method of diagnosis, it lacks sensitivity early during infection due to absence of detectable levels of antibodies and may also lack specificity due to cross-reactive antibodies (8). Furthermore, demonstration of pathogen-specific antibodies does not differentiate between current infection and past exposure. In contrast, PCR assays are highly sensitive and specific. However, use of single or multiplex PCR assays may result in missed detection of non-targeted or unknown etiologies and therefore strategies targeting multiple pathogens have been attempted with limited success (9). In this context, Next Generation Sequencing (NGS)-based metagenomic approach has a potential for the detection of diverse microbial pathogens and discovery of novel/unknown etiologies of infectious diseases (10–12). However, limited studies have examined the feasibility of using NGS-based metagenomic analysis for the diagnosis of tick-borne diseases in either humans or animals (13, 14).

In this study, we investigated use of metagenomic based NGS analysis of blood microbiome from horses with suspected tick-borne disease and compared it to apparently healthy horses. The study established the feasibility of NGS-based metagenomic shot gun approach for the detection of tick-borne pathogens in blood samples.

MATERIALS AND METHODS
Blood Sample and Extraction of Total Genomic DNA

A subset of blood samples ($n = 10$) were randomly selected for metagenomic analysis from a larger cohort of horses suspected of having tick-borne diseases (TBD) recruited for studying prevalence of *Anaplasma phagocytophilum* and *Borrelia burgdorferi* infections during 2017–2019. In addition, blood samples ($n = 5$) from apparently healthy horses that were not part of the TBD study cohort were included in the metagenomic study. The horses with suspected tick-borne illnesses often had history of tick exposure and showed clinical signs such as fever, depression, petechiae, and inappetence. The reported clinical signs among the horses included in the study are listed in **Table 1**

and horses suspected with tick-borne infection with clinical signs are referred as "sick group."

Blood samples were collected in EDTA vacutainer tubes (BD Bioscience, San Jose, CA). The total genomic DNA from blood samples were extracted using the Blood or Body Fluids Spin Protocol (QIAmp DNA extraction mini kit, Qiagen, Germantown, MD) following the manufacturer's instructions. The extracted DNA was not treated with RNAase and the quality and quantity of the DNA were analyzed by spectrophotometry (Nanodrop, Thermo Fisher Scientific, Waltham, MA) and fluorometric method (Qubit, Thermo Fisher Scientific, Waltham, MA), respectively.

Microbial DNA Enrichment

Microbial DNA from the horse blood samples was enriched using the Illustra DNA enrichment kit (Biolabs, New England, MA). Briefly, up to 1 µg of total nucleic acid extracted from blood samples was subjected to illustra DNA enrichment protocol, which binds and removes a proportion of mammalian genomic DNA. These enriched DNA were then amplified using Genomiphi DNA amplification kit (GE Healthcare, UK) and the quantity of enriched and amplified blood DNA was estimated using Qubit.

Sequencing

Between 100 to 500 ng of enriched and amplified genomic DNA samples were used to prepare library for NGS using Nextera DNA Flex Library Preparation Kit (Illumina, San Diego, CA) according to the manufacturer's protocol. The quantity and the fragment size of libraries were measured using Qubit and Bioanalyzer (Agilent, Santa Clara, CA), respectively. The individual libraries were normalized according to the manufacturer's protocol and then pooled (5–6 samples per pool) before loading into MiSeq instrument (Illumina, San Diego, CA). MiSeq Reagent Kit v2 (2 × 150; 2 × 250 cycles) was used for sequencing the DNA libraries.

Bioinformatics Analysis

The MiSeq run quality was checked using Illumina Sequencing Analysis Viewer. The trimmed reads from MiSeq runs were collected as fastaq files, analyzed in cloud based BaseSpace (Illumina) platform and the quality was analyzed using Quast application (quast.sourceforge.net). Samples that contained good quality reads (Quast default standards) were further analyzed for the taxonomic identification using Kraken metagenomic analysis application v2.0.1 that uses an exact-alignment database queries of k-mers from each read (15). A subset of reads categorized as unidentified by Kraken were mapped to determine the taxa using nucleotide blast search in NCBI. The detection threshold for microbial DNA reads was set at 1% of total microbial reads and microbial phylum/families/genera/species reads that constitute > 1% of the respective microbial taxonomy were considered for further analyses. The Shannon indices for richness and diversity and Simpson's index for evenness of microbial families/genera/species (16) were estimated using online statistical tools (datanalytics.org.uk; easycalculation.com). Hutchinson's *t*-test was used to estimate the statistical significance of diversity index between healthy and sick groups. Average percent of each microbial family/genus/species were

TABLE 1 | Demographic, clinical and laboratory analyses for horses included in the study.

Sample ID*	Age (years)	Temperature (°C)	Metagenome analysis	PCR	Presence of morulae	Clinical parameters and history
SAMN18751441	3	39.66	0	0	No	Inappetence, Tick exposure.
SAMN18751440	21	38.94	1	1	Yes	Depression; edema.
SAMN18751442	18	40.33	1	1	Yes	Depression, petechiae and inappetence, low hematocrit values.
SAMN18751435	25	40	0	0	No	Depression, petechiae, inappetence.
SAMN18751436	21	40	0	0	No	Inappetence.
SAMN18751437	22	40.33	1	1	No	Depression, inappetence, tick exposure, edema and petechiae.
SAMN18751439	NA	40.56	0	1	No	Depression and tick exposure.
SAMN18751438	7	NA	1	1	Yes	Low hematocrit values.
SAMN18751447	18	40.56	1	0	No	Depression, petechiae and inappetence.
SAMN18751443	1	NA	0	1	No	None reported.
SAMN18751444	17	37.22	0	0	No	Healthy
SAMN18751445	15	37.22	0	0	No	Healthy
SAMN18751446	9	37.22	0	0	No	Healthy
SAMN18751448	22	37.22	0	0	No	Healthy
SAMN18751449	25	37.22	0	0	No	Healthy

*The metagenome data can be accessed at https://www.ncbi.nlm.nih.gov/sra/PRJNA722464.
NA, not available; PCR and Next-Generation Metagenomic analyses: 0 - negative and 1 - positive.

TABLE 2 | The composition (%) of major circulating microbial DNA present in healthy and sick equine blood samples.

	Healthy (n = 5)	Sick (n = 10)
Bacteria	0.80	0.72 ± 0.06 (0.5–1.0)
Virus	0.01 ± 0.004 (0.01–0.03)	0.01
Fungi	0.16 ± 0.02 (0.1–0.2)	0.29 ± 0.13 (0.11–1.5)
Apicomplexa	0.14 ± 0.02 (0.1–0.16)	0.24 ± 0.12 (0.1–1.3)
Archaea	0.03	0.02
# of reads*	386,375 ±113,142 (139,595–753,414)	653,318 ± 188,828 (80,491–1,965,941)

The percentages and standard errors were estimated out of total number of reads (for fungi and apicomplexa out of total number of domain eukaryote reads). The values in the parenthesis indicate the range; n = number of samples.
*The mean number of reads with standard error of mean and the range are included.

estimated for both healthy and sick groups and the prominent microbial families/genera/species that are relevant to equine infections are discussed more in details.

Anaplasma Phagocytophilum Real-Time PCR

A. phagocytophilum msp2 gene was amplified and detected using a real-time PCR as described previously (17).

RESULTS

NGS Data Analysis and Quality Control

A total of 8,826,219 good quality reads were generated with an average of 0.4–0.6 million reads per sample from apparently healthy horses ($n = 5$) and horses with suspected tick-borne

infection ($n = 10$). The sequence data of this project were submitted to NCBI, BioProject reference number PRJNA722464 (https://www.ncbi.nlm.nih.gov/sra/PRJNA722464). Overall, 95–97% of the reads from each sample were considered belonging to host DNA. Microbial reads contributed to 1.1 and 1.3% of total reads from healthy and sick samples, respectively (**Table 2**). The remaining non-host genome reads were mapped to microbes from other Eukarya and plant kingdom (data not shown). Approximately 97 to 98% of the microbial reads were assigned to bacteria, virus, fungi and apicomplexan groups. Overall, no differences were noted in the percentages of total microbial and host reads between these two groups of animals.

Microbial Content of Blood Samples

Analysis of microbial reads using Shannon and Simpson diversity indices showed presence of a diverse population of microbial DNA comprising apicomplexan parasites, bacteria, viruses and fungi in both healthy and sick horses ($P > 0.01$). Notably, the low (below 0.5) Simpson's evenness index was suggestive of uneven distribution of the microbial genera in both sick and healthy horses (**Supplementary Table 1**).

Bacterial Diversity in Equine Blood

Most of the bacterial reads (~91%) from horses with suspected tick-borne infection and apparently healthy group were assigned to the phyla belonging to Firmicutes, Proteobacteria, Bacteroidetes, Actinobacteria, Cyanobacteria and Tenericutes (**Figure 1**). Bacterial Phyla that represented <2% of total bacterial reads were not included for analysis. Notably, a higher level of Proteobacteria was found in horses with suspected tick-borne infection compared to apparently healthy horses. In

Detection of Anaplasma Phagocytophilum in Horses with Suspected Tick-Borne Disease...

9

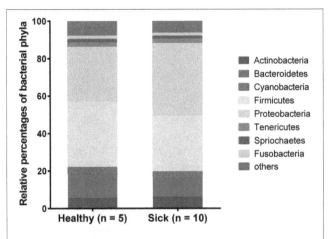

FIGURE 1 | Relative abundance of circulating bacterial phyla reads from horses with suspected tick-borne infection (sick) and apparently healthy animals. The percentages were estimated out of total bacterial reads.

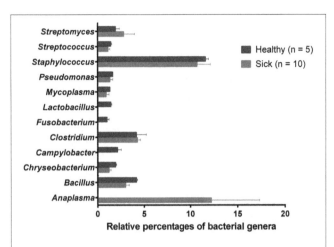

FIGURE 2 | Relative abundance (average percentage + standard error) of bacterial genera. No difference (P-value = 0.54) in the diversity of bacterial genera between healthy (H = 2.28) and sick (H = 2.18) groups. Simpson's evenness scores show uneven distribution of bacterial species in both apparently healthy (0.42) and sick (0.33) groups.

contrast, a higher proportion of Bacteroidetes and Firmicutes genomes were found in apparently healthy horses compared to sick horses.

Analysis of bacterial reads at genus level showed a diverse composition [Shannon diversity index (H) > 2 for both apparently healthy and sick groups, **Supplementary Table 1**] of microbial population comprising multiple genera (**Figure 2**). *Anaplasma* was the most abundant genus in 5 of the 10 samples (range 10–42.5%) from sick horses and was only present in the samples from sick horses. Notably, four out of five samples containing *Anaplasma phagocytophilum* reads by metagenomic analysis were also positive by a *A. phagocytophilum* PCR. One animal from the sick group that was positive for *A. phagocytophilum* reads by metagenomic analysis tested negative by PCR. Two animals from the sick group that tested positive for *A. phagocytophilum* by PCR did not have any *Anaplasma* sp. reads by metagenomic analysis (**Table 1**). Genera *Bacillus* and *Chryseobacterium* were relatively more abundant in apparently healthy horses and reads for genera *Campylobacter*, *Fusobacterium*, and *Lactobacillus* were found exclusively in healthy horses (**Figure 2**). Overall, *A. phagocytophilum* was the most abundant bacterial species found in animals with suspected tick-borne infection (**Table 3**).

Distribution of Viruses, Fungi and Apicomplexa

The viral reads represented a very small proportion, ~0.01% of total reads analyzed (**Table 2**), belonging mainly to DNA viruses. Even with very small percentages of reads, no significant differences were observed in the major viral families between the two groups of horses. Similarly, no significant differences were observed in the percentages of fungal or Apicomplexa reads between the sick and healthy groups. These findings were considered of no significance due to low read counts.

TABLE 3 | Major bacterial species detected with equine blood metagenomic analysis.

Bacterial species	Percentage of bacterial reads	
	Healthy (*n* = 5)	Sick (*n* = 10)
Anaplasma phagocytophilum	0	12.2 ± 5.1
Staphylococcus aureus	9.0 ± 0.4	7.9 ± 1.7
Staphylococcus simulans	0	1.4 ± 0.7
Streptomyces sp. ICC1	0	1.4 ± 0.9

The percentages and standard error were estimated out of total number of bacterial reads. n = number of samples.

DISCUSSION

Recent advances in Next Generation Sequencing (NGS)-based metagenomic analysis have potential clinical applications including diagnosis of infectious diseases, host microbiome analysis, host immune response analysis and oncology (10, 11). NGS-based metagenomic analysis can involve either targeted amplicon sequencing such as 16S ribosomal RNA genes or shotgun sequencing. Shotgun sequencing allows unbiased analysis of partial or complete microbial genomes, transcriptomes and viromes from diagnostic specimens. However, NGS-based metagenomic shotgun sequencing is more expensive, requires greater sequencing depth for the detection of rare or less abundant targets and generates greater amounts of data that requires advanced computational tools for storage and bioinformatic analysis compared to targeted sequencing (11). Metagenomic approach for infectious diseases diagnostics has the potential for diagnosis of mixed infections, detection of associated virulence and antimicrobial resistance genes and discovery of novel/unknown etiologies (18).

In the present study, we used metagenomic based shotgun NGS for analysis of blood microbiome in sick horses with clinical suspicion of tick-borne disease and compared it with the blood microbiome of apparently healthy horses. The proportion of microbial (~1.1%) reads, especially bacterial reads (0.8%) detected out of total genomic reads in horse blood were comparable to those found in the blood of humans with acute leukemia (19). A key observation of our study is that while the proportion of the microbial DNA was comparable between healthy and sick horses, there were differences in the composition of the microbial DNA in blood between these two groups.

The higher proportion of phyla proteobacteria detected in horses with suspected tick-borne infection compared to apparently healthy group directly correlated with the detection of *Anaplasma phagocytophilum* reads in the former group. This finding was further confirmed by a PCR targeted to detect *A. phagocytophilum* and also correlated with the history of tick-bite and with one or more clinical signs including fever, anorexia, depression, petechial hemorrhage on conjunctival membrane and icterus or detection of morulae in blood smears. Genus *Anaplasma* is classified under *Alphaproteobacteria*, and *Anaplasma phagocytophilum* is an important tick-borne bacterium causing disease in horses (20). Currently, PCR for the detection of *A. phagocytophilum* DNA in blood and demonstration of a 4-fold or greater increase in the antibody titer by an Indirect Fluorescent Antibody (IFA) test are commonly employed for diagnosis of equine granulocytic anaplasmosis (5). The finding of one blood sample from the sick group showing presence of *A. phagocytophilum* by metagenomic analysis but negative by PCR was possibly due to PCR inhibition. The two samples from the sick group that were positive by PCR but negative by metagenomic analysis was likely due to lower sensitivity of NGS metagenomic method compared to amplification-based assays (21).

Non-detection of any other significant pathogen by metagenomic analysis is likely due to small sample size and sampling bias as the sick animals included in the study were selected based on high index of suspicion for tick-borne diseases. It is worth noting that *A. phagocytophilum* and *Borrelia burgdorferi* are prevalent tick-borne pathogens in the region where the study was conducted (3, 5). Rarity of detection of *B. burgdorferi* in blood of infected animals may explain non-detection of *B. burgdorferi* reads by metagenomic analysis (22, 23). Our results suggest that sequencing of microbial DNA from blood using NGS can be used as a diagnostic tool for unbiased detection of blood-borne pathogens and is consistent with a previous study that reported detection of vector-borne pathogens in five out of eight known positive human blood samples using metagenomic shotgun sequencing method (13). Recent studies have demonstrated utility of targeted amplicon NGS metagenomic approach for the detection vector-borne bacteria and protozoan haemoparasites in canine blood samples (24, 25).

The distribution of viral, fungal and apicomplexan families/genera/species did not differ significantly among healthy and sick horses and significance of these findings is uncertain due to low read counts. Blood has traditionally been considered devoid of microbes in healthy individuals. However, recent metagenomic studies provide evidence for the presence of signature fragments of bacterial, viral and other microbial nucleic acids in blood of healthy human beings (26). Presence of

phyla including Proteobacteria, Actinobacteria, Firmicutes and Bacteroidetes in blood of healthy human beings has also been reported based on analysis of DNA and RNA (27). In addition, some studies demonstrated the presence of viable bacteria in blood of healthy human beings (28).

A major advantage of sequencing is that the method can identify mutant and variant microbes (strain level identification), particularly important for viruses, that PCR assays might fail to identify. Furthermore, sequencing can also provide valuable insights for studying pathogen evolution, which is not possible with PCR-based methods. However, application of NGS metagenomics in microbial diagnostics is still limited due to high cost, complexity of data, potential for contamination, difficulty in discerning clinical relevance of sequencing data and need for standardization of NGS methods for diagnostic applications (18, 29).

NGS based testing is still an evolving field and some of the challenges we encountered during this study were choosing an appropriate platform for the analyses of the millions of sequenced reads, setting a threshold value to parse the lowest abundant taxa, deciding the appropriate enrichment strategy of microbial genomes and exclusion of host DNA. In the current study we used Kraken metagenomics analysis application from Basespace (Illumina Inc., San Diego, CA). The Kraken metagenomics analysis uses long exact sequence matches alignment when classifying short-read sequences and label almost all the reads sequenced that has exact matches unlike programs which label sequences that are most abundant (15). These qualities of chosen analytical platform may be essential to identify the lowest abundant microbial taxa. In this study we used 1% of specific reads out of total respective microbial reads as a threshold for a phylum/genus/species to be included in the analysis. We recognize that there is a potential risk of excluding low abundant but important microbial reads with such a strategy (29). Lastly, our study focus was on establishing a methodology with a small sample set. Expanding the study to a large population and including variety of disease conditions besides tick borne illness would be valuable.

Overall, the findings of metagenomics analysis of blood samples from apparently healthy horses and horses with suspected tick-borne infection suggest that the approach can be used to detect blood borne pathogens. Additional studies to establish a baseline of potential circulating background microbial DNA in healthy animals would be useful to parse the non-significant microbial sequences.

ETHICS STATEMENT

Ethical review and approval was not required for the animal study because the study involves a specimen set that were already collected as part of State survey for monitoring animal diseases for disease investigation authorized in the State of Pennsylvania. A subset of stored samples from this survey meeting qualifications were investigated in this study at an official State veterinary diagnostic facility.

AUTHOR CONTRIBUTIONS

MS carried out the study, analyzed data, and wrote manuscript. NT managed the study and wrote the manuscript. DTh helped in selecting samples. SK, BJ, and DTe coordinated and conceptualized the study and reviewed manuscript.

All authors contributed to the article and approved the submitted version.

ACKNOWLEDGMENTS

We thank Julia Livengood and Corey Zellers for their technical support.

REFERENCES

1. Sonenshine DE. Range expansion of tick disease vectors in north America: implications for spread of tick-borne Disease. *Int J Environ Res Public Health*. (2018) 15:478. doi: 10.3390/ijerph15030478
2. Rochlin I, Toledo A. Emerging tick-borne pathogens of public health importance: a mini-review. *J Med Microbiol*. (2020) 69:781–91. doi: 10.1099/jmm.0.001206
3. Divers TJ, Gardner RB, Madigan JE, Witonsky SG, Bertone JJ, Swinebroad EL, et al. Borrelia burgdorferi infection and lyme Disease in North American horses: a consensus statement. *J Vet Intern Med*. (2018) 32:617–32. doi: 10.1111/jvim.15042
4. Tirosh-Levy S, Gottlieb Y, Fry LM, Knowles DP, Steinman A. Twenty years of equine piroplasmosis research: global distribution, molecular diagnosis, and phylogeny. *Pathogens*. (2020) 9:926. doi: 10.3390/pathogens9110926
5. Pusterla N, Madigan JE. Equine granulocytic anaplasmosis. *J Equine Vet Sci*. (2013) 33:493–6. doi: 10.1016/j.jevs.2013.03.188
6. Lecollinet S, Pronost S, Coulpier M, Beck C, Gonzalez G, Leblond A, et al. Viral equine encephalitis, a growing threat to the horse population in Europe? *Viruses*. (2019) 12:23. doi: 10.3390/v12010023
7. Pace EJ, O'Reilly M. Tickborne Diseases: diagnosis and management. *Am Fam Physician*. (2020) 101:530–40.
8. Tokarz R, Mishra N, Tagliafierro T, Sameroff S, Caciula A, Chauhan L, et al. A multiplex serologic platform for diagnosis of tick-borne diseases. *Sci Rep*. (2018) 8:3158. doi: 10.1038/s41598-018-21349-2
9. Livengood J, Hutchinson ML, Thirumalapura N, Tewari D. Detection of babesia, borrelia, anaplasma, and rickettsia spp. In Adult Black-Legged Ticks (Ixodes scapularis) from Pennsylvania, United States, with a Luminex Multiplex Bead Assay. *Vector Borne Zoonotic Dis*. (2020) 20:406–11. doi: 10.1089/vbz.2019.2551
10. Chiu CY, Miller SA. Clinical metagenomics. *Nat Rev Genet*. (2019) 20:341–55. doi: 10.1038/s41576-019-0113-7
11. Dekker JP. Metagenomics for clinical infectious disease diagnostics steps closer to reality. *J Clin Microbiol*. (2018) 56:e00850-18. doi: 10.1128/JCM.00850-18
12. Charalampous T, Kay GL, Richardson H, Aydin A, Baldan R, Jeanes C, et al. Nanopore metagenomics enables rapid clinical diagnosis of bacterial lower respiratory infection. *Nat Biotechnol*. (2019) 37:783–92. doi: 10.1038/s41587-019-0156-5
13. Vijayvargiya P, Jeraldo PR, Thoendel MJ, Greenwood-Quaintance KE, Esquer Garrigos Z, Sohail MR, et al. Application of metagenomic shotgun sequencing to detect vector-borne pathogens in clinical blood samples. *PLoS ONE*. (2019) 14:e0222915. doi: 10.1371/journal.pone.0222915
14. Kingry L, Sheldon S, Oatman S, Pritt B, Anacker B, Bjork J, et al. Targeted metagenomics for clinical detection and discovery of bacterial tick-borne pathogens. *J Clin Microbiol*. (2020) 58:e00147-20. doi: 10.1128/JCM.00147-20
15. Wood DE, Salzberg SL. Kraken: ultrafast metagenomic sequence classification using exact alignments. *Genome Biol*. (2014) 15:R46. doi: 10.1186/gb-2014-15-3-r46
16. Li K, Bihan M, Yooseph S, Methe BA. Analyses of the microbial diversity across the human microbiome. *PLoS ONE*. (2012) 7:e32118. doi: 10.1371/journal.pone.0032118
17. Courtney JW, Kostelnik LM, Zeidner NS, Massung RF. Multiplex real-time PCR for detection of anaplasma phagocytophilum and borrelia burgdorferi. *J Clin Microbiol*. (2004) 42:3164–8. doi: 10.1128/JCM.42.7.3164-3168.2004
18. Dulanto Chiang A, Dekker JP. From the pipeline to the bedside: advances and challenges in clinical metagenomics. *J Infect Dis*. (2020) 221:S331–40. doi: 10.1093/infdis/jiz151
19. Gyarmati P, Kjellander C, Aust C, Song Y, Ohrmalm L, Giske CG. Metagenomic analysis of bloodstream infections in patients with acute leukemia and therapy-induced neutropenia. *Sci Rep*. (2016) 6:23532. doi: 10.1038/srep23532
20. Dziegiel B, Adaszek L, Kalinowski M, Winiarczyk S. Equine granulocytic anaplasmosis. *Res Vet Sci*. (2013) 95:316–20. doi: 10.1016/j.rvsc.2013.05.010
21. Perlejewski K, Bukowska-Osko I, Rydzanicz M, Pawelczyk A, Caraballo Corts K, Osuch S, et al. Next-generation sequencing in the diagnosis of viral encephalitis: sensitivity and clinical limitations. *Sci Rep*. (2020) 10:16173. doi: 10.1038/s41598-020-73156-3
22. Lee SH, Yun SH, Choi E, Park YS, Lee SE, Cho GJ, et al. Serological detection of borrelia burgdorferi among horses in Korea. *Korean J Parasitol*. (2016) 54:97–101. doi: 10.3347/kjp.2016.54.1.97
23. Schutzer SE, Body BA, Boyle J, Branson BM, Dattwyler RJ, Fikrig E, et al. Direct diagnostic tests for lyme disease. *Clin Infect Dis*. (2019) 68:1052–7. doi: 10.1093/cid/ciy614
24. Huggins LG, Koehler AV, Ng-Nguyen D, Wilcox S, Schunack B, Inpankaew T, et al. A novel metabarcoding diagnostic tool to explore protozoan haemoparasite diversity in mammals: a proof-of-concept study using canines from the tropics. *Sci Rep*. (2019) 9:12644. doi: 10.1038/s41598-019-49118-9
25. Huggins LG, Koehler AV, Ng-Nguyen D, Wilcox S, Schunack B, Inpankaew T, et al. Assessment of a metabarcoding approach for the characterisation of vector-borne bacteria in canines from Bangkok, Thailand. *Parasit Vectors*. (2019) 12:394. doi: 10.1186/s13071-019-3651-0
26. Paisse S, Valle C, Servant F, Courtney M, Burcelin R, Amar J, et al. Comprehensive description of blood microbiome from healthy donors assessed by 16S targeted metagenomic sequencing. *Transfusion*. (2016) 56:1138–47. doi: 10.1111/trf.13477
27. Whittle E, Leonard MO, Harrison R, Gant TW, Tonge DP. Multi-method characterization of the human circulating microbiome. *Front Microbiol*. (2018) 9:3266. doi: 10.3389/fmicb.2018.03266
28. Damgaard C, Magnussen K, Enevold C, Nilsson M, Tolker-Nielsen T, Holmstrup P, et al. Viable bacteria associated with red blood cells and plasma in freshly drawn blood donations. *PLoS ONE*. (2015) 10:e0120826. doi: 10.1371/journal.pone.0120826
29. Couto N, Schuele L, Raangs EC, Machado MP, Mendes CI, Jesus TF, et al. Critical steps in clinical shotgun metagenomics for the concomitant detection and typing of microbial pathogens. *Sci Rep*. (2018) 8:13767. doi: 10.1038/s41598-018-31873-w

3

A Multi-Epitope Fusion Protein-Based p-ELISA Method for Diagnosing Bovine and Goat Brucellosis

Dehui Yin[1†], Qiongqiong Bai[1†], Xiling Wu[1], Han Li[2], Jihong Shao[1], Mingjun Sun[3*] and Jinpeng Zhang[1*]

[1] Key Lab of Environment and Health, School of Public Health, Xuzhou Medical University, Xuzhou, China, [2] Department of Infection Control, The First Hospital of Jilin University, Changchun, China, [3] Laboratory of Zoonoses, China Animal Health and Epidemiology Center, Qingdao, China

*Correspondence:
Mingjun Sun
sunmingjun@cahec.cn
Jinpeng Zhang
xiaopangpeng@126.com

[†] These authors have contributed equally to this work

In recent years, the incidence of brucellosis has increased annually, causing tremendous economic losses to animal husbandry in a lot of countries. Therefore, developing rapid, sensitive, and specific diagnostic techniques is critical to control the spread of brucellosis. In this study, bioinformatics technology was used to predict the B cell epitopes of the main outer membrane proteins of *Brucella*, and the diagnostic efficacy of each epitope was verified by an indirect enzyme-linked immunosorbent assay (iELISA). Then, a fusion protein containing 22 verified epitopes was prokaryotically expressed and used as an antigen in paper-based ELISA (p-ELISA) for serodiagnosis of brucellosis. The multi-epitope-based p-ELISA was evaluated using a collection of brucellosis-positive and -negative sera collected from bovine and goat, respectively. Receiver operating characteristic (ROC) curve analysis showed that the sensitivity and specificity of detection-ELISA in diagnosing goat brucellosis were 98.85 and 98.51%. The positive and the negative predictive values were 99.29 and 98.15%, respectively. In diagnosing bovine brucellosis, the sensitivity and specificity of this method were 97.85 and 96.61%, with the positive and negative predictive values being identified as 98.28 and 97.33%, respectively. This study demonstrated that the B cell epitopes contained in major antigenic proteins of *Brucella* can be a very useful antigen source in developing a highly sensitive and specific method for serodiagnosis of brucellosis.

Keywords: brucellosis, p-ELISA, serodiagnosis, B cell epitope, bioinformatics technology

INTRODUCTION

Brucellosis, as a re-emerging zoonosis, not only puts human health at risk but also causes tremendous losses in animal husbandry around the world, especially in developing countries (1). Human brucellosis is mainly caused by direct contact with *Brucella*-infected animals or consuming contaminated food (2). In humans, due to the lack of specific clinical manifestations, brucellosis is easily misdiagnosed as other febrile diseases, such as dengue fever, malaria, or viral bleeding diseases (3, 4). In animals, this disease is often neglected as there are no symptoms at the early stage of infection. Therefore, application of diagnostic methods is very important for accurate and early detection of this disease in human and animal populations.

Among the many techniques currently used for diagnosing brucellosis, serological diagnosis methods are the most widely used. It is worth pointing out that accurate serological diagnosis requires highly specific and sensitive antigens (5). However, the current most commonly used antigens for diagnosing brucellosis mainly depend on *Brucella* whole cell and lipopolysaccharide (LPS), which can cross-react with the antibodies aroused by other bacteria, such as *Yersinia enterocolitica* serotype O:9 and *Escherichia coli* O:157. Therefore, it is still meaningful to develop new diagnostic antigens to improve the specificity and sensitivity of serological diagnostic methods for brucellosis (6).

Quite a number of studies showed that the *Brucella* outer membrane proteins (Omps) have good immunogenicity, which can be potentially used as new diagnostic antigens to substitute for LPS (7–9). In this study, B cell epitopes were predicted from these Omps with the help of an online bioinformatics tool, and their capacity in identifying brucellosis-positive sera was further verified. Subsequently, a novel fusion protein containing multiple predicted epitopes was obtained as a candidate antigen for the serodiagnosis of brucellosis. At the same time, using the fusion protein as an antigen, a rapid paper-based enzyme-linked immunosorbent assay (p-ELISA) was constructed and evaluated for its possible use in detecting small ruminant and cattle brucellosis (10).

METHODS

Serum Samples

A total of 194 goat serum samples (brucellosis-positive sera = 140; brucellosis-negative sera = 54) and 191 bovine sera (brucellosis-positive sera = 116; brucellosis-negative sera = 75) were provided by the China Animal Health and Epidemiology Center (Qingdao, China). All brucellosis-positive sera were confirmed by the Rose Bengal plate agglutination test (RBPT) and tube agglutination test (SAT) according to the national standard for animal brucellosis diagnosis. Negative serum samples were originated from a brucellosis-free area in China. All experiments involving animals or animal samples were fully compliant with ethical approval granted by the Animal Care and Ethics Committee of Xuzhou Medical University (ethical approval no.: 201801W005).

Prediction and Synthesis of Peptide Epitopes

The amino acid sequences of *Brucella* outer membrane proteins Omp16, Omp25, Omp31, Omp2b, and BP26 were downloaded from NCBI (https://www.ncbi.nlm.nih.gov/protein/). The conserved amino acid sequences were assessed and selected by BLAST. Prediction of B cell epitopes was carried out by online B cell epitope prediction tool BepiPred Linear Epitope Prediction at IEDB (http://tools.iedb.org/bcell/). The predicted B cell epitope peptides were synthesized by Sangon Biotech (Shanghai, China) and coupled to keyhole limpet hemocyanin (KLH) with a productive purity of more than 90%.

Epitope Verification

Forty-five bovine and goat sera, which were positive for brucellosis, were randomly selected to verify the capability of the predicted peptides in identifying brucellosis through an indirect enzyme-linked immunosorbent assay (iELISA). In addition, KLH was used as negative control and LPS was used as the positive antigen control. For the procedure, in a 96-well microtiter plate (NUNC, Denmark), 100 μL of peptide (30 μg/mL in carbonate buffer solution (CBS), pH 9.6) was added to each well and incubated overnight at 4°C. The wells were blocked with 300 μL/well of 5% skimmed milk powder (Sangon, Shanghai) at 37°C for 2 h, then 100 μL/well of serum was added (1:400 dilution with PBS) and incubated at 37°C for 1 h. HRP-labeled protein G (diluted 1:5,000, PBS) (Thermo, USA) was added and incubated at room temperature for 30 min. After that, an EL-TMB kit was utilized (Sangon) for the coloring step. Optical density was measured at 450 nm (OD450) using an ELISA plate reader (BioTek, USA). During the whole process, plates were washed three times with PBST before each reagent was added.

Preparation of the Fusion Protein

The effective peptides were connected in random order, and adjacent peptides were linked by the 'GGGS' linker. For the concatenated amino acid sequence, the molecular weight (https://web.expasy.org/compute_pi/), spatial conformation (http://zhanglab.ccmb.med.umich.edu/I-TASSER/), and other parameters were predicted. According to the concatenated sequence, the corresponding codon was designated and optimized for prokaryotic expression. The full length of nucleic acid sequence coding for the multi-epitope fusion protein was synthesized and subcloned into expression vector pET30a (Beijing Protein Innovation, Beijing). The vector was then transferred into competent BL21 cells for IPTG-induced expression. Specifically, competent cells (BL21 cells) (100 μL), stored at−80°C, were slowly thawed on ice, after which the ligation product was added to the cells and mixed well; the cells were then placed on ice for 30 min, heat shocked at 42°C for 90 s, and then incubated in an ice bath for 2 min. Subsequently, 800 μL of non-resistant LB medium was added, incubated at 37°C for 45 min, and centrifuged at 5,000 rpm for 3 min. The majority of the supernatant was discarded, leaving approximately 100–150 μL, which was used to resuspend the cell pellet. The resuspended cells were added to LB plates with the corresponding resistance antibiotic and spread over plates, which were air-dried and cultured upside down and placed in an incubator at 37°C overnight. Then, the transformed BL21 cells were selected and cultured in 1.5 ml of LB liquid medium at 37°C and shaken at 200 rpm. The cells were incubated until OD600 = 0.6, at which time they were induced by IPTG (0.5 mm) and cultured for 2 h at 37°C. 1 ml of induced bacterial solution was centrifuged at 12,000 rpm for 1 min, the supernatant was discarded, and the precipitate was resuspended in 50–100 μL of 10 mM Tris-HCl (pH 8.0) solution (the amount of added buffer was dependent on the amount of bacteria). Loading buffer equal to twice the volume of the resuspended precipitate was added, after which the sample was boiled at 100°C for 5 min and then assessed by SDS-PAGE electrophoresis.

When OD600 of bacterial culture reached 0.6–0.8, IPTG was added to the culture to a final concentration of 0.5 mM and incubated overnight at 16°C. After centrifugation at 6,000 rpm for 5 min, the supernatant was discarded and the precipitation was resuspended in 10 mM of Tris-HCl (pH 8.0) solution. The resuspended bacteria was lysed by ultrasonication (500 W, 60 times, 10 s/each time, 15 s /intervals). The ultrasonic-treated bacterial solution was then centrifuged at 12,000 rpm for 10 min. The supernatant was transferred into another container, and the precipitation was resuspended in 10 mM of Tris-HCl (pH 8.0) solution and assessed by SDS-PAGE electrophoresis.

Purification of Fusion Protein

The nickel column (Ni Sepharose 6 Fast Flow, GE Healthcare, Uppsala, Sweden) was washed with deionized water at pH 7.0. The nickel column was adjusted to pH 2~3. The column was washed with deionized water at pH 7.0. The nickel column was equilibrated with 10 mM of Tris-HCl (pH 8.0) solution (~100 mL). Then, the nickel column was equilibrated with 10 mM of Tris-HCl (pH 8.0) solution containing 0.5 M of sodium chloride (~50 mL). The diluted sample was loaded. The sample contained sodium chloride at a final concentration of 0.5 M. After loading, the column was washed with 10 mm of Tris-HCl (pH 8.0) solution containing 0.5 M of sodium chloride. The proteins were eluted with 10 mm of Tris-HCl (pH 8.0) (containing 0.5 M of sodium chloride) solution containing 15 mm of imidazole, 60 mM of imidazole, and 300 mm of imidazole, and the protein peaks were collected separately. SDS-PAGE electrophoresis was used to assess the protein purity.

Antigenicity Assessment of the Fusion Protein

iELISA was used to assess the capability of purified protein in identifying brucellosis-positive sera. In a 96-well ELISA plate (NUNC, Denmark), 100 μL of fusion protein (2.5 μg/mL

in CBS) and 100 μL of LPS (1 μg/mL in CBS) as the positive antigen control were added to the wells, respectively, and incubated overnight at 4°C. In the blocking step, 300 μL of 5% skimmed milk (PBS) was added per well and incubated at 37°C for 2 h. Then, 100 μL of serum (1:400 dilution in PBS) was added and incubated at 37°C for 1 h. After that, 100 μL of HRP-labeled protein G (diluted 1:8,000 in PBS) was added and incubated at room temperature for 30 min. When the coloring step was finished with the EL-TMB kit, the absorbance of the wells was measured at OD450. After each step, the plates were washed three times with PBST.

In addition, rabbit sera confirmed to be infected with *Yersinia enterocolitica* O:9, *Escherichia coli* O157:H7, *Salmonella, Vibrio cholerae, Vibrio parahaemolyticus,* and *Listeria monocytogenes* were used to assess the specificity of the fusion protein antigen. All these rabbit sera were purchased from Tianjin Biochip Corporation (Tianjin, China). The verification method was the same as iELISA described above except a 1:10,000 dilution of HRP-labeled goat anti-rabbit secondary antibody (Bioworld, USA) was used in this assay.

Establishment of the p-ELISA Method

A round sheet with a diameter of 10 mm was punched from Whatman No. 1 filter paper, and a small hole (6 mm diameter) was punched out of A4 plastic packaging paper. The 10 mm filter paper was placed in the center of the 6 mm hole in the plastic packaging paper, and a laminating machine was used to join the filter sheet and packaging paper together, and then the combined papers were fixed and cut into small strips with three holes in each strip. The following steps were conducted according to the literature (11): 5 μl of chitosan in deionized water (0.25 mg/ml) was added to the round holes with Whatman No. 1 filter paper and dried at room temperature; then, 5 μl of 2.5% glutaraldehyde solution in PBS was added and incubated at room

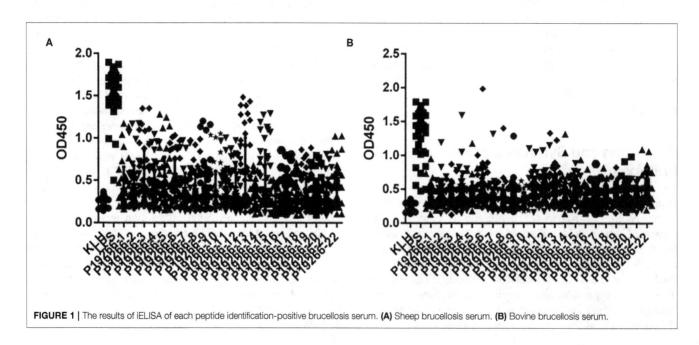

FIGURE 1 | The results of iELISA of each peptide identification-positive brucellosis serum. **(A)** Sheep brucellosis serum. **(B)** Bovine brucellosis serum.

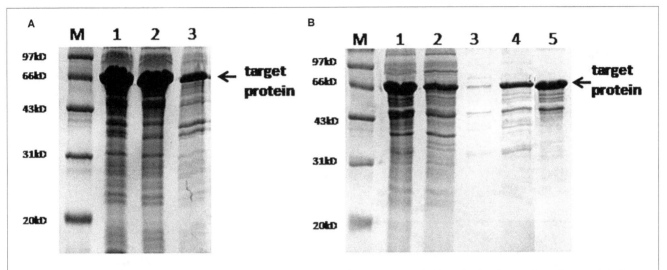

FIGURE 2 | SDS-PAGE analysis of the fusion protein. **(A)** Protein expression results. M, marker; lane 1, whole bacteria after ultrasound; lane 2, supernatant after ultrasound; lane 3, precipitation after ultrasound. **(B)** SDS-PAGE after protein purification. M, marker; lane 1, the original protein before purification; lane 2, flow-through solution; lane 3, 15 mm of imidazole elution fraction; lane 4, 60 mm of imidazole elution fraction; lane 5, 300 mm of imidazole elution fraction.

temperature for 2 h. After washing three times with 20 µl of deionized water, 5 µl of fusion protein solution (2.5 µg/ml in PBS) was added to each well and incubated at room temperature for 30 min. After another three washes with 20 µl of deionized water, 20 µl of 5% skimmed milk powder was added and incubated at room temperature for 15 min. Subsequently, 5 µl of serum (1:400 dilution) and 5 µl of HRP-labeled protein G (1:8,000 dilution) were added in order and washed three times with PBST at intervals. Finally, 5 µl of TMB substrate solution was added and incubated for 10 min, then a HP Laser Jet Pro MFP M227 was used to scan the samples to obtain images. ImageJ software was used to perform gray intensity analysis for quantitation. The cattle and goat serum samples were assessed according to the established p-ELISA method, and ROC curves were used to analyze the diagnostic effect of the established method.

Statistical Analysis

Dot plot and receiver operating characteristic curve (ROC) analyses were performed using GraphPad Prism version 6.05 for Windows. The significance of gray intensity differences was determined by Student's t-test (unpaired t-test). Differences were considered statistically significant when $P < 0.05$.

RESULTS

B Cell Epitope Peptide Prediction and Antigenicity Verification

From 5 Omps, a high number of epitopes were predicted by BepiPred software with the length of peptides ranging from 1 to 28. Empirically, only peptides longer than six amino acids were chosen as candidate epitopes. Thus, a total of 22 B cell epitopes were selected and synthesized for subsequent

verification analysis, including six peptides from BP26, two from Omp16, five from Omp25 and Omp31 respectively, and four from Omp2b (**Supplementary Table 1**). Indirect ELISA results showed that all 22 peptides demonstrated some extent of capability in identifying animal-sourced brucellosis-positive sera (**Figure 1**).

Preparation of the Multi-Epitope Fusion Protein

The full sequence of the fusion protein containing 22 epitopes and 'GGGS' linker is listed in **Supplementary Figure 1**. This fusion protein was successfully expressed in the soluble form in the prokaryotic system. SDS-PAGE electrophoresis showed that the molecular weight of the purified fusion protein was ∼66 kd. Mass spectrometry analysis confirmed that the sequence of the purified protein was identical to the designed target. Gray intensity analysis showed that the purity of the purified protein was ∼90% (**Figure 2**).

Antigenicity Assessment of the Fusion Protein

The ability of the fusion protein in diagnosing goat brucellosis was evaluated using 140 sera with a known *Brucella* infection background and 54 sera negative control sera by the method of iELISA. According to ROC curve analysis, the area under the ROC curve was 0.9799 (95% CI, 0.9654 to 0.9944), and the cutoff value calculated by the Youden index was 0.4675. In this case, the diagnostic sensitivity was 87.14% (95% CI, 0.8044 to 0.9220), and the specificity was 100.0% (95% CI, 0.9340 to 1.000). The positive predictive value was 100.0%, and the negative predictive value was 75.00% (**Figure 3** and **Table 1**). In LPS control experiments, the area under the ROC curve was 0.9514 (95% CI, 0.9191 to 0.9836), and the cutoff value

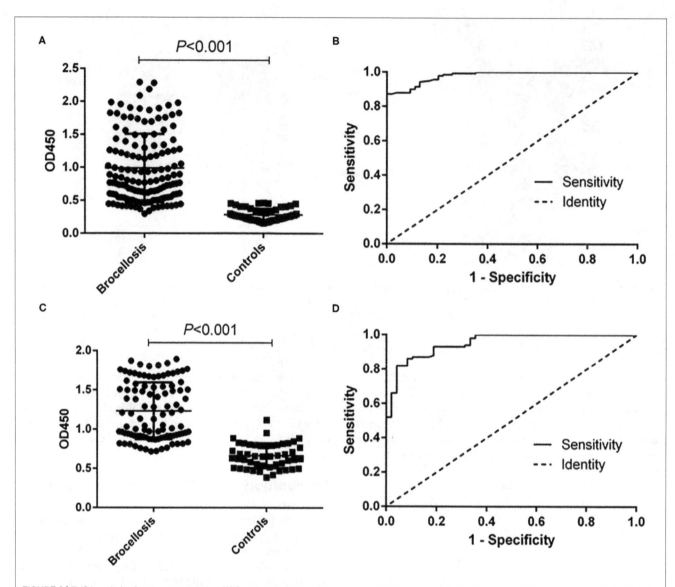

FIGURE 3 | ELISA analysis of goat serum samples. **(A)** Dot plot of the fusion protein ELISA assay. **(B)** ROC analysis of fusion protein iELISA assay results. **(C)** Dot plot of the LPS antigen ELISA assay. **(D)** ROC analysis of LPS antigen ELISA assay results.

TABLE 1 | Positive and negative predictive values of the test calculated for different cutoff values.

Cutoff value	Positive		Negative		PPV (%)	NPV (%)
	TP	FN	TN	FP		
≥0.4675 (fusion protein)[a]	122	18	54	0	100.0	75.00
≥0.8890 (LPS)a	122	18	52	2	98.39	74.29
≥0.4530 (fusion protein)[b]	103	13	70	5	95.37	84.34
≥0.8105 (LPS)[b]	107	9	68	7	93.86	88.31
≥34.12 (p-ELISA)[a]	139	1	53	1	99.29	98.15
≥30.21 (p-ELISA)[b]	114	2	73	2	98.28	97.33

a, goat sera; b, cattle sera. TP, true positives; TN, true negatives; FP, false positives; FN, false negatives; PPV, positive predictive value (TP/TP+FP)×100; NPV, negative predictive value (TN/TN+FN) ×100.

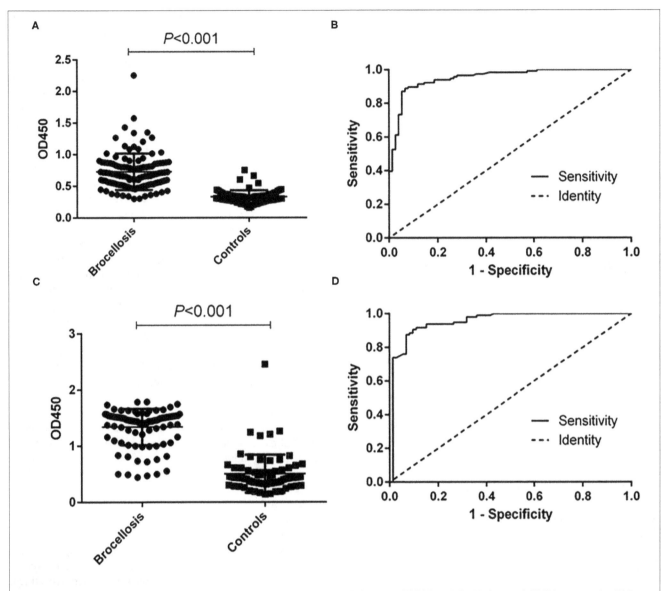

FIGURE 4 | ELISA analysis of cattle serum samples. **(A)** Dot plot of the fusion protein ELISA assay. **(B)** ROC analysis of fusion protein iELISA assay results. **(C)** Dot plot of the LPS antigen ELISA assay. **(D)** ROC analysis of LPS antigen ELISA assay results.

was 0.8890. At this cutoff value, the diagnostic sensitivity was 82.00% (95% CI, 0.7305 to 0.8897) and the specificity was 95.83% (95% CI, 0.8575 to 0.9949). The positive predictive value was 98.39%, and the negative predictive value was 74.29% (**Figure 3**, **Table 1**).

In the cattle brucellosis experiment using 191 cattle sera with a known infection background, the area under the ROC curve was 0.9518 (95% CI, 0.9224 to 0.9812), and the cutoff value calculated by the Youden index was 0.4530. In this case, the diagnostic sensitivity was 88.79% (95% CI, 0.8160 to 0.9390), and the specificity was 93.33% (95% CI, 0.8512 to 0.9780) (**Figure 4** and **Table 1**). The positive predictive value was 95.37%, and the negative predictive value was 84.34%. When using LPS as the antigen, the area under the ROC curve was 0.9528 (95% CI,

0.9187 to 0.9868) and the cutoff value was 0.8105. In this case, the diagnostic sensitivity was 90.63% (95% CI, 0.8295 to 0.9562) and the specificity was 90.28% (95% CI, 0.8099 to 0.9600). The positive predictive value was 93.86%, and the negative predictive value was 88.31% (**Figure 4**, **Table 1**).

Determining the Cross-Reactivity With the Fusion Protein

To verify whether the fusion protein as a diagnostic antigen showed cross-reactivity with other bacteria, we selected six zoonotic pathogens for a cross-reactivity test. The results showed that the fusion protein did not cross-react with other bacteria according to an S/N (OD450, sample/negative) > 2.1,

TABLE 2 | Specific cross-reactivity test results of the indirect ELISA diagnostic method for the fusion protein.

Rabbit sample	OD450	S/N
Vibrio parahaemolyticus	0.1230	1.64
Escherichia coli O157:H7	0.0457	0.61
Salmonella	0.1267	1.69
Vibrio cholerae	0.0598	0.80
*Yersinia enterocolitica*O9	0.0443	0.59
Listeria monocytogenes	0.0758	1.01
Negative	0.0751	-

which indicated that the fusion protein antigen had better specificity (**Table 2**).

Evaluation of the Diagnostic Ability of the p-ELISA

The effectiveness of the established p-ELISA method in detecting animal brucellosis was also evaluated. When it was used for diagnosing goat sera, the area under the ROC curve was 0.9986 (95% CI, 0.9957 to 1.002). The cutoff value was 34.12, at which the diagnostic sensitivity was 98.85% (95% CI, 0.9376 to 0.9997) and the specificity was 98.51% (95% CI, 0.9196 to 0.9996). The positive predictive value was 99.29% and the negative predictive value was 98.15% (**Table 1**). When it was used for diagnosing cattle brucellosis, the area under the ROC curve was 0.9964 (95% CI, 0.9910 to 1.002), and the cutoff value calculated by the Youden index was 30.21. In this case, the diagnostic sensitivity was 97.85% (95% CI, 0.9245 to 1.002) and the specificity was 96.61% (95% CI, 0.8829 to 0.9959). The positive predictive value was 98.28%, and the negative predictive value was 97.33% (**Figure 5, Table 1**).

DISCUSSION

Brucellosis is a serious zoonotic disease. Bovine and small ruminants are the most susceptible animals (12). Currently, culling infected animals is an effective strategy to prevent this disease from spreading (13). Thus, accurate diagnosis would be very important to pick out truly *Brucella*-infected animals and reduce unnecessary economic losses. Particularly in China, where a large number of bovine and goat are raised, fast and efficient methods for brucellosis are of great significance (14). Serological diagnostic techniques are mainly used for brucellosis detection, including the agglutination test, complement fixation test (CFT), ELISA, immunochromatographic diagnostic test (ICDT), and fluorescence polarization assay (FPA) (15, 16). But, these methods normally use *Brucella*-derived LPS as the diagnostic antigen, and a false positive result can be easily produced as *Brucella* LPS shares a common antigenic epitope with other pathogens such as *Escherichia coli* O157:H7 and *Yersinia enterocolitica* O9 (17). In addition, LPS antigen is only obtained by culturing live *Brucella*, which greatly

reduces its availability. Therefore, seeking more specific and easily accessible antigens is still meaningful for brucellosis diagnostics research.

ELISA is currently the most widely studied serological diagnosis method, even as diagnostic confirmation in brucellosis (16). The main problem with using ELISAs for the diagnosis of brucellosis is the choice of antigen, but to date, ELISA-based diagnoses lack a single standard antigen (18). Currently, the most commonly used diagnostic antigens used in ELISA are whole bacteria or extracts. These diagnostic antigens are prone to cross-reactivity with other bacteria, have poor specificity, and have considerable defects. Therefore, the development of new diagnostic antigens is key to improving the diagnostic effect of ELISAs.

The *Brucella* Omps are a group of proteins with various molecular weights (19). Some Omps have been identified to be able to arouse strong immune responses in infected animals, including Omp16, Omp25, BP26, Omp2b, and Omp31. In this study, Omp16, Omp25, BP26, Omp2b, and Omp31 were selected for prediction of B cell epitopes and construction of a new diagnostic antigen. Omp16 is a lipoprotein that can elicit immune response and can be potentially used in diagnostics and vaccine development (8, 20). Omp25 plays an important role in Brucella pathogenesis during infection, and exhibits strong immunogenicity (21). A subunit vaccine comprising BP26 triggers a mixed Th1/Th2 immune response in a mice model (7), and it has been also used in diagnosis of brucellosis (22). Animal experiments indicated that Omp31 can not only elicit a strong humoral immune response in mice, but also protects mice against *Brucella* infection (23, 24). Omp2b is another important candidate for brucellosis diagnostics and vaccine research (25, 26). The data in this paper proved that the shorter linear peptides contained in these Omps are also effective in detecting brucellosis-positive sera. In addition, better effectivity can be achieved by using multiple epitopes, as data showed that a single epitope only identified partial serum samples while a multi-epitope fusion protein detected almost all the positive sera. More importantly, the specificity of a multi-epitope protein antigen was higher than that of LPS, implying that the method using the multi-epitope antigen can be used as a confirmatory diagnosis method for brucellosis. It is worth pointing out that bioinformatics tools applied in this study are very helpful to predict effective antigens (27, 28), in the future, more novel antigens can be prepared using this strategy.

The p-ELISA method using paper as the solid-phase carrier is a new technology developed based on the traditional ELISA method (11, 29). Compared with the traditional ELISA method, p-ELISA is faster, less reagent is required, and no special instruments are needed (30). Currently, the most commonly used paper-processing method for p-ELISA involves preparing hydrophilic and hydrophobic areas through wax-printing technology. This method requires expensive printers, which limits the application of this method. We used plastic-encapsulated paper to prepare a hydrophobic area, punched small holes in it, and filled the small holes with hydrophilic

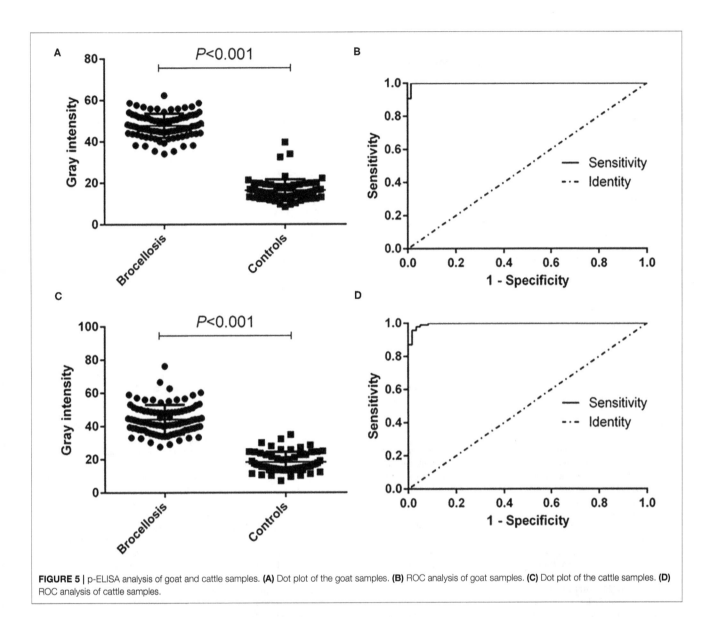

FIGURE 5 | p-ELISA analysis of goat and cattle samples. **(A)** Dot plot of the goat samples. **(B)** ROC analysis of goat samples. **(C)** Dot plot of the cattle samples. **(D)** ROC analysis of cattle samples.

paper sheets to make a sandwich structure. This modification greatly reduced the production cost. Combing the multi-epitope-based fusion protein as the antigen, our *p*-ELISA demonstrated improved sensitivity and specificity in diagnosing cattle and small ruminant brucellosis. This newly developed p-ELISA method is more suitable for rural areas where animal brucellosis is highly epidemic and experiment equipment is unavailable.

In China, animal immunization by *Brucella* vaccine has been carried out in some provinces. A serological method for distinguishing infected from vaccinated animals (DIVA) is urgently needed. As the sera used in this study were collected from wild-type *Brucella*-infected animals, the DIVA ability of the multi-epitope-based p-ELISA is not known. Further research will be carried out to determine whether this method can be

applied to test other animal or human brucellosis or used for DIVA purposes.

ETHICS STATEMENT

The animal study was reviewed and approved by Animal Care and Ethics Committee of Xuzhou Medical University.

AUTHOR CONTRIBUTIONS

DY and QB analyzed the data and drafted the manuscript. QB, XW, and HL performed the assays. JS reviewed and made improvements in the manuscript. DY, MS, and JZ conceived and designed the study. All authors read and approved the final version of the paper.

ACKNOWLEDGMENTS

We thank the China Animal Health and Epidemiology Center (Qingdao, China) for their gift of animal serum samples and LPS antigens.

REFERENCES

1. Pappas G, Papadimitriou P, Akritidis N, Christou L, Tsianos EV. The newglobal map of human brucellosis. *Lancet Infect Dis.* (2006) 6:91–9. doi: 10.1016/S1473-3099(06)70382-6

2. Olsen SC, Palmer MV. Advancement of knowledge of Brucella over the past 50years. *Vet Pathol.* (2014) 51:1076–89. doi: 10.1177/0300985814540545

3. Deng Y, Liu X, Duan K, Peng Q. Research progress on brucellosis. *Curr Med Chem.* (2019) 26:5598–608. doi: 10.2174/0929867325666180510125009

4. Franco MP, Mulder M, Gilman RH, Smits HL. Human brucellosis. *Lancet Infect Dis.* (2007) 7:775–86. doi: 10.1016/S1473-3099(07)70286-4

5. Araj GF. Update on laboratory diagnosis of human brucellosis. *Int J Antimicrob Agents.* (2010) 36:12–7. doi: 10.1016/j.ijantimicag.2010.06.014

6. Yagupsky P, Morata P, Colmenero JD. Laboratory diagnosis of humanbrucellosis. *Clin Microbiol Rev.* (2019) 33:e00073-19. doi: 10.1128/CMR.00073-19

7. Gupta S, Singh D, Gupta M, Bhatnagar R. A combined subunit vaccine comprisingBP26, Omp25 and L7/L12 against brucellosis. *Pathog Dis.* (2019) 77:ftaa002. doi: 10.1093/femspd/ftaa002

8. Rezaei M, Rabbani-Khorasgani M, Zarkesh-Esfahani SH, Emamzadeh R, Abtahi H. Prediction of the Omp16 epitopes for the development of an epitope-based vaccineagainst brucellosis. *Infect Disord Drug Targets.* (2019) 19:36–45. doi: 10.2174/1871526518666180709121653

9. Verdiguel-Fernández L, Oropeza-Navarro R, Ortiz A, Robles-Pesina MG, Ramírez-Lezama J, Castañeda-Ramírez A, et al. Brucella melitensis omp31 mutant is attenuated and confers protection against virulent brucella melitensis challenge in BALB/c mice. *J Microbiol Biotechnol.* (2020) 30:497–504. doi: 10.4014/jmb.1908.08056

10. Cheng CM, Martinez AW, Gong J, Mace CR, Phillips ST, Carrilho E, et al. Paper-based ELISA. *Angew Chem Int Ed Engl.* (2010) 49:4771–4. doi: 10.1002/anie.201001005

11. Wang S, Ge L, Song X, Yu J, Ge S, Huang J, et al. Paper-based chemiluminescence ELISA: lab-on-paper based on chitosan modified paper device and wax-screen-printing. *Biosens Bioelectron.* (2012) 31:212–8. doi: 10.1016/j.bios.2011.10.019

12. Zheng R, Xie S, Lu X, Sun L, Zhou Y, Zhang Y, et al. A systematic review andmeta-analysis of epidemiology and clinical manifestations of human brucellosis in China. *Biomed Res Int.* (2018) 2018:5712920. doi: 10.1155/2018/5712920

13. Zhang N, Huang D, Wu W, Liu J, Liang F, Zhou B. et al. Animal brucellosiscontrol or eradication programs worldwide: a systematic review of experiencesand lessons learned. *Prev Vet Med.* (2018) 160:105–15. doi: 10.1016/j.prevetmed.2018.10.002

14. Zhong Z, Yu S, Wang X, Dong S, Xu J, Wang Y, et al. Humanbrucellosis in the people's republic of China during 2005-2010. *Int J Infect Dis.* (2013) 17:e289–92. doi: 10.1016/j.ijid.2012.12.030

15. Khan MZ, Zahoor M. An overview of brucellosis in cattle and humans, and itsserological and molecular diagnosis in control strategies. *Trop Med Infect Dis.* (2018) 3:65. doi: 10.3390/tropicalmed3020065

16. Xu N, Wang W, Chen F, Li W, Wang G. ELISA is superior to bacterial culture and agglutination test in the diagnosis of brucellosis in an endemic area in China. *BMC Infect Dis.* (2020) 20:11. doi: 10.1186/s12879-019-4729-1

17. Chart H, Okubadejo OA, Rowe B. The serological relationship between *Escherichia coli* O157 and yersinia enterocolitica O9 using sera from patients with brucellosis. *Epidemiol Infect.* (1992) 108:77–85. doi: 10.1017/S0950268800049529

18. Ducrotoy MJ, Muñoz PM, Conde-Álvarez R, Blasco JM. Moriyón I. A systematic review of current immunological tests for the diagnosis of cattle brucellosis. *Prev Vet Med.* (2018) 151:57–72. doi: 10.1016/j.prevetmed.2018.01.005

19. Cloeckaert A, Vizcaíno N, Paquet JY, Bowden RA. Elzer PH. Major outer membrane proteins of *Brucella* spp: past, present and future. *Vet Microbiol.* (2002) 90:229–47. doi: 10.1016/S0378-1135(02)00211-0

20. Huy TXN, Nguyen TT, Reyes AWB, Vu SH, Min W, Lee HJ, et al. Immunization with a combination of four recombinant *Brucella abortus* proteins Omp16, Omp19, Omp28, and L7/L12 Induces T helper 1 immune response against virulent *B. abortus* 544 infection in BALB/c mice. *Front Vet Sci.* (2021) 7:577026. doi: 10.3389/fvets.2020.577026

21. Zhang J, Guo F, Huang X, Chen C, Liu R, Zhang H, et al. A novel Omp25-binding peptide screened by phage display can inhibit *Brucella abortus* 2308 infection *in vitro* and *in vivo*. *J Med Microbiol.* (2014) 63:780–7. doi: 10.1099/jmm.0.069559-0

22. Xin T, Yang H, Wang N, Wang F, Zhao P, Wang H, et al. Limitations of the BP26 protein-based indirect enzyme-linked immunosorbent assay for diagnosis of Brucellosis. *Clin Vaccine Immunol.* (2013) 20:1410–7. doi: 10.1128/CVI.00052-13

23. Ghasemi A, Jeddi-Tehrani M, Mautner J, Salari MH, Zarnani AH. Simultaneous immunization of mice with Omp31 and TF provides protection against *Brucella melitensis* infection. *Vaccine.* (2015) 33:5532–8. doi: 10.1016/j.vaccine.2015.09.013

24. Zheng WY, Wang Y, Zhang ZC, Yan F. Immunological characteristics of outer membrane protein omp31 of goat brucella and its monoclonal antibody. *Genet Mol Res.* (2015) 14:11965–74. doi: 10.4238/2015.October.5.10

25. Vatankhah M, Beheshti N, Mirkalantari S, Khoramabadi N, Aghababa H, Mahdavi M. Recombinant Omp2b antigen-based ELISA is an efficient tool for specific serodiagnosis of animal brucellosis. *Braz J Microbiol.* (2019) 50:979–84. doi: 10.1007/s42770-019-00097-z

26. Sung KY, Jung M, Shin MK, Park HE, Lee JJ, Kim S, et al. Induction of immune responses by two recombinant proteins of brucellaabortus, outer membrane proteins 2b porin and Cu/Zn superoxide dismutase, in mouse model. *J Microbiol Biotechnol.* (2014) 24:854–61. doi: 10.4014/jmb.1312.12063

27. D'Annessa I, Di Leva FS, La Teana A, Novellino E, Limongelli V, Di Marino D. Bioinformatics and biosimulations as toolbox for peptides and peptidomimetics design: where are we? *Front Mol Biosci.* (2020) 7:66. doi: 10.3389/fmolb.2020.00066

28. Agyei D, Tsopmo A, Udenigwe CC. Bioinformatics and peptidomics approaches to the discovery and analysis of food-derived bioactive peptides. *Anal Bioanal Chem.* (2018) 410:3463–72. doi: 10.1007/s00216-018-0974-1

29. Pang B, Zhao C, Li L, Song X, Xu K, Wang J, et al. Development of a low-cost paper-based ELISA method forrapid *Escherichia coli* O157:H7 detection. *Anal Biochem.* (2018) 542:58–62. doi: 10.1016/j.ab.2017.11.010

30. Hsu MY, Hung YC, Hwang DK, Lin SC, Lin KH, Wang CY, et al. Detection of aqueous VEGF concentrations before and after intravitrealinjection of anti-VEGF antibody using low-volume sampling paper-based ELISA. *Sci Rep.* (2016) 6:34631. doi: 10.1038/srep34631

4

Novel Application of Nanofluidic Chip Digital PCR for Detection of African Swine Fever Virus

Rui Jia[1], Gaiping Zhang[1], Hongliang Liu[2], Yumei Chen[1,2], Jingming Zhou[1], Yankai Liu[2], Peiyang Ding[1], Yanwei Wang[2], Weimin Zang[2] and Aiping Wang[1*]

[1] School of Life Sciences, Zhengzhou University, Zhengzhou, China, [2] Henan Zhongze Biological Engineering Co. LTD, Zhengzhou, China

*Correspondence:
Aiping Wang
pingaw@126.com

African swine fever virus (ASFV) gives rise to a grievous transboundary and infectious disease, African swine fever (ASF), which has caused a great economic loss in the swine industry. To prevent and control ASF, once suspicious symptoms have presented, the movement of animal and pork products should be stopped, and then, laboratory testing should be adopted to diagnose ASF. A method for ASFV DNA quantification is presented in this research, which utilizes the next-generation PCR platform, nanofluidic chip digital PCR (cdPCR). The cdPCR detection showed good linearity and repeatability. The limit of detection for cdPCR is 30.1995 copies per reaction, whereas no non-specific amplification curve was found with other swine viruses. In the detection of 69 clinical samples, the cdPCR showed significant consistency [91.30% (63/69)] to the Office International des Epizooties-approved quantitative PCR. Compared with the commercial quantitative PCR kit, the sensitivity of the cdPCR assay was 86.27% (44/50), and the specificity was 94.44% (17/18). The positive coincidence rate of the cdPCR assay was 88% (44/50). The total coincidence rate of the cdPCR and kit was 89.86% (62/69), and the kappa value reached 0.800 ($P < 0.0001$). This is the first time that cdPCR has been applied to detecting ASFV successfully.

Keywords: African swine fever virus, chip digital PCR, sensitive detection, application, nanofluidic

INTRODUCTION

African swine fever (ASF) was first reported in Kenya, Eastern Africa, in 1921 and then gradually swept across the globe to this day (1, 2). With the death rate of the swine approaching 100%, ASF is putting downward pressure on the global economy and is a disaster for the pig industry (3, 4). African swine fever virus (ASFV), the pathogen causing ASF, is a large double-stranded DNA virus with an envelope and is the only member of the *Asfivirus* genus in the *Asfarviridae* family (5). The genome size of ASFV is from 170 to 190 kb, so it belongs to the nucleocytoplasmic large DNA viruses (6, 7).

Domestic pigs with ASFV infections have serious clinical manifestations such as acute hemorrhagic fever, dyspnea, serous or mucopurulent conjunctivitis, bloody dysentery, vomiting, among others (8). Currently, there are no effective treatments, and vaccine research is progressing slowly. Once suspicious symptoms of ASF presented, the most valid measurements are to firstly stop all circulation of animals and pork products, for example, *via* animal isolation and traffic restriction (9–11). ASF can then be confirmed by a laboratory test (12).

The laboratory diagnostic approaches of ASF are mainly divided into two groups: one includes isolating the virus, detecting virus antigens and genomic DNA, whereas the other aims at detecting an antibody (12, 13). Polymerase chain reaction (PCR) technique is the most mature molecular method for determining virus genomic DNA/RNA. Conventional PCR (14) and fluorescent quantitative PCR (qPCR) (15) have been applied in testing ASFV. Several PCR technologies have been established to achieve quantitative analysis for the concentration of virus DNA during amplification. Real-time fluorogenic qPCR is the most frequently used form of qPCR, in which concentrations of samples are calculated from initial concentrations of standard sample templates. Currently, although qPCR has been used in ASFV detection studies to measure the virus genomic DNA (16–21), digital PCR is getting increasingly popular because it realizes absolute quantification without reliance on external standards, standard curves, and the cycle within the amplification process that the reporter dye signal exceeds a threshold [cycle threshold (CT) value] (22).

Nanofluidic chip digital PCR (cdPCR), a type of digital PCR supported by QuantStudio 3D (Applied Biosystems, US), adopts a sealed chip that partitions samples into thousands of reaction wells to run independent PCR amplifications. When amplifications are finished, the concentration of the target gene in the original sample is calculated by counting and converting positive wells, which have positive amplification of the viral target gene using the Poisson model correction coefficient (22, 23). Another superiority of cdPCR is the high sensitivity, which makes it a dream platform for studying (24, 25) low-level pathogen detection (26, 27) as well as absolute quantification of viral load (28).

This study focuses on the application of cdPCR, in which ASFV is detected by designing a pair of primers and the minor groove binder (MGB) probe in the portion sequence of the ASFV B646L gene. Applicability of this new ASFV diagnosis methods is evaluated in terms of sensitivity, specificity, and coincidence rate with qPCR approved by the Office International des Epizooties (OIE) and commercial qPCR kits.

MATERIALS AND METHODS

Probe and Primers

We designed a set of the MGB probe [5′-(FAM)-ACTGGGACAACCAAAC-3′-(MGB)], upstream primer (ASFV-For: 5′-ACGTTTCCTCGCAACGGATA-3′) and downstream primer (ASFV-Back: 5′-CGTGTAAACGGCGCCCTCTAA-3′), which aimed at the B646L gene (Genebank: MK128995.1) using PRIMER EXPRESS software (version 1.5, Applied Biosystems, USA). The size of the target gene was approximately 63 bp. Primers and the probe sequences were compared with genes of some various ASFV strains sequences in the GenBank database (**Table 1**).

Construction of Standard Plasmid

A 1,941 bp complete fragment of ASFV B646L gene-encoded p72 protein and the ASFV B646L gene with EcoRI/XbaI restriction enzyme cutting site were obtained from the pUC57-p72 plasmid (synthesized by Sangon, Shanghai) by PCR using primers p72-Fwd: 5′-CGGAATTCATGGCATCAGGAGGAGC-3′ and p72-Rev: 5′-GCTCTAGATTAATGATGATGATGATGATGGGTACTGTAACG-3′. Then, the B646L gene was recombined with pFastBacI vector (Promega, USA) and transformed into DH5α (Takara, Dalian, China). The recombinant plasmid, pFastBacI-p72 plasmid, was extracted using Omega Plasmid mini kit (Omega, US). Restriction enzyme digestion and sequencing were used to determine whether the target fragment could be inserted correctly.

Samples Preparation

The protocols of standard templates and clinical sample preparations were as follows. The concentration of the standard plasmid constructed in Section Construction of Standard Plasmid was detected using the NanoDrop One (ThermoFisher, US, AZY1812131) and diluted to the appropriate copy number, which began with 10^{10} copies/ml to 10-fold dilution. Copy number calculating formulas was shown as below.

$$\text{Copy number} \ (copies/ml)$$
$$= \frac{6.02 \times 10^{23} \ (copies/mol) \times C \ (g/ml)}{n \ (bp) \times (1.096 \times 10^{-23} g/bp) \ (g/mol)}$$

where C (g/ml) means the concentration of standard templates, and n (bp) means the genome size in base pairs.

Plasmids ranged from 10^{10} to 10^0 copies/ml were as templates and positive controls for subsequent experiments. Inactivated clinical serum samples were obtained from the Henan Animal Husbandry Bureau and pig farms in Henan province, China. ASFV genomic DNA of clinical samples was extracted from swine serum samples by DNA Extraction Kit (Takara MiniBEST Viral DNA/RNA Extraction Kit, Takara, Dalian, China).

Optimal Conditions of Quantitative PCR

An ABI 7500 Real-time PCR system (Applied Biosystems, USA) was used as a fluorescence quantification platform in this study. The reaction system was 10 μl, including 5 μl TaqMan Universal Master Mix II with uracil-N-glycosylase (purchased from Applied Biosystems, USA), 0.4 μl sense primer (ASFV-For), 0.4 μl anti-sense primer (ASFV-Back), 0.4 μl of probe, 1.8-μl nuclease-free water (Promega, USA), and 2 μl of template. The optimal concentrations of primers and the probe were then measured when the ASFV pFastBacI-p72 plasmid was 1×10^8 copies/ml. Primers with optimal concentration were determined by 12.5, 25, 50, and 100 μM; meanwhile, the probe with optimal concentration was selected by 1.25, 2.5, 5, and 10 μM. The qPCR program was carried out as follows: initial denaturation at 95°C for 10 min, and at 95°C for 15 s, cycling 40 times, and at 60°C holding for 45 s. Negative and positive controls were set at the same time in a run.

Digital PCR

QuantSudio™ 3D Digital PCR System (ThermoScientific, US) was used as a cdPCR amplification platform. The volume of the reaction mixture was 20 μl, containing 10 μl 2× QuantSudio™

TABLE 1 | The primers and MGB probe were aligned with 53 ASFV epidemic strains and 5 other swine pathogenes.

ASFV isolate	GeneBank accession number	Target sequence
ASFV/pig/China/CAS19-01/2019	MN172368.1	ACGTTTCCTCGCAACGGATATGACTGGGACAACCAAACACCCTTAGAGGGCGCCGTTTACACG
ASFV/LT14/1490	MK628478.1	ACGTTTCCTCGCAACGGATATGACTGGGACAACCAAACACCCTTAGAGGGCGCCGTTTACACG
CzechRepublic 2017/1	LR722600.1	ACGTTTCCTCGCAACGGATATGACTGGGACAACCAAACACCCTTAGAGGGCGCCGTTTACACG
taibntMoldova2017/1	LR722599.1	ACGTTTCCTCGCAACGGATATGACTGGGACAACCAAACACCCTTAGAGGGCGCCGTTTACACG
ASFV-wbBS01	MK645909.1	ACGTTTCCTCGCAACGGATATGACTGGGACAACCAAACACCCTTAGAGGGCGCCGTTTACACG
Belgium2018/1	LR536725.1	ACGTTTCCTCGCAACGGATATGACTGGGACAACCAAACACCCTTAGAGGGCGCCGTTTACACG
ASFV-SY18	MH713612.1	ACGTTTCCTCGCAACGGATATGACTGGGACAACCAAACACCCTTAGAGGGCGCCGTTTACACG
Georgia 2007/1	NC_044959.1	ACGTTTCCTCGCAACGGATATGACTGGGACAACCAAACACCCTTAGAGGGCGCCGTTTACACG
47/Ss/2008	NC_044955.1	ACGTTTCCTCGCAACGGATATGACTGGGACAACCAAACACC**T**TTAGAGGGCGCCGTTTACACG
ETH/1a	KT795359.1	ACGTTTCCTCGCAACGGATATGACTGGGACAACCAAACACCCTT**G**GAGGGCGCCGTTTACACG
AnhuiXCGQ	MK128995.1	ACGTTTCCTCGCAACGGATATGACTGGGACAACCAAACACCCTTAGAGGGCGCCGTTTACACG
ETH/2a	KT795358.1	ACGTTTCCTCGCAACGGATATGACTGGGACAACCAAACACCCTT**G**GAGGGCGCCGTTTACACG
POL/2015/Podlaskie	MH681419.1	ACGTTTCCTCGCAACGGATATGACTGGGACAACCAAACACCCTTAGAGGGCGCCGTTTACACG
R7	MH025917.1	ACGTTTCCTCGCAACGGATATGACTGGGACAACCAAACACC**TTG**GAGGGCGCCGTTTACACG
ETH/1	KT795354.1	ACGTTTCCTCGCAACGGATATGACTGGGACAACCAAACACCCTTGGAGGGCGCCGTTTACACG
ETH/AA	KT795353.1	ACGTTTCCTCGCAACGGATATGACTGGGACAACCAAACACCCTT**G**GAGGGCGCCGTTTACACG
BA71	NC_044942.1	ACGTTTCCTCGCAACGGATATGACTGGGACAACCAAACACC**T**TTAGAGGGCGCCGTTTACACG
Ken05/Tk1	NC_044945.1	ACGTTTCCTCGCAACGGATATGACTGGGACAACCAAACACC**T**TTAGAGGGCGCCGTTTACACG
NHV	NC_044943.1	ACGTTTCCTCGCAACGGATATGACTGGGACAACCAAACACC**T**TTAGAGGGCGCCGTTTACACG
L60	NC_044941.1	ACGTTTCCTCGCAACGGATATGACTGGGACAACCAAACACC**T**TTAGAGGGCGCCGTTTACACG
BA71V	U18466.2	ACGTTTCCTCGCAACGGATATGACTGGGACAACCAAACACC**T**TTAGAGGGCGCCGTTTACACG
E75	NC_044958.1	ACGTTTCCTCGCAACGGATATGACTGGGACAACCAAACACC**T**TTAGAGGGCGCCGTTTACACG
OURT 88/3	NC_044957.1	ACGTTTCCTCGCAACGGATATGACTGGGACAACCAAACACC**T**TTAGAGGGCGCCGTTTACACG
Benin 97/1	NC_044956.1	ACGTTTCCTCGCAACGGATATGACTGGGACAACCAAACACC**T**TTAGAGGGCGCCGTTTACACG
BEN/1/97	EF121428.1	ACGTTTCCTCGCAACGGATATGACTGGGACAACCAAACACC**T**TTAGAGGGCGCCGTTTACACG
Za	AY578708.1	ACGTTTCCTCGCAACGGATATGACTGGGACAACCAAACACC**T**TTAGAGGGCGCCGTTTACACG
Wb	AY578707.1	ACGTTTCCTCGCAACGGATATGACTGGGACAACCAAACACC**T**TTAGAGGGCGCCGTTTACACG
Wart	AY578706.1	ACGTTTCCTCGCAACGGATATGACTGGGACAACCAAACACC**T**TTAGAGGGCGCCGTTTACACG
Vic	AY578705.1	ACGTTTCCTCGCAACGGATATGACTGGGACAACCAAACACC**T**TTAGAGGGCGCCGTTTACACG
Ten	AY578704.1	ACGTTTCCTCGCAACGGATATGACTGGGACAACCAAACACC**T**TTAGAGGGCGCCGTTTACACG
Pr5	AY578703.1	ACGTTTCCTCGCAACGGATATGACTGGGACAACCAAACACC**T**TTAGAGGGCGCCGTTTACACG
Pr4	AY578702.1	ACGTTTCCTCGCAACGGATATGACTGGGACAACCAAACACC**T**TTAGAGGGCGCCGTTTACACG
o1	AY578701.1	ACGTTTCCTCGCAACGGATATGACTGGGACAACCAAACACC**T**TTAGAGGGCGCCGTTTACACG
Mk	AY578700.1	ACGTTTCCTCGCAACGGATATGACTGGGACAACCAAACACC**T**TTAGAGGGCGCCGTTTACACG
M1	AY578699.1	ACGTTTCCTCGCAACGGATATGACTGGGACAACCAAACACC**T**TTAGAGGGCGCCGTTTACACG
Ker	AY578697.1	ACGTTTCCTCGCAACGGATATGACTGGGACAACCAAACACC**T**TTAGAGGGCGCCGTTTACACG
K1	AY578696.1	ACGTTTCCTCGCAACGGATATGACTGGGACAACCAAACACC**T**TTAGAGGGCGCCGTTTACACG
F6	AY578694.1	ACGTTTCCTCGCAACGGATATGACTGGGACAACCAAACACC**T**TTAGAGGGCGCCGTTTACACG
E70	AY578692.1	ACGTTTCCTCGCAACGGATATGACTGGGACAACCAAACACC**T**TTAGAGGGCGCCGTTTACACG
cro3.5	AY578691.1	ACGTTTCCTCGCAACGGATATGACTGGGACAACCAAACACC**T**TTAGAGGGCGCCGTTTACACG
Cam	AY578689.1	ACGTTTCCTCGCAACGGATATGACTGGGACAACCAAACACC**T**TTAGAGGGCGCCGTTTACACG
Warthog	AY261366.1	ACGTTTCCTCGCAACGGATATGACTGGGACAACCAAACACC**T**TTAGAGGGCGCCGTTTACACG
Warmbaths	AY261365.1	ACGTTTCCTCGCAACGGATATGACTGGGACAACCAAACACC**T**TTAGAGGGCGCCGTTTACACG
Tengani 62	AY261364.1	ACGTTTCCTCGCAACGGATATGACTGGGACAACCAAACACC**T**TTAGAGGGCGCCGTTTACACG
Pretorisuskop/96/4	AY261363.1	ACGTTTCCTCGCAACGGATATGACTGGGACAACCAAACACC**T**TTAGAGGGCGCCGTTTACACG
Mkuzi 1979	AY261362.1	ACGTTTCCTCGCAACGGATATGACTGGGACAACCAAACACC**T**TTAGAGGGCGCCGTTTACACG
26544/OG10	NC_044947.1	ACGTTTCCTCGCAACGGATATGACTGGGACAACCAAACACC**T**TTAGAGGGCGCCGTTTACACG
R35	MH025920.1	ACGTTTCCTCGCAACGGATATGACTGGGACAACCAAACACC**TTT G**GAGGGCGCCGTTTACACG
N10	MH025919.1	ACGTTTCCTCGCAACGGATATGACTGGGACAACCAAACACC**TTT G**GAGGGCGCCGTTTACACG

(Continued)

TABLE 1 | Continued

ASFV isolate	GeneBank accession number	Target sequence
Ken06.Bus	NC_044946.1	ACGTTTCCTCGCAACGGATATGACTGGGACAACCAAACACC**TTTG**GAGGGCGCCGTTTACACG
UgH03	EF121429.1	ACGTTTCCTCGCAACGGATATGACTGGGACAACCAAACACC**TTTG**GAGGGCGCCGTTTACACG
Kn	AY578698.1	ACGTTTCCTCGCAACGGATATGACTGGGACAACCAAACACC**TTTG**GAGGGCGCCGTTTACACG
RSA_2_2008	MN336500.1	ACGTTTCCTCGCAACGGATATGACTGGGACAACCAAACACC**TG**TAGAGGGCGCCGTTTACACG
CSFV	AF092448	No matches
PPV	AY583318.1	No matches
PRRSV	MH500776.1	No matches
PEDV	KY496315.1	No matches
PCV2	MK604485	No matches

The left grey sequence is sense primer, the right grey sequence is anti-sense primer, and the middle grey sequence is MGB probe. Moreover, the bold letters indicate the mutated bases.

3D Digital PCR Master Mix (v2), 1.8 μl of each primer with optimal concentration determined by qPCR, 1.8 μl of the probe with optimal concentration determined by qPCR, 2.6 μl nuclease-free water (ThermoScientific, US), and 2 μl of DNA template. After sufficient mixed and briefly centrifuged, the 14.5 μl cdPCR reaction mixture was immediately loaded to the chips. Negative control and positive control were set for each test. Three replicates of the standard plasmid template were performed in each run. The program was in operation at 96°C for 10 min as a predenaturation step, at 60°C for 2 min, and at 98°C for 30 s, cycling 39 times, and finally, at 60°C for 2 min as a final elongation step.

Limit of Detection for Chip Digital PCR

The limit of detection (LOD) for cdPCR was determined by the continuous dilution method. At the same time, the same templates were used for qPCR, approved by OIE (12) to compare the LOD between the two methods. The two amplification methods were repeated three times, and the data were analyzed statistically by logistic regression (Statistica 64, USA) (29).

Specificity Analysis

In this analysis, the classical swine fever virus strain Shimen (AF092448), the porcine circovirus 2 strain HN-LB-16 (MK604485), the porcine reproductive and respiratory syndrome virus strain NADC30 (MH500776.1), and the porcine parvovirus strain China (AY583318.1) were kindly provided by Henan Agricultural University (Zhengzhou, Henan, China), and the porcine epidemic diarrhea virus strain CH/hubei/2016 (KY496315.1) was kindly provided by Jilin University (Changchun, Jilin, China). All these pathogens were detected by the nanofluidic cdPCR assay as nucleic acid templates.

Repeatability Evaluation

The repeatability of cdPCR was evaluated by using the continuous dilution of ASFV standard plasmid containing 10^0, 10^1, 10^2, 10^3, and 10^4 copies/ml as templates. On different days, three experiments were carried out, and each template in each experiment was repeated three times. The coefficient of variation (CV) was measured to analyze repeatability.

Comparison of Chip Digital PCR With Quantitative PCR Approved by Office International des Epizooties and Commercial Kits

Comprehensive comparisons of cdPCR with qPCR approved by OIE and commercial kit (VetMAX™ African Swine Fever Virus Detection Kit, Thermofisher, US) were carried on by detecting 69 clinical samples. SPSS (version 21.0, IBM, USA) software and GraphPad Prism software (version 7.04; LA Jolla, California, USA) were used for statistical analysis, including the compliance rate, Bland and Altman analyses, and linear regression with the confidence limit of 95% ($P < 0.05$).

RESULTS

Construction of Standard Plasmid and Identification of Target Gene

The standard plasmid, pFastBacI-p72, was successfully constructed and identified by PCR and sequencing (**Figure 1**). The recombination process of objective gene ASFV p72 (B646L) and vector pFastBacI is shown in **Figure 1A**. The target gene, ASFV B646L, was amplified by PCR with 1,941 bp (**Figure 1B**) and spliced into two cleavage sites of restriction enzyme EcoRI and XbaI of vector pFastBacI. As shown in **Figure 2A**, double-stranded DNA sequences of the MGB probe and primers were marked in different colors within the conserved region of ASFV B646L. The size of the target gene amplified by cdPCR was ~63 bp. A single band of approximately 63 bp was obtained from PCR amplification products *via* 1% agarose gel electrophoresis (**Figure 2B**).

Reaction Conditions of Quantitative PCR

The optimum reaction condition for qPCR was detected *via* using a series of different concentrations of primers and the probe. The optimal concentration of primers was 12.5 μM, and the optimal concentration of the probe was 10 μM, at that time the C_T value was minimum (**Figure 3A**). The optimum reaction system and the program are shown in **Figures 3B,C**.

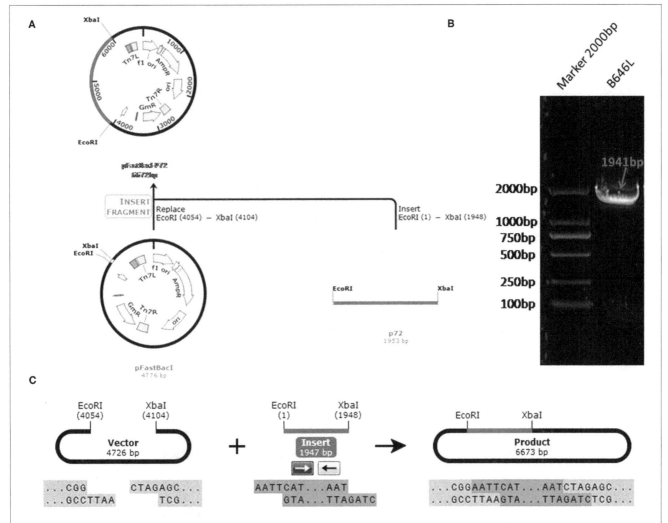

FIGURE 1 | The strategy for the standard plasmid construction. **(A)** The recombination process of objective gene ASFV VP72 (B646L) and vector pFastBacI. **(B)** The size of target gene, ASFV B646L, was 1,941 bp on 1% agarose gel electrophoresis. **(C)** The cleavage sites of the recombination process is EcoR I/Xba I.

Linear Standard Curve of Chip Digital PCR Assay

Using 10-fold diluted ASFV standard plasmid of 10^4-10^{-1} copies/ml as templates, the standard curve of cdPCR was established. At the same time, the standard curve of qPCR confirmed by OIE was created by the same standard plasmid of 10^9-10^0 copies/ml. The trend line was highly linear with the assumed concentration for both cdPCR (**Figure 4A**) and qPCR (**Figure 4B**). The cdPCR assay proved greater linearity with an R^2 of 0.9985 than the qPCR assay with an R^2 of 0.9881 (**Figure 4**).

Limit of Detection of Curve of Chip PCR Assay

The LODs for both cdPCR and qPCR approved by OIE were determined using the same set of primers and the probe with ASFV standard plasmid diluted 10 times as templates. The results are shown in **Figure 5**. Using the least-squares modeling approach and logistic regression analysis, the LOD$_{95\%}$ of the

cdPCR assay was 1.48 Log10 copies per reaction, that is, 30.1995 copies per reaction (**Figures 5A,C**), and the LOD$_{95\%}$ of the qPCR assay was estimated as three Log10 copies per reaction, that is, 1,000 copies per reaction (**Figures 5B,D**). Hence, the LOD$_{95\%}$ of cdPCR assay was approximately 33 times higher than that of the qPCR assay. The cdPCR assay was more sensitive than the qPCR assay.

Specificity Analysis

To analyze the specificity of cdPCR, DNA and complementary DNA, extracted from other swine viruses containing classical swine fever virus, porcine parvovirus, porcine circovirus 2, porcine reproductive and respiratory syndrome virus, and porcine epidemic diarrhea virus, were used as templates, and ASFV pFastBacI-p72 standard plasmid was used as a positive control in specificity assay. The standard plasmid was positive, but nucleic acid templates of the other five pathogens were negative (**Figure 6** and **Table 2**). The result was strongly in line with our theorized expectations that the sequences of primers and probe for the ASFV cdPCR

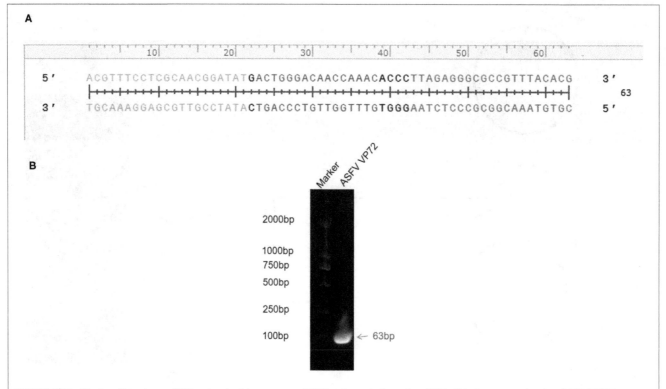

FIGURE 2 | Identification of target gene. (A) Target nucleotide sequences of MGB probe and primers for cdPCR within the conserved region of ASFV B646L gene. Forward primer was marked in orange, reverse primer was marked in red and the probe was marked in purple. (B) Amplification products were analyzed by agarose gel electrophoresis.

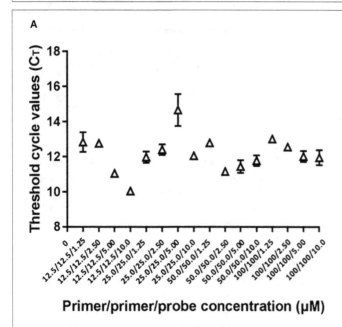

B **The optimum reaction system**

Components	Volume (μL)
nuclease-free water	1.8 μl
(2×conc.) TaqMan® PCR Universal Master Mixer II with UNG	5 μl
forward primer (12.5 μM)	0.4 μl
reserve primer (12.5 μM)	0.4 μl
MGB probe (10 μM).	0.4 μl
Template	2μl
Total volume	10μl

c **The operational procedure of qPCR**

Steps	Temprature (℃)	Time	Cycle numbers
Holding	50	2min	0
Holding	95	10min	0
Cycling	95	15s	40
	60	1min	

FIGURE 3 | The optimum reaction condition for qPCR. (A) Influence of different concentrations PCR primers and probe with use of 108 copies/μl ASFV standard plasmid. (B) The optimum reaction system of qPCR. (C) The operational procedure of qPCR.

did not match with the nucleic acid sequences of any other swine pathogens (**Table 1**). All results mentioned earlier demonstrated that the ASFV cdPCR detection method had good specificity.

Repeatability Analysis

Using serially diluted standard plasmids as templates for cdPCR amplification, three independent experiments were performed by different operators at different times. The cdPCR assay displayed

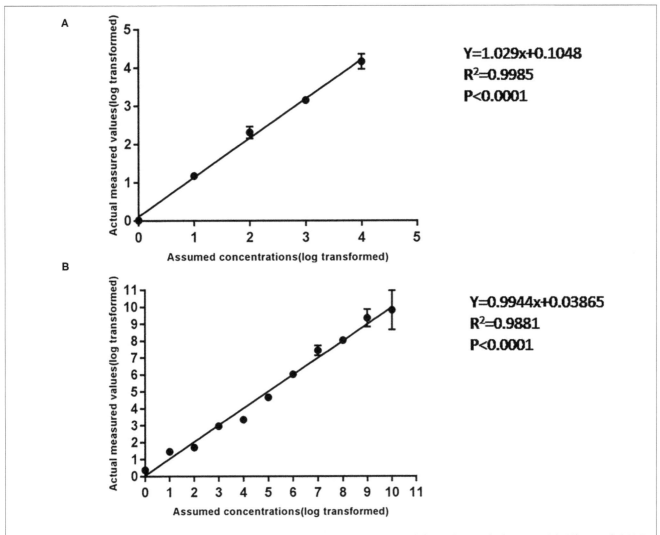

FIGURE 4 | The standard curve of cdPCR and qPCR. **(A)** The standard curve of cdPCR. The slope of this linear fitting equation is 1.029 and the Y-intercept is 0.1048. **(B)** The standard curve of qPCR. The slope of this linear fitting equation is 0.9944 and the Y-intercept is 0.03865.

good repeatability and a low coefficient of variation between most dilution points (**Figure 7**). The cdPCR assay had an average CV% of 9.56%, which was lower than the average CV of 12.67% of qPCR approved by OIE, resulting in an average decrease in CV% of 26.99% (**Figure 7**).

Analysis With Clinical Samples

To calculate the coincidence rate of the cdPCR method to detect ASFV, we compared, respectively, the cdPCR method established in this study with the qPCR approved by OIE and commercial qPCR kit (VetMAX™ African Swine Fever Virus Detection Kit, Thermofisher, US), by testing 69 swine serum samples.

As shown in **Table 3A**, the cdPCR and qPCR approved by OIE have, respectively, detected 50 and 48 positive samples in the clinical diagnosis of 69 domestic pigs. The sensitivity of the cdPCR assay was 95.83% (46/48), and the specificity was 94.44% (17/21). The positive coincidence rate of the cdPCR assay was 92% (46/50). The total coincidence rate of the two methods was 91.30% (63/69), and the kappa value reached 0.789 ($P <$

0.0001). There was significant consistency between the two from the results. Furthermore, quantitation of the correlation between the two was analyzed by Pearson correlation and linear regression analysis on 46 positive samples (**Figure 8**). The quantitative analysis of the correlation between the two showed that they had a good correlation because the R^2 value of linear regression was 0.984 ($P < 0.0001$) (**Figure 8A**). The standard deviation of cdPCR was lower than that of qPCR by Mann–Whitney U test (**Figure 8B**). Bland and Altman analyses plots (**Figure 8C**) demonstrated that 5.797% (4/69) dots were outside the region between 95% lower limit of agreement and 95% upper limit of agreement, and the bias value for this agreement's range was 1,381 copies/ml ($P < 0.05$) by Graphpad Prism 7.04.

The data in **Table 3B** show that 45 of 69 samples were judged to be positive by VetMAX™ African Swine Fever Virus Detection Kit. The sensitivity of the cdPCR assay was 86.27% (44/50), and the specificity was 94.44% (17/18). Furthermore, the positive coincidence rate and the overall coincidence rate of the cdPCR assay were 88% (44/50) and 89.86% (62/69),

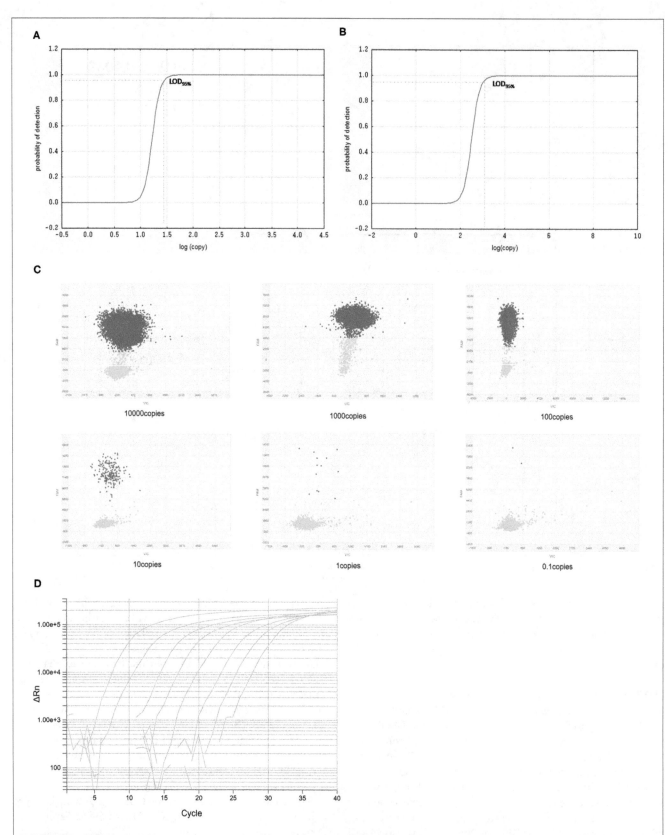

FIGURE 5 | The LOD$_{95\%}$ of cdPCR and qPCR assay. Logit analysis plots of the cdPCR **(A)** and qPCR **(B)** used in the study show the LOD$_{95\%}$, which are the minimum amounts of DNA detectable with a 95% probably. The amplification curve of cdPCR **(C)** and qPCR **(D)** is obtained with 10-fold diluted standard plasmids.

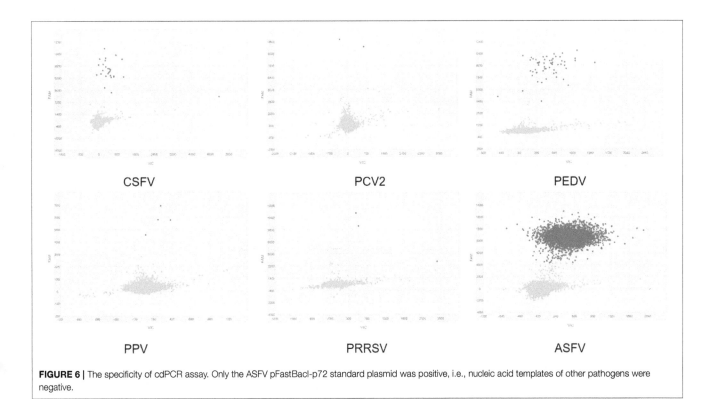

FIGURE 6 | The specificity of cdPCR assay. Only the ASFV pFastBacI-p72 standard plasmid was positive, i.e., nucleic acid templates of other pathogens were negative.

respectively, and the kappa value was 0.800 ($P < 0.0001$). Those seven samples with inconsistent results between two assays were tested with cdPCR three times to exclude false-positive events, and negative and positive controls were included in all trials. All seven samples were declared as positive samples by cdPCR tests. In addition, the quantitative agreements were evaluated using Pearson correlation and linear regression analysis on 44 positive samples. The quantitative analysis of the correlation between the two showed that they had a good correlation because the R^2 value of linear regression was 0.864 ($P < 0.0001$) (**Figure 8D**). The standard deviation of cdPCR was lower than that of the kit (**Figure 8E**). Bland and Altman analyses plots (**Figure 8F**) demonstrated that 1.449% (1/69) dots were outside the region between 95% lower limit of agreement and 95% upper limit of agreement with that of the bias value. Within the consistency limit, the absolute value of the difference between the concentration of the sample to be measured by cdPCR and qPCR was 1,762.59 copies/ml (the top point in **Figure 8F**), and the average value of the difference was 54.85 copies/ml determined by Graphpad Prism 7.04.

Above all, the cdPCR technology developed in this study had comparable performances with the qPCR approved by OIE as well as VetMAX™ African Swine Fever Virus Detection Kit in terms of detecting ASFV clinical samples.

DISCUSSION

ASFV has been widely spreading outside Africa to Europe (30, 31) and most recently to Georgia (32), China (33), Cambodia (12), South America (21, 34, 35), and so on, even to reach

TABLE 2 | Concentration of CSFV, PPV, PCV2, PRRSV, and PEDV, and ASFV standard plasmid by cdPCR assay.

Isolation virus	Mean concentration (copies/μl)
CSFV	1.027
PPV	0.616
PRRSV	0.532
PEDV	1.391
PCV2	0.692
ASFV	845.11

almost every corner of the world, which is a significant transboundary and emerging virus (36, 37). ASF is a serious and highly contagious disease with high mortality, causing acute hemorrhagic fever in domestic pigs and wild boars (38–40). Hence, ASF was the biggest threat to the world pork industry (41). Although vaccination is the preferred method for controlling the disease, the development of safe vaccines to protect pigs from ASFV has not achieved significant success since the first isolation of ASFV (42). Because there are no safe and efficacious vaccines, the key of current surveillance and control measures against ASF is firstly to cut off the transmission of the pathogen once ASFV clinical symptoms are observed. Then, diagnosis and confirmation of ASFV require laboratory testing. The traditional method of diagnosing ASFV is using qPCR to measure the ASFV genomic DNA. However, the quality of the standard curve affects the accuracy quantification of qPCR. If the standard curve is unstable, ASFV DNA quantification will

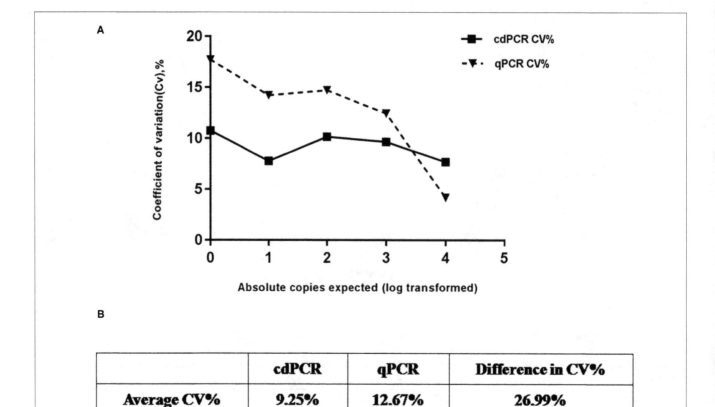

FIGURE 7 | Repeatability analysis. **(A)** Trend line comparing coefficient of variation (CV%) for cdPCR and qPCR at different concentration points. The square with the full line stands for CV % of cdPCR and the triangle with the dotted line indicated as the CV% of qPCR. **(B)** Table shows that average CV% value of cdPCR (9.25%) is lower than that of qPCR (12.67%).

be inexact (43). Additionally, CT values in qPCR related to amplification efficiencies are obtained from the amplification of standards and the samples. Also, several factors, such as inhibitors, amount of total DNA, and variations between the primers and the probe, may cause the false amplification of the templates, resulting in the CT values going up. Digital PCR as a novel approach to nucleic acid quantification has been used in several aspects with equal or superior performance to qPCR.

Digital PCR can realize an absolute target quantification without standards and the standard curve. Nanofluidic cdPCR running on QuantStudio 3D digital PCR platform (Applied Biosystems) has been applied as a useful tool for sensitive and accurate detection of norovirus low-copy targets (28), quantification of bacterial pathogens (44), quantifying microRNAs in infarction patients (45), and detection of enterotoxigenic *Bacteroides fragilis* (46). Although droplet digital PCR has been reported being applied to detecting ASFV (47), in this paper, we applied nanofluidic cdPCR on QuantStudio 3D digital PCR platform to diagnose ASF for the first time and assess the applicability of detection ASFV by using cdPCR on aspects such as sensitivity, specificity, reproducibility, among others.

The 53 complete ASFV genome sequences in the GenBank database were aligned, and a suite of primers and an MGB probe were designed based on a highly conserved fragment of the B646L gene coded p72 protein. Various properties of cdPCR assays, such

TABLE 3A | Testing of clinical samples by cdPCR and qPCR assay approved by OIE.

Samples		qPCR approved by OIE		Summary
		Positive	Negative	
cdPCR	Positive	46	4	50
	Negative	2	17	19
Summary		48	21	69

TABLE 3B | Testing of clinical samples by cdPCR and commercial kit.

Samples		qPCR (commercial kit)		Summary
		Positive	Negative	
cdPCR	Positive	44	6	50
	Negative	1	18	19
Summary		45	24	69

as sensitivity, repeatability, and coincidence rate, were evaluated after optimizing reaction conditions. The linearity analysis of cdPCR detection was performed using 10-fold diluted ASFV standard plasmid as templates, with initial concentration of 10^4

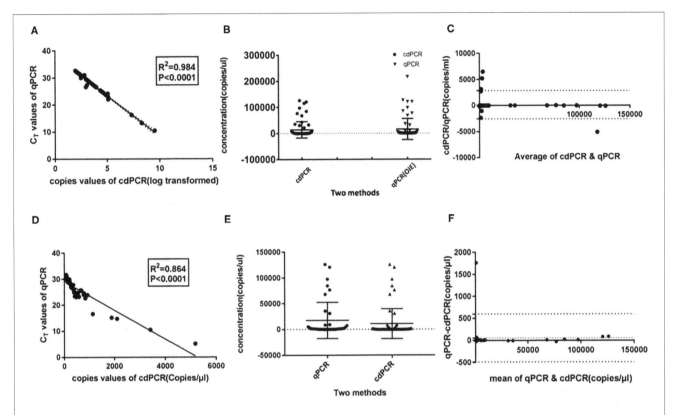

FIGURE 8 | Statistical analysis for cdPCR in testing clinical blood samples. Pearson correlation and linear regression analysis showed well-consistency between qPCR approved by OIE ($R^2 = 0.864$) **(A)** as well as between cdPCR and commercial qPCR kit ($R^2 = 0.864$) **(D)**. The standard deviation of cdPCR is lower than that of qPCR approved by OIE **(B)** and that of commercial qPCR kit **(E)**. **(C)** Bland and Altman analyses plots for cdPCR and qPCR approved by OIE demonstrated that 5.797% (4/69) dots were outside the region between 95% lower limit of agreement and 95% upper limit of agreement, and the bias value for this agreement's range was 1,381 copies/ml ($P < 0.05$) by Graphpad Prism 7.04. **(F)** Bland and Altman analyses plots for cdPCR and the kit demonstrated that 1.449% (1/69) dots were outside the region between 95% lower limit of agreement and 95% upper limit of agreement with that of the bias value.

to 10^{-1} copies/ml. The results showed that the limit detection of cdPCR [30.1995 copies per reaction ($n = 3$)] was approximately 33 times higher than that of qPCR approved by OIE (1,000 copies per reaction) (12). Also, the limit detection of cdPCR did correlate well with that of an improved new real-time PCR assay established by Tignon et al. (5.7–57 copies per reaction) (21). The sensitivity of the cdPCR detection method has been significantly improved.

The statistics offer further support in that cdPCR is a perfect tool to detect ASFV. Detecting 69 inactivated clinical serum samples by cdPCR and other techniques showed good consistency with cdPCR and qPCR approved by OIE as well as VetMAX™ African Swine Fever Virus Detection Kit (Thermofisher, US). The positive detection rate of the cdPCR method established in this study was 72.46% (50/69), which had a better performance than both qPCR approved by OIE [69.57% (48/69)] and VetMAX™ African Swine Fever Virus Detection Kit [65.22% (45/69)]. Additionally, the cdPCR assay did not react with other swine viruses. Both Bland and Altman analyses and line regression analysis exhibited that cdPCR carried out comparably better than the other two methods.

There are some limitations of the novel cdPCR. That specific equipment is required for nanofluidic cdPCR, which makes

it hard to popularize and be widely applied. A specialized nanofluidic chip that accompanies QuantStudio 3D digital PCR platform is a little bit expensive. So, qPCR assay is more economical than cdPCR. Also, cdPCR can only amplify a maximum of 24 samples in a single run, 72 samples fewer than qPCR for a single run. Although this shortcoming of cdPCR can be overcome by adding the number of the ProFlex™ 2× Flat PCR System or Dual Flat Block GeneAmp™ PCR System (Applied Biosystem, US), the cost is too high. Therefore, qPCR is more applicable in detecting large numbers of clinical samples than cdPCR. However, cdPCR is suitable for the quantification of low copy numbers, especially when the laboratory standard of quantification qPCR for virus genomic DNA/RNA is limited (44). Taken together, the method of using cdPCR to detect ASFV in serum samples has been established and feasible. The cdPCR, as a good tool, can be applied to the absolute quantification of ASFV.

ETHICS STATEMENT

Ethical statement is not applicable because sample collection has been gathered. Written informed consent was obtained from the owners for the participation of their animals in this study.

AUTHOR CONTRIBUTIONS

AW contributed to study design, laboratory supervision, and manuscript editing. RJ contributed to study design, doing experiments, data analysis and manuscript drafting, editing, and writing. HL contributed significantly to the collection of laboratory data. YC, JZ, YW, and WZ contributed to laboratory quality control and data collection. YL polished the language of the manuscript. PD helped perform the analysis with constructive discussions. GZ and AW contributed to study design, laboratory supervision, and manuscript editing. All authors contributed to the article and approved the submitted version.

ACKNOWLEDGMENTS

We thank Dr. Yilin Bai of Northwest Agriculture and Forestry University in helping us contact the instrument. Also, we thank Ms. Xiaolian Hu, the technician of Themofisher, for the instruction of the experiment.

REFERENCES

1. Olesen A, Belsham G, Bruun Rasmussen T, Lohse L, Bødker R, Halasa T, et al. Potential routes for indirect transmission of African swine fever virus into domestic pig herds. *Transbound Emerg Dis.* (2020) 67:1472–84. doi: 10.1111/tbed13538

2. Li C, Chai Y, Song H, Weng C, Qi J, Sun Y, et al. Crystal structure of African swine fever virus dUTPase reveals a potential drug target. *mBio.* (2019) 10:1–11. doi: 10.1128/mBio02483-19

3. He Q, Yu D, Bao M, Korensky G, Chen J, Shin M, et al. High-throughput and all-solution phase African Swine Fever Virus (ASFV) detection using CRISPR-Cas12a and fluorescence based point-of-care system. *Biosens Bioelectron.* (2020) 154:112068. doi: 10.1016/j.bios.2020112068

4. Yoon H, Hong S, Lee I, Yoo D, Jung C, Lee E, et al. Clinical symptoms of African swine fever in domestic pig farms in the Republic of Korea, 2019. *Transbound Emerg Dis.* (2020) 67:2245–8. doi: 10.1111/tbed13552

5. Meng XY, Zhang H, Luo Y, Sun Y, Li Y, Abid M, et al. Cross-priming amplification combined with immunochromatographic strip for rapid on-site detection of African swine fever virus. *Sens Actuators B Chem.* (2018) 274:304–5. doi: 10.1016/j.snb.2018.07164

6. Galindo I, Alonso C. African swine fever virus: a review. *Viruses.* (2017) 9:103. doi: 10.3390/v9050103

7. Liu Q, Ma B, Qian N, Zhang F, Tan X, Lei J, et al. Structure of the African swine fever virus major capsid protein p72. *Cell Res.* (2019) 29:953–5. doi: 10.1038/s41422-019-0232-x

8. Boer CJD, Hess WR, Dardiri AH. African swine fever. *Adv Vet Med.* (2019) 8:191–4. doi: 10.1016/S0166-3542(98)00015-1

9. Gaudreault NN, Richt JA. Subunit vaccine approaches for African swine fever virus. *Vaccines.* (2019) 7:56. doi: 10.3390/vaccines70 20056

10. Sánchez EG, Pérez-Núñez D, Revilla Y. Development of vaccines against African swine fever virus. *Virus Res.* (2019) 265:150–5. doi: 10.1016/j.virusres.2019.03022

11. Revilla Y, Pérez-Núñez D, Richt JA. African swine fever virus biology and vaccine approaches. *Adv Virus Res.* (2018) 100:41. doi: 10.1016/bs.aivir.2017.10002

12. OIE-WAHID. *World Animal Health Information Database (Wahid). World Organisation for Animal Health (OIE).* (2017). [Cited World Animal Health Information System (WAHIS)]. Available online at: http://www.Oie.Int/wahis/public.Php?Page=home (accessed on March 27, 2017).

13. Mehlhorn H. *World Organisation for Animal Health (OIE).* Berlin Heidelberg: Springer (2015).

14. Agüero M, Fernández J, Romero L, Mascaraque CS, Arias M, SánchezVizcaíno JM. Highly sensitive PCR assay for routine diagnosis of African swine fever virus in clinical samples. *J Clin Microbiol.* (2003) 41:4431–4. doi: 10.1128/JCM.41.9.4431-44342003

15. King DP, Reid SM, Hutchings GH, Grierson SS, Wilkinson PJ, Dixon LK, et al. Development of a TaqMan† PCR assay with internal amplification control for the detection of African swine fever virus. *J Virol Methods.* (2003) 107:9. doi: 10.1016/S0166-0934(02)00189-1

16. Wang A, Jia R, Liu Y, Zhou J, Zhang G. Development of a novel quantitative real-time PCR assay with lyophilized powder reagent to detect African swine fever virus in blood samples of domestic pigs in China. *Transbound Emerg Dis.* (2019) 67:284–97. doi: 10.1111/tbed13350

17. Shi X, Liu X, Wang Q, Das A, Ma G, Xu L, et al. A multiplex real-time PCR panel assay for simultaneous detection and differentiation of 12 common swine viruses. *J Virol Methods.* (2016) 236:258–65. doi: 10.1016/j.jviromet.2016.08005

18. Giammarioli M, Pellegrini C, Casciari C, Mia GMD. Development of a novel hot-start multiplex PCR for simultaneous detection of classical swine fever virus, African swine fever virus, porcine circovirus type 2, porcine reproductive and respiratory syndrome virus and porcine parvovirus. *Vet Res Commun.* (2008) 32:255–62. doi: 10.1007/s11259-007-9026-6

19. Erickson A, Fisher M, Furukawa-Stoffer T, Ambagala A, Hodko D, Pasick J, et al. A multiplex reverse transcription PCR and automated electronic microarray assay for detection and differentiation of seven viruses affecting swine. *Transbound Emerg Dis.* (2018) 65:e272–83. doi: 10.1111/tbed.12749

20. Fernández-Pinero J, Gallardo C, Elizalde M, Robles A, Gómez C, Bishop R, et al. Molecular diagnosis of African swine fever by a new real-time PCR using universal probe library. *Transbound Emerg Dis.* (2013) 60:48–58. doi: 10.1111/j.1865-1682.2012.01317x

21. Tignon M, Gallardo C, Iscaro C, Hutet E, Van der Stede Y, Kolbasov D, et al. development and inter-laboratory validation study of an improved new real-time PCR assay with internal control for detection and laboratory diagnosis of African swine fever virus. *J Virol Methods.* (2011) 178:161–70. doi: 10.1016/j.jviromet.2011.09007

22. Hindson B, Ness K, Masquelier D, Belgrader P, Heredia N, Makarewicz A, et al. High-throughput droplet digital PCR system for absolute quantitation of DNA copy number. *Anal Chem.* (2011) 83:8604–10. doi: 10.1021/ac202028g

23. Ahmed FE, Ahmed NC, Gouda MM. Quantification of MicroRNAs for the diagnostic screening of colon cancer in human stool by absolute digital(d) PCR. *Surg Case Stud Open Access J.* (2018) 1:110–8. doi: 10.32474/SCSOAJ.2019.01000125

24. Maynard CL, Wong WKM, Hardikar AA, Joglekar MV. Droplet digital PCR for measuring absolute copies of gene transcripts in human islet-derived progenitor cells. *Methods Mol Biol.* (2019) 37–48. doi: 10.1007/978-1-4939-9631-5_4

25. Handschuh L, Kazmierczak M, Milewski MC, Goralski M, Luczak M, Wojtaszewska M, et al. Gene expression profiling of acute myeloid leukemia samples from adult patients with AML-M1 and -M2 through boutique microarrays, real-time PCR and droplet digital PCR. *Int J Oncol.* (2018) 52:656–78. doi: 10.3892/ijo.20174233

26. Strain MC, Lada SM, Luong T, Rought SE, Gianella S, Terry VH, et al. Highly precise measurement of HIV DNA by droplet digital PCR. *PLoS ONE.* (2013) 8:e55943. doi: 10.1371/journal.pone0055943

27. Taylor SC, Laperriere G. Germain H. Droplet Digital PCR versus qPCR for gene expression analysis with low abundant targets: from variable nonsense to publication quality data. *Sci Rep.* (2017) 7:1–8. doi: 10.1038/s41598-017-02217-x

28. Monteiro S, Santos R. Nanofluidic digital PCR for the quantification of Norovirus for water quality assessment. *PLoS ONE.* (2017) 12:e0179985. doi: 10.1371/journal.pone0179985

29. Burns M, Valdivia H. Modelling the limit of detection in real-time quantitative PCR. *Eur Food Res Technol.* (2008) 226:1513–24. doi: 10.1007/s00217-007-0683-z

30. Wozniakowski G, Kozak E, Kowalczyk A, Lyjak M, Pomorska-Mol M, Niemczuk K, et al. Current status of African swine fever virus in a population

of wild boar in eastern Poland (2014-2015). *Arch Virol.* (2016) 161:189–95. doi: 10.1007/s00705-015-2650-5

31. Pejsak Z, Truszczyński M, Niemczuk K, Kozak E, Markowska-Daniel I. Epidemiology of African swine fever in Poland since the detection of the first case. *Pol J Vet Sci.* (2014) 17:665–72. doi: 10.2478/pjvs-2014-0097

32. Sánchez-Cordón P, Montoya M, Reis A, Dixon L. African swine fever: a re-emerging viral disease threatening the global pig industry. *Vet J.* (2018) 233:41–8. doi: 10.1016/j.tvjl.2017.12025

33. Zhou X, Li N, Luo Y, Liu Y, Miao F, Chen T, et al. Emergence of African swine fever in China, 2018. *Transbound Emerg Dis.* (2018) 65:1482–4. doi: 10.1111/tbed12989

34. Wormington JD, Golnar A, Poh KC, Kading RC, Martin E, Hamer SA. Risk of african swine fever virus sylvatic establishment and spillover to domestic swine in the united states. *Vector Borne Zoonotic Dis.* (2019) 19:506–11. doi: 10.1089/vbz.20182386

35. Golnar AJ, Martin E, Wormington JD, Kading RC, Teel PD, Hamer SA. Reviewing the potential vectors and hosts of african swine fever virus transmission in the united states. *Vector Borne Zoonotic Dis.* (2019) 7:197. doi: 10.1089/vbz.20182387

36. Karger A, Pérez-Núñez D, Urquiza J, Hinojar P, Alonso C, Freitas F, et al. An update on African swine fever virology. *Viruses.* (2019) 11:864. doi: 10.3390/v11090864

37. Arabyan E, Kotsynyan A, Hakobyan A, Zakaryan H. Antiviral agents against African swine fever virus. *Virus Res.* (2019) 270:197669. doi: 10.1016/j.virusres.2019197669

38. Simões M, Freitas F, Leitão A, Martins C, Ferreira F. African swine fever virus replication events and cell nucleus: new insights and perspectives. *Virus Res.* (2019) 270:197667. doi: 10.1016/j.virusres.2019197667

39. James H, Ebert K, McGonigle R, Reid S, Boonham N, Tomlinson J, et al. Detection of African swine fever virus by loop-mediated isothermal amplification. *J Virol Methods.* (2010) 164:68–74. doi: 10.1016/j.jviromet.2009.11.034

40. Hübner A, Petersen B, Keil G, Niemann H, Mettenleiter T, Fuchs W. Efficient inhibition of African swine fever virus replication by CRISPR/Cas9 targeting of the viral p30 gene (CP204L). *Sci Rep.* (2018) 8:1449. doi: 10.1038/s41598-018-19626-1

41. Sánchez-Cordón P, Nunez A, Neimanis A, Wikström-Lassa E, Montoya M, Crooke HD. Gavier-Widén. African swine fever: disease dynamics in wild boar experimentally infected with ASFV isolates belonging to genotype I and II. *Viruses.* (2019) 11:852. doi: 10.3390/v110 90852

42. Sang H, Miller G, Lokhandwala S, Sangewar N, Waghela S, Bishop R, et al. Progress toward development of effective and safe African swine fever virus vaccines. *Front Vet Sci.* (2020) 7:84. doi: 10.3389/fvets.2020 00084

43. Busby E, Whale AS, Ferns RB, Grant PR, Garson JA. Instability of 8E5 calibration standard revealed by digital PCR risks inaccurate quantification of HIV DNA in clinical samples by qPCR. *Sci Rep.* (2017) 7:1209. doi: 10.1038/s41598-017-01221-5

44. Ricchi M, Bertasio C, Boniotti MB, Vicari N, Russo S, Tilola M, et al. Comparison among the quantification of bacterial pathogens by qPCR, dPCR, and cultural methods. *Front Microbiol.* (2017) 8:1174. doi: 10.3389/fmicb.2017.01174

45. Robinson S, Follo M, Haenel D, Mauler M, Stallmann D, Tewari M. Chip-based digital pcr as a novel detection method for quantifying micrornas in acute myocardial infarction patients. *Acta Pharmacol Sin.* (2017) 257:247–54. doi: 10.1038/aps.2017136

46. Purcell RV, Pearson J, Frizelle FA, Keenan JI. Comparison of standard, quantitative and digital PCR in the detection of enterotoxigenic Bacteroides fragilis. *Sci Rep.* (2016) 6:34554. doi: 10.1038/srep34554

47. Wu X, Xiao L, Lin H, Chen S, Yang M, An W, et al. Development and application of a droplet digital polymerase chain reaction (ddPCR) for detection and investigation of African swine fever virus. *Can J Vet Res.* (2018) 82:70–74. doi: 10.1016/j.meegid.2017.10019

5

Development Real-Time PCR Assays to Genetically Differentiate Vaccinated Pigs from Infected Pigs with the Eurasian Strain of African Swine Fever Virus

Lauro Velazquez-Salinas [1,2]*, Elizabeth Ramirez-Medina [1], Ayushi Rai [1,3], Sarah Pruitt [1], Elizabeth A. Vuono [1,4], Nallely Espinoza [1], Douglas P. Gladue [1]* and Manuel V. Borca [1]*

[1] Agricultural Research Service, United States Department of Agriculture, Plum Island Animal Disease Center, Greenport, NY, United States, [2] Department of Anatomy and Physiology, Kansas State University, Manhattan, KS, United States, [3] Oak Ridge Institute for Science and Education (ORISE), Oak Ridge, TN, United States, [4] Department of Pathobiology and Population Medicine, Mississippi State University, Mississippi, MS, United States

*Correspondence:
Lauro Velazquez-Salinas
lauro.velazquez@usda.gov
Douglas P. Gladue
douglas.gladue@usda.gov
Manuel V. Borca
manuel.borca@usda.gov

Currently, African swine fever virus (ASFV) represents one of the most important economic threats for the global pork industry. Recently, significant advances have been made in the development of potential vaccine candidates to protect pigs against this virus. We have previously developed attenuated vaccine candidates by deleting critical viral genes associated with virulence. Here, we present the development of the accompanying genetic tests to discriminate between infected and vaccinated animals (DIVA), a necessity during an ASFV vaccination campaign. We describe here the development of three independent real-time polymerase chain reaction (qPCR) assays that detect the presence of MGF-360-12L, UK, and I177L genes, which were previously deleted from the highly virulent Georgia strain of ASFV to produce the three recombinant live attenuated vaccine candidates. When compared with the diagnostic reference qPCR that detects the p72 gene, all assays demonstrated comparable levels of sensitivity, specificity, and efficiency of amplification to detect presence/absence of the ASFV Georgia 2007/1 strain (prototype virus of the Eurasian lineage) from a panel of blood samples from naïve, vaccinated, and infected pigs. Collectively, the results of this study demonstrate the potential of these real-time PCR assays to be used as genetic DIVA tests, supporting vaccination campaigns associated with the use of ASFV-ΔMGF, ASFV-G-Δ9GL/ΔUK, and ASFV-ΔI177L or cell culture adapted ASFV-ΔI177LΔLVR live attenuated vaccines in the field.

Keywords: ASFV, ASF real time PCR, genetic DIVA test, live attenuated vaccine, phylogenetics

INTRODUCTION

African swine fever virus (ASFV), an arbovirus, and unique member of the *Asfarviridae* family, is a double-stranded DNA virus with a varying genome length that ranges between 170 and 193 kbp, encoding for between 150 and 167 open reading frames (1). ASFV is the causal agent of African swine fever (ASF), a reportable highly contagious disease of pigs and wild boar that represents a significant socio-economic threat for the pork industry worldwide (2).

A recent report of the World Organization for Animal Health (https://www.oie.int/app/uploads/2021/03/report-47-global-situation-asf.pdf) regarding the global situation of ASFV between 2016 and 2020 indicates that ASFV is endemic in most Sub-Saharan African countries and is causing outbreaks throughout Europe and Asia resulting in the loss of more than 6,000,000 domestic pigs, representing 82% of global losses to ASF during this time period.

In this context, the increased number of cases currently reported out of Africa are mostly attributed to the emergence of the Eurasian ASFV lineage (genotype II) (3), one of 23 ASFV genotypes (4). ASFV genotype II was first reported in the Republic of Georgia in 2007 and has subsequently spread to different countries in Asia and Europe (3, 5). Just recently (07/15/2021), The Friedrich-Loeffler-Institute reported the first cases of ASFV in domestic pigs in Germany (https://www.fli.de/en/news/animal-disease-situation/african-swine-fever), and (7/28/2021) The U.S. Department of Agriculture's (USDA) Foreign Animal Disease Diagnostic Laboratory confirmed the presence of ASFV in Dominican Republic, being this first report of this genotype in the Americas (https://www.aphis.usda.gov/aphis/newsroom/news/sa_by_date/sa-2021/asf-confirm).

Experimental infection of domestic pigs and wild boars with ASFV genotype II produced 100% mortality around 7 days post-infection (6–8), confirming the devastating effect of this virus to swine production. The latest epizootic has devastated swine industries across many countries in Europe and Asia, making development of an effective vaccine and a complementary diagnostic test that differentiates infected from vaccinated animals (DIVA) an international priority (9).

Currently, there is no commercial vaccine for ASFV, despite decades of work and multiple developmental strategies (3). Recently, experimental evaluation of three potential vaccine candidates obtained by deleting seven genes belonging to the MGF360 and MGF 505 families (ASFV-ΔMGF) (10), 9GL and UK (ASFV-G-Δ9GL/ΔUK) (11) or I177L (ASFV-ΔI177L) (12) demonstrated protection against challenge with the highly virulent ASFV Georgia 2007/1 strain. Recently, we published the adaptation of the recombinant ASFV-ΔI177L to grow in an established cell line (ASFV-ΔI177LΔLVR) and its potential to be used as a live attenuated vaccine (13). All four live attenuated vaccine candidates are in the process of being licensed in the U.S, with future possibility of commercialization. We developed genetic DIVA tests to support the use of these three vaccines in the field. For this purpose, three independent qPCR assays that detect the presence of MGF-360-12L, I177L and UK genes of ASFV were developed and validated. The results of this study are discussed in terms of the impact that these genetic DIVA marker tests may have in an outbreak situations as well as to support future experimental studies in pigs to evaluate the dynamic of the infection in vaccinated pigs challenged with the homologous virulent ASFV.

MATERIALS AND METHODS
Viruses and Cells
Recombinant viruses ASFV-ΔMGF, ASFV-G-Δ9GL/ΔUK ASFV-ΔI177L and ASFV-ΔI177LΔLVR, all previously developed in our laboratory (10–13), as well as the parental virus ASFV Georgia 2007/1 strain (ASFV-G), a field isolate kindly provided by Nino Vepkhvadze from the Laboratory of the Ministry of Agriculture (LMA) in Tbilisi, Republic of Georgia were used to conduct this study.

Primary swine macrophage cell cultures were prepared from defibrinated blood as previously described (14).

Primers and Probes Design
To detect target sequences of MGF-360-12L, I177L, and UK genes of ASFV, primers and probes were developed using the RealTime qPCR Assay tool from Integrated DNA Technologies (https://www.idtdna.com/scitools/Applications/RealTimePCR/).

All primers and probes were designed based on the reference sequence of ASFV Georgia 2007/1 strain (GenBank data base NC_044959.2), considering the boundaries of the deletion of each gene as described in the publication of each vaccine candidate (10–12). The sequences of primers and probes are provided in **Figure 1**.

Additionally, to support the validation, specific primers and probes were designed for the detection of genes that code for fluorescent proteins present in each recombinant virus. For the detection of the mCherry gene, the sequence of the expression vector precB5R.1 (NCBI accession number: LC325569) was used as a reference sequence for the design of primers: forward, 5′-GCT TCT TGG CCT TGT AGG TG-3′, reverse, 5′-CAG AGG CTG AAG CTGAAG GA-3′, and probe, 5′-FAM-CGG CGG CCA CTA CGA CGC TG-MGB NFQ-3′.

The sequence of Gateway positive vector pENTR-gus (LC588893.1) was used for the design of primers and probe for the detection of the GUS gene encoding the protein beta-glucuronidase (β-GUS): forward, 5′-TCT ACT TTA CTG GCT TTG GTC G-3′, reverse, 5′-CGT A AG GGT AAT GCG AGG TAC, and probe, 5′-FAM-AGG ATT CGA TAA CGT GCT GAT GGT GC-MG B NFQ-3′.

Standard Plasmid Control
A standard plasmid (pCloneEZ-NRS-Blunt-Amp) containing sequences of targeted regions of primers and probes from all designs was developed to support the validation of real-time PCRs. This plasmid was developed by Epoch Life Sciences, Missouri City, TX, USA.

DNA Extraction
DNA extraction was conducted using a KingFisher automated extraction and purification system (ThermoFisher Scientific), using the MagMAX™ Pathogen RNA/DNA kit following the manufacturer instructions for 200 µl of sample.

Real-Time PCR Performance
Real-time PCR assays were performed using an Applied Biosystems™ 7500 Real-time PCR system, using the TaqMan™ Universal PCR Master Mix (Applied Biosystems Catalog No. 4305719). Briefly, master mix was prepared in a final volume of 25 µl as follows: Universal mix 12.5 µl, primer forward (50 µM) 0.1 µl, primer reverse (50 µM) 0.1 µl, probe (10 µM) 0.25 µl, water 7.05 µl, and DNA sample 5 µl. Amplification conditions were

qPCR	Primers and Probes	Sequence 5'-3'	Position in the reference strain	Sense	TM(°C)	GC(%)		Dimer		
							Hairpin	Forward	Reverse	Probe
I177L	Forward	GAACTGGAAAAAACTTTAACGGC	175529-175551	Positive	61.20	39.10	0.00	-4.00	-5.01	-4.84
	Reverse	CCATTACCGGCAAGCTAGG	175606-175588	Negative	62.10	57.90	0.00		-7.85	-4.08
	Probe	6FAM-ACGGATCCCCCTTCGCATTTGA-MGB-NFQ	175580-175559	Negative	68.00	54.50	-0.10			-7.16
MGF360-12L	Forward	CATACCCTTCCCCTAAAGCTG	30504-30524	Positive	61.90	52.40	0.00	-4.80	-4.26	-4.97
	Reverse	CTACTGCTATGTCCTGGGC	30646-30628	Negative	61.20	57.90	0.00		-4.48	-5.92
	Probe	6FAM-ACCCTCTTCGAAAACATCAGCCCC-MGB-NFQ	30529-30552	Positive	68.20	54.20	0.00			-6.77
UK	Forward	TGGATAATGCACCCGAGAAAC	185412-185432	Positive	55.10	47.60	0.34	-7.05	-6.60	-8.26
	Reverse	TCATTTCCACGTTTTATACCTTTCC	185529-185505	Negative	53.60	36.00	0.86		-6.30	-3.61
	Probe	VIC-CATATACCTGAGAAGTCGGCCCGC-MGF-NFQ	185447-185470	Positive	61.10	58.30	-0.44			-6.68

FIGURE 1 | Sequences of primers and probes used in the qPCR reactions as well as multiple parameters calculated during these developments. Hairpin and dimer values are expressed in standard Gibbs free energy (ΔG kcal/mole). Designs were carried out using the RealTime qPCR Assay tool. Probes were labeled at 5' with FAM (Fluorescein amidites) or VIC (Victoria) dyes and at 3' with MGB-NFQ (Minor groove binder-non fluorescent quencher).

as follows: Uracil N-glycosylase enzyme activation at 50°C for 2 min, polymerase activation at 95°C for 10 min; PCR of 40 cycles of 95°C for 15 s and 60°C for 1 min. Based on the validation, qPCR amplification of the I177L and UK targets was reduced to 37 cycles, and analysis used a manual threshold set at 0.1, with exception of the I177L target that utilized a 0.2 threshold.

As a gold standard to evaluate the performance of qPCRs designed in this study, we used the validated p72 qPCR, a reference test for the diagnosis of ASFV (15).

In silico Primer and Probe Evaluation

To evaluate the potential of the qPCRs designed in this study to detect all ASFV genotypes, different primers and probes were assessed using the BLASTN tool, version 2.1.12.0 (16).

The results of this analysis were visualized in a phylogenetic tree. Full-length genomes that had 100% coverage of target areas were downloaded from GenBank. Sequence alignments were conducted using CLC Genomics Workbench, using a slow algorithm (very accurate) based on the progressive alignment method (17). MEGA X was used to construct the phylogenetic tree, using the neighbor-joining maximum likelihood method, with a bootstrap of 1,000 replicates (18).

Amplification Efficiency (ε) and Analytical Sensitivity

To calculate the amplification efficiency (ε) of each qPCR, defined as the consistent increase in amplicon per cycle (19), 10-fold serial dilutions of the standard plasmid were produced using nuclease-free water. Average C_T values of each dilution were used to determine the amplification efficiency using the following equation:

$$\varepsilon = 100 \times (10^{-1/slope} - 1)$$

Also, amplification efficiency was expressed as linearity (R^2) (20).

Analytical sensitivity, defined as the smallest amount of the target template in the sample that can precisely be measured by qPCR (21), was calculated using the 10-fold serial dilutions of the standard plasmid, with the nucleic acid concentration previously calculated using the copy number calculator for real-time PCR (http://www.scienceprimer.com/copy-number-calculator-for-realtime-pcr). Values were calculated at the last

dilution where different tests got the limit of detection, being 6/6 replicates detected. Final values for each test were expressed as target copy numbers.

Two additional experiments were performed to evaluate the analytical sensitivity of qPCR. To evaluate the analytical sensitivity of each test expressed as hemoadsorbing doses 50% per milliliter (HAD/$_{50}$ doses/mL), multiple 10-fold dilutions were prepared from a viral stock of ASFV-G with a known titer of 1×10^8 HAD/$_{50}$ doses/mL. DNA from each dilution was extracted as previously described and qPCRs were performed in six replicates. The final dilution where 6/6 replicates produced C_T values was used to determine the limit of detection.

To assess the ability of each assay to detect low concentrations of ASFV-G in the presence of high concentrations of recombinant viruses, 10-fold dilutions made from a viral stock of ASFV-G were mixed with constant concentrations of different vaccine candidate stocks. DNA extractions and PCR reactions were performed using multiple mixes. Also, to evaluate how virus isolation can improve the sensitivity of the developed real-time PCRs, different mixes were used to infect primary swine macrophages, using plates containing 1×10^7 cells per well. Based on the number of cells per well, the multiplicity of infection (MOI) for each recombinant virus in the mix was calculated as follows; ASFV-ΔI177L = 1, ASFV-G-Δ9GL/ΔUK = 0.003, and ASFV-ΔMGF = 0.01, while for ASFV-G the MOIs ranged between 0.01 and 0.000001. In all cases the initial concentration of the recombinant virus in the mix was determined based on the concentration of the original stock.

Briefly, cells were infected with 1 mL of the virus mixture, after 1 h of adsorption at 37°C the inoculum was removed, and cells were rinsed twice with PBS and then incubated at 37°C for 24 h. Finally, DNA was extracted, and qPCR reactions were performed and compared with the ones using the original mixes.

Diagnostic Specificity

To calculate the diagnostic specificity, defined as the percentage of pigs that are not infected by ASFV and are identified by qPCR as negative for that condition (21), a total of 153 blood samples were evaluated. For this, two different sample sources were used. A total of 108 blood samples came from naïve pigs used in multiple previous ASFV experiments at PIADC (8–10;

19–23; (13)). An additional 45 blood samples were obtained from an unpublished experiment at PIADC that assessed the safety of different ASFV vaccine candidates. In this context, samples were collected from groups of three pigs inoculated with each of the vaccine candidates at 0, 7, 14, 21, and 49-days post inoculation ($n = 15$ samples per group).

Final values were expressed as a false positive rate using the following equation (20): False positive rate = (100 × number of misclassified known negative samples)/ (total number of negative samples).

Diagnostic Sensitivity

To calculate the diagnostic sensitivity, defined as the percentage of pigs that are infected by ASFV and are correctly identified as positive for the presence of this virus by qPCR (21), 30 blood samples collected from pigs experimentally infected by intramuscular inoculation with ASFV-G ($\sim 1 \times 10^2$ HAD/$_{50}$ doses) and collected between 4 ($n = 15$) and 7 ($n = 15$) days post-challenge were used to evaluate the different qPCR tests (7, 8, 10–13, 22–24).

The capability of different qPCRs to detect minimal quantities of the desired DNA target was evaluated using serial 10-fold dilutions of the standard plasmid and from a virus stock with a known titer of ASFV Georgia strain. The averages of six independent repetitions were used to determine the limit of detection (LOD) of each of the developed real-time PCRs. LOD was expressed as DNA copy number and HAD$_{50}$ doses.

Final values were expressed as a false negative rate using the following equation (20): False negative rate = (100 × number of misclassified known positive samples)/ (total number of positive samples).

Virus Titrations

The virus titer from blood samples of viremic pigs was determined using primary swine macrophage cell cultures in 96-well plates, using hemadsorption (HA) as evidence of the presence of ASFV. After 7 days of incubation at 37°C, the Reed and Muench method was applied to determine the final virus titers (25).

RESULTS AND DISCUSSION

The prevention and control of ASFV is a major challenge for the global pork industry. In this context, during the last decade our research has been focused on the identification of essential virulence genes of ASFV. This research has led to the development of three promising vaccine candidates to promote the control of the Eurasian strain of ASFV (10–13). Herein, we present the development of three independent qPCRs to be used as complementary genetic DIVA tests, supporting the use of our vaccines in the field. The use of genetic DIVA tests has been applied to other swine diseases like classical swine fever, where this approach has been successfully used to differentiate animals vaccinated with the C-strain virus from animals infected with field strains (26).

Real-Time PCR Design and *in silico* Evaluation

Using the sequence of the ASFV Georgia 2007/1 strain, we focused on the development of three independent qPCRs to target genes MGF360-12L, UK and I177L; these three genes were independently deleted to develop vaccine candidates ASFV-ΔMGF, ASFV-G-Δ9GL/ΔUK and ASFV-ΔI177L, respectively. Results obtained using the RealTime qPCR Assay tool are presented in **Figure 1**. Overall, *in silico* evaluation of different primers and probes reveled that all oligonucleotides had values of standard Gibbs free energy (ΔG kcal/mole) higher than −9 kcal/mol, a desired condition that may prevent excessive formation of hairpins and dimers that can interfere with amplification conditions (**Figure 1**).

We then assessed the genetic coverage of the different real-time PCRs designed in this study. Primers and probes were evaluated using the software BLASTN. As expected, all oligonucleotides shared 100% nucleotide identity with the viral sequence of the ASFV Eurasian strain (genotype II). This was consistent with the results of our phylogenetic analysis that demonstrated high nucleotide conservation of the Eurasian strain after more than 12 years of circulation, appearing in the tree as a highly conserved monophyletic lineage (**Figure 2**). This result supported previous studies using the B646L gene as a genetic marker for the phylogenetic analysis (27, 28), suggesting that the genetic stability of this strain may favor the use of genetic DIVA tests as part of a control strategy.

Although the main goal of our study was to design different qPCRs to efficiently detect the Eurasian strain of ASFV (genotype II), our analysis would also demonstrate the ability to detect additional genotypes of ASFV with the developed assays. It would include the ability of MGF360-12L and UK designs to match 100% with viral strains associated with genotypes V and I, respectively (**Figure 2**). The I177L design appeared to detect strains associated with genotypes I and VII. However, while the I177L reverse primer and the probe were 100% identical, the forward primer was 95.6% identical due to a single mismatch.

Interestingly, the ASFV LIV 13/33 isolate, one of the strains potentially covered by the I177L design and classified as genotype I based on the B646L gene (29), was genetically distant from multiple strains of genotype I viruses using full-length sequences, suggesting the potential ability of the qPCR I177L to detect viral strains other than I, II and VII genotypes. Also, considering the high bootstrap values that support our analysis, our results agree with previous studies (29, 30) that suggest potential differences in the genotype classification of ASFV strains, dependent on selection of gene-specific or full-length genome sequence used for phylogenetic analysis.

Amplification Efficiency and Analytical Sensitivity Determinations

Part of the *in vitro* validation of the qPCRs was the calculation of their amplification efficiency and analytical sensitivity parameters. For this purpose, serial 10-fold dilutions of a standard plasmid containing all different PCR targets was used for the determinations. As a gold standard for this validation, we

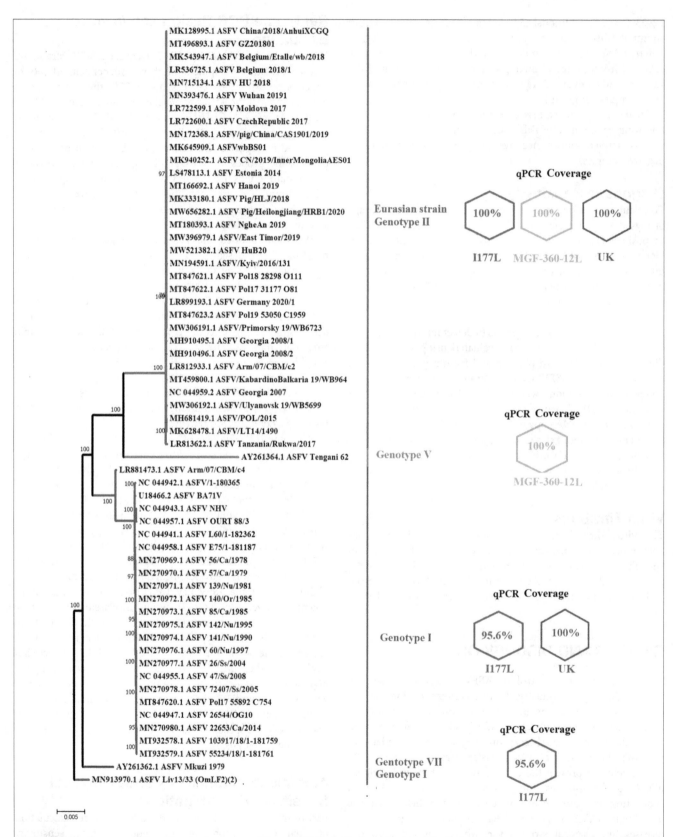

FIGURE 2 | Graphic representation of the genetic coverage of different qPCR tests. The figure shows a phylogenetic analysis reconstructed by neighbor-joining using full-length sequences of multiple ASFV strains which may be potentially detected by different qPCRs designed in this study. Next to each clade representing multiple genotypes are expressed the identity of different primers and probes included in each qPCR. Values of 100% indicate no differences between viral sequences and different oligonucleotides. A value of 95.65%, for one I177L real-time PCR primer, is due to the presence of one mismatch between the forward primer and sequences of different genotypes. Numbers along the branches represent the bootstrap support values.

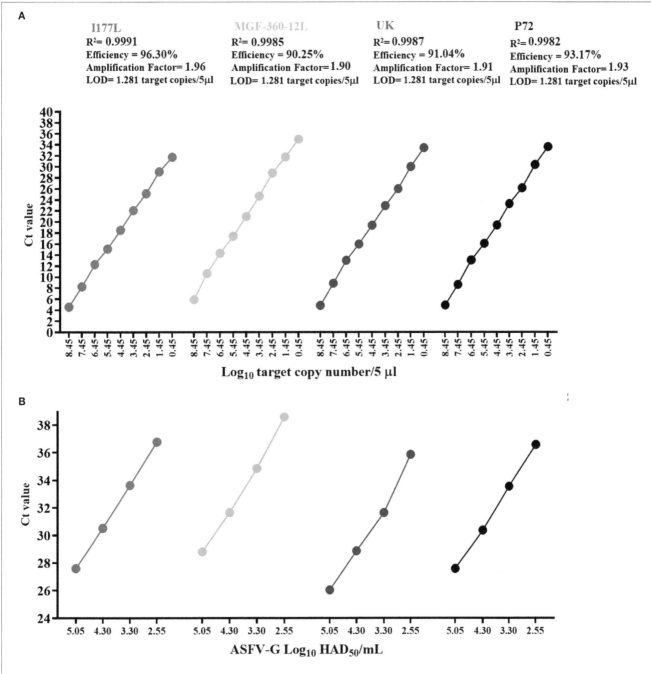

FIGURE 3 | Amplification efficiency and analytical sensitivity determinations. **(A)** Ten-fold dilutions of a standard plasmid representing variable amounts of all gene targets were used to calculate the amplification efficiency and analytical sensitivity of multiple qPCRs. **(B)** Ten-fold dilutions of a stock of ASFV-G with a known titer was used to establish parameters of analytical sensitivity in terms of the capability of different qPCRs to detect minimal amounts of infectious ASFV. Amount of infectious virus is expressed as HAD_{50}/mL units. In all cases results represent the average value of six replicates.

included the previously validated qPCR for the detection of the B646L gene (p72 protein), a standard assay for field diagnosis of ASFV (15).

Overall, all three real-time PCRs designed in this study had comparable values of amplification efficiency when compared with the p72 qPCR (**Figure 3A**). These results agree with the previously proposed accepted standard values for amplification

efficiency based on the determination of an amplification factor (between 80 and 120%), expressed as linearity (R^2), where the acceptable values for each target should be ≥ 0.98 (20).

Analytical sensitivity of all three qPCRs, like the p72 qPCR, demonstrated the capability to detect 1.28 copies of each of the gene targets (**Figure 3A**). The limit of detection for all assays was achieved with C_T values < 36, increasing the chances to obtain

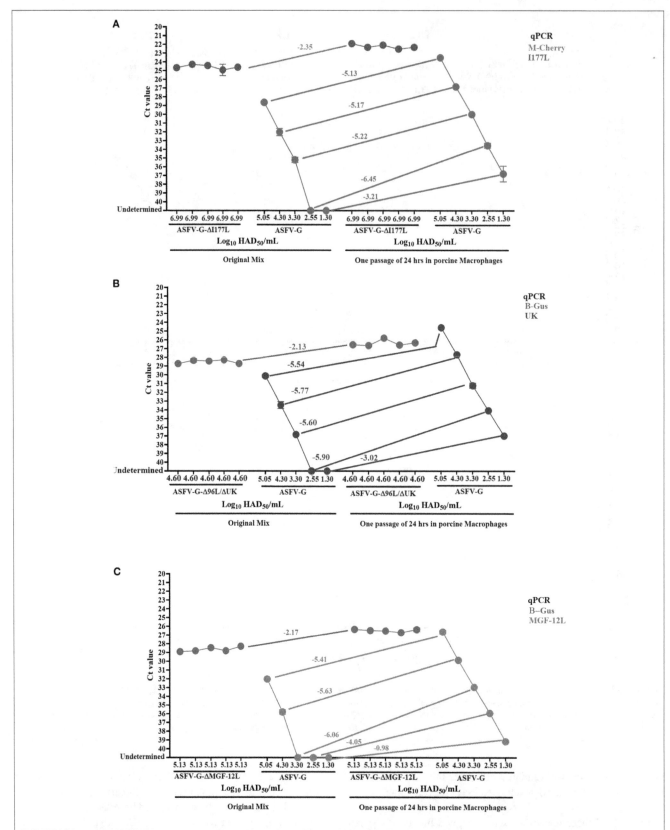

FIGURE 4 | Detection of ASFV-G in the presence of recombinant viruses. The sensitivity of different real-time PCRs was evaluated using mixes obtained from combined infections using constant concentrations of recombinant viruses and variable amount of ASFV-G **(A)** ASFV-ΔI177L, **(B)** ASFV-G-Δ9GL/ΔUK, and **(C)** ASFV-ΔMGF. This evaluation was carried out in both the original virus mixes and after being passed once in porcine macrophage. The detection of recombinant viruses was conducted using specific qPCRs to detect the gene encoding the markers M-cherry (ASFV-ΔI177L) and β-Gus (ASFV-G-Δ9GL/ΔUK and ASFV-ΔMGF).

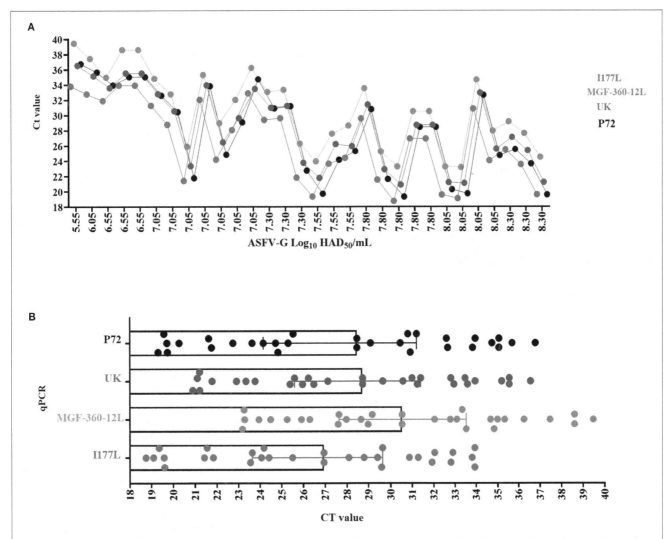

FIGURE 5 | Diagnostic sensitivity. of the different qPCRs assessed using a set of blood samples with different viral titers (expressed in HAD50/ml) collected from pigs experimentally infected with ASFV-G **(A)**. Comparative average C_T values among the different qPCRs in the detection of viremic blood samples obtained from pigs infected with ASFV-G **(B)**.

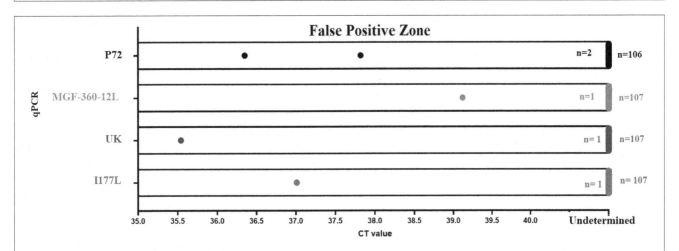

FIGURE 6 | Diagnostic specificity. The diagnostic specificity of different qPCRs was assessed using a set of 108 blood samples collected from naïve pigs. Results from different tests represent the detection of nonspecific reactions after 40 (p72 and MGF-360-12L) or 37 (I177L and UK) cycles of amplification.

consistent levels of the repeatability during the performance of these assays (31). Also, when compared to other designs, our results were similar to a previously reported qPCR developed to detect the MGF505 gene of ASFV (3 copies of the target gene) (31), supporting the robustness of our assays to detect minimal amounts of ASFV from pig samples collected in the field.

Furthermore, when analytical sensitivity was assessed in terms of the ability of different designs to detect minimal amounts of infectious virus quantified as HAD_{50}/mL, the detection was consistent with the results showed by the standard diagnostic p72 qPCR (2.55 HAD_{50}/mL) (**Figure 3B**). Interestingly, all these calculations were consistent with the values obtained in the original validation of the p72 real-time PCR (15), supporting the reliability of our results.

Assessing the Presence of ASFV-G in a Combined Infection With Different Recombinant Viruses

We evaluated the performance of multiple qPCRs to detect different concentrations of ASFV-G in the presence of constant levels of the three different recombinant viruses. The presence of both viruses circulating in the blood of vaccinated and infected pigs is a possible field scenario, since experimental evidence has shown the absence of sterile immunity in a proportion of pigs vaccinated with ASFV-ΔMGF or ASFV-G-Δ9GL/ΔUK (10, 11).

Interestingly, in the presence of the recombinant viruses the qPCR detection of ASFV-G decreased its levels of analytical sensitivity by ten- (I177L and UK) (**Figures 4A,B**) or 100-fold (MGF-360-12L) (**Figure 4C**). However, after one 24-h passage in cell culture of porcine macrophages, all qPCRs restored and improved their levels of analytical sensitivity to detect samples with original titers as low as $10^{1.30}$ HAD_{50}/mL. After this passage in porcine macrophages, there was a reduction in average C_T values of all three qPCRs used to detect ASFV-G when compared with the C_T values obtained by qPCRs targeting the florescent markers in the recombinant viruses (**Figure 4**).

It is possible that the overall loss of analytical sensitivity of all qPCRs may be impacted by the extraction method used in this study, where the higher concentrations of recombinant virus present in all mixes might have favored the attachment of the DNA from this virus to the magnetic beads. This possibility highlights the necessity to explore alternative extraction methods to improve the performance of these tests (32). Regarding the increased loss of analytical sensibility seen from the MGF-360-12L design, it may be explained by the lowest level of amplification efficiency showed by this test in comparison with the other qPCRs designed in this study (**Figure 3**).

Therefore, the combined use of virus isolation and qPCR may be an alternative to consider in order to improve the performance of genetic DIVA tests to rule out the presence of ASFV in pigs vaccinated with recombinant viruses in the field. Experimental evidence indicates that in pigs vaccinated with ASFV-ΔMGF and ASFV-G-Δ9GL/ΔUK the infection with ASFV-G were asymptomatic, so that low levels of viremia are expected (10, 11). ASFV isolation typically requires the use of primary cell cultures of swine macrophages, however the recently identified adapted cell line MA-104 may be an alternative to

be considered for this purpose particularly when primary cell cultures are not available (33).

Diagnostic Sensitivity

The diagnostic sensitivity of different qPCRs was evaluated using a set of blood samples from viremic pigs infected with an average of 10^2 $HAD/_{50}$ doses of ASFV-G and collected between days 4 and 7 post-infection. In general, all qPCRs were able to detect 100% of the samples tested for this validation, producing a false positive rate = 0% (**Figure 5A**). The average C_T values for the detection of all samples were consistent with the levels of amplification efficiency calculated for each qPCR, with the lowest values associated with the I177L test and the highest with the MGF-360-12L test (**Figure 5B**). Interestingly, we found an absence of a positive linear correlation between the viral titer and the C_T values produced by all qPCRs, including p72, which may be explained by the presence of PCR inhibitors in the samples decreasing the diagnostic sensitivity of these tests. In blood the presence of inhibitors may be associated with substances like antibodies (IgG), hemoglobin, lactoferrin, heparin, hormones, and some antiviral agents (34, 35).

In this context, the use of alternative sample types, like nasal, oral swabs, and the collection of oral fluids may represent a good alternative to maintain optimal levels of diagnostic sensitivity in these tests (15, 36). Further studies will involved the evaluation of different types of clinical samples, as oral, rectal and nasal swabs.

In light of these results, we can state that despite the apparent loss of analytical sensitivity produced by blood inhibitors, the high levels of viremia that are expected in domestic or wild pigs during clinical infection with the highly virulent Eurasian strain of ASFV (6, 24) may help to ensure the proper levels of diagnostic sensitivity of these tests when used in the field. However, it is important to consider the recent reports regarding the circulation of low virulent genotype II ASFV strains (37, 38), a situation that may affect the diagnostic sensitivity of these tests considering that blood is used as a primary sample for the performance of these tests. Interestingly, experimental infections comparing the pathogenesis among ASFV isolates (genotype II) of disparate levels of virulence have shown that blood can be isolated from pigs infected with strains with low and moderate levels of virulence as late as 19- and 44-days post-infection respectively, thus supporting the use of blood as a valuable sample for the detection of ASFV genotype II (37).

Furthermore, consistent with the original publications [8–10; (13)], the evaluation of blood collected from pigs (n = 5 per group) vaccinated and then challenged 21 days later, the qPCRs designed herein did not produce positive results in pigs vaccinated with ASFV-ΔI177L, a fact consistent with the previously described ability of this vaccine to produce sterile immunity in vaccinated pigs. Conversely, one out of five animals (20%) vaccinated with ASFV-ΔMGF had a positive result by qPCR, while 3 out of 5 pigs (60%) vaccinated with ASFV-G-Δ9GL/ΔUK had positive results.

Diagnostic Specificity

Finally, we assessed the diagnostic specificity of the designed real-time PCR tests. We evaluated a total of 108 negative blood samples collected from naïve pigs. Similar results were seen

A

Blood sample	Pig number	Collection day	Viral titer Log $_{10}$HAD $_{50}$/mL	Ct value P72	Ct value M-cherry	Ct value I177L	Ct value P72	Ct value M-cherry	Ct value I177L
1	Pig 1	0	0	Und	Und	Und	Und	Und	Und
2	Pig 2	0	0	Und	Und	Und	Und	Und	Und
3	Pig 3	0	0	Und	Und	Und	Und	Und	Und
4	Pig 1	7	4.05	35.24	36.33	Und	25.38	26.50	Und
5	Pig 2	7	6.55	29.26	30.35	Und	23.11	24.54	Und
6	Pig 3	7	3.05	Und	Und	Und	26.28	27.30	Und
7	Pig 1	14	3.05	36.43	36.9	Und	26.38	26.90	Und
8	Pig 2	14	6.3	31.11	32.31	Und	23.50	24.50	Und
9	Pig 3	14	2.08	Und	Und	Und	29.70	29.92	Und
10	Pig 1	21	1.8	Und	Und	Und	32.52	33.05	Und
11	Pig 2	21	5.3	32.97	32.46	Und	22.95	23.95	Und
12	Pig 3	21	1.8	Und	Und	Und	36.78	37.50	Und
13	Pig 1	49	0	Und	Und	Und	Und	Und	Und
14	Pig 2	49	1.8	Und	Und	Und	36.50	37.70	Und
15	Pig 3	49	0	Und	Und	Und	Und	Und	Und

B

Blood sample	Pig number	Collection day	Viral titer Log $_{10}$HAD $_{50}$/mL	Ct value P72	Ct value B-Gus	Ct value MGF	Ct value P72	Ct value B-Gus	Ct value MGF
1	Pig 1	0	0	Und	Und	Und	Und	Und	Und
2	Pig 2	0	0	Und	Und	Und	Und	Und	Und
3	Pig 3	0	0	Und	Und	Und	Und	Und	Und
4	Pig 1	7	0	Und	Und	Und	Und	Und	Und
5	Pig 2	7	0	Und	Und	Und	Und	Und	Und
6	Pig 3	7	6.3	32.84	33.82	Und	21.06	21.6	Und
7	Pig 1	14	0	Und	Und	Und	Und	Und	Und
8	Pig 2	14	3.05	Und	Und	Und	22.94	24.22	Und
9	Pig 3	14	5.55	35.22	35.32	Und	20.67	20.94	Und
10	Pig 1	21	5.3	35.32	34.69	Und	20.93	20.69	Und
11	Pig 2	21	1.8	Und	Und	Und	Und	Und	Und
12	Pig 3	21	5.55	35.34	36.96	Und	20.61	20.92	Und
13	Pig 1	49	3.05	Und	Und	Und	19.82	21.4	Und
14	Pig 2	49	0	Und	Und	Und	Und	Und	Und
15	Pig 3	49	1.8	Und	Und	Und	23.29	23.96	Und

C

Blood sample	Pig number	Collection day	Viral titer Log $_{10}$HAD $_{50}$/mL	Ct value P72	Ct value B-Gus	Ct value UK	Ct value P72	Ct value B-Gus	Ct value UK
1	Pig 1	0	0	Und	Und	Und	Und	Und	Und
2	Pig 2	0	0	Und	Und	Und	Und	Und	Und
3	Pig 3	0	0	Und	Und	Und	Und	Und	Und
4	Pig 1	7	0	Und	Und	Und	Und	Und	Und
5	Pig 2	7	4.8	36.85	36.49	Und	24.32	23.53	Und
6	Pig 3	7	1.8	Und	Und	Und	37.13	37.1	Und
7	Pig 1	14	0	Und	Und	Und	Und	Und	Und
8	Pig 2	14	4.3	37.08	35.91	Und	30.84	29.93	Und
9	Pig 3	14	1.8	Und	Und	Und	28.25	27.69	Und
10	Pig 1	21	0	Und	Und	Und	Und	Und	Und
11	Pig 2	21	1.8	38.92	39.21	Und	28.77	28.76	Und
12	Pig 3	21	2.05	Und	Und	Und	34.08	33.41	Und
13	Pig 1	49	0	Und	Und	Und	Und	Und	Und
14	Pig 2	49	0	Und	Und	Und	Und	Und	Und
15	Pig 3	49	0	Und	Und	Und	Und	Und	Und

FIGURE 7 | Evaluation the capability of qPCRs to differentiate vaccinated pigs with (A) ASFV-ΔI177L, (B) ASFV-G-Δ9GL/ΔUK, and (C) ASFV-ΔMGF from those infected with ASFV-G. Blood samples collected from pigs at different time points of vaccination were tested before and after (green boxes) one passage of 72 h in swine macrophage cell cultures. M-cherry and β-Gus q PCRs were used for the detection of the recombinant viruses, while p72 assay was used as a marker for the presence of ASFV.

between p72 and all qPCRs developed in this study. The overall false positive rate was estimated to be less than 1%, due to 1/108 positive result (**Figure 6**). The amplification profile of this sample was characterized by the amplification of just one of the two replicates evaluated; considering that none of the samples were positive by two different tests, we determined this was a nonspecific detection.

It is important to mention that in the case of real-time PCRs I177L and UK, we noticed that a small percentage of samples (5%) reported a nonspecific amplification in one of the 2 replicates, with C_T values >38. Interestingly, as mentioned above, none of these blood samples had a positive amplification in two different real-time PCRs. In this context and based on the parameters of analytical and diagnostic sensitivity displayed by the I177L and UK tests, amplification protocol for these tests was set at 37 amplification cycles instead of 40, producing in this way the presence of just one sample showing a nonspecific amplification in one out of the two repetitions (**Figure 6**).

At this point, we cannot rule out the possibility that the increased number of nonspecific reactions recorded using the I177L and UK qPCRs might have been the result of dimer formation between different primers, so that alternative primer technology like the use of cooperative primers may be explored in future studies to improve this condition (39). Furthermore, negative results were recorded when multiple qPCR's were performed in the presence of other viral swine diseases like classical swine fever virus (CSFV), vesicular stomatitis virus (VSV) and foot and mouth disease virus (FMDV).

Alternatively, to estimate the diagnostic specificity of different designs in samples containing variable concentrations of recombinant viruses, we evaluated blood samples collected at different time points post-vaccination from groups of viremic pigs ($n = 3$ animals per group) inoculated with different recombinant viruses. Overall, positive results were obtained by p72, M-cherry and β-Gus qPCRs in blood collected from all groups at different time points, denoting the presence of different recombinant viruses in the blood of vaccinated pigs. The number of positive results increased in all groups of pigs after passing these samples once in cell cultures of porcine macrophages (**Figure 7**). Negative results were found in all blood samples when evaluated by I177L, MGF-360-12L, and UK qPCRs, confirming the absence of ASFV-G in the samples, confirming the ability of these tests to differentiate infected and vaccinated pigs.

In conclusion, we present the design of three independent genetic DIVA tests for use in the field in the presence of recombinant vaccines ASFV-ΔMGF, ASFV-G-Δ9GL/ΔUK, ASFV-ΔI177L and ASFV-DI177LDLVR. Future studies are being planned to conduct a full validation under field conditions and confirm the accuracy of the validation parameters established here. The qPCR DIVA tests developed here are a promising option to support the control and eradication of the ASFV-G strain during a potential vaccination program. In addition to the vaccine strains tested here, these qPCR tests would also be appropriate for experimental vaccines developed by other groups using Chinese strains of ASFV. The qPCR DIVA test for UK could identify ASFV-SY18-ΔCD2v/UK (40), the MGF qPCR DIVA test could be used to detect HLJ/18-6GD (41) and HLJ/18-7GD (41) since in all of these experimental vaccine candidates the viral sequence is 100% homologous to the primer sets tested here in this study making the qPCR DIVA tests potentially useful in areas where a potential vaccine program may use one of the experimental vaccines.

ETHICS STATEMENT

The animal study was reviewed and approved by Animal experiments were performed under biosafety level 3 conditions in the animal facilities at Plum Island Animal Disease Center, following a strict protocol approved by the Institutional Animal Care and Use Committee (225.01-16-R approved on 09-07-16).

AUTHOR CONTRIBUTIONS

LV-S, MB, and DG conceived and designed the experiments and analyzed the data. LV-S, ER-M, AR, SP, EV, and NE performed the experiments. LV-S, MB, DG, ER-M, AR, SP, EV, and NE wrote the manuscript. All authors contributed to the article and approved the submitted version.

ACKNOWLEDGMENTS

We would like to thank Melanie Prarat for editing the manuscript.

REFERENCES

1. Dixon LK, Chapman DA, Netherton CL, Upton C. African swine fever virus replication and genomics. *Virus Res.* (2013) 173:3–14. doi: 10.1016/j.virusres.2012.10.020
2. Tonsor GT, Schulz LL. Will an incentive-compatible indemnity policy please stand up? livestock producer willingness to self-protect. *Transbound Emerg Dis.* (2020) 67:2713–30. doi: 10.1111/tbed.13626
3. Gaudreault NN, Madden DW, Wilson WC, Trujillo JD, Richt JA. African Swine Fever Virus: An Emerging DNA Arbovirus. *Front Vet Sci.* (2020) 7:215. doi: 10.3389/fvets.2020.00215
4. Malogolovkin A, Kolbasov D. Genetic and antigenic diversity of African swine fever virus. *Virus Res.* (2019) 271:197673. doi: 10.1016/j.virusres.2019.197673
5. Cwynar P, Stojkov J, Wlazlak K. African swine fever status in Europe. *Viruses.* (2019) 11:310. doi: 10.3390/v11040310
6. Blome S, Gabriel C, Beer M. Pathogenesis of African swine fever in domestic pigs and European wild boar. *Virus Res.* (2013) 173:122–30. doi: 10.1016/j.virusres.2012.10.026
7. Ramirez-Medina E, Vuono EA, Rai A, Pruitt S, Silva E, Velazquez-Salinas L, et al. The C962R ORF of African swine fever strain georgia is non-essential and not required for virulence in swine. *Viruses.* (2020) 12:676. doi: 10.3390/v12060676
8. Ramirez-Medina E, Vuono EA, Velazquez-Salinas L, Silva E, Rai A, Pruitt S, et al. The MGF360-16R ORF of African swine fever virus strain georgia encodes for a nonessential gene that interacts with host proteins SERTAD3 and SDCBP. *Viruses.* (2020) 12:60. doi: 10.3390/v12010060

9. Arias M, de la Torre A, Dixon L, Gallardo C, Jori F, Laddomada A, et al. Approaches and perspectives for development of African swine fever virus vaccines. *Vaccines.* (2017) 5:35. doi: 10.3390/vaccines5040035

10. O'Donnell V, Holinka LG, Gladue DP, Sanford B, Krug PW, Lu X, et al. African swine fever virus Georgia isolate harboring deletions of MGF360 and MGF505 genes is attenuated in swine and confers protection against challenge with virulent parental Virus. *J Virol.* (2015) 89:6048–56. doi: 10.1128/JVI.00554-15

11. O'Donnell V, Risatti GR, Holinka LG, Krug PW, Carlson J, Velazquez-Salinas L, et al. Simultaneous deletion of the 9GL and UK genes from the African swine fever virus Georgia 2007. Isolate offers increased safety and protection against homologous challenge. *J Virol.* (2017) 91:e01760-16. doi: 10.1128/JVI.01760-16

12. Borca MV, Ramirez-Medina E, Silva E, Vuono E, Rai A, Pruitt S, et al. Development of a highly effective African swine fever virus vaccine by deletion of the I177L gene results in sterile immunity against the current epidemic Eurasia strain. *J Virol.* (2020) 94:e02017-19. doi: 10.1128/JVI.02017-19

13. Borca MV, Rai A, Ramirez-Medina E, Silva E, Velazquez-Salinas L, Vuono E, et al. A Cell culture-adapted vaccine virus against the current African swine fever virus pandemic strain. *J Virol.* (2021) 95:e0012321. doi: 10.1128/JVI.00123-21

14. Borca MV, Berggren KA, Ramirez-Medina E, Vuono EA, Gladue DP. CRISPR/Cas gene editing of a large DNA virus: African swine fever virus. *Bio-Protocol.* (2018) 8:e2978. doi: 10.21769/BioProtoc.2978

15. Zsak L, Borca MV, Risatti GR, Zsak A, French RA, Lu Z, et al. Preclinical diagnosis of African swine fever in contact-exposed swine by a real-time PCR assay. *J Clin Microbiol.* (2005) 43:112–9. doi: 10.1128/JCM.43.1.112-119.2005

16. Altschul SF, Madden TL, Schaffer AA, Zhang J, Zhang Z, Miller W, et al. Gapped BLAST and PSI-BLAST: a new generation of protein database search programs. *Nucleic Acids Res.* (1997) 25:3389–402. doi: 10.1093/nar/25.17.3389

17. Feng D-F, Doolittle RF. [21] Progressive alignment of amino acid sequences and construction of phylogenetic trees from them. *Methods Enzymol.* (1996) 266:368–82. doi: 10.1016/S0076-6879(96)66023-6

18. Kumar S, Stecher G, Li M, Knyaz C, Tamura K. MEGA X: Molecular evolutionary genetics analysis across computing platforms. *Mol Biol Evol.* (2018) 35:1547–9. doi: 10.1093/molbev/msy096

19. Ruijter JM, Ramakers C, Hoogaars WM, Karlen Y, Bakker O, van den Hoff MJ, et al. Amplification efficiency: linking baseline and bias in the analysis of quantitative PCR data. *Nucleic Acids Res.* (2009) 37:e45. doi: 10.1093/nar/gkp045

20. Shehata HR, Ragupathy S, Shanmughanandhan D, Kesanakurti P, Ehlinger TM, Newmaster SG. Guidelines for validation of qualitative real-time PCR methods for molecular diagnostic identification of probiotics. *J AOAC Int.* (2019) 102:1774–8. doi: 10.5740/jaoacint.18-0320

21. Saah AJ, Hoover DR. "Sensitivity" and "specificity" reconsidered: the meaning of these terms in analytical and diagnostic settings. *Ann Intern Med.* (1997) 126:91–4. doi: 10.7326/0003-4819-126-1-199701010-00026

22. Gladue DP, O'Donnell V, Ramirez-Medina E, Rai A, Pruitt S, Vuono EA, et al. Deletion of CD2-Like (CD2v) and C-type lectin-like (EP153R) genes from African swine fever virus Georgia-9GL abrogates its effectiveness as an experimental vaccine. *Viruses.* (2020) 12:1185. doi: 10.3390/v12101185

23. Vuono E, Ramirez-Medina E, Pruitt S, Rai A, Silva E, Espinoza N, et al. Evaluation in Swine of a recombinant Georgia 2010. African swine fever virus lacking the I8L gene. *Viruses.* (2020) 13:39. doi: 10.3390/v13010039

24. Ramirez-Medina E, Vuono E, Pruitt S, Rai A, Silva E, Espinoza N, et al. Development and *in vivo* evaluation of a MGF110-1L deletion mutant in African swine fever strain Georgia. *Viruses.* (2021) 13:286. doi: 10.3390/v13020286

25. Reed LJ, Muench HA. Simple method of estimating fifty percent endpoints. *Am J Hyg.* (1938) 27:493–7. doi: 10.1093/oxfordjournals.aje.a118408

26. Blome S, Wernike K, Reimann I, Konig P, Moss C, Beer M. A decade of research into classical swine fever marker vaccine CP7_E2alf (Suvaxyn((R)) CSF Marker): a review of vaccine properties. *Vet Res.* (2017) 48:51. doi: 10.1186/s13567-017-0457-y

27. Gallardo C, Fernandez-Pinero J, Pelayo V, Gazaev I, Markowska-Daniel I, Pridotkas G, et al. Genetic variation among African swine fever genotype II viruses, eastern and central Europe. *Emerg Infect Dis.* (2014) 20:1544–7. doi: 10.3201/eid2009.140554

28. Mazloum A, van Schalkwyk A, Shotin A, Igolkin A, Shevchenko I, Gruzdev KN, et al. Comparative analysis of full genome sequences of African swine fever virus isolates taken from wild boars in Russia in 2019. *Pathogens.* (2021) 10:521. doi: 10.3390/pathogens10050521

29. Aslanyan L, Avagyan H, Karalyan Z. Whole-genome-based phylogeny of African swine fever virus. *Vet World.* (2020) 13:2118–25. doi: 10.14202/vetworld.2020.2118-2125

30. de Villiers EP, Gallardo C, Arias M, da Silva M, Upton C, Martin R, et al. Phylogenomic analysis of 11 complete African swine fever virus genome sequences. *Virology.* (2010) 400:128–36. doi: 10.1016/j.virol.2010.01.019

31. Guo Z, Li K, Qiao S, Chen XX, Deng R, Zhang G. Development and evaluation of duplex TaqMan real-time PCR assay for detection and differentiation of wide-type and MGF505-2R gene-deleted African swine fever viruses. *BMC Vet Res.* (2020) 16:428. doi: 10.1186/s12917-020-02639-2

32. Cankar K, Stebih D, Dreo T, Zel J, Gruden K. Critical points of DNA quantification by real-time PCR–effects of DNA extraction method and sample matrix on quantification of genetically modified organisms. *BMC Biotechnol.* (2006) 6:37. doi: 10.1186/1472-6750-6-37

33. Rai A, Pruitt S, Ramirez-Medina E, Vuono EA, Silva E, Velazquez-Salinas L, et al. Identification of a continuously stable and commercially available cell line for the identification of infectious African swine fever virus in clinical samples. *Viruses.* (2020) 12:820. doi: 10.3390/v12080820

34. Schrader C, Schielke A, Ellerbroek L, Johne R. PCR inhibitors - occurrence, properties and removal. *J Appl Microbiol.* (2012) 113:1014–26. doi: 10.1111/j.1365-2672.2012.05384.x

35. Sidstedt M, Hedman J, Romsos EL, Waitara L, Wadso L, Steffen CR, et al. Inhibition mechanisms of hemoglobin, immunoglobulin G, and whole blood in digital and real-time PCR. *Anal Bioanal Chem.* (2018) 410:2569–83. doi: 10.1007/s00216-018-0931-z

36. Goonewardene KB, Chung CJ, Goolia M, Blakemore L, Fabian A, Mohamed F, et al. Evaluation of oral fluid as an aggregate sample for early detection of African swine fever virus using four independent pen-based experimental studies. *Transbound Emerg Dis.* (2021) 68:2867–77. doi: 10.1111/tbed.14175

37. Gallardo C, Soler A, Nurmoja I, Cano-Gomez C, Cvetkova S, Frant M, et al. Dynamics of African swine fever virus (ASFV) infection in domestic pigs infected with virulent, moderate virulent and attenuated genotype II ASFV European isolates. *Transbound Emerg Dis.* (2021) 68:2826–41. doi: 10.1111/tbed.14222

38. Sun E, Zhang Z, Wang Z, He X, Zhang X, Wang L, et al. Emergence and prevalence of naturally occurring lower virulent African swine fever viruses in domestic pigs in China in 2020. *Sci China Life Sci.* (2021) 64:752–65. doi: 10.1007/s11427-021-1904-4

39. Satterfield, B. C. (2014). Cooperative primers: 2.5 million-fold improvement in the reduction of nonspecific amplification. *J Mol Diagn* 16:163–173. doi: 10.1016/j.jmoldx.2013.10.004

40. Teklue T, Wang T, Luo Y, Hu R, Sun Y, Qiu HJ. Generation and evaluation of an African swine fever virus mutant with deletion of the CD2v and UK genes. *Vaccines (Basel).* (2020) 8:763. doi: 10.3390/vaccines8040763

41. Chen W, Zhao D, He X, Liu R, Wang Z, Zhang X, et al. A seven-gene-deleted African swine fever virus is safe and effective as a live attenuated vaccine in pigs. *Sci China Life Sci.* (2020) 63:623–34. doi: 10.1007/s11427-020-1657-9

A Multiplex Real-Time Reverse Transcription Polymerase Chain Reaction Assay with Enhanced Capacity to Detect Vesicular Stomatitis Viral Lineages of Central American Origin

Kate Hole[1], Charles Nfon[1], Luis L. Rodriguez[2] and Lauro Velazquez-Salinas[2]*

[1] National Centre for Foreign Animal Disease, Canadian Food Inspection Agency, Winnipeg, MB, Canada, [2] Foreign Animal Disease Research Unit, Plum Island Animal Disease Center, United States Department of Agriculture-Agricultural Research Service, Greenport, NY, United States

Correspondence:
Lauro Velazquez-Salinas
lauro.velazquez@usda.gov

Vesicular stomatitis virus (VSV) causes a disease in susceptible livestock that is clinically indistinguishable from foot-and-mouth disease. Rapid testing is therefore critical to identify VSV and rule out FMD. We previously developed and validated a multiplex real-time reverse transcription polymerase chain reaction assay (mRRT-PCR) for detection of both VS New Jersey virus (VSNJV) and VS Indiana virus (VSIV). However, it was subsequently apparent that this assay failed to detect some VSNJV isolates in Mexico, especially in genetic group II, lineage 2.1. In order to enhance the sensitivity of the mRRT-PCR for VSNJV, parts of the assay were redesigned and revalidated using new and improved PCR chemistries. The redesign markedly improved the assay by increasing the VSNJV detection sensitivity of lineage 2.1 and thereby allowing detection of all VSNJV clades. The new assay showed an increased capability to detect VSNJV. Specifically, the new mRRT-PCR detected VSNJV in 100% (87/87) of samples from Mexico in 2006-2007 compared to 74% for the previous mRRT-PCR. Furthermore, the analytical sensitivity of the new mRRT-PCR was enhanced for VSNJV. Importantly, the modified assay had the same sensitivity and specificity for VSIV as the previously published assay. Our results highlight the challenges the large genetic variability of VSV pose for virus detection by mRRT-PCR and show the importance of frequent re-evaluation and validation of diagnostic assays for VSV to ensure high sensitivity and specificity.

Keywords: vesicular stomatitis, real time PCR, diagnostic, genetic diversity, epidemic lineage

INTRODUCTION

Vesicular stomatitis virus (VSV) is an arbovirus and prototype of the *Rhabdovirus* viral family and *vesiculovirus* genus from which vesicular stomatitis Indiana virus (VSIV) and vesicular stomatitis New Jersey virus (VSNJV) constitute the main serotypes (1). VSV has a single-stranded negative-sense RNA genome structured in five different genes, encoding five structural proteins: nucleoprotein (N), phosphoprotein (P), matrix (M), glycoprotein (G) and the large RNA-dependent polymerase (L) (2).

The genetic diversity of VSNJV has been associated with at least six different phylogenetic clades, which are directly linked to the geographical regions where these viruses are typically circulating (3). The homology among VSNJV has been calculated between 79.56 and 85.16% and 91.04 and 94.66% at the nucleotide and amino acid levels, respectively (3).

In southern Mexico, where VSV is endemic, clinical cases are recorded on an annual basis (4). These VSV endemic zones are colonized by multiple lineages belonging to North American Clade I (3). Most VSV outbreaks recorded in the United States have been linked to endemic ancestors from these regions (4–6).

Between 2005 and 2011 two interesting epidemiological events occurred in Mexico. The emergence of a highly virulent epidemic lineage 1.1 (7), which affected central and northern Mexico was reported, and was subsequently isolated in the US in 2012 (4). Concurrently, an incursion of multiple lineages belonging to the Central America clade II were described for the first time in Mexico (4). Although these lineages were initially found to produce clinical infections in livestock in southern Mexico, by 2011 clinical cases associated with these lineages were detected in central Mexico. This implies that VSV may spread from Central America into the US via Mexico.

VSV clinical manifestations, such as epithelial lesions, resemble the ones produced by foot and mouth disease virus (FMDV), one of the most economically devastating livestock diseases worldwide (8). As such, the differential diagnosis of VSV is performed on a regular basis. Real-time reverse transcription polymerase chain reaction (rRT-PCR) is one of the quickest diagnostic and most valuable tests for this purpose (9–12). In this context, we consider it imperative to have continuous validation of this diagnostic mRRT-PCR assay to ensure the accuracy and reliability over time, especially given the genetic heterogeneity of VSV and the possibility for sequence mutations within the target gene.

We initially published the development and the validation of a mRRT-PCR that targets a specific region of the L gene; an assay capable of detecting and serotyping VSIV and VSNJV strains from field samples in a single reaction (13). This was followed by a reevaluation and subsequent validation using representative strains of different VSNJV genetic groups (3), to extend its range of detection associated with genetic groups II, IV, V, and VI (10).

Herein, we are presenting the results of the second redesign and validation of our mRRT-PCR assay to enhance the detection of VSNJV associated with the genetic group II. We aimed to evaluate the performance of our mRRT-PCR assay to detect samples from both the Central American lineage 2.1 recently introduced in Mexico and the epidemic lineage 1.1. The results of this study are discussed in terms of the importance of maintaining a continuous validation program of the mRRT-PCR protocols used in the detection of VSV. This highlights the relevance of molecular epidemiology studies using multiple methods to promote the detection of new lineages of this virus and the consequent improvement of routine diagnostic tools.

METHODS

Sample Collection

A total of 17 tissue suspensions from epithelial samples collected during 2008 from naturally infected cows in eight different states of Mexico were obtained from the Mexico-United States Commission for Prevention of Foot-and-Mouth Disease and other Animal Exotic Diseases (CPA). These samples represent the genetic diversity of VSNJV in Mexico from 2005 to 2011 and include VSNJV associated with genetic clades I including a sample representing the endemic lineages in Mexico, as well as samples from lineages 1.1 and 1.2 (the most recent common endemic ancestor of lineage 1.1) ($n = 6$) and lineage 2.1 ($n = 11$) (**Figure 1A**). These samples were from a molecular epidemiology study conducted in Mexico and were previously determined to be positive for VSNJV by double antibody sandwich ELISA (DAS ELISA) for VSV antigen detection, viral isolation, conventional RT-PCR, and sanger sequencing (4). Specific details about these samples are presented in **Figure 1**.

RNA Extraction and mRRT-PCR Performance

Viral RNA was extracted using the MagMax™-96 viral RNA isolation kit (AM1836, Applied Biosystems) and a KingFisher automated extraction system (ThermoFisher Scientific) following the manufacturer's instructions. The presence of VSNJV by mRRT-PCR was evaluated using an Applied Biosystems 7500 real-time PCR platform. Initially, samples were evaluated using the 2010 protocol and conditions (10). Briefly, master mix preparation was carried out using the Platinum Quantitative RT-PCR Thermoscript One-Step System kit (Applied Biosystems #11731015), in a final volume of 25 ul. Amplification conditions were as follows: one cycle of reverse transcription for 30 min at 50°C, followed by 1 min at 95°C, and 45 cycles of 95°C for 15 s, 54°C for 30 s, and 72°C for 1 min (Data collection). Additionally, to evaluate the potential effect of the master mix kit in the reaction, we performed this protocol using the TaqMan™ Fast Virus 1-Step Master Mix kit (Applied Biosystems #4444434) in a final volume of 25 ul. Amplification conditions for this kit are as follows: For reverse transcription 1 cycle of 5 min at 50°C followed by 95°C for 20 s, and 45 cycles of 95°C for 15 s and 60°C for 45 s (Data collection).

Primers, Probes and Amplification Conditions Developed for the 2021 Protocol

The set of primers and probes included in the 2021 protocol for the VSIV component, produce a predicted amplicon size of 227 bp. The nucleotide locations in the L gene are based on the VSIV strain Mudd-Summers (GenBank: MN164438.1). Primers are described as: 7230F 5'-TGATACAGTACAATTATTTTGGGAC-3' (7230-7254 nucleotides), and 7456R 5'-GAGACTTTCTGTTACGGGATCTGG-3' (7456-7433). The probe IN 22 was labeled at the 5'-end with the reporter dye VIC and MGB (minor groove binder) was incorporated at the 3'-end. 5'-VIC-ATGATGCATGATCCTGCTCTTC-MGB-3' (7274-7295). The primers and probes included in the VSNJV

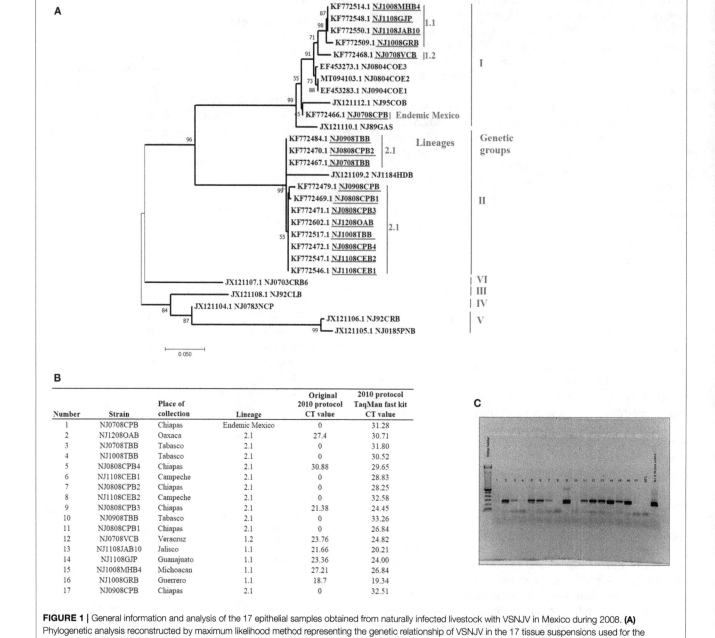

FIGURE 1 | General information and analysis of the 17 epithelial samples obtained from naturally infected livestock with VSNJV in Mexico during 2008. **(A)** Phylogenetic analysis reconstructed by maximum likelihood method representing the genetic relationship of VSNJV in the 17 tissue suspensions used for the validation of this study (highlighted in red). The analysis was enhanced using VSNJV isolates representing different genetic groups of this serotype. **(B)** Results of the comparison of the 2010 protocol using different master mix kits. **(C)** Gel visualization of the amplicons from the mRRT-PCR reactions using the original 2010 protocol.

component produce a predicted amplicon size of 266 bp. The nucleotide locations in the gene L are based on the VSNJV strain NJ0612NME6 (GenBank: MG552609.1) Primers were described as: 7230F-1: 5'-TGATTCAATATAATTATTTTGGGAC-3' (7133-7157), 7230F-2: 5'-TGATTCAATATAATTACTTTGGAAC-3 (7133-7154) and REV2: 5'-AGGCTCAGAGGCATGTTCAT-3' (7398-7379). Probes were labeled at the 5'end with the reporter dye FAM and MGB was incorporated at the 3'end. These were identified as: M1 5'-FAM-TTTATGCATGATCCCGCAATACG-MGB-3' (7177-7199), M2

5'-FAM-TTTATGCATGACCCTGCCATAAG-MGB-3' (7177-7199), and short probe 5'-FAM-TTGCACACCAGAACAT-MGB-3' (7237-7252). Details about the development of the 2021 protocol are presented in the results and discussion sections.

The master mix for the reaction was made with the TaqMan™ Fast Virus 1-Step Master Mix kit in a final volume of 25 ul. Final 1× mix included: RNase-Free Water 12.25 μl, 4× TaqMan Fast Virus 1-step Master Mix 6.25 μl, Forward primer mix (7230F +7230F-1 +7230F-2: 0.2 μM each) 0.5 μl, reverse primer mix (7456R + REV2: 0.2/0.8μM, respectively) 0.5 μl, and probe mix (short + M1+ M2 + IN 22: 0.1, 0.05, 0.05, 0.1μM, respectively) 0.5 μl, and RNA template 5 μl. Amplification conditions were as described above for the TaqMan™ Fast Virus 1-Step Master Mix kit. More information about this is available in the **Supplementary File 1**.

Amplification Efficiency, Analytical Sensitivity and Diagnostic Specificity

The determination of amplification efficiency and analytical sensitivity of the new protocol were performed as previously described (14). Several 10-fold dilutions of a known titer of either VSNJV or VSIV reference strains (Ogden and San Juan, respectively) were prepared and triplicates of each dilution were assessed by mRRT-PCR to ascertain the limit of detection, defined as the last dilution where all repetitions were positive in all three replicates. To assess the accuracy of the results, this experiment was performed three times.

For the diagnostic specificity a total of 80 negative cattle epithelial tissues were evaluated, as well as different viruses associated with the production of vesicular lesions in livestock. This analysis comprised of six FMDV strains including serotypes A, O, Asia 1, SAT 1, SAT 2 and SAT 3, two strains of swine vesicular disease virus (SVDV) and two strains of Senecavirus A (SVA).

Phylogenetic Analysis

To evaluate the genetic relationship between the 17 viruses included in this study and the six genetic groups of VSNJV, a phylogenetic analysis was reconstructed by Maximum likelihood method under the general time reversible model, with a bootstrap analysis of 1,000 replicates to assess the accuracy of the reconstruction. Analysis was conducted on the software MEGA X (15). Alignments were conducted with Jalview version 2.11.1.3 using the Clustal W algorithm.

Sanger Sequencing

Primers used for the purpose of sequencing were the previously described 7230F-1 and REV2 located in the gene L. PCR products were purified using QIAquick PCR purification kits (Qiagen). Sanger sequencing of these products was performed using a BigDye Terminator Cycle Sequencing kit (Applied Biosystems). Sequencing reactions were run on a 3500xL genetic analyzer (Applied Biosystems) and the raw data was analyzed using Geneious Prime version 2021.0.3 (Biomatters Ltd.).

RESULTS AND DISCUSSION

The results indicated that our 2010 protocol was unable to detect 8 out of the 11 samples associated with clade II lineage 2.1 and one sample associated with endemic lineages of Mexico (**Figure 1B**). Conversely, this protocol was able to detect all samples associated with clade I lineages 1.1 and 1.2. When PCR products were visualized by agarose gel electrophoresis, amplification products matching the expected size of VSNJV amplicon were observed in most of the mRRT-PCR negative reactions indicating failure of VSNJV detection in these samples by mRRT-PCR might be associated with mismatches in the probes. In addition, the presence of weak bands (low amount of amplicons) observed in some samples was potentially due to issues with the primers (**Figure 1C**). We then evaluated the potential effect of the TaqMan™ Fast Virus 1-Step Master Mix kit and the new cycling conditions on the performance of the 2010 protocol. Interestingly, the use of this new kit and amplification conditions allowed for the detection of all samples, albeit at suspicious or high Ct values and weak curves (**Figure 1B**), demonstrating the positive effect that the use of this kit and amplification conditions have for this protocol.

To assess the presence of mutations potentially causing specific mismatches between regions of the L gene and the primers and probes of this assay, Sanger sequencing was conducted using the forward and reverse primers described in our 2010 protocol (10). Consistent with the results observed in the analysis of negative reactions in the agarose gel, a total of seven mutations were present in all samples associated with the lineage 2.1 viruses in both the primers and probe regions; mismatches at forward primer ($n = 3$), probe 1 ($n = 3$) and reverse primer ($n = 1$) (**Figure 2A**). Though using TaqMan fast enabled the 2010 mRRT-PCR to detect VSNJV in all samples tested, we hypothesized that the mismatches in the primers and probes diminished the overall performance of the assay, especially the analytical sensitivity. Based on these results, and to improve the assay to better detect VSNJV from a Central America origin, primers and probes were modified based on the sequences obtained from the Mexico isolates and were further evaluated. Overall, we included a new forward primer (NJ-7230F-2), replaced the 2010 probe 1 with probes M1 and M2 (representing clades I and II), and substituted probe 2 with a shorter probe at the same location (**Figure 2A**). For the VSIV component of the assay, the only modification in relation to the 2010 protocol, was the addition of five nucleotides at the 3' end of the IN 22 probe to promote the stability of this reagent in the reaction. Blast analysis of IN 22 probe showed 100% of identity with all VSIV isolates reported in GenBank database including all isolates reported from the most recent VSIV outbreak in the USA (16).

To evaluate the effect of the newly designed primers and probes in the detection of lineage 2.1, the 2010 protocol was performed using either the original primers and probe set or a combination including some of the original assay and the newly designed primers and probes (see Methods section for exact information about this mix. Both versions were performed using the TaqMan™ Fast Virus 1-Step Master Mix kit.

Compared to the results obtained using the 2010 protocol with the original set of primers and probes, the 11 samples associated with lineage 2.1 showed a statistically significant ($p < 0.05$) decrease in the Ct values (between −10.25 and −11.88), producing a significant 3.5-4 $\log_{10}$ improvement in terms of diagnostic sensitivity for this lineage when using a combination primer and probe mix containing some of the original set and the new set (**Figure 2B**). Conversely, no statistically significant differences were found in the six samples associated with lineages 1.1, 1.2 and endemic Mexico (**Figure 2C**). Furthermore, the increase in the diagnostic sensitivity for the detection of samples from lineage 2.1 was evidenced when the performance of the 2010

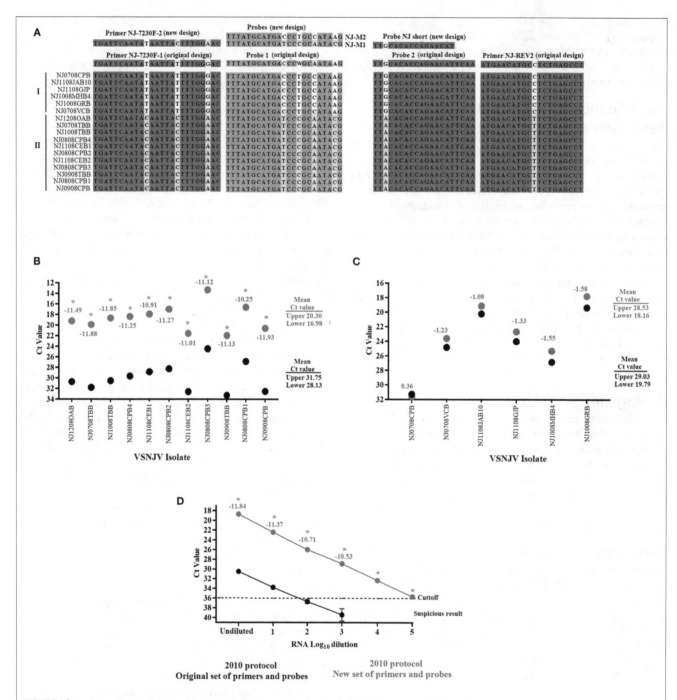

FIGURE 2 | Development and validation of the new set of primers and probes for the VSVNJ component. **(A)** Detection of mutations associated with viruses from lineage 2.1 in the target region of the L gene. The sequence of new primers and probes designed to update the 2010 protocol are shown. The performance of the 2010 protocol using either the original or with a combination between some of the original and the new designed primerson **(B)** 11 samples from Central American lineage 2.1, and **(C)** 6 samples representing 1.1, 1.2 and endemic lineages from Mexico. **(D)** Comparison in the analytical sensitivity between the two versions of the 2010 protocol using several 10-fold dilutions of RNA extraction from a representative virus of lineage 2.1.Upper and lower means were calculated using JMP PRO software with the standard error set at $p < 0.05$. Numbers under different symbols represents the differences in the Ct values between samples evaluated by the two versions of the 2010 protocol. Asterisks represent statistically significant values ($p < 0.05$) obtained by the paired T-test conducted in GraphPad 9.0.0; symbols represent the average of three replicates.

protocol was compared again using either the original or a mix containing both new and old primers and probes (Both using the TaqMan™ Fast Virus 1-Step Master Mix kit) using multiple 10-fold serial dilutions of viral RNA from a sample belonging to the 2.1 lineage (NJ1008TBB) (**Figure 2D**). Although both assays exhibited comparable amplification efficiency R^2 values (~0.99),

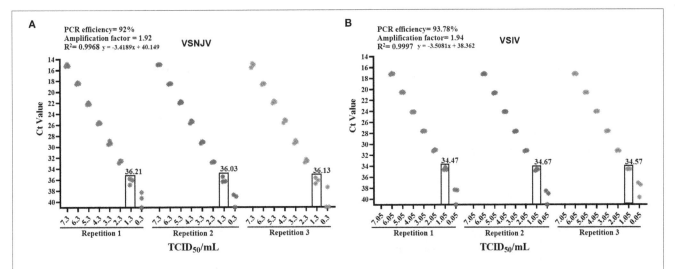

FIGURE 3 | Determination of the amplification efficiency and the analytical sensitivity values of the 2021 protocol using reference strains of each serotype. Initial validation of the 2021 protocol was conducted on the **(A)** VSNJV and **(B)** VSIV components of this protocol. In each graphic are depicted values of PCR efficiency, amplification factor, and R² correlation values associated with the PCR efficiency. The analytical sensitivity of each component is shown in the rectangle that corresponds to the last dilution where all three replicates were detected.

the 2010 protocol using a mix between the original and new set of primers and probes appeared statistically ($p < 0.05$) 1,000 times more sensitive than the same protocol using the original set of primers and probes, showing the positive effect that the new set of primers and probes have in the detection of lineage 2.1 (**Figure 2D**).

Based on the results expressed above, we changed the conditions of our 2010 protocol to include a primer-probe mix containing a combination of some of the original set and the newly designed set of primers and probes. We also incorporated the TaqMan™ Fast Virus 1-Step Master Mix kit and the amplification conditions for this kit to establish the improved assay referred to as the 2021 protocol.

To get a better perspective of the overall performance of the 2021 protocol, a validation testing was performed. The validation analysis showed that the 2021 protocol is highly sensitive for the detection of VSNJV and VSIV serotypes (1.3 and 1.05 $TCID_{50}$/ml, respectively), both the PCR efficiency and amplification factor parameters were found to be optimal (17) (**Figures 3A,B**). No positive reactions were obtained after 45 cycles of amplification when negative epithelial samples were tested, resulting in a diagnostic specificity of 100%. In addition, no cross-reactivity was observed when representative isolates of FMDV, SVDV and SVA were evaluated with this protocol. Based on these results, samples were considered positive with Ct values < 36, suspicious between Cts 36-40 and negative with a Ct > 40. Furthermore, comparability testing of the 2021 protocol on additional real-time PCR machines including the CFX96 Touch (BIO RAD) and the QuantStudio 7 Pro (Applied Biosystems) gave similar results indicating the robustness of this assay across platforms.

To further validate the performance of the 2021 assay, a historical collection of VSV samples stored at the NCFAD were tested and compared to previous results. These samples included

VSNJV samples from Mexico ($n = 87$) collected between 2006 and 2007, Colombia ($n = 78$), VSIV from Colombia ($n = 74$) collected between 1996 and 2002 as well as multiple VSNJV samples ($n = 11$) (representative of all six genetic groups) and VSIV ($n = 4$) representing multiple lineages from the Americas received from PIADC.

Interestingly, with the VSNJV samples from Mexico, we observed an overall slight decrease in the mean of the Ct values between the original 2010 protocol (10), and the newly established 2021 protocol (**Figure 4A**). Within this group, a statistically significant ($p < 0.05$) decrease in the Ct values was recorded in a total of 20 samples, showing an improvement in analytical sensitivity for these samples. The 2021 protocol was also able to detect 100% of the samples (87/87) compared with a detection rate of 74.1 % (65/87) using the 2010 protocol. This represents an increase of 25.9% in the diagnostic sensitivity for detection of lineages circulating in Mexico. Similar results were found in the overall mean Cts during the evaluation of VSNJV samples from Colombia (**Figure 4B**). In this context, we saw a significant ($p < 0.05$) decrease in Ct values in a total of 25 samples and an increase in the diagnostic sensitivity of 1.2% for the detection of all samples. Conversely, a slight increase in the overall mean of Ct values was seen in the 2021 protocol when compared with the 2010 protocol during the evaluation of VSIV from Colombia (**Figure 4C**). Furthermore, we recorded an improvement in the diagnostic sensitivity for VSIV, from 94.5% (70/74) to 100% when using the 2021 protocol.

Finally, similar to the 2010 protocol, the 2021 protocol was able to detect not only all reference VSNJV isolates representing all genetic groups of this serotype, but also all isolates associated with VSIV (**Figure 4D**). In case of VSNJV, there was a slight decrease in the Ct values for isolates representing the genetic groups III, IV, V, and VI. We observed a slight increase in the Ct value for the detection of the isolate associated with

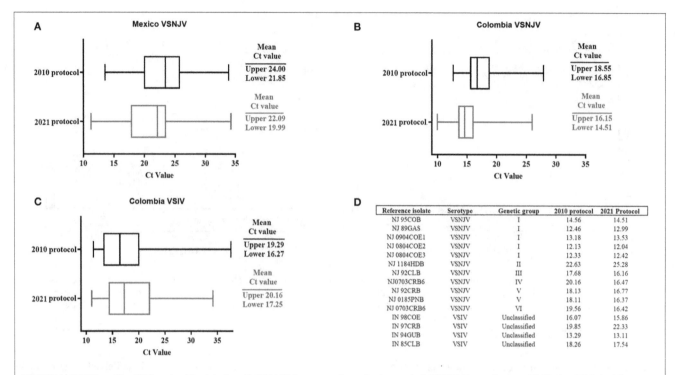

FIGURE 4 | Validation of the 2021 protocol for detection of VSV. Validation was performed using a set of VSNJV field samples from **(A)** Mexico, **(B)** Colombia, and VSIV field samples from **(C)** Colombia. **(D)** Isolates representing the different genetic groups of VSNJV and VSIV. Comparisons were established using historical values obtained during the validation of the 2010 protocol. Upper and lower means of Cts were calculated using JMP PRO software with the standard error set at $p < 0.05$.

the genetic group II. VSIV isolate IN97CRB, also had an increased Ct (**Figure 4D**). Furthermore, low Ct values (Cts of 18-19) were obtained with the 2021 protocol, detecting viral isolates NJ0612NME6, and IN0919WYB1 associated with the 2012 VSNJV and 2019 VSIV outbreaks in the US, respectively (16, 18). Interestingly, during the revision process of this manuscript, we were able to evaluate the ability of the 2021 protocol to detect a group of five representative isolates (NJ0911CPB7, NJ0911CPB1, NJ1011TBP3, NJ0911TBB3, NJ0911CPB10) of the central American lineage 2.2 circulating in Mexico during 2011 (4), confirming the ability of this protocol to detect additional VSNJV lineages from central America (Ct values ranged between 17 and 19).

Overall, our data shows that the updating the primers and probes for VSV mRRT-PCR and using TaqMan™ Fast Virus 1-Step Master Mix kit substantially improves the detection of the Central America VSNJV lineage 2.1. This new assay is a vast improvement over previous ones for the detection of VSNJV group II which has high genetic variability. As lineage 2.1 has the potential to cause outbreaks in northern Mexico and the southern USA (4), it could be readily identified using this assay thereby making it an important diagnostic tool. Currently, studies are being conducted in Mexico to determine the molecular epidemiology of this lineage.

We think that the combination of two main factors contributed to the improved performance of the 2021 protocol. The most important changes were the sequence of the primers and probes that were redesigned in the new assay to accommodate mutations in the mRRT-PCR target on the L gene. The other important change was the TaqMan™ Fast Virus 1-Step Master Mix kit in place of the Platinum Quantitative RT-PCR Thermoscript One-Step System kit. The effect of this variable was evidenced by the overall improvement of the 2010 protocol. However, the inclusion of the new set of primers and probes in the VSNJV component of this assay was clearly a key factor to improve the detection of the central American lineage 2.1 Regarding the improvement in the sensitivity of the VSIV component of the assay, the most likely explanation may be associated with the use of the new amplification kit and conditions. However, at this point, we can't rule out the potential positive effect that the increase in the length of probe IN 22 might have in the performance of this component of the assay.

Considering the absence of sequencing information from the historical Mexican samples (2006-2007), we cannot rule out the possibility that some of these samples were associated with central America lineages, as they were identified in Mexico in 2005 (4). This may therefore explain improvement in the diagnostic sensitivity observed with the 2021 protocol for VSNJV samples from Mexico. Along with the molecular changes to the assay and based on the information provided by the manufacturer, one of the features of the TaqMan™ Fast Virus 1-Step Master Mix kit is its ability to better handle PCR inhibitors which may explain the added improvement this chemistry also provides to the assay. This feature may be especially important considering that the main target of this protocol is the use of clinical samples mostly represented by epithelial tissues.

The results presented in this study show the difficulties involved in the diagnosis of VSV by mRRT-PCR assay due to the heterogeneity of VSNJV. Based on these findings, we consider it imperative to perform continuous molecular epidemiology studies to increase the knowledge regarding the tremendous genetic diversity associated with this virus. In this context, although we demonstrate the capability of our protocol to detect VSNJV from all genetic groups, we consider that one of the main limitations of this study is the reduced number of samples used to support the development of the new primers and probes presented herein. Thus, we consider it imperative to conduct future validations using a vast number of samples to deeply cover the genetic variability within the different genetic groups.

Furthermore, this study exposes the necessity to keep a continuous validation program in diagnostic laboratories to ensure the correct performance of VSV mRRT-PCR using recent field isolates and the evaluation of new master mix kits.

In conclusion, we consider that the 2021 protocol presented herein, represents an excellent option not only for diagnostic purposes, but also for research laboratories that perform various studies with VSV (19–21).

AUTHOR CONTRIBUTIONS

KH and LV-S conceived and designed the experiments and analyzed the data. KH performed the experiments. KH, CN, LR, and LV-S wrote the manuscript. All authors contributed to the article and approved the submitted version.

FUNDING

This work was supported by the Canadian Food Inspection Agency (WIN-A-1302) and the USDA Research Service CRIS Project No. 8064-32000-059-00D.

ACKNOWLEDGMENTS

We thank the authorities of the Mexico-United States Commission for Prevention of Foot-and-Mouth Disease and other Animal Exotic Diseases in Mexico (CPA laboratory) for kindly providing the samples to conduct this study.

REFERENCES

1. Rodriguez LL. Emergence and re-emergence of vesicular stomatitis in the United States. *Virus Res.* (2002) 85:211–9. doi: 10.1016/S0168-1702(02)00026-6

2. Dietzgen RG. Morphology genome organization, transcription replication of rhabdoviruses. In: Kuzmin RGDaIV, editor. *Rhabdoviruses*. Norfolk; England: Caister Academic Press (2012). p. 5–11.

3. Pauszek SJ, Rodriguez LL. Full-length genome analysis of vesicular stomatitis New Jersey virus strains representing the phylogenetic and geographic diversity of the virus. *Arch Virol.* (2012) 157:2247–51. doi: 10.1007/s00705-012-1420-x

4. Velazquez-Salinas L, Pauszek SJ, Zarate S, Basurto-Alcantara FJ, Verdugo-Rodriguez A, Perez AM, et al. Phylogeographic characteristics of vesicular stomatitis New Jersey viruses circulating in Mexico from 2005 to 2011 and their relationship to epidemics in the United States. *Virology.* (2014) 449:17–24. doi: 10.1016/j.virol.2013.10.025

5. Rainwater-Lovett K, Pauszek SJ, Kelley WN, Rodriguez LL. Molecular epidemiology of vesicular stomatitis New Jersey virus from the 2004-2005 US outbreak indicates a common origin with Mexican strains. *J Gen Virol.* (2007) 88:2042–51. doi: 10.1099/vir.0.82644-0

6. Rodriguez LL, Bunch TA, Fraire M, Llewellyn ZN. Re-emergence of vesicular stomatitis in the western United States is associated with distinct viral genetic lineages. *Virology.* (2000) 271:171–81. doi: 10.1006/viro.2000.0289

7. Velazquez-Salinas L, Pauszek SJ, Stenfeldt C, O'Hearn ES, Pacheco JM, Borca MV, et al. Increased virulence of an epidemic strain of vesicular stomatitis virus is associated with interference of the innate response in pigs. *Front Microbiol.* (2018) 9:1891. doi: 10.3389/fmicb.2018.01891

8. Mwiine FN, Velazquez-Salinas L, Ahmed Z, Ochwo S, Munsey A, Kenney M, et al. Serological and phylogenetic characterization of foot and mouth disease viruses from Uganda during cross-sectional surveillance study in cattle between 2014 and 2017. *Transbound Emerg Dis.* (2019) 66:2011–24. doi: 10.1111/tbed.13249

9. Fernandez J, Aguero M, Romero L, Sanchez C, Belak S, Arias M, et al. Rapid and differential diagnosis of foot-and-mouth disease, swine vesicular disease, and vesicular stomatitis by a new multiplex RT-PCR assay. *J Virol Methods.* (2008) 147:301–11. doi: 10.1016/j.jviromet.2007.09.010

10. Hole K, Velazquez-Salinas L, Clavijo A. Improvement and optimization of a multiplex real-time reverse transcription polymerase chain reaction assay for the detection and typing of Vesicular stomatitis virus. *J Vet Diagn Invest.* (2010) 22:428–33. doi: 10.1177/104063871002200315

11. Lung O, Fisher M, Beeston A, Hughes KB, Clavijo A, Goolia M, et al. Multiplex RT-PCR detection and microarray typing of vesicular disease viruses. *J Virol Methods.* (2011) 175:236–45. doi: 10.1016/j.jviromet.2011.05.023

12. Wilson WC, Letchworth GJ, Jimenez C, Herrero MV, Navarro R, Paz P, et al. Field evaluation of a multiplex real-time reverse transcription polymerase chain reaction assay for detection of Vesicular stomatitis virus. *J Vet Diagn Invest.* (2009) 21:179–86. doi: 10.1177/104063870902100201

13. Hole K, Clavijo A, Pineda LA. Detection and serotype-specific differentiation of vesicular stomatitis virus using a multiplex, real-time, reverse transcription-polymerase chain reaction assay. *J Vet Diagn Invest.* (2006) 18:139–46. doi: 10.1177/104063870601800201

14. Velazquez-Salinas L, Ramirez-Medina E, Rai A, Pruitt S, Vuono EA, Espinoza N, et al. Development real-time PCR assays to genetically differentiate vaccinated pigs from infected pigs with the eurasian strain of african swine fever virus. *Front Vet Sci.* (2021) 8:768869. doi: 10.3389/fvets.2021.768869

15. Kumar S, Stecher G, Li M, Knyaz C, Tamura K. MEGA X: molecular evolutionary genetics analysis across computing platforms. *Mol Biol Evol.* (2018) 35:1547–9. doi: 10.1093/molbev/msy096

16. O'Donnell VK, Pauszek SJ, Xu L, Moran K, Vierra D, Boston T, et al. Genome sequences of vesicular stomatitis indiana viruses from the 2019 outbreak in the Southwest United States. *Microbiol Resour Announc.* (2020) 9:e00894-20. doi: 10.1128/MRA.00894-20

17. Shehata HR, Ragupathy S, Shanmughanandhan D, Kesanakurti P, Ehlinger TM, Newmaster SG. Guidelines for validation of qualitative real-time PCR methods for molecular diagnostic identification of probiotics. *J AOAC Int.* (2019) 102:1774–8. doi: 10.5740/jaoacint.18-0320

18. Velazquez-Salinas L, Pauszek SJ, Verdugo-Rodriguez A, Rodriguez LL. Complete genome sequences of two vesicular stomatitis New Jersey viruses representing the 2012 U.S. epidemic strain and its closest relative endemic strain from Southern Mexico. *Genome Announc.* (2018) 6:e00049-18. doi: 10.1128/genomeA.00049-18

19. Morozov I, Davis AS, Ellsworth S, Trujillo JD, McDowell C, Shivanna V, et al. Comparative evaluation of pathogenicity of three isolates of vesicular stomatitis virus (Indiana serotype) in pigs. *J Gen Virol.* (2019) 100:1478–90. doi: 10.1099/jgv.0.001329

20. Velazquez-Salinas L, Naik S, Pauszek SJ, Peng KW, Russell SJ, Rodriguez LL. Oncolytic recombinant vesicular stomatitis virus (VSV) is nonpathogenic and nontransmissible in pigs, a natural host of VSV. *Hum Gene Ther Clin Dev.* (2017) 28:108–15. doi: 10.1089/humc.2017.015

21. Velazquez-Salinas L, Pauszek SJ, Holinka LG, Gladue DP, Rekant SI, Bishop EA, et al. A single amino acid substitution in the matrix protein (M51R) of vesicular stomatitis New Jersey virus impairs replication in cultured porcine macrophages and results in significant attenuation in pigs. *Front Microbiol.* (2020) 11:1123. doi: 10.3389/fmicb.2020.01123

Discrepancy between In-Clinic and Haemagglutination-Inhibition Tests in Detecting Maternally-Derived Antibodies against Canine Parvovirus in Puppies

Paola Dall'Ara[1], Stefania Lauzi[1], Joel Filipe[1*], Roberta Caseri[1], Michela Beccaglia[2], Costantina Desario[3], Alessandra Cavalli[3], Giulio Guido Aiudi[3], Canio Buonavoglia[3] and Nicola Decaro[3]

[1] Department of Veterinary Medicine, University of Milan, Lodi, Italy, [2] Ambulatorio Veterinario Beccaglia, Lissone, Italy, [3] Department of Veterinary Medicine, University of Bari, Bari, Italy

*Correspondence:
Joel Filipe
joel.soares@unimi.it

Canine parvovirus (CPV) is one of the most common causes of mortality in puppies worldwide. Protection against CPV infection is based on vaccination, but maternally-derived antibodies (MDA) can interfere with vaccination. The aim of this study was to evaluate the applicability of an in-clinic ELISA test to assess the CPV MDA in unvaccinated puppies and CPV antibodies in bitches, comparing the results with the gold standard haemagglutination inhibition (HI) test. Serum samples of 136 unvaccinated puppies were tested, along with sera of 16 vaccinated bitches. Five unvaccinated puppies were retested after vaccination. Both assays showed that the 16 vaccinated bitches had protective antibody levels against CPV. Conversely, significant discrepancies were observed for the MDA titers in unvaccinated puppies. Protective MDA titers were observed in 91.9% puppies using HI and in 40.4% by the in-clinic ELISA test, and only the latter one showed a decrease of MDA titers and percentages of protected puppies after the first weeks of age. Vaccination of five puppies with high HI and low in-clinic ELISA MDA titers resulted in seroconversion. Our results confirm the reliability of the in-clinic ELISA test in determining protective antibodies against CPV in adult dogs. Our findings also suggest that the in-clinic ELISA test kit may also be a useful tool to detect and quantify CPV MDA, thus allowing prediction of the best time to vaccinate puppies and reduction of the rate of vaccination failures due to interference by maternally-derived antibodies.

Keywords: canine parvovirus, dog, haemagglutination inhibition test, in-clinic ELISA test, maternally-derived antibodies, vaccination

INTRODUCTION

Canine parvovirus (CPV) is one of the most common causes of mortality in puppies (1). The virus is highly contagious and relatively stable in the environment, causing high morbidity in dogs worldwide. Dogs can be infected at any age, but puppies between 6 weeks and 6 months of age are more commonly infected, showing a more severe disease (1). In puppies, maternally-derived antibody (MDA) titers $\geq$1:80 are considered protective against CPV infection in the first weeks of life (2–4). After the first weeks of age, vaccination is the main method to control the disease worldwide (5).

The World Small Animal Veterinary Association (WSAVA) "Guidelines for vaccination of dogs and cats" recommend that all dogs should be vaccinated, whenever possible, not only to prevent individual infections but also to assure herd immunity and to reduce the prevalence of the disease (6). However, several factors can interfere with an adequate immune response and result in vaccination failure. In puppies, MDA are one of the major factors that can interfere with an immune response to vaccination. According to previous studies, MDA titers $\geq$1:20 are reported to cause a vaccination failure against CPV (2, 7–9).

CPV MDA vanish with a linear decrease during the post-birth period and their half-life is about 9–10 days (2, 10, 11). In most puppies, MDA decline by 8–12 weeks of age to a level that allows vaccination. Absence of MDA is reported by 10–14 weeks of age (2, 12).

It is not possible to accurately predict the first vaccination time because different MDA titers and kinetics have been reported in puppies, depending on vaccination status of bitches, magnitude of colostrum intake and environmental infective pressure (11, 13). To overcome MDA vaccination interference, administration of initial core vaccination in puppies at 6–8 weeks of age, then every 3–4 weeks until 16 weeks of age or older is recommended by WSAVA guidelines (6). Optimization of vaccination protocols in puppies is recommended and should rely on each puppy's individual needs (11, 14).

It would be important to know MDA titers in puppies in order to reduce interference with vaccination and consequently vaccination failures or, on the other hand, avoid unnecessary vaccinations. Serological testing has been introduced in veterinary practices to determine CPV seroprotection in dogs to assess revaccination requirements (3, 15). The gold standard test for detection and titration of CPV post-infection and/or post-vaccination antibodies in adult dogs is the haemagglutination inhibition (HI) test that has to be performed in specialist diagnostic laboratories (16). Recently, the WSAVA guidelines also support the use of simple in-practice tests for determination of seroprotection in dogs (6). These kits are quick and easy to use in clinics for the determination of immunity duration in vaccinated and/or infected dogs (17–19) but are not licensed to quantify MDA in unvaccinated puppies.

Given the usefulness of testing CPV MDA titers in unvaccinated puppies and the availability of in-practice test kits, the aim of this study was to evaluate the applicability of an in-clinic ELISA test to determine CPV MDA titers in unvaccinated puppies during their first weeks of life and CPV antibody titers in bitches, comparing the results with the gold standard HI test.

MATERIALS AND METHODS

Animals and Sample Collection

Unvaccinated puppies and vaccinated bitches were included after owner's consent to participate in the study, which was approved by Ethics Committee of the Department of Veterinary Medicine, University of Bari (approval number 10/17).

One-hundred and thirty-six puppies and 16 bitches (8 were mothers of the tested puppies) were analyzed in this study, for a total of 152 dogs. Puppies were from 40 litters, ranging from 1 to 11 puppies per litter. Sixty puppies were females and 76 were males. Sixteen animals were <40 days of age, 76 were between 40 and 50 days of age and 44 were >50 days of age. The median age was 47 days. Puppies were from 21 different breeds. Puppies were from small ($n = 19$), medium ($n = 51$), and large ($n = 66$) breed sizes. All the 136 puppies had never been vaccinated. Moreover, 5 unvaccinated puppies were retested after being vaccinated with a trivalent MLV vaccine (Nobivac CEP, MSD) (against CPV, CDV, and CAdV-1 infections). Vaccine was administered to the puppies on the first day of sample collection.

Bitches ($n = 16$) were between 1 and 8 years of age. The median age was 3 years. They were from 12 different breeds and from small ($n = 3$), medium ($n = 5$), and large ($n = 8$) breed sizes. Fourteen bitches were tested between 40 and 50 days of gestation while the other two were tested during the post-partum period with their puppies. All 15 bitches were repeatedly vaccinated starting from 5 months (end of the initial puppy vaccination) till 4 years of age, generally once a year. One cross-breed bitch from a kennel had never been vaccinated and was infected by CPV one week post-partum. Her puppies ($n = 6$), were promptly taken away and remained healthy. Their sera (mother and puppies) were collected 45 days post-partum.

When possible, puppies were retested after the first vaccination. Animals were sampled during 2017 by veterinarians in different Italian clinics, breeding kennels, and animal shelters. Data pertaining to vaccination history and other relevant clinical details were recorded for each dog. Puppies were classified in three age categories: <40 days of age, 40–50 days of age, and >50 days of age. Breeds were classified in small (<10 kg), medium (10–25 kg), and large (>25 kg) size.

Blood samples (1 mL) were collected by cephalic venepuncture from each animal. Samples were immediately centrifuged (1,000 × g for 10 min) and sera were separated and stored at −20°C until analysis.

In-clinic ELISA Test

Each serum sample was tested using an in-clinic ELISA test (Canine VacciCheck Antibody Test Kit, Biogal, supplied in Italy by Agrolabo), following the manufacturer's instruction. The kit is a rapid dot-ELISA-based system licensed to determine the titer of antibodies against canine adenovirus type 1 (CAdV-1), canine parvovirus (CPV), and canine distemper virus (CDV) antigens. The test kit has been approved by some official agencies and has been used in UK, Israel, and India to evaluate CPV antibodies in dogs (18–21).

The concentration of CPV antibodies in serum samples was defined by the color intensity of the spots measured in "S" units, on a scale from 0 to 6. An S value of 3 (S3) was standardized by the manufacturer to be the equivalence of a 1:80 CPV serum antibody titer by the HI test. As per the information provided by the manufacturer, S units from 0 to 6 corresponds to <1:20, 1:20,

1:40, 1:80, 1:160, 1:320, and 1:640 titer, respectively. Antibody titers ≥1:80 were indicative of protective levels of antibodies to CPV.

Haemagglutination Inhibition (HI) Test

Serum samples were also subjected to the HI test. Antibody testing was carried out as previously described, with minor modifications (16). The tests were performed at +4°C in 96-well V-plates, using 6–8 haemagglutination units of CPV-2b antigen (22) and 1% porcine erythrocytes. Serial 2-fold serum dilutions were made in phosphate-buffered saline, starting from a 1:10 dilution. Results were read after about 2–4 h at +4°C. The HI titer was indicated as the highest serum dilution completely inhibiting viral haemagglutination. Antibody titers ≥1:80 were indicative of protective levels of antibodies to CPV. As positive controls sera we used known sera from another work already published (23).

Data Analysis

Statistical analysis was performed using Graph Pad Prism 6, GraphPad Software (La Jolla, CA, USA), and EpiTools Epidemiological Calculators[1] (24). To compare the validity of in-clinic ELISA with that of haemagglutination inhibition a Spearman correlation test (for not normally distributed data; Shapiro-Wilk test) was used, considering statistically significant value of $p < 0.05$, and a linear regression analyses was also performed. A Pearson's Chi-square test was used to assess the relationship between the presence of protective MDA titers (obtained by in-clinic ELISA or by HI tests) and independent variables such as gender, age, and breed size. A $p < 0.05$ was considered as statistically significant. The relative sensitivity and specificity of in-clinic ELISA were determined with Epitools epidemiological calculators software (epitools.ausvet.com.au) by comparison with the results of HI test (gold standard).

Results of the gold standard (HI) assays were compared with results of the in-clinic ELISA to determine measures of the diagnostic performance of the assay.

RESULTS

CPV Antibody Titers and Comparison Between In-clinic ELISA and HI Tests

Considering a MDA titer ≥1:80 as indicative of protection against CPV infection in both tests, the overall percentage of puppies with protective MDA was 40.4% (55/136) using in-clinic ELISA test and 91.9% (125/136) using HI test. Comparison of protective results (MDA titer ≥1:80) obtained in unvaccinated puppies by in-clinic ELISA and HI testing are reported in **Table 1**.

The results of HI and in-clinic ELISA are given in **Table 2** and relationship exist between these two tests analyzed by ROC is depicted in **Figure 1**.

MDA titers displayed large variability among puppies and between the two tests. MDA titers ranged from <1:20 to 1:320 using in-clinic ELISA test and from 1:10 to 1:2,560 using HI test (**Figure 2**). However, the two tests appear to be strictly correlated ($p < 0.0001$).

[1] Freely available at http://epitools.ausvet.com.au

TABLE 1 | Comparison of in-clinic ELISA test and HI test in detecting MDA (titer ≥1:80) in unvaccinated puppies.

	Positive HI test	Negative HI test	Total
Positive in-clinic ELISA test	52	3	55 (40.4%)
Negative in-clinic ELISA test	73	8	81 (59.6%)
Total puppies	125 (91.9%)	11 (8.1%)	136

TABLE 2 | Relative sensitivity and specificity of in-clinic ELISA in comparison to HI test.

		HI	
		Positive	Negative
VacciCheck	**Positive**	68	3
	Negative	69	12

Sensitivity = 49.64%.
Specificity = 80%.

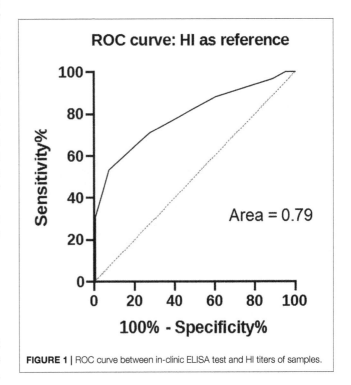

FIGURE 1 | ROC curve between in-clinic ELISA test and HI titers of samples.

The results of protected puppies (MDA titer ≥1:80) and antibody titers according to gender, age, and breed size are reported in **Table 3**.

Different MDA titers in puppies from the same litter were observed in majority of the litters. In 11 and 9 litters, puppies from the same litter had the same MDA titer as detected by both HI and in-clinic ELISA test. Both tests always reported different MDA titers between bitches and their offspring.

HI test revealed significant differences in the presence of protective MDA between male and female puppies, with male puppies being significantly more protected than female puppies

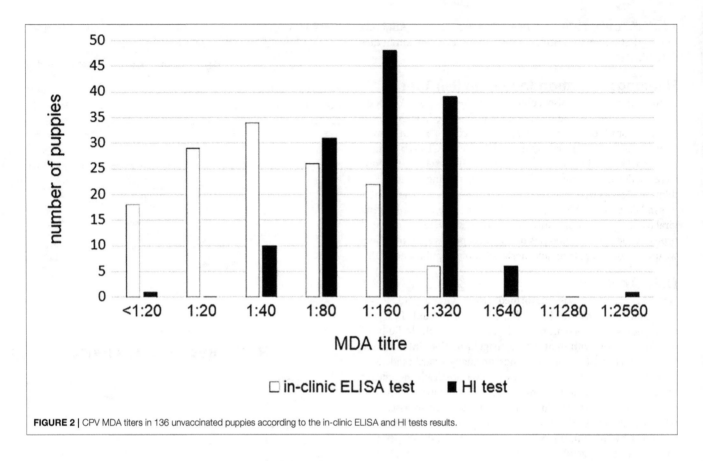

FIGURE 2 | CPV MDA titers in 136 unvaccinated puppies according to the in-clinic ELISA and HI tests results.

TABLE 3 | Puppies with protective CPV MDA titer (≥1:80) and mean CPV MDA titer detected using in-clinic ELISA test and HI test according to gender, age, and breed size.

| | No. puppies | No. puppies with protective MDA titer (%) | |
		In-clinic ELISA test	HI test
Gender			
Female	60	24 (40)	51 (85)[a]
Male	76	31 (40)	74 (97)[a]
Age			
<40 days old	16	4 (25)	16 (100)
40-50 days old	76	35 (46)	65 (85)[b]
>50 days old	44	16 (36)	44 (100)[b]
Breed size			
Small	19	3 (16)	19 (100)
Medium	51	24 (47)	46 (90)[c]
Large	66	28 (42)	66 (100)[c]

[a,b,c] Significant difference between categories of the same variable (p < 0.05).

TABLE 4 | CPV MDA and active antibody titers detected using in-clinic ELISA test and HI test before and after administration of the first vaccination in 5 puppies.

| | Before vaccination MDA titer | | Post-vaccination Antibody titer | |
Puppy ID	In-clinic-ELISA	HI	In-clinic ELISA	HI
1	<1:20	1:160	>1:640	1:2,560
2	1:20	1:320	1:80	1:2,560
3	1:20	1:160	1:160	1:1,280
4	1:20	1:640	1:320	1:1,280
5	1:20	1:640	1:80	1:1,280

($p = 0.021$). Presence of HI protective MDA were significantly lower in 40–50 days old puppies compared with older (>50 days old) puppies ($p = 0.02$). Presence of HI protective MDA were significantly lower in puppies from medium size breeds compared with large size breed ($p = 0.032$). No other significant differences were observed for HI test results. No significant

differences were observed between the result of the in-clinic ELISA test and the variables analyzed (gender, age, and breed size) (**Table 3**).

The MDA and active antibody titers obtained by both tests in 5 puppies tested before and after their first vaccination are shown in **Table 4**. Before the first vaccination, no puppy had protective titers (all of them presented titers ≤1:20) by the in-clinic ELISA test, and this result was in contrast with HI test, which estimated a percentage of 100% of protected puppies. After the first vaccination all puppies seroconverted and became protected as assessed by both tests.

All the 16 bitches in the study resulted highly protected by both assays. Antibody titers ranged from 1:80 to 1:640 using in-clinic ELISA test and from 1:160 to 1:5,120 using HI test.

The antibody titers of the unvaccinated kennel bitch that was infected with CPV one week post-partum and the MDA titers of her offspring obtained by both tests are shown in **Table 5**. Forty-five days post-partum, the bitch presented a protective CPV antibody titer due to the previous CPV infection, as detected by both tests; conversely, no puppy was positive using the in-clinic-ELISA test, while 5 of 6 puppies resulted protected by HI.

DISCUSSION

MDA are known to be a two-edged sword in puppies. MDA are essential for protection against CPV infection but in high concentrations it may cause vaccination failures in puppies. In this study, we evaluated the applicability of an in-clinic ELISA test to assess MDA level in puppies under field conditions in comparison with the gold standard HI test.

Both VacciCheck and HI titers are considered protective if ≥1:80. As stated by Taguchi et al. (25), it is possible to consider a protective titer ≥1:40 using CPV-2b in HI test, as demonstrated in a challenge infection study using a Japanese CPV-2b-based vaccine (Rescamune). In our study, only 10 out of 136 puppies displayed HI MDA titers of 1:40, and according to Taguchi et al. (25) even these puppies could be considered protected against infection by a CPV field strain, thus resulting in a total of 135/136 animals with protective levels of MDA as assessed by HI test (the last one had a titer of 1:10 and then was surely unprotected). However, in the recent review of Chastant and Mila (26) regarding passive immune transfer (PIT) in puppies, adequate PIT was defined as IgG concentration >2.3 g/L for general immunity and CPV-2-antibody titer >1:80 for specific immunity evaluation, independently of CPV-2 strain (26).

The in-clinic ELISA test is commonly used to detect specific CPV post-vaccination/infection antibodies in dogs. In the analyzed bitches, the 100% overall accuracy of the in-clinic ELISA test compared to the HI test to detect protective titers in all the vaccinated adult dogs was expected, since the dogs had been vaccinated within a maximum 4 year-period prior sampling. Vaccination administered within 3-years is considered protective in adult dogs and protective antibody titers have been reported

in dogs even after longer periods (19, 27). The results of this study confirm previous findings that indicate the reliability of the in-clinic ELISA test for detection of protective antibodies against CPV in adult dogs (18). Even if antibody titers were not perfectly the same, the higher antibody titers detected using HI test compared to in-clinic ELISA test were previously reported for the HI titers >1:1,280 (17). The in-clinic ELISA test was not able to determine antibody titers in the HI range ≥1:640, indicating that the gold standard test is more reliable in detecting very high antibody titers in dogs after vaccination and/or infection. This limitation is not considered important because titers in the high range indicate protective levels of immunity (17). As reported by Thomas et al. (28), quite low and high HI titers may not have good correlations with any other serological test for the quantification of CPV specific antibodies. This was taken into account while analyzing our results, but in our case no differences were found when those values were eliminated.

Although HI internal control was used, a possible incorrect control titration could have been a bias in the subsequent antibody titration. In fact, as suggested by Senda et al. (29) also small changes in the technique could strongly affect results. Consequently, our HI test might be overestimating puppy antibody titers and be the main cause of the observed discrepancy. Only using true negative sera, it would be possible to increase HI accuracy.

The high percentage (91.9%) of protection and the high MDA titers (1:2,560) by HI test were not expected in puppies, considering the linear decrease of MDA in the first weeks of age (11, 30). Moreover, results obtained by HI test showed a constantly and unexpected highly significant protection of puppies in older age groups (100% puppies >50 days of age with protective MDA titers). According to the expected decline of MDA in the first weeks after birth (2, 10, 11), only the in-clinic ELISA test showed a decrease of MDA titers and percentages of protected puppies starting from 40 days of age (corresponding to ≥6 weeks old puppies).

Compared to older puppies, higher protective MDA titers and prevalence of protected puppies were expected in younger ones (<40 days of age, corresponding to ≤6 weeks old puppies). HI test identified 100% of puppies <40 days old as MDA protected. However, protection of all the puppies after 6 weeks from birth is not likely, as demonstrated by lower prevalence previously reported in 6 weeks old puppies (11). The lower protection in puppies ≤6 weeks old (<40 days) compared to older ones, as observed by the in-clinic ELISA test, may be due to puppies' features. Anamnestic data revealed that the 16 puppies <40 days old were Dobermanns, Rottweilers and Bull Terriers. These breeds are suspected to be genetically low-responder breeds, thus failing to develop an antibody response after repeated revaccination (6, 31). It is possible that these puppies did not receive adequate MDA because of the low quality of colostrum produced by the bitches due to the inability to develop an adequate antibody response after vaccination. Unfortunately, comparison with puppies <40 days old of other breeds and/or with older Dobermanns, Rottweilers and Bull Terriers puppies was not possible because they were not sampled in this work and further investigations are needed.

TABLE 5 | Antibody titers against CPV of 6 puppies and their unvaccinated mother.

Dog ID	In-clinic ELISA titer	HI titer
Bitch A	1:160	1:320
Puppy A1	<1:20	1:80
Puppy A2	<1:20	1:80
Puppy A3	<1:20	1:80
Puppy A4	<1:20	1:40
Puppy A5	<1:20	1:80
Puppy A6	1:20	1:80

The bitch was infected in kennel by CPV one week post-partum and puppies were promptly separated from the dam and remained healthy. Blood samples were collected 45 days post-partum from the puppies and the bitch.

The significantly higher percentage of male puppies with protective HI MDA compared to females was not expected and gender being a factor linked to differences in maternal colostrum ingestion in the first day of life has not been reported. The significantly higher percentage of large size breed puppies with protective HI MDA compared to medium size breed was unexpected. An in direct correlation between the duration of MDA and the growth rate of the animal was previously observed, with slow-growth breeds (small and medium size breeds) eliminating their MDA more slowly than rapid growth-breeds (large and giant size breeds) (7).

Differences in MDA titers in bitches and puppies from the same litter were previously reported (17), probably linked to differences in colostrum intake among puppies (7).

CPV antibody titers of the puppies of the unvaccinated bitch infected by CPV one week after delivery also showed discrepancies between the two tests. Puppies were promptly separated from their mother and remained healthy. As expected, by in-clinic ELISA test all puppies presented MDA titers below the protective titer, whereas the HI test showed that 5 of the 6 puppies had protective MDA titers against CPV. Regarding the dam, as a consequence of the CPV infection, specific antibodies protective titers were detected by both tests at 45 days post-partum. The results of the in-clinic-ELISA test seem to be more reliable because these puppies, promptly taken away from the infected mother, remained healthy and did not shed CPV, so that they could not have neither MDA from their unvaccinated mother nor protective antibody titers due to an active immunization.

Discrepancies in results of the two tests in the 5 puppies tested before and after vaccination were also observed. Before the first vaccination the in-clinic ELISA test showed the absence of protective MDA titers in puppies, whereas HI estimated a 100% of puppies having protective MDA. After the first vaccination, all puppies seroconverted and protective antibodies were observed by both tests. Post-vaccination titers seem to support the reliability of the in-clinic ELISA test: in fact, according to previous studies, only puppies with low MDA titers (<1:20) are supposed to develop an appropriate immunity after the first vaccination (2, 7). However, in some circumstances, CPV seroconversion has been observed even in the presence of higher MDA levels (32). Even though the sample is too small, the final result gives a clear indication of the importance of both tests, and further studies are needed.

Overall, our results are indicative of the reliability of the in-clinic ELISA test to detect MDA in puppies and at the same time account for a lower specificity of HI test in determining MDA levels.

Regardless the serological test used, a practical approach may be suggested to overcome the difficulties and expensiveness related to the theoretical possibility to repeatedly sample and test young puppies in order to monitor the decline of MDA and decide the first vaccination time. Instead of repeated sampling, puppies might be tested once for MDA titers, at an age of 6 weeks. Decline of MDA may be subsequently estimated considering a CPV antibody half-life of 9–10 days and vaccination may therefore be scheduled when MDA estimated titers are <1:20 (33).

CONCLUSIONS

The present study reveals the utility of an in-clinic ELISA test in detecting protective antibodies against CPV in adult dogs in comparison with the gold standard HI test. However, discrepancy could be observed between the tests in determining the CPV MDA antibodies in puppies. Only the in-clinic ELISA test showed a decline in MDA titers in older puppies as compared with HI, thus suggesting that this in-clinic ELISA test can be used as a specific and sensitive tool to determine MDA in unvaccinated puppies. This allows the prediction of the best time of vaccination, thus reducing the rate of vaccination failures.

AUTHOR CONTRIBUTIONS

PDA and ND designed this study. PDA, SL, RC, MB, CD, AC, GA, and CB performed the experimental analysis. JF performed the statistical analysis. JF, RC, PDA, and ND drafted and revised the manuscript. All authors read and approved the final manuscript.

ACKNOWLEDGMENTS

We are grateful to Mrs. Stefania Rizzi and Mr. Omar Machich (Cocker House—Allevamento dei Machich, Mola di Bari, Italy), Mr. Sergio Severgnini (Allevamento St. John, Misinto, Italy), Mr. Stefano Piva (Allevamento Bluveil, Monza), Mrs. Gabriella Caneparo (Allevamento Madamadorè, Cesano Maderno), Mrs. Cecilia Dal Molin and Dr. Elisa Finucci (Allevamento Moonnala Kennel) and all other breeders for collaboration, and to Dr. Gianpiero Ventrella and Dr. Valeria Bove (Centro Veterinario 2000, Putignano, Italy) for sampling animals and providing sera. Preliminary results were presented as an Abstract at the LXXII SISVet Congress, Turin, 20–22 June 2018.

REFERENCES

1. Decaro N, Buonavoglia C. Canine parvovirus - a review of epidemiological and diagnostic aspects, with emphasis on type 2c. *Veterinary Microbiol.* (2012) 155:1–12. doi: 10.1016/j.vetmic.2011.09.007

2. Pollock RVH, Carmichael LE. Maternally derived immunity to canine parvovirus infection: transfer, decline and interference with vaccination. *J Am Veterinary Med Assoc.* (1982) 180:37–42.

3. Twark L, Dodds J. Clinical use of serum parvovirus and distemper virus antibody titers for determining revaccination strategies in healthy dogs. *J Am Veterinary Med Assoc.* (2000) 217:1021–4. doi: 10.2460/javma.2000.21 7.1021

4. Decaro N, Campolo M, Desario C, Elia G, Martella V, Lorusso E, et al. Maternally derived antibodies in pups and protection from canine parvovirus infection. *Biologicals.* (2005) 33:261–7. doi: 10.1016/j.biologicals.2005. 06.004

5. Miranda C, Thompson G. Canine parvovirus: the worldwide occurrence of antigenic variants. *J General Virol.* (2016) 97:2043–57. doi: 10.1099/jgv.0.000540

6. Day MJ, Horzinek MC, Schultz RD, Squires RA. Vaccination Guidelines Group (VGG) of the World Small Animal Veterinary Association (WSAVA). WSAVA guidelines for the vaccination of dogs and cats. *J Small Animal Practice.* (2016) 57:E1–45. doi: 10.1111/jsap.12431

7. Chappuis G. Neonatal immunity and immunisation in early age: lessons from veterinary medicine. *Vaccine.* (1998) 16:1468–72. doi: 10.1016/S0264-410X(98)00110-8

8. Pratelli A, Cavalli A, Normanno G, De Palma MG, Pastorelli G, Martella V, et al. Immunization of pups with maternally derived antibodies to canine parvovirus (CPV) using a modified-live variant (CPV-2b). *J Veterinary Med.* (2000) 47:273–6. doi: 10.1046/j.1439-0450.2000.00340.x

9. De Cramer KGM, Styliandes E, Van Vuuren M. Efficacy at 4 and 6 weeks in the control of canine parvovirus. *Veterinary Microbiol.* (2011) 149:126–32. doi: 10.1016/j.vetmic.2010.11.004

10. Decaro N, Desario C, Campolo M, Cavalli A, Ricci D, Martella V, et al. Evaluation of lactogenic immunity to canine parvovirus in pups. *New Microbiol.* (2004) 27:375–9.

11. Mila H, Grellet A, Desario C, Feugier A, Decaro N, Buonavoglia C, et al. Protection against canine parvovirus type 2 infection in puppies by colostrum-derived antibodies. *J Nutritional Sci.* (2014) 3:e54:1–4. doi: 10.1017/jns.2014.57

12. Friedrich K, Truyen U. Untersuchung der wirksamkeit von parvovirussimpfstoffen und der effektivitat zweier impfschemata. *Der Praktische Tierarzt.* (2000) 81:988–94.

13. Macartney L, Thompson H, McCandlish IA, Cornwell HJ. Canine parvovirus: interaction between passive immunity and virulent challenge. *Veterinary Rec.* (1988) 122:573–6. doi: 10.1136/vr.122.24.573

14. Wilson S, Siedek E, Thomas A, King,V., Stirling C, Plevová E, et al. Influence of maternally-derived antibodies in 6-week old dogs for the efficacy of a new vaccine to protect dogs against virulent challenge with canine distemper virus, adenovirus or parvovirus. *Trials Vaccinol.* (2014) 3:107–13. doi: 10.1016/j.trivac.2014.06.001

15. Heayns BJ, Baugh S. Survey of veterinary surgeons on the introduction of serological testing to assess revaccination requirements. *Veterinary Rec.* (2012) 170:74–8. doi: 10.1136/vr.100147

16. Carmichael LE, Joubert JC, Pollock VH. Hemagglutination by canine parvovirus: serologic studies and diagnostic application. *Am J Veterinary Res.* (1980) 4:784–91.

17. Waner T, Naveh A, Wudovsky I, Carmichael LE. Assessment of maternal antibody decay and response to canine parvovirus vaccination using a clinic-based enzyme-linked immunosorbent assay. *J Veterinary Diagn Invest.* (1996) 8:427–32. doi: 10.1177/104063879600800404

18. Waner T, Mazar S, Keren-Kornblatt E. Application of a dot enzyme-linked immunosorbent assay for evaluation of the immune status to canine parvovirus and distemper virus in adult dogs before revaccination. *J Veterinary Diagnostic Invest.* (2006) 18:267–70. doi: 10.1177/104063870601800306

19. Killey R, Mynors C, Pearce R, Nell A, Prentis A, Day MJ. Long-lived immunity to canine core vaccine antigens in UK dogs as assessed by an in-practice test kit. *J Small Animal Practice.* (2018) 59:27–31. doi: 10.1111/jsap.12775

20. Adam JM, Asgarali Z, Singh SM, Ezeokoli CD. A serological study of canine parvovirus (CPV-2) and distemper virus (CDV) in stray dogs in North Trinidad, West Indies. *West Indian Veterinary J.* (2011) 11:1–4.

21. Belsare AV, Vanak AT, Gompper ME. Epidemiology of viral pathogens of free-ranging dogs and Indian foxes in a human-dominated landscape in central India. *Transboundary Emerg Dise.* (2014) 61(Suppl. 1):78–86. doi: 10.1111/tbed.12265

22. Buonavoglia C, Pratelli A, Tempesta M, Martella V, Normanno G. Valutazione delle caratteristiche di innocuitaʿ e immunogenicitaʿ di una variante 2b di parvovirus del cane (CPV-2b). *Veterinaria.* (1998) 6:55–8.

23. Cavalli A, Martella V, Desario C, Camero M, Bellacicco AL, De Palo P, et al. Evaluation of the antigenic relationships among canine parvovirus type 2 variants. *Clin Vaccine Immunol.* (2008)15:534–9. doi: 10.1128/CVI.00444-07

24. Sergeant ESG. *Epitools Epidemiological Calculators.* Ausvet Pty Ltd (2018). Available online at: http://epitools.ausvet.com.au (accessed February 17, 2021).

25. Taguchi M, Namikawa K, Maruo T, Orito K, Lynch J, Sahara H. Antibody titers for canine parvovirus type-2, canine distemper virus, and canine adenovirus type-1 in adult household dogs. *Can Vet J.* (2011) 52:983–6.

26. Chastant S., Mila H. Passive immune transfer in puppies. *Anim Reproduct Sci.* (2019) 207:162–70. doi: 10.1016/j.anireprosci.2019.06.012

27. Schultz RD. Duration of immunity for canine and feline vaccines: a review. *Vet Microbiol.* (2006) 117:75–9. doi: 10.1016/j.vetmic.2006.04.013

28. Thomas J, Singh M, Goswami TK, Glora P, Chakravarti S, Chander V, et al. Determination of immune status in dogs against CPV-2 by recombinant protein based latex agglutination test. *Biologicals.* (2017) 49:51–6. doi: 10.1016/j.biologicals.2017.06.009

29. Senda M, Hirayama N, Yamamoto H, Kurata K. An improved hemagglutination test for study of canine parvovirus. *Veterinary Microbiol.* (1986) 12:1–6. doi: 10.1016/0378-1135(86)90035-0

30. Day MJ. Immune system development in the dog and cat. *J Compar Pathol.* (2007) 137(Suppl. 1):S10–5. doi: 10.1016/j.jcpa.2007.04.005

31. Kennedy LJ, Lunt M, Barnes A, McElhinney L, Fooks AR, Baxter DN, et al. Factors influencing the antibody response of dogs vaccinated against rabies. *Vaccine.* (2007) 25:8500–7. doi: 10.1016/j.vaccine.2007.10.015

32. Martella V, Cavalli A, Decaro N, Elia G, Desario C, Campolo M, et al. Immunogenicity of an intranasally administered modified live canine parvovirus type 2b vaccine in pups with maternally derived antibodies. *Clin Diagnostic Lab Immunol.* (2005) 12:1243–5. doi: 10.1128/CDLI.12.10.1243-1245.2005

33. Greene CE, Decaro N. Canine viral enteritis. In: Greene CE, editor. *Infectious Diseases of the Dog and Cat.* 4th edn. St. Louis, MO: Saunders Elsevier (2012). p. 67–80.

Establishment of a Multiplex RT-PCR Method for the Detection of Five Known Genotypes of Porcine Astroviruses

Xin Liu [1†], Wenchao Zhang [1†], Dongjing Wang [2], Xinyue Zhu [1], Ying Chen [1], Kang Ouyang [1], Zuzhang Wei [1], Huan Liu [3*] and Weijian Huang [1*]

[1] College of Animal Science and Technology, Guangxi University, Nanning, China, [2] Institute of Animal Husbandry and Veterinary Medicine, Tibet Academy of Agriculture and Animal Husbandry Science, Lhasa, China, [3] Department of Scientific Research, The First Affiliated Hospital of Guangxi University of Chinese Medicine, Nanning, China

*Correspondence:
Weijian Huang
huangweijian-1@163.com
Huan Liu
liuchujie@yeah.net

[†] These authors have contributed equally to this work

Porcine astroviruses (PAstVs) are prevalent in pigs worldwide, and five genotypes have been reported to circulate in China. However, little is known about the coinfection status of PAstVs. For differential and simultaneous diagnoses of these five genotypes of PAstVs, a multiplex RT-PCR method was established on the basis of the *ORF2* gene of type 1 PAstV, and the *ORF1ab* genes of type two to five PAstVs. This quintuple PCR system was developed through optimization of multiplex PCR and detection sensitivity and specificity. The results showed that this multiplex RT-PCR method could specifically detect all the five PAstV genotypes without cross-reaction to any other major viruses circulating in Chinese pig farms. The detection limit of this method was as low as 10 pg of standard plasmids of each PAstV genotype. In addition, a total of 275 fecal samples collected from different districts of Guangxi, China, between April 2019 and November 2020, were tested by this newly established multiplex RT-PCR. Moreover, the sensitivity and specificity of monoplex and multiplex RT-PCR methods were compared by detecting the same set of clinical positive samples. The results revealed that PAstV1 (31/275), PAstV2 (49/275), PAstV3 (36/275), PAstV4 (41/275), and PAstV5 (22/275) were all detected, and dual (PAstV1+PAstV2, PAstV1+PAstV3, PAstV2+PAstV3, PAstV2+PAstV4, PAstV3+PAstV4, and PAstV4+PAstV5) or triple genotypes (PAstV1+PAstV2+PAstV3 and PAstV2+PAstV3+PAstV4) of coinfections were also unveiled in this study. The detection result of multiplex PCR was consistent with that of monoplex PCR. Compared with monoplex PCR, this multiplex PCR method showed obvious advantages such as time and cost efficiency and high sensitivity and specificity. This multiplex RT-PCR method offered a valuable tool for the rapid and accurate detection of PAstV genotypes circulating in pig herds and will facilitate the surveillance of PAstV coinfection status.

Keywords: porcine astrovirus, multiplex RT-PCR, co-infection, genotype differentiation, epidemiology, Guangxi, China

INTRODUCTION

Astroviruses are non-enveloped, positive-sense, single-stranded RNA (+ssRNA) viruses whose genomes are 6–7 kb in length and contain three open reading frames (ORFs), namely, ORF1a, ORF1b, and ORF2 (1). Astrovirus could infect a wide range of hosts from birds to mammals including humans, causing diseases from asymptomatic to systematic such as diarrhea, vomiting, and virus-associated hepatitis in birds or encephalitis in human and mammals (2, 3). In 1980, porcine astrovirus (PAstV) was firstly discovered from pig feces by electron microscopy (4). Since then, PAstV was generally considered as a diarrhea-associated agent and circulated in many countries worldwide (5–7). However, polioencephalomyelitis cases have emerged in pig herds in recent years, indicating the neuro-pathogenicity and neuro-invasiveness of PAstVs (8–10). Based on the full-length ORF2 sequences, PAstV could be divided into five distinct genotypes (PAstV1–PAstV5), suggesting different genetic evolutionary ancestors of PAstV (11). The overall prevalence rates and the dominant genotypes of PAstV in different countries or districts varied on geographic locations. Xiao et al. (7) reported that 64% of fecal samples collected from US farms were detected to be positive for PAstV, and 97.2% of PAstV-positive pigs were shown to be infected by PAstV4; 80% of healthy finisher pigs from a Canadian province were found harboring PAstV at slaughter (12). In addition, 70.4% of pigs were detected to be PAstV4 positive in five European countries (13). Till now, all the five known PAstV genotypes have been detected in China (6, 14), and the overall prevalence rate ranged from 17.5% in Sichuan Province to 56.4% in Guangxi Province (6, 15, 16). Meanwhile, the prevalence rates in Thailand (6.5%) (17) and India (17.6%) (5) were lower than in other countries. Moreover, coinfections of two more PAstV genotypes or PAstV with other pig viruses were also observed (7, 14, 15). PAstV2 and PAstV5 were found in the brains of newborn piglets suffering congenital tremors (18). PAstV2 and PAstV4 were detected from the blood and fecal samples, causing viremia and circulate in pig herds (19). It is worth noting that genetic recombination events among PAstVs or other astrovirus species were frequently reported, which may contribute to the genetic diversity and evolution of PAstVs (19–24). Multiple genotypes of PAstV coinfections will further accelerate the genetic variation

of this virus and bring challenges to the monitoring of PAstVs. In addition, the interspecies barrier of PAstV may not be strict. Results of genetic evolution analysis suggest that PAstV may have crossed the interspecies barrier between humans and other animals (23, 25, 26).

Considering the error-prone RNA polymerase, multi-genotype coinfections, frequent recombination events, and the zoonotic potential of PAstV, a comprehensive PAstV diagnosis method is in urgent need. It is necessary to establish an efficient and fast detection method to clarify the infection and genetic variation status of PAstV in pigs. However, the detection methods used currently are usually time-consuming and expensive. In this study, a multiplex PCR detection method was established and showed good specificity and high sensitivity. Additionally, this assay was employed to analyze a total of 275 swine fecal samples collected from different districts of Guangxi. These results provided us with a detailed PAstV infection status of swine herds in Guangxi and will facilitate the virus evolution monitoring and the development of accurate prevention strategies for PAstV.

MATERIALS AND METHODS

Porcine Astrovirus and Major Swine Viruses

All the five genotypes of PAstV-positive samples were collected and identified by our laboratory previously and preserved at −80°C (6). The complete or partial genomic sequences of these positive samples are available in GenBank under following accession numbers: NC_025379 for PAstV1, KY412124 for PAstV2, KY412129 for PAstV3, KY412125 for PAstV4, and MH064173 for PAstV5. Porcine enterovirus G (EV-G), porcine Seneca virus [Seneca Valley virus (SVV)] (27), porcine pseudorabies virus (PRV), classical swine fever virus (CSFV), porcine reproductive and respiratory syndrome virus (PRRSV) (28), porcine epidemic diarrhea virus (PEDV) (29), porcine transmissible gastroenteritis virus (TGEV), and porcine rotavirus (PoRV) were all isolated and identified by our laboratory and stored at −80°C. The total RNA was extracted using TRIzol reagent (Takara, Dalian, China) and subjected to reverse transcription for first cDNA synthesis with the PrimeScript RT reagent (Takara, Dalian, China) following the manufacturer's

TABLE 1 | Multiplex primers used in this study.

Genotype	Primer name	Sequence (5′-3′)	GenBank accession	Product size (bp)	Target gene	Position
PAstV1	PAstV1-F	GGCCGTGGCAGGAGCAGATC	NC_025379	124	ORF2	4,300–4,424
	PAstV1-R	GACTGAGGTTTACCCCGTCT				
PAstV2	PAstV2-F	ACCACCGCGCAGGAGG	NC_023674	573	ORF1ab	2,537–3,109
	PAstV2-R	TGTTGYTCAAGRGCAGC				
PAstV3	PAstV3-F	GATGTGATGACCCTCTATGGG	NC_019494	175	ORF1ab	3,879–4,053
	PAstV3-R	GCCGGTCAAGCATCTCATCAG				
PAstV4	PAstV4-F	TGGGGTCCTGAAGCATTTGC	JF713713	485	ORF1ab	2,777–3,261
	PAstV4-R	AATGGGGACCATCCACA				
PAstV5	PAstV5-F	AATGTGCGKGTGAAAGA	JX556693	305	ORF1ab	3,319–3,623
	PAstV5-R	TGAAATGTGACTTCACCTGA				

TABLE 2 | Detection primers used for specificity analysis.

Viruses	Sequence (5′-3′)	Target genes	Product size (bp)	Reference
PRV	F: CGGCTTCCACTCGCAGCTCTTCTC	gE	388	MN443981.1
	R: TCTGGGTCATCACGAGCACGTACAGC			
CSFV	F: ACAGCCACGATTTGCAACTGTATG	E2	347	FJ598612.1
	R: TCTCAGAGTTGTTGGGCTCACTGC			
PoRV	F: GATGCTAG GACAAAATTG	VP6	309	MG066585.1
	R: CGCTTCAGATTGCGGAGCTAC			
TGEV	F: GACAAACTCGCTATCGCATGGTG	N	638	KU981074.1
	R: CACAGATGGAACACATTCAGCCAG			
PEDV	F: ATTCGCTGGCGCATGCGCCGTGGTG	N	509	JN601062.1
	R: ACAGCAGCCACCAGATCATCGCGTG			
EV-G	F: AGACTGGAGCTAGCTCCACTGCTAG	VP1	302	MT274669.1
	R: GACCTGGACTTGAACTGGGTGCTGT			
SVV	F: CACCTGACTGCCCACAGAGTCCCTGT	VP1	813	MK039162.1
	R: CCGCCACGTGCTTTACAGCGGTGCTT			
PRRSV	F: TGTATCGTGCCGTTCTATCTTGCTGT	ORF5	547	EF635006.1
	R: AGAGACGACCCCATTGTTCCGCTG			

instructions. The genomic DNA of PRV was extracted by TIANamp Virus DNA/RNA Kit (TIANGEN, Beijing, China) according to the Kit instructions. The obtained cDNAs and viral genomic DNA were stored at −80°C until use.

Experimental Design

In this study, we designed a multiplex RT-PCR method to identify the five known genotypes of PAstV in a single reaction tube. In short, the total RNA of fecal samples was extracted, and then the cDNA was synthesized by reverse transcription using hexamer random primers. The cDNAs and the primers specific for PAstV1, PAstV2, PAstV3, and PAstV4 and PAstV5 were added into the PCR mixture. PCR products were observed under UV light after 1.5% agarose gel electrophoresis. The genotypes were identified according to the length of PCR fragments.

Primer Design and Standard Preparation

Based on the highly conserved regions of PAstV representative strains in GenBank, genotype-specific primer sets targeting the OFR2 gene of PAstV1, and the ORF1ab genes of PAstV2, PAstV3, PAstV4, and PAstV5 were designed by Oligo 6.0 along with National Center for Biotechnology Information (NCBI) primer-BLAST comparison. All these primers were synthesized by Shanghai Sangon Biotech Co., Ltd. (Shanghai, China) and diluted with distilled deionized water (ddH$_2$O) to a concentration of 10 μmol/L and stored at −20°C for later utilization. The primer sequences and the respective amplification lengths are shown in **Table 1**.

In order to build detection standards of the multiplex PCR assay, the synthesized cDNAs obtained from PAstV-positive samples were used as templates and mixed with the primer sets for the individual genotypes to amplify all the fragments of the five genotypes. A 50 μl PCR system was built as follows: 25 μl 2× Premix Taq (Takara, Dalian, China), 2.5 μl cDNA template (about 100 ng/μl), primer sets at a final

concentration of 1.0 μmol/L, and ddH$_2$O were added to a final volume of 50 μl. The PCRs were conducted according to the manufacturer's instructions. PCR products were stained with ethidium bromide (EB), separated by 1.5% agarose gel electrophoresis, and visualized under UV light. The PCR products were further gel purified and cloned into pMD18-T vector (Takara, Dalian, China) according to manufacturer's instructions. These constructed plasmids were transformed into competent Escherichia coli DH5α for propagation. The recombinant plasmid DNAs were extracted and purified by TIANprep Mini Plasmid Kit (TIANGEN, Beijing, China) according to kit instructions and sequenced with M13 primers. The plasmid DNAs were quantified spectrophotometrically by NanoDrop 2000 (Thermo Fisher Scientific, Waltham, MA, USA) and diluted to 100 ng/μl. Subsequently, the standards were 10-fold diluted in ddH$_2$O, resulting a concentration gradient of 10 ng/μl, 1 ng/μl, 100 pg/μl, 10 pg/μl, 1 pg/μl, and 0.1 pg/μl and used as templates to evaluate the analytic sensitivity of the monoplex and multiplex RT-PCR assays.

Establishment of Multiplex PCR

For the multiplex RT-PCR assay development, a duplex PCR was firstly established with the primer sets for type 1 and type 2 PAstVs, using the corresponding standards as templates (100 ng each). A 20 μl PCR system was built as follows: 10 μl 2× Premix Taq, 1 μl standards (~100 ng), primer sets at a final concentration of 1.0 μmol/L, and ddH$_2$O were added to a final volume of 20 μl. The PCRs were conducted under the following conditions: 30 cycles of 10 s at 98°C; 30 s at 55°C, 1 min at 72°C, and final extension of 45 s at 72°C The primer sets of type three to five PAstV and its standards were added to the former established duplex (PAstV1–2), triplex (PAstV1–3), and quadruple (PAstV1–4) PCR assays one by one to establish the final quintuple PCR to detect all the genotypes. For a better output of the multiplex PCR assay, the reactions conditions were optimized by varying a

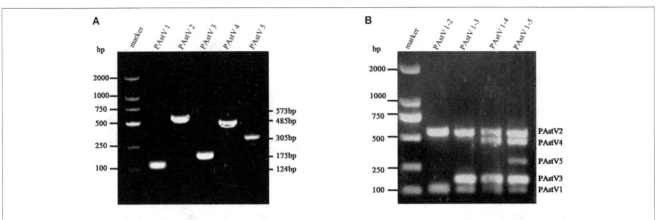

FIGURE 1 | The multiplex RT-PCR assay is well-established. **(A)** Total RNA was extracted from the clinical positive samples with TRIzol reagent and subjected to reverse transcription with hexamer random primer. The cDNAs were amplified with primers targeting genes of each genotype described in **Table 1**. **(B)** Multiplex RT-PCR was developed for the detection of all these five known porcine astrovirus (PAstV) genotypes. The prepared standard plasmids and corresponding primer sets were added one by one, constituting duplex, triplex, quadruple, and quintuple PCR mixtures.

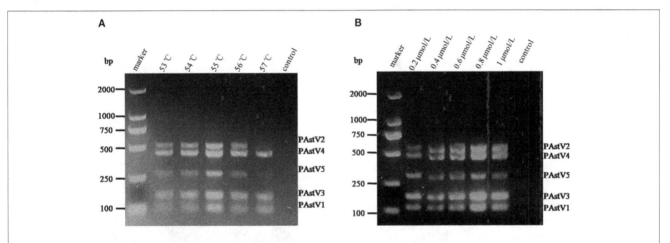

FIGURE 2 | Optimization of the multiplex RT-PCR conditions. **(A)** The standard plasmids of each porcine astrovirus (PAstV) genotype (10 ng each) were mixed and used as template for PCR amplification with combined primer sets at a final concentration of 1 μmol/L. **(B)** The standard plasmids (10 ng each) were combined with the primer sets at different concentrations (0.2–1.0 μmol/L) and amplified at an annealing temperature of 55°C.

single parameter, while other parameters were fixed as described by Ding et al. (30). The primer concentration for each target ranged from 0.2 to 1.0 μmol/L The annealing temperatures (53–57°C) were also tested. In this way, the primer concentration and annealing temperature were optimized. All PCR amplifications were carried out under the optimized conditions in one tube, and the PCR products were visualized on 1.5% agarose gel.

The Sensitivity of the Multiplex RT-PCR

The sensitivity of multiplex RT-PCR detection was evaluated by detecting 10-fold (10 ng, 1 ng, 100 pg, 10 pg, 1 pg, and 0.1 pg) diluted standard plasmids of PAstV1, PAstV2, PAstV3, PAstV4, and PAstV5, respectively. The same amounts of standards of each genotype were combined and used as templates for PCR with the optimized reaction system. In addition, the sensitivity of the monoplex RT-PCR was also tested. The standards of

each genotype were added to a separate RT-PCR tube as an amplification template.

The Specificity Test of Multiplex PCR

The established RT-PCR system was used to amplify the cDNAs or DNA templates of EV-G, SVV, PRRSV, PEDV, TGEV, PoRV, CSFV, and PRV-positive samples. Primer sets targeting these viruses were used as internal control. The primer sequences and the respective amplification lengths are shown in **Table 2**. The specificity of the method was verified using the mixed standards (100 ng each) as a positive control.

Detection of Clinical Samples

A total of 275 fecal samples were collected from Nanning, Chongzuo, Liuzhou, and Guigang in Guangxi Province between April 2019 and November 2020. All these samples (about 100 mg each) were mixed with 500 μl of sterile phosphate-buffered saline (PBS) and centrifuged at 2,000 ×g for 20 min at 4°C. About

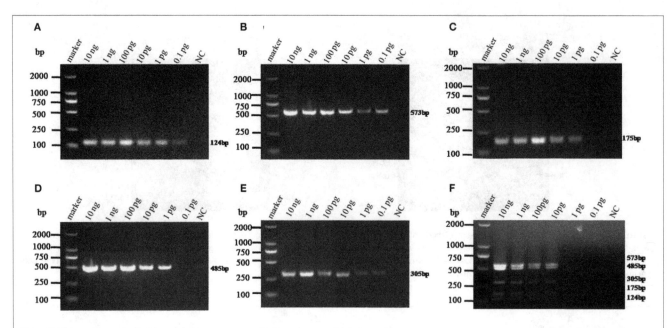

FIGURE 3 | Sensitivity analysis of the monoplex and multiplex PCR method established in this study. Equal amounts of standards of each genotype (10 ng–0.1 pg) were added to the single or multiplex PCR mixture and amplified at the optimized thermo cycle condition. **(A–E)** Monoplex PCR sensitivity analysis of PAstV1, PAstV2, PAstV3, PAstV4, and PAstV5, respectively. **(F)** Multiplex PCR sensitivity analysis.

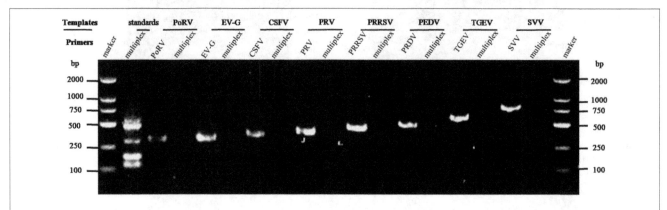

FIGURE 4 | Specificity analysis of the multiplex RT-PCR method established in this study. The cDNA or DNA obtained from common swine viruses circulating in Chinese pig herds was used as templates to validate the specificity of the multiplex RT-PCR assay. The porcine astrovirus (PAstV) standards were mixed and used as positive control. Primers specific to other individual viruses were employed as internal controls. Primer sequences are shown in **Table 2**.

300 µl of the supernatants was collected and subjected to RNA extraction by TRIzol reagent and following cDNA synthesis as manufacturer's instructions. The cDNAs (about 100 ng/µl) were then subjected to PCR amplification by the established multiplex and monoplex in a 20 µl reaction mixture: 10 µl 2× Premix Taq, 3 µl cDNA, primer sets at a final concentration of 0.8 µmol/L, and ddH$_2$O were added to a final volume of 20 µl. The detection results were compared to evaluate the detection consistency between monoplex and multiplex PCR methods established in this study. The standard plasmids were used as a positive control and determination criteria of the multiplex PCR results.

RESULTS

Establishment of Multiplex RT-PCR Method

The monoplex RT-PCR result showed that the fragments at expected sizes of each genotype (124 bp for PAstV1, 573 bp for PAstV2, 175 bp for PAstV3, 485 bp for PAstV4, and 305 bp for PAstV5) were successfully amplified from the stored positive samples (**Figure 1A**). In addition, neither non-specific bands nor primer dimers appeared on the agarose gel, indicating high amplification quality and specificity of these primer sets (**Figure 1A**). Next, the standards and primer sets of type one to five PAstVs were added to the reaction tube one by one, and the results demonstrated that all these target genes were well-amplified without any interference, indicating good amplification and high efficacy of this multiplex RT-PCR method (**Figure 1B**).

Optimization of the Multiplex RT-PCR Conditions

With the use of the standard plasmids (10 ng each) as templates, the PCR annealing temperatures and primer concentrations were optimized in this study. On equal conditions, annealing temperature at 55°C could obtain the best detection result (**Figure 2A**). Meanwhile, the optimal primer concentration was revealed to be 0.8 μmol/L (**Figure 2B**).

The Sensitivity of the Multiplex RT-PCR

The sensitivity of monoplex RT-PCR to each genotype was firstly investigated. The results showed that the standards of PAstV1, PAstV2, and PAstV5 were detectable with a minimum amount of 0.1-pg standards, while the standards of PAstV3 and PAstV4 could be detected as low as 1 pg (**Figures 3A–E**), indicating high sensitivity of the designed primer sets to each genotype. When the sensitivity of multiplex RT-PCR is measured, all the primers are mixed at the optimal concentration to prepare a PCR mixture, which was used to detect pooled standards of each genotype at the indicated amounts (10 ng–0.1 pg). The results showed that the detection limit of this method was as low as 10-pg standards of all the five genotypes of PAstVs (**Figure 3F**), indicating high sensitivity of the multiplex RT-PCR for PAstV detection.

The Specificity of the Multiplex RT-PCR

The cDNAs of EV-G, PRRSV, SVV, CSFV, PEDV, PoRV, TGEV, and the DNA template of the PRV samples were used to detect specificity by the established RT-PCR method. The results showed that five target fragments were obtained when standard plasmids were used as template. Meanwhile, no bands were detected if templates were replaced by other common viruses' cDNA or DNA (**Figure 4**). This method did not cross-react with other major swine pathogens, indicating good specificity of this multiplex PCR method.

Detection of Field Samples Using the Multiplex RT-PCR

The 275 fecal samples from different districts of Guangxi Province were detected by this newly established multiplex RT-PCR method. The results showed that the overall positive rate of PAstV infection was 46.9% (129/275); and PAstV1 (31/275), PAstV2 (49/275), PAstV3 (36/275), PAstV4 (41/275), and PAstV5 (22/275) were all found circulating in pig herds in Guangxi Province (**Figure 5**). In addition, dual-genotype infections such as PAstV1+PAstV2 (3/275), PAstV2+PAstV3 (10/275), PAstV3+PAstV4 (8/275), and PAstV4+PAstV2 (4/275) and even triple genotype of PAstV infections, such as PAstV1+PAstV2+PAstV3 (2/275) and PAstV2+PAstV3+PAstV4 (1/275), were also detected (**Figure 5**). Moreover, as shown in **Table 3**, the infection rate of sucking piglets (77.8%) is much higher than that of other age groups, indicating that the younger groups are more susceptible to PAstVs infection. Meanwhile, the overall infection rates of

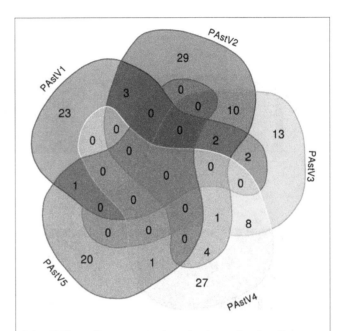

FIGURE 5 | Venn diagram showing the total and proportion of positive samples for each porcine astrovirus (PAstV) genotype. The overlapping areas indicate the total samples that were positive in one to three different genotypes by multiplex RT-PCR.

PAstV2 (17.8%, 49/275) and PAstV4 (14.9%, 41/275) were moderately higher than those of other types, indicating the dominance of these genotypes in Guangxi. cDNAs of the same set of positive samples were used as temples for detection consistency analysis. As shown in **Figure 6**, the detection result of multiplex PCR is in concordance with that of monoplex PCR, indicating good reliability of this method.

DISCUSSION

PAstV has been circulating in many countries around the world. In the recent decade, with the aid of improved sequencing techniques such as high-throughput sequencing, increasing novel clades of astroviruses have been discovered (31). For quite some time, PAstV was considered as a low-pathogenic virus causing a short-term mild diarrhea (32, 33). However, emerging cases of PAstV associated enteritis or polioencephalomyelitis were reported and attracted public attention in recent years (8, 9, 34, 35). As an enteric virus, PAstVs were more frequently detected in the pig herds, and the prevalent rates of PAstV were usually reported much higher than those of other diarrheal viruses such as PEDV, TGEV, and porcine deltacoronavirus (PDCoV) (30, 36). Besides, the high genetic variability and possible recombination events of PAstVs further remind people to develop comprehensive methods for astrovirus diagnosis and epidemiological investigation (23, 37).

At present, methods used for PAstV diagnosis mostly stay at the level of single RT-PCR or quantitative RT-PCR detection (6, 38). Although more advanced detection methods such as nanofluidic PCR, microarrays, or high-throughput

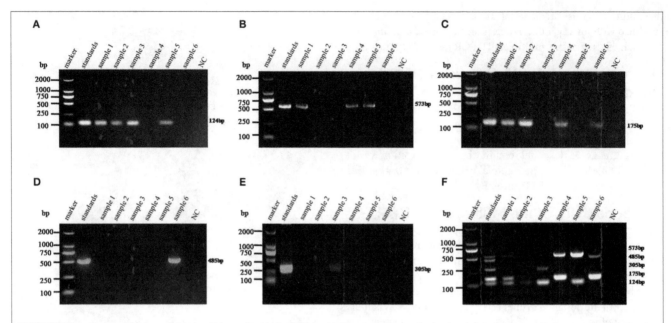

FIGURE 6 | Detection consistency analysis of multiplex and monoplex PCR used in this study. The standards of each genotype were mixed as a template pool and used as a positive control. The cDNAs of selected samples were used as templates for monoplex and multiplex PCR in the optimized PCR system. **(A–E)** Porcine astrovirus (PAstV) one to five genotype monoplex PCR results of the selected positive samples. **(F)** Multiplex PCR result of the selected positive samples. The indicated sizes of each genotype are shown in the right panel.

TABLE 3 | Results of field samples detected by the multiplex RT-PCR.

Age groups	Sample number	Positive rate (positive number)	Number of positive samples				
			PAstV1	PAstV2	PAstV3	PAstV4	PAstV5
Suckling pig	45	77.8% (35)	5	13	16	16	1
Nursery pigs	45	48.8% (22)	10	12	15	10	1
Growing and fattening pigs	35	57.1% (20)	3	10	5	7	0
Lactating sow	80	53.7% (43)	5	14	0	7	20
Pregnant sow	40	10% (4)	3	0	0	1	0
Backup pigs	30	16.6% (5)	5	0	0	0	0
Total	275	46.9% (129)	31	49	36	41	22

sequencing are valuable assets for the diagnosis of astrovirus (39), there are some disadvantages such as being expensive and time-consuming and requiring instruments and experimenters, limiting their popularization and field application. Multiplex PCR/RT-PCR is still widely used in veterinary diagnostic centers at present. This was mainly owing to its cost-efficiency, simple procedures, and time-efficiency. In addition, multiplex PCR technology can detect multiple pathogens at the same time, which is of great value in differential diagnosis, especially in veterinary medicine.

As mentioned previously, coinfections of multiple genotypes of PAstVs in a pig farm, even in an individual pig, were reported (7, 16). Moreover, five known genotypes of PAstVs were detected in China (6, 14, 40). However, the methods used in those studies could not differentiate the genotypes at the first time. Based on genotype-specific primer sets, multiplex

RT-PCR method was built in this study and showed good performance in PAstV genotype differentiation. The detection limit of the multiplex PCR method established in this experiment for PAstV1, PAstV2, PAstV3, PAstV4, and PAstV5 is 10 pg of standard plasmids, indicating high sensitivity and good field applicability. Of the 275 collected fecal samples, all five known genotypes of PAstV were detected, and dual or triple genotypes of PAstV coinfections were also unveiled in this study (**Figure 5**). Meanwhile, PAstV2 and PAstV4 were shown to be the dominant genotypes in Guangxi, which is consistent to our lab's previously results (6). As for humans, infant and young children were major victims of astrovirus infection (41, 42). In this study, the infection rates of pigs at lactation and nursery stage were also higher than those of grown pigs (**Table 2**). Pathogenic studies have shown that PAstV infection could cause diarrhea and growth retardation, which could lead to economic losses and cannot be ignored in large-scale pig industries (32, 33). Moreover, coinfections of PAstV with other swine viruses were also reported, which pointed out that PAstVs were more intended to co-infect with other viruses, and immunosuppressive viruses such as CSFV could benefit from the replication of PAstV (13, 14, 43). All this reminds us that PAstV infections could be a landmine if it is not well-controlled. However, comprehensive understanding of all types of PAstV epidemiology, which is of great value for infectious disease control, is not available. The multiplex RT-PCR method developed in this study specifically targets all types of PAstVs and performed well in detection specificity and sensitivity, providing a valuable tool for PAstV clinical diagnosis and understanding the full picture of PAstV infections.

ETHICS STATEMENT

The animal study was reviewed and approved by Ethics Committee of Animal Experiments of Guangxi University (protocol number: GXU2018-044).

AUTHOR CONTRIBUTIONS

HL and WH designed the experiments. XL and WZ are major contributors for experimental implementation. XZ is mainly responsible for sample collection and helped perform some experiments. HL and XL wrote the manuscript. All authors have read and approved the final manuscript.

REFERENCES

1. Mendez E, Arias CF. Astroviruses. In: *Fields Virology*. 6th ed. New York, NY: Lippincott Williams &Wilkins (2013). p. 609–28.
2. Cortez V, Meliopoulos VA, Karlsson EA, Hargest V, Johnson C, Schultz-Cherry S. Astrovirus biology and pathogenesis. *Annu Rev Virol*. (2017) 4:327–48. doi: 10.1146/annurev-virology-101416-041742
3. Johnson C, Hargest V, Cortez V, Meliopoulos VA, Schultz-Cherry S. Astrovirus pathogenesis. *Viruses*. (2017) 9:22. doi: 10.3390/v9010022
4. Bridger JC. Detection by electron microscopy of caliciviruses, astroviruses and rotavirus-like particles in the faeces of piglets with diarrhoea. *Vet Rec*. (1980) 107:532–3.
5. Kattoor JJ, Malik YS, Saurabh S, Sircar S, Vinodhkumar OR, Bora DP, et al. First report and genetic characterization of porcine astroviruses of lineage 4 and 2 in diarrhoeic pigs in India. *Transbound Emerg Dis*. (2019) 66:47–53. doi: 10.1111/tbed.13058
6. Qin Y, Fang Q, Li X, Li F, Liu H, Wei Z, et al. Molecular epidemiology and viremia of porcine astrovirus in pigs from Guangxi province of China. *BMC Vet Res*. (2019) 15:471. doi: 10.1186/s12917-019-2217-x
7. Xiao CT, Giménez-Lirola LG, Gerber PF, Jiang YH, Halbur PG, Opriessnig T. Identification and characterization of novel porcine astroviruses (PAstVs) with high prevalence and frequent co-infection of individual pigs with multiple PAstV types. *J Gen Virol*. (2013) 94:570–82. doi: 10.1099/vir.0.048744-0
8. Matias Ferreyra FS, Bradner LK, Burrough ER, Cooper VL, Derscheid RJ, Gauger PC, et al. Polioencephalomyelitis in domestic swine associated with porcine astrovirus type 3. *Vet Pathol*. (2020) 57:82–9. doi: 10.1177/0300985819875741
9. Arruda B, Arruda P, Hensch M, Chen Q, Zheng Y, Yang C, et al. Porcine astrovirus type 3 in central nervous system of swine with polioencephalomyelitis. *Emerg Infect Dis*. (2017) 23:2097–100. doi: 10.3201/eid2312.170703
10. Boros A, Albert M, Pankovics P, Biro H, Pesavento PA, Phan TG, et al. Outbreaks of neuroinvasive astrovirus associated with encephalomyelitis, weakness, and paralysis among weaned pigs, Hungary. *Emerg Infect Dis*. (2017) 23:1982–93. doi: 10.3201/eid2312.170804
11. Wu H, Bao Z, Mou C, Chen Z, Zhao J. Comprehensive analysis of codon usage on porcine astrovirus. *Viruses*. (2020) 12:991. doi: 10.3390/v12090991
12. Luo Z, Roi S, Dastor M, Gallice E, Laurin MA, L'Homme Y. Multiple novel and prevalent astroviruses in pigs. *Vet Microbiol*. (2011) 149:316–23. doi: 10.1016/j.vetmic.2010.11.026
13. Zhou W, Ullman K, Chowdry V, Reining M, Benyeda Z, Baule C, et al. Molecular investigations on the prevalence and viral load of enteric viruses in pigs from five European countries. *Vet Microbiol*. (2016) 182:75–81. doi: 10.1016/j.vetmic.2015.10.019
14. Su M, Qi S, Yang D, Guo D, Yin B, Sun D. Coinfection and genetic characterization of porcine astrovirus in diarrheic piglets in china from 2015 to 2018. *Front Vet Sci*. (2020) 7:462. doi: 10.3389/fvets.2020.00462

15. Cai Y, Yin W, Zhou Y, Li B, Ai L, Pan M, et al. Molecular detection of Porcine astrovirus in Sichuan Province, China. *Virol J*. (2016) 13:6. doi: 10.1186/s12985-015-0462-6
16. Xiao CT, Luo Z, Lv SL, Opriessnig T, Li RC, Yu XL. Identification and characterization of multiple porcine astrovirus genotypes in Hunan province, China. *Arch Virol*. (2017) 162:943–52. doi: 10.1007/s00705-016-3185-0
17. Kumthip K, Khamrin P, Saikruang W, Kongkaew A, Vachirachewin R, Ushijima H, et al. Detection and genetic characterization of porcine astroviruses in piglets with and without diarrhea in Thailand. *Arch Virol*. (2018) 163:1823–9. doi: 10.1007/s00705-018-3806-x
18. Blomström AL, Ley C, Jacobson M. Astrovirus as a possible cause of congenital tremor type AII in piglets? *Acta veterinaria Scandinavica*. (2014) 56:82. doi: 10.1186/s13028-014-0082-y
19. Brnić D, Prpić J, Keros T, Roić B, Starešina V, Jemeršić L. Porcine astrovirus viremia and high genetic variability in pigs on large holdings in Croatia. *Infect Genet Evol J Mol Epidemi Evol Genet Infect Dis*. (2013) 14:258–64. doi: 10.1016/j.meegid.2012.12.027
20. Ito M, Kuroda M, Masuda T, Akagami M, Haga K, Tsuchiaka S, et al. Whole genome analysis of porcine astroviruses detected in Japanese pigs reveals genetic diversity and possible intra-genotypic recombination. *Infect Genet Evol J Mol Epidemi Evol Genet Infect Dis*. (2017) 50:38–48. doi: 10.1016/j.meegid.2017.02.008
21. Lv SL, Zhang HH, Li JY, Hu WQ, Song YT, Opriessnig T, et al. High genetic diversity and recombination events of porcine astrovirus strains identified from ill and asymptomatic pigs in 2017, Hunan Province, China. *Virus Genes*. (2019) 55:673–681. doi: 10.1007/s11262-019-01692-w
22. Amimo JO, Machuka EM, Abworo EO, Vlasova AN, Pelle R. Whole genome sequence analysis of Porcine astroviruses reveals novel genetically diverse strains circulating in East African smallholder pig farms. *Viruses*. (2020) 12:1262. doi: 10.3390/v121 11262
23. Ulloa JC, Gutiérrez MF. Genomic analysis of two ORF2 segments of new porcine astrovirus isolates and their close relationship with human astroviruses. *Can J Microbiol*. (2010) 56:569–77. doi: 10.1139/W10-042
24. Lan D, Ji W, Shan T, Cui L, Yang Z, Yuan C, et al. Molecular characterization of a porcine astrovirus strain in China. *Arch Virol*. (2011) 156:1869–75. doi: 10.1007/s00705-011-1050-8
25. Pankovics P, Boros Á, Kiss T, Delwart E, Reuter G. Detection of a mammalian-like astrovirus in bird, European roller (*Coracias garrulus*). *Infect Genet Evol J Mol Epidemi Evol Genet Infect Dis*. (2015) 34:114–21. doi: 10.1016/j.meegid.2015.06.020
26. Mor SK, Chander Y, Marthaler D, Patnayak DP, Goyal SM. Detection and molecular characterization of *Porcine astrovirus* strains associated with swine diarrhea. *J Vet Diagn Invest*. (2012) 24:1064–7. doi: 10.1177/1040638712458781
27. Wang H, Niu C, Nong Z, Quan D, Chen Y, Kang O, et al. Emergence and phylogenetic analysis of a novel Seneca Valley virus strain in the Guangxi Province of China. *Res Vet Sci*. (2020) 130:207–11. doi: 10.1016/j.rvsc.2020.03.020

28. Wang J, Lin S, Quan D, Wang H, Huang J, Wang Y, et al. Full genomic analysis of new variants of porcine reproductive and respiratory syndrome virus revealed multiple recombination events between different lineages and sublineages. *Front Vet Sci*. (2020) 7:603. doi: 10.3389/fvets.2020.00603

29. Lu Y, Su X, Du C, Mo L, Ke P, Wang R, et al. Genetic diversity of Porcine epidemic diarrhea virus with a naturally occurring truncated ORF3 gene found in Guangxi, China. *Frontiers Vet. Sci*. (2020) 7:435. doi: 10.3389/fvets.2020.00435

30. Ding G, Fu Y, Li B, Chen J, Wang J, Yin B, et al. Development of a multiplex RT-PCR for the detection of major diarrhoeal viruses in pig herds in China. *Transbound Emerg Dis*. (2020) 67:678–85. doi: 10.1111/tbed.13385

31. Donato C, Vijaykrishna D. The broad host range and genetic diversity of mammalian and avian astroviruses. *Viruses*. (2017) 9:102. doi: 10.3390/v9050102

32. Fang Q, Wang C, Liu H, Wu Q, Liang S, Cen M, et al. Pathogenic characteristics of a Porcine astrovirus strain isolated in China. *Viruses*. (2019) 11:1156. doi: 10.3390/v11121156

33. Indik S, Valicek L, Smid B, Dvorakova H, Rodak L. Isolation and partial characterization of a novel porcine astrovirus. *Vet Microbiol*. (2006) 117:276–83. doi: 10.1016/j.vetmic.2006.06.020

34. Opriessnig T, Xiao CT, Halbur PG. Porcine astrovirus type 5-associated enteritis in pigs. *J Comp Pathol*. (2020) 181:38–46. doi: 10.1016/j.jcpa.2020.09.014

35. Rawal G, Ferreyra FM, Macedo NR, Bradner LK, Harmon KM, Allison G, et al. Ecology of Porcine astrovirus type 3 in a herd with associated neurologic disease. *Viruses*. (2020) 12:992. doi: 10.3390/v12090992

36. Shi Y, Li B, Tao J, Cheng J, Liu H. The complex co-infections of multiple porcine diarrhea viruses in local area based on the luminex xTAG multiplex detection method. *Front Vet Sci*. (2021) 8:602866. doi: 10.3389/fvets.2021.602866

37. Zhao C, Chen C, Li Y, Dong S, Tan K, Tian Y, et al. Genomic characterization of a novel recombinant porcine astrovirus isolated in northeastern China. *Arch Virol*. (2019) 164:1469–73. doi: 10.1007/s00705-019-04162-8

38. Goecke NB, Hjulsager CK, Kongsted H, Boye M, Rasmussen S, Granberg F, et al. No evidence of enteric viral involvement in the new neonatal porcine diarrhoea syndrome in Danish pigs. *BMC Vet Res*. (2017) 13:315. doi: 10.1186/s12917-017-1239-5

39. Pérot P, Lecuit M, Eloit M. Astrovirus diagnostics. *Viruses*. (2017) 9:10. doi: 10.3390/v9010010

40. Chu DK, Poon LL, Guan Y, Peiris JS. Novel astroviruses in insectivorous bats. *J Virol*. (2008) 82:9107–14. doi: 10.1128/JVI.00857-08

41. Olortegui MP, Rouhani S, Yori PP, Salas MS, Trigoso DR, Mondal D, et al. Astrovirus infection and diarrhea in 8 countries. *Pediatrics*. (2018). 141:e20171326. doi: 10.1542/peds.2017-1326

42. Naficy AB, Rao MR, Holmes JL, Abu-Elyazeed R, Savarino SJ, Wierzba TF, et al. Astrovirus diarrhea in Egyptian children. *J Infect Dis*. (2000) 182:685–90. doi: 10.1086/315763

43. Mi S, Guo S, Xing C, Xiao C, He B, Wu B, et al. Isolation and characterization of porcine astrovirus 5 from a classical swine fever virus-infected specimen. *J Virol*. (2020) 95:e01513–20. doi: 10.1128/JVI.01513-20

9

Dynamics of Salivary Adenosine Deaminase, Haptoglobin and Cortisol in Lipopolysaccharide-Challenged Growing Pigs

Virpi Sali[1]*, Christina Veit[2], Anna Valros[3], Sami Junnikkala[4], Mari Heinonen[1,3] and Janicke Nordgreen[2]

[1] Department of Production Animal Medicine, University of Helsinki, Mäntsälä, Finland, [2] Department of Paraclinical Sciences, Norwegian University of Life Sciences, Oslo, Norway, [3] Department of Production Animal Medicine, Research Centre for Animal Welfare, University of Helsinki, Mäntsälä, Finland, [4] Department of Veterinary Biosciences, Faculty of Veterinary Medicine, University of Helsinki, Helsinki, Finland

*Correspondence:
Virpi Sali
virpi.sali@helsinki.fi

Infectious and inflammatory conditions are common especially in growing pigs. Lipopolysaccharide (LPS) is an important antigenic structure of Gram-negative bacteria and can be used to induce inflammation experimentally. As pigs are usually group-housed in commercial conditions, it is difficult to detect sick individuals, particularly at an early stage of illness. Acute phase proteins such as haptoglobin (Hp) are known indicators of an activated innate immune system whereas adenosine deaminase (ADA) is a relatively novel inflammatory biomarker in pigs. Both parameters can be measured in saliva and could be used as indicators of inflammation. Compared with blood sampling, saliva sampling is a less stressful procedure that is rapid, non-invasive and easy to perform both at group and at individual level. In this blinded randomized clinical trial, 32 female pigs at their post-weaning phase were allocated to one of four treatments comprising two injections of the following substance combinations: saline-saline (SS), ketoprofen-saline (KS), saline-LPS (SL), and ketoprofen-LPS (KL). First, ketoprofen or saline was administered intramuscularly on average 1 h before either LPS or saline was given through an ear vein catheter. In all groups, saliva was collected prior to injections (baseline) and at 4, 24, 48, and 72 h post-injection for determination of ADA, Hp, and cortisol concentrations. A multivariate model was applied to describe the dynamics of each biomarker. Pairwise relationships between ADA, Hp, and cortisol responses from baseline to 4 h post-injection within the SL group were studied with Spearman correlations. A significant increase in the SL group was seen in all biomarkers 4 h post-injection compared to baseline and other time points (pairwise comparisons, $p < 0.01$ for all) and ketoprofen alleviated the LPS effect. We found a significant positive correlation between ADA and Hp within the SL group ($r = 0.86$, $p < 0.05$). The primary and novel findings of the present study are the response of ADA to LPS, its time course and alleviation by ketoprofen. Our results support the evidence that ADA and Hp can be used as inflammatory biomarkers in pigs. We suggest further studies to be conducted in commercial settings with larger sample sizes.

Keywords: pig, LPS, ADA, haptoglobin, cortisol, saliva, experimental

INTRODUCTION

In commercial pig production, infectious and inflammatory conditions are common (1–3). Growing pigs are housed in groups of variable size, which potentially hinders the detection of sick individuals by herd employees. Moreover, sub-clinical illness poses a risk for disease transmission and can result in a reduced performance of pigs (4). In order to prevent disease outbreaks within herds and minimize production losses, it would be advantageous to detect problems as early as possible. Therefore, sampling methods that are easy to perform for a group of animals under practical farm conditions (4–6) would be of great value in pig herd health evaluation. Several biomarkers circulating in the bloodstream are detectable in saliva as well (6–9), and saliva sampling is also a less stressful alternative to blood sampling.

Lipopolysaccharide (LPS), also known as endotoxin, is an important antigenic structure of the cell wall in Gram-negative bacteria (10). It can be used experimentally to induce a systemic inflammation (11), which includes innate immune system activation (10) followed by an acute inflammatory response (10, 12) accompanied by sickness behavior (13). The key mediators during the inflammatory process are pro-inflammatory cytokines that trigger acute-phase protein (APP) production in the liver (12).

Haptoglobin (Hp) is an important APP in pigs (14, 15). It is primarily synthetized in the liver (12) yet some evidence about local Hp production in salivary gland exists (16). Serum Hp concentration is known to increase in pigs suffering from infectious diseases (5, 17, 18) or acute inflammatory processes (17, 18). Salivary Hp is elevated by systemic disease in pigs (19) and some evidence indicates that it is a more sensitive and specific biomarker for the detection of certain porcine diseases than serum Hp (9). It is also suitable for the detection of sub-clinical illness in pigs (5). Measurement of several APPs has been shown to improve diagnostic sensitivity (18), and increasing evidence supports determination of a panel of biomarkers with different triggers (7, 12, 17, 18) and dynamics (8, 20) instead of single ones.

Adenosine deaminase (ADA) is an enzyme involved in normal purine metabolism (21) and it is expressed in most tissues at some levels (22). Its expression, however, is highest in lymphoid organs indicating the role of ADA in immune activation (21) and ADA has been additionally proposed as a potential inflammatory biomarker in pigs (6, 19). Cortisol, which is usually perceived as a stress biomarker, is an indicator of activation of the hypothalamic-pituitary-adrenal (HPA) axis (8). Its release from the adrenal cortex happens within a few minutes under various stressful situations (8), including LPS injection (23), after which it is spread via the bloodstream.

Haptoglobin has been investigated previously in combination with ADA (6, 24) and cortisol (7, 20). To the authors' knowledge, neither the magnitude nor time course of the ADA response under a controlled immune challenge nor ADA's relation to Hp and cortisol in that setting have been described previously. Former reports have primarily been either cross-sectional (6, 19, 25) or longitudinal studies with sampling intervals of days or weeks (5, 7, 20, 24, 26) and conducted under farm conditions (5, 6, 24).

Ketoprofen is a commonly used non-steroidal anti-inflammatory drug (NSAID) in veterinary medicine and has been established as a potent anti-inflammatory drug in pigs (27, 28). NSAIDs target cyclo-oxygenase enzymes 1 and 2 (COX 1-2) and reduce pain, fever, and inflammation through inhibition of prostaglandin synthesis (29). Ketoprofen administration prior to LPS injection was recently shown to diminish the effect of LPS on cortisol and attenuated the behavioral signs of sickness in challenged pigs (30). An alleviating effect of an NSAID on an LPS-induced increase in one or more inflammatory biomarkers will strengthen the evidence for those biomarkers being sensitive indicators of pig health.

The aim of this experimental study was therefore to investigate the dynamics of salivary biomarkers of systemic inflammation in LPS – challenged growing pigs and to test whether an NSAID could alleviate the effect of LPS. We predicted that porcine salivary ADA, Hp, and cortisol would increase in response to LPS and that ketoprofen would alleviate the effect of LPS. In addition, we wanted to describe the correlations between the responses of salivary (1) ADA and Hp, (2) ADA and cortisol, and (3) Hp and cortisol in pigs injected with saline and LPS.

MATERIALS AND METHODS
Ethical Statement
The Norwegian animal research authority approved the experiment (FOTS id 15232).

Animals and Housing
The experiment took place in two blocks between April and May 2018 at the Livestock Production Research Center of the Norwegian University of Life Sciences (NMBU), campus Ås. Thirty-two female pigs (Norwegian Landrace), henceforth referred to as experimental pigs, were used in the study and comprised a subset of the pigs investigated by Veit et al. (30). The experimental pigs were 68–85 days (median 83 days) old at the beginning of the study. All pigs were kept in one room and group-housed in pens containing four experimental and two companion male pigs in order to increase the stocking density up to 1.3 m^2

per pig. Pigs had visual and limited tactile contact with other pigs in the adjoining pen. One half of the pen (2.4 × 1.6 m) consisted of a solid lying area and the other half of slatted floor. Each pen had three nipple drinkers and pelleted feed (IDEAL S Die Ekstra, produced by Norgesfôr, Mysen, Norway) was provided for the pigs *ad libitum* at an animal-to-feeding place ratio of 3:1. The animal caretakers provided two handfuls of wood shavings and a handful of grass silage per pen on the lying area twice per day. Additionally, one handful of grass silage was placed in a rack. Each pen was equipped with a water sprinkler, which turned on every 10 min for 20 s. Lights were on between 6 am and 10 pm and the room was dimmed with night-lights during the night. Average ambient temperature in the unit was set to 20°C.

Experimental Procedures

Within each pen, the four experimental pigs were randomly allocated to one of four treatments that were made up of four substance combinations: saline-saline (SS), ketoprofen-saline (KS), saline-LPS (SL), and ketoprofen-LPS (KL). The numbers of pigs per treatment were nine for SS and KL, and seven for KS and SL. The weight of the pigs was measured one the day before treatment and the pigs weighed between 16.3 and 50.7 kg (median 41 kg). The LPS dose used was determined according to previous research (23, 31) and for ketoprofen, the dosing was according to Fosse et al. (32). Ketoprofen (Romefen vet 100 mg/ml, Ceva Santé Animale, France) or saline were administered intramuscularly (i.m.) behind the ear. LPS (Serotype 0111: B4 of *Escherichia coli* dissolved in 0.9% sterile saline to a concentration of 100 μg/ml, produced by Sigma, Germany) or saline (sodium chloride 9 mg/ml) were administered intravenously (i.v.) through an ear vein catheter on average 61 ± 16 min after the first substance. The ear vein catheter was used only for injection, and removed immediately afterwards. The ketoprofen dose was 6 mg/kg, and the LPS dose 1.2 μg/kg. The pigs injected with LPS were observed closely in the hours after injection in order to detect individuals reacting stronger or for a longer time period than expected.

Repeated saliva samples were collected from individual pigs before any substance administration (baseline) and at 4, 24, 48, and 72 h after the intravenous injection. All baseline saliva samples were taken between 08:30 and 10:45 a.m. Each pig was allowed to chew a dental cotton pad suspended on a dental cord until it was moistened [modified from (33)]. Saliva was extracted by centrifuging the pad for 5 min at 1,000 × g. Saliva was pipetted to 2 ml Eppendorf tubes and stored on dry ice until it was moved to a −80°C freezer at the end of each sampling day.

Salivary ADA, Hp, and Cortisol Measurements

Salivary ADA and Hp were measured in collaboration with a Spanish laboratory (Department of Animal Medicine and Surgery, Faculty of Veterinary Medicine, University of Murcia, Spain). A commercial automatized assay (Adenosine-Glutamate Dehydrogenase, BioSystems S.A., Barcelona, Spain) was used for ADA quantification according to the manufacturer's instructions. The method of the assay is based on the measurement of the decrease in absorbance (OD) per minute of a coupled

TABLE 1 | Median (min–max) values of adenosine deaminase (ADA), haptoglobin (Hp), and cortisol in saliva across 32 experimental pigs at different time points.

Biomarker	Baseline $n = 31$	4 h p.i. $n = 31$	24 h p.i. $n = 30$	48 h p.i. $n = 27$	72 h p.i. $n = 29$
ADA, U/L	118.0 (46.7–258.6)	115.3 (46.7–850.6)	137.0 (46.7–301.3)	112.7 (35.3–596.6)	108.7 (54.7–338.6)
Hp, μg/ml	0.33 (0.08–1.61)	0.31 (0.05–1.65)	0.45 (0.09–0.98)	0.37 (0.06–1.27)	0.23 (0.03–0.80)
Cortisol, ng/ml	0.32 (0.11–0.45)	0.33 (0.10–2.28)	0.30 (0.11–0.69)	0.22 (0.08–1.35)	0.20 (0.08–0.48)

p.i., post-injection.

reaction initially catalyzed by ADA (OD/min × 3,333 = U/L). The reaction is measured at 340 nm. Salivary Hp concentration was quantified by using an in-house time-resolved immunofluorometric assay, previously validated by Gutiérrez et al. (34). The assay is a non-competitive sandwich immunoassay based on the fluorescence of lanthanide chelate labels that provides a minimal background, lack of any sample interference, and an in-house highly specific monoclonal antibody against porcine Hp. Salivary cortisol concentration was measured using an enzyme immunoassay kit (DetectX®, Catalogue Number K0033-H5W, Arbor Assays, MI, USA) according to the manufacturer's protocol. Processing of saliva samples prior to cortisol analysis and the protocol itself are described in detail elsewhere (30).

Statistical Analysis

SPSS (IBM SPSS Statistics 25) was used for statistical analysis of the data. Pig was used as experimental unit in all statistical analyses. In all statistical analyses, *p*-values below 0.05 were considered as significant and *p*-values of $0.05 \leq 0.1$ as tendency. Data normality was tested visually and with a Shapiro-Wilk test. Because none of the biomarkers studied met the normal distribution criteria, results are presented as median with range (see **Table 1** in Results section).

To ensure normality of residuals and homogeneity of variance, all parameters were root-transformed prior to the statistical analysis. A multivariate approach was used to test the effect of LPS and ketoprofen on salivary ADA, Hp, and cortisol. Individual pigs were included as subjects and saliva sampling time point (0–72 h) as repeated measures. Saliva sampling time point and treatment and their interaction were added as fixed factors. Pre-planned pairwise comparisons were performed for all treatments at time point t4 and between different time points for the SL group using a Bonferroni correction. For the cortisol model, one pig belonging to the SS group was discarded from the analysis because it had exceptionally high salivary cortisol concentration at time point t4.

Non-parametric Spearman correlation was used to investigate whether ADA, Hp, and cortisol responses correlate between baseline (t0) and 4 h post-injection (t4). For this purpose, new outcome variables for each biomarker were generated for each individual in the SL group by calculating the difference in measured concentrations between time points t4 and t0.

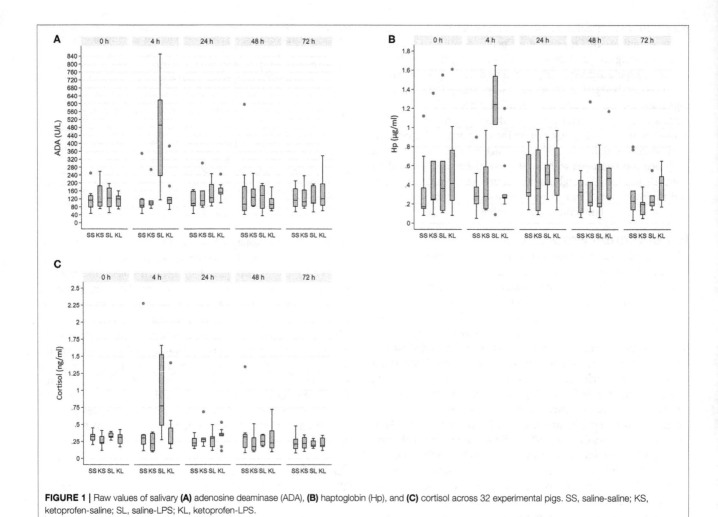

FIGURE 1 | Raw values of salivary **(A)** adenosine deaminase (ADA), **(B)** haptoglobin (Hp), and **(C)** cortisol across 32 experimental pigs. SS, saline-saline; KS, ketoprofen-saline; SL, saline-LPS; KL, ketoprofen-LPS.

RESULTS

Dynamics of Salivary Biomarkers

Descriptive results of salivary ADA, Hp, and cortisol measurements by sampling time point are shown in **Table 1**. Altogether seven ADA, seven Hp, and five cortisol samples were discarded from the analyses due to erroneous interpretation of the tube labeling in the laboratory. Raw values of each biomarker separated by time point are shown in **Figure 1**.

There was a significant interaction between time point and treatment for ADA ($F_{12,58} = 2.8$, $p = 0.01$). ADA was clearly increased in SL 4 h post-injection compared with other treatment groups (pairwise comparisons, $p < 0.01$ for all). Moreover, ADA within the SL group at t4 was significantly increased relative to baseline and all other time points (pairwise comparisons, $p < 0.001$ for all). For Hp, the interaction between time point and treatment was not significant ($F_{12,55.6} = 1.7$, $p = 0.10$). Overall, Hp concentration tended to be increased in the SL group compared with the SS group (pairwise comparisons, $p = 0.06$). However, 4 h post-injection Hp was significantly increased in the SL group compared with t48 and t72 (pairwise comparisons, $p < 0.01$ for both), but not with baseline or t24.

Cortisol response was similar to that of ADA and Hp, with a significant interaction between time point and treatment ($F_{12,68.4} = 1.9$, $p = 0.04$). A significant increase in salivary cortisol concentration occurred at t4 in SL compared with SS and KS (pairwise comparison, $p < 0.01$ for both), and it tended to be higher than KL (pairwise comparison, $p = 0.05$). In the SL, salivary cortisol was significantly increased at t4 relative to baseline and all other time points (pairwise comparisons, $p < 0.01$ for all).

Correlations Between Salivary Biomarkers

Across all experimental pigs, ADA, Hp, and cortisol did not correlate (Spearman correlation, $p > 0.05$ for all) at baseline. The response values calculated between baseline and t4 in the SL group showed a significant correlation for ADA and Hp ($r = 0.86$, $p < 0.05$). Although no significant correlations were found between ADA and cortisol or between Hp and cortisol, the correlation coefficients were moderate for both ($r = 0.64$ and $r = 0.57$, respectively).

DISCUSSION

As predicted, LPS injection resulted in an increase in salivary ADA and Hp as well as in salivary cortisol. A significant elevation in all studied biomarkers occurred at 4 h post-injection in LPS-challenged pigs. In other treatment groups, including the KL group, their concentrations remained relatively stable during the study period. Based on this, pre-treatment with ketoprofen was able to alleviate the LPS effect. The response of ADA and Hp showed positive significant correlations in the SL group indicating their parallel dynamics under the influence of bacterial LPS.

Increased salivary ADA concentrations have been reported in pigs suffering from clinically evident infectious and inflammatory conditions (6) and in stressed sheep (35). Several pig studies have investigated concentrations of Hp induced by viral (5, 9, 17, 18, 36) or bacterial (17, 18, 37) pathogens. Stressful occasions can increase serum Hp concentration (38, 39) as well. In this experiment, basal Hp concentration in saliva varied considerably between individual pigs with a range of: 0.08–1.61 µg/ml. For serum, high inter-individual variation has been reported previously (40–42). As a strong positive correlation between serum and salivary Hp concentrations exists (5), serum and salivary Hp dynamics are comparable to each other. Moreover, we observed high Hp concentration in one pig per treatment group at baseline. All of these pigs were among the pigs of lowest weight within the respective groups. Gutierrez et al. (6) did not find an increase in salivary Hp, ADA in growth retarded pigs. Even though we did not examine the study pigs clinically, all experimental pigs appeared healthy both prior to and during the experiment. There might be, however, differences in stress responsivity or subclinical conditions that could explain our findings.

Administration of E. coli LPS mimics an endotoxemic state that is known to induce a systemic inflammatory response (43). The pigs in this study were a subset of those in Veit et al. (30), where the behavioral signs of illness were reported. While the clinical onset of acute inflammatory response was not confirmed [for details, see (30)], an earlier report with the same E. coli strain and LPS dose indicates a strong activation of the innate immune system already 1 h after LPS injection (23). The rapid increase in the concentrations of all biomarkers in this paper is in line with this. The concentrations of all biomarkers returned to baseline levels by 24 h post-injection. To the best knowledge of the authors, previous pig studies have not investigated either short-term dynamics of salivary ADA, or ADA concentrations of pigs under a controlled immune challenge.

Previous research has shown that when triggered by an infectious agent serum Hp remains high for several days in pigs (18, 20, 44, 45). Heegaard et al. (18) reported differing dynamics of serum Hp depending on the disease causative agent, including bacterial, viral, and parasitic ones, and compared with aseptic inflammation. The rapid decline in salivary Hp in the present study might have been caused by the use of a single low-dose of synthetically purified LPS, which was likely to be eliminated from the body faster than LPS during natural infection. Escribano et al. (20) reported a three-fold increase in salivary Hp after LPS treatment, which remained high throughout the 7-day study period in growing pigs. In contrast to our study, they used a different E. coli strain (O55:B5), about 30 times higher LPS dose and repeated LPS injections (20). Moreover, the LPS dose was raised between the consecutive injections (20). As predicted, salivary cortisol of LPS-injected pigs not pre-treated with ketoprofen peaked at 4 h after injection, confirming the findings of others measuring cortisol from saliva and serum (23, 30, 45, 46). These results are in line with those of Escribano et al. (20) and Nordgreen et al. (23), who reported that salivary and plasma cortisol was elevated for only a short period of time following LPS challenge.

Our results indicated that intramuscularly administered ketoprofen was able to inhibit the effect of LPS, when given 1 h prior to LPS injection. Others have shown a similar effect of orally administered ketoprofen pigs (27). Moreover, the bioavailability of oral and intramuscularly administered ketoprofen has been reported to be similar (28). The appropriate dose of oral ketoprofen was set at 2 mg/kg (27), which is a third of the dose administered to KS and KL pigs in the present study. Mustonen et al. (46) reported that the effect of oral ketoprofen was seen immediately after its administration and that the effect lasted for ∼7 h.

Because the concentration of all biomarkers peaked at the same time point in the SL group, we wanted to test whether the increases from baseline to 4 h post injection were correlated. A significant correlation was found only between ADA and Hp. Gutiérrez et al. (25) reported a significant positive correlation between salivary ADA and Hp in healthy finishing pigs. In addition, their study population contained both female and male pigs (25) and therefore the comparison between the results of these two studies is not straightforward. Neither ADA nor Hp correlated with cortisol in the SL group. Contreras-Aguilar et al. (35) reported a significant correlation between salivary ADA and cortisol concentrations in sheep caused by either shearing stress or being frightened by a dog. Although we found no significant correlations between these, the correlation coefficients were at least moderate compared with Contreras-Aguilar et al. (35), who reported low correlation coefficients (0.34 and 0.19, respectively).

The present study was conducted in experimental conditions, with a possibility to optimize the management and housing conditions of the experimental pigs. The sampling occurred in pre-defined times during each day in order to avoid potential bias caused by a circadian rhythm as reported for cortisol (47) and Hp (48). To the best of our knowledge, no circadian pattern has been reported for ADA. The experimental pigs were of same age, breed and sex thus the potential bias caused by those factors (24) was supposed to be negligible. However, further studies including both genders as well as pigs at different stages of production should be conducted to investigate the dynamics of salivary biomarkers more thoroughly and to extrapolate the results to be applied in commercial settings.

CONCLUSIONS

The salivary concentration of ADA, Hp and cortisol increased rapidly after LPS challenge and they followed a similar pattern, and ketoprofen was able to alleviate the LPS effect. The results indicate that the selected salivary parameters, are indicative of systemic inflammatory response in pigs at an early stage. Primary and novel findings of the study are the response of ADA to LPS, its time course, and alleviation by ketoprofen. The usefulness of these biomarkers should be validated in a larger sample and in practical farm conditions.

ETHICS STATEMENT

The animal study was reviewed and approved by the Norwegian Animal Research Authority (FOTS id 15232).

AUTHOR CONTRIBUTIONS

VS drafted the manuscript, prepared the raw data, performed statistical analyses, and assisted in sample collection. CV processed the manuscript together with VS and participated in planning the experiment and sample collection. JN planned the experiment and performed sample collection. AV participated in experiment planning and statistical analyses. JN, MH, and SJ were actively involved in the manuscript writing process together with VS, CV, and AV. All authors contributed to the article and approved the submitted version.

REFERENCES

1. Jensen VF, Emborg HD, Aarestrup FM. Indications and patterns of therapeutic use of antimicrobial agents in the Danish pig production from 2002 to 2008. *J Vet Pharmacol Ther.* (2012) 35:33–46. doi: 10.1111/j.1365-2885.2011.01291.x
2. van Rennings L, von Münchhausen C, Ottilie H, Hartmann M, Merle R, Honscha W, et al. Cross-sectional study on antibiotic usage in pigs in Germany. *PLoS ONE.* (2015) 10:e0119114. doi: 10.1371/journal.pone.0119114
3. Lekagul A, Tangcharoensathien V, Yeung S. Patterns of antibiotic use in global pig production: a systematic review. *Vet Anim Sci.* (2019) 7:100058. doi: 10.1016/j.vas.2019.100058
4. Goecke NB, Kobberø M, Kusk TK, Hjulsager CK, Pedersen KS, Kristensen CS, et al. Objective pathogen monitoring in nursery and finisher pigs by monthly laboratory diagnostic testing. *Porc Heal Manag.* (2020) 6:23. doi: 10.1186/s40813-020-00161-3
5. Gutiérrez AM, Cerón JJ, Fuentes P, Montes A, Martínez-Subiela S. Longitudinal analysis of acute-phase proteins in saliva in pig farms with different health status. *Anim An Int J Anim Biosci.* (2012) 6:321–6. doi: 10.1017/S1751731111001662
6. Gutiérrez AM, De La Cruz-Sánchez E, Montes A, Sotillo J, Gutiérrez-Panizo C, Fuentes P, et al. Easy and non-invasive disease detection in pigs by adenosine deaminase activity determinations in saliva. *PLoS ONE.* (2017) 12:e0179299. doi: 10.1371/journal.pone.0179299
7. Ott S, Soler L, Moons CPH, Kashiha MA, Bahr C, Vandermeulen J, et al. Different stressors elicit different responses in the salivary biomarkers cortisol, haptoglobin, and chromogranin A in pigs. *Res Vet Sci.* (2014) 97:124–8. doi: 10.1016/j.rvsc.2014.06.002
8. Martínez-Miró S, Tecles F, Ramón M, Escribano D, Hernández F, Madrid J, et al. Causes, consequences and biomarkers of stress in swine: an update. *BMC Vet Res.* (2016) 12:171. doi: 10.1186/s12917-016-0791-8
9. Gutiérrez AM, Martínez-Subiela S, Soler L, Pallarés FJ, Cerón JJ. Use of saliva for haptoglobin and C-reactive protein quantifications in porcine respiratory and reproductive syndrome affected pigs in field conditions. *Vet Immunol Immunopathol.* (2009) 132:218–23. doi: 10.1016/j.vetimm.2009.06.013
10. Mayeux PR. Pathobiology of lipopolysaccharide. *J Toxicol Environ Health.* (1997) 51:415–35. doi: 10.1080/00984109708984034
11. Seemann S, Zohles F, Lupp A. Comprehensive comparison of three different animal models for systemic inflammation. *J Biomed Sci.* (2017) 24:1–17. doi: 10.1186/s12929-017-0370-8
12. Murata H, Shimada N, Yoshioka M. Current research on acute phase proteins in veterinary diagnosis: an overview. *Vet J.* (2004) 168:28–40. doi: 10.1016/S1090-0233(03)00119-9
13. Hart BL. Biological basis of the behavior of sick animals. *Neurosci Biobehav Rev.* (1988) 12:123–37. doi: 10.1016/S0149-7634(88)80004-6

14. Eckersall PD, Bell R. Acute phase proteins: biomarkers of infection and inflammation in veterinary medicine. *Vet J.* (2010) 185:23–7. doi: 10.1016/j.tvjl.2010.04.009
15. Pradeep M. Application of acute phase proteins as biomarkers in modern veterinary practice. *Ind J Vet Anim Sci.* (2014) 43:1–13.
16. Gutiérrez AM, Yelamos J, Pallarés FJ, Gómez-Laguna J, Cerón JJ. Local identification of porcine haptoglobin in salivary gland and diaphragmatic muscle tissues. *Histol Histopathol.* (2012) 27:187–96. doi: 10.14670/HH-27
17. Parra MD, Fuentes P, Tecles F, Martínez-Subiela S, Martínez JS, Muñoz A, et al. Porcine acute phase protein concentrations in different diseases in field conditions. *J Vet Med Ser B Infect Dis Vet Public Heal.* (2006) 53:488–93. doi: 10.1111/j.1439-0450.2006.01002.x
18. Heegaard PMH, Stockmarr A, Piñeiro M, Carpintero R, Lampreave F, Campbell FM, et al. Optimal combinations of acute phase proteins for detecting infectious disease in pigs. *Vet Res.* (2011) 42:1–13. doi: 10.1186/1297-9716-42-50
19. Gutiérrez AM, Nöbauer K, Soler L, Razzazi-Fazeli E, Gemeiner M, Cerón JJ, et al. Detection of potential markers for systemic disease in saliva of pigs by proteomics: a pilot study. *Vet Immunol Immunopathol.* (2013) 151:73–82. doi: 10.1016/j.vetimm.2012.10.007
20. Escribano D, Campos PHRF, Gutiérrez AM, Le Floc'h N, Cerón JJ, Merlot E. Effect of repeated administration of lipopolysaccharide on inflammatory and stress markers in saliva of growing pigs. *Vet J.* (2014) 200:393–7. doi: 10.1016/j.tvjl.2014.04.007
21. Bradford KL, Moretti FA, Carbonaro-Sarracino DA, Gaspar HB, Kohn DB. Adenosine deaminase (ADA) -deficient severe combined immune deficiency (SCID): molecular pathogenesis and clinical manifestations. *J Clin Immunol.* (2017) 37:626–37. doi: 10.1007/s10875-017-0433-3
22. Widar J, Ansay M. Adenosine deaminase in the pig: tissue-specific patterns and expression of the silent ADA0 allele in nucleated cells. *Anim Blood Groups Biochem Genet.* (1975) 6:109–16. doi: 10.1111/j.1365-2052.1975.tb01357.x
23. Nordgreen J, Munsterhjelm C, Aae F, Popova A, Boysen P, Ranheim B, et al. The effect of lipopolysaccharide (LPS) on inflammatory markers in blood and brain and on behavior in individually-housed pigs. *Physiol Behav.* (2018) 195:98–111. doi: 10.1016/j.physbeh.2018.07.013
24. Sánchez J, García A, Ruiz JM, Montes AM, Cabezas-Herrera J, Ros-Lara S, et al. Porcine breed, sex, and production stage influence the levels of health status biomarkers in saliva samples. *Front Vet Sci.* (2019) 6:32. doi: 10.3389/fvets.2019.00032
25. Gutiérrez AM, Montes A, Gutiérrez-Panizo C, Fuentes P, De La Cruz-Sánchez E. Gender influence on the salivary protein profile of finishing pigs. *J Proteomics.* (2018) 178:107–113. doi: 10.1016/j.jprot.2017.11.023
26. Martín de la Fuente AJ, Carpintero R, Rodríguez Ferri EF, Álava MA, Lampreave F, Gutiérrez Martín CB. Acute-phase protein response in pigs experimentally infected with *Haemophilus parasuis.* *Comp Immunol Microbiol Infect Dis.* (2010) 33:455–65. doi: 10.1016/j.cimid.2008.11.001

27. Mustonen K, Banting A, Raekallio M, Heinonen M, Peltoniemi OAT, Vainio O. Dose-response investigation of oral ketoprofen in pigs challenged with *Escherichia coli* endotoxin. *Vet Rec.* (2012) 171:70. doi: 10.1136/vr.100431

28. Raekallio MR, Mustonen KM, Heinonen ML, Peltoniemi OAT, Säkkinen MS, Peltoniemi SM, et al. Evaluation of bioequivalence after oral, intramuscular, and intravenous administration of racemic ketoprofen in pigs. *Am J Vet Res.* (2008) 69:108–13. doi: 10.2460/ajvr.69.1.108

29. Vane JR, Botting RM. Mechanism of action of nonsteroidal anti-inflammatory drugs. *Am J Med.* (1998) 104:2S–8S. doi: 10.1016/S0002-9343(97)00203-9

30. Veit C, Janczak AM, Ranheim B, Vas J, Valros A, Sandercock DA, et al. The effect of LPS and ketoprofen on cytokines, brain monoamines, and social behavior in group-housed pigs. *Front Vet Sci.* (2021) 7:617634. doi: 10.3389/fvets.2020.617634

31. Munsterhjelm C, Nordgreen J, Aae F, Heinonen M, Valros A, Janczak AM. Sick and grumpy: changes in social behaviour after a controlled immune stimulation in group-housed gilts. *Physiol Behav.* (2019) 198:76–83. doi: 10.1016/j.physbeh.2018.09.018

32. Fosse TK, Toutain PL, Spadavecchia C, Haga HA, Horsberg TE, Ranheim B. Ketoprofen in piglets: enantioselective pharmacokinetics, pharmacodynamics and PK/PD modelling. *J Vet Pharmacol Ther.* (2011) 34:338–49. doi: 10.1111/j.1365-2885.2010.01236.x

33. Munsterhjelm C, Brunberg E, Heinonen M, Keeling L, Valros A. Stress measures in tail biters and bitten pigs in a matched case-control study. *Anim Welf.* (2013) 22:331–8. doi: 10.7120/09627286.22.3.331

34. Gutiérrez AM, Martínez-Subiela S, Cerón JJ. Evaluation of an immunoassay for determination of haptoglobin concentration in various biological specimens from swine. *Am J Vet Res.* (2009) 70:691–6. doi: 10.2460/ajvr.70.6.691

35. Contreras-Aguilar MD, Escribano D, Quiles A, López-Arjona M, Cerón JJ, Martínez-Subiela S, et al. Evaluation of new biomarkers of stress in saliva of sheep. *Animal.* (2019) 13:1278–86. doi: 10.1017/S1751731118002707

36. Grau-Roma L, Heegaard PMH, Hjulsager CK, Sibila M, Kristensen CS, Allepuz A, et al. Pig-major acute phase protein and haptoglobin serum concentrations correlate with PCV2 viremia and the clinical course of postweaning multisystemic wasting syndrome. *Vet Microbiol.* (2009) 138:53–61. doi: 10.1016/j.vetmic.2009.03.005

37. Sorensen NS, Tegtmeier C, Andresen LO, Piñeiro M, Toussaint MJM, Campbell FM, et al. The porcine acute phase protein response to acute clinical and subclinical experimental infection with *Streptococcus suis.* *Vet Immunol Immunopathol.* (2006) 113:157–68. doi: 10.1016/j.vetimm.2006.04.008

38. Piñeiro M, Piñeiro C, Carpintero R, Morales J, Campbell FM, Eckersall PD, et al. Characterisation of the pig acute phase protein response to road transport. *Vet J.* (2007) 173:669–74. doi: 10.1016/j.tvjl.2006.02.006

39. Piñeiro C, Piñeiro M, Morales J, Carpintero R, Campbell FM, Eckersall PD, et al. Pig acute-phase protein levels after stress induced by changes in the pattern of food administration. *Animal.* (2007) 1:133–9. doi: 10.1017/S1751731107283909

40. Hennig-Pauka I, Menzel A, Boehme TR, Schierbaum H, Ganter M, Schulz J. Haptoglobin and C-reactive protein-non-specific markers for nursery conditions in swine. *Front Vet Sci.* (2019) 6:92. doi: 10.3389/fvets.2019.00092

41. Petersen HH, Dideriksen D, Christiansen BM, Nielsen JP. Serum haptoglobin concentration as a marker of clicinal signs in finishing pigs. *Vet Rec.* (2002) 151:85–9. doi: 10.1136/vr.151.3.85

42. Piñeiro C, Piñeiro M, Morales J, Andrés M, Lorenzo E, Pozo M del, et al. Pig-MAP and haptoglobin concentration reference values in swine from commercial farms. *Vet J.* (2009) 179:78–84. doi: 10.1016/j.tvjl.2007.08.010

43. Tuchscherer M, Kanitz E, Otten W, Tuchscherer A. Effects of prenatal stress on cellular and humoral immune responses in neonatal pigs. *Vet Immunol Immunopathol.* (2002) 86:195–203. doi: 10.1016/S0165-2427(02)00035-1

44. Webel DM, Finck BN, Baker DH, Johnson RW. Time course of increased plasma cytokines, cortisol, and urea nitrogen in pigs following intraperitoneal injection of lipopolysaccharide. *J Anim Sci.* (1997) 75:1514–20. doi: 10.2527/1997.7561514x

45. Terenina E, Sautron V, Ydier C, Bazovkina D, Sevin-Pujol A, Gress L, et al. Time course study of the response to LPS targeting the pig immune gene networks. *BMC Genomics.* (2017) 18:988. doi: 10.1186/s12864-017-4363-5

46. Mustonen K, Ala-Kurikka E, Orro T, Peltoniemi O, Raekallio M, Vainio O, et al. Oral ketoprofen is effective in the treatment of non-infectious lameness in sows. *Vet J.* (2011) 190:55–9. doi: 10.1016/j.tvjl.2010.09.017

47. Ruis MAW, Te Brake JHA, Engel B, Ekkel ED, Buist WG, Blokhuis HJ, et al. The circadian rhythm of salivary cortisol in growing pigs: effects of age, gender, and stress. *Physiol Behav.* (1997) 62:623–30. doi: 10.1016/S0031-9384(97)00177-7

48. Gutiérrez AM, Escribano D, Fuentes M, Cerón JJ. Circadian pattern of acute phase proteins in the saliva of growing pigs. *Vet J.* (2013) 196:167–70. doi: 10.1016/j.tvjl.2012.10.003

10

Establishment of a Blocking ELISA Detection Method for against African Swine Fever Virus p30 Antibody

Xuexiang Yu [1,2,3], Xianjing Zhu [1,2,3], Xiaoyu Chen [1,2,3], Dongfan Li [1,2,3], Qian Xu [1,2,3], Lun Yao [1,2,3], Qi Sun [1,2,3], Ahmed H. Ghonaim [1,3,4], Xugang Ku [1,3], Shengxian Fan [1], Hanchun Yang [5] and Qigai He [1,2,3]*

[1] College of Veterinary Medicine, Huazhong Agricultural University, Wuhan, China, [2] State Key Laboratory of Agricultural Microbiology, Wuhan, China, [3] The Cooperative Innovation Center for Sustainable Pig Production, Wuhan, China, [4] Desert Research Center, Cairo, Egypt, [5] College of Veterinary Medicine, China Agricultural University, Beijing, China

Correspondence:
Qigai He
he628@mail.hzau.edu.cn

African swine fever (ASF) is a highly lethal hemorrhagic viral disease of domestic pigs caused by African swine fever virus (ASFV). A sensitive and reliable serological diagnostic assay is required, so laboratories can effectively and quickly detect ASFV infection. The p30 protein is abundantly expressed early in cells and has excellent antigenicity. Therefore, this study aimed to produce and characterize p30 monoclonal antibodies with an ultimate goal of developing a monoclonal antibody-based enzyme-linked immunosorbent assay (ELISA) for ASFV antibody detection. Three monoclonal antibodies against p30 protein that were expressed in *E. coli* were generated, and their characterizations were investigated. Furthermore, a blocking ELISA based on a monoclonal antibody was developed. To evaluate the performance of the assay, 186 sera samples (88 negative and 98 positive samples) were analyzed and a receiver-operating characteristic (ROC) analysis was applied to determine the cutoff value. Based on the ROC analysis, the area under the curve (AUC) was 0.997 (95% confidence interval: 99.2 to 100%). Besides, a diagnostic sensitivity of 97.96% (95% confidence interval: 92.82 to 99.75%) and a specificity of 98.96% (95% confidence interval: 93.83 to 99.97%) were achieved when the cutoff value was set to 38.38%. Moreover, the coefficients of inter- and intra-batches were <10%, indicating the good repeatability of the method. The maximum dilution of positive standard serum detected by this ELISA method was 1:512. The blocking ELISA was able to detect seroconversion in two out of five pigs at 10 Dpi and the p30 response increasing trend through the time course of the study (0–20 Dpi). In conclusion, the p30 mAb-based blocking ELISA developed in this study demonstrated a high repeatability with maximized diagnostic sensitivity and specificity. The assay could be a useful tool for field surveillance and epidemiological studies in swine herd.

Keywords: African swine fever virus, blocking ELISA, diagnosis, monoclonal antibodies, p30

INTRODUCTION

African swine fever (ASF), caused by African swine fever virus (ASFV), is a highly contagious hemorrhage lethal disease of domestic and wild pigs and is responsible for serious economical losses, international trading, and adverse sociophysical impacts (1–6). It is causing a serious deterioration and incalculable economic impact due to its fast spread. The disease was first reported in Kenya in the 1910s, and 51 countries are currently affected by African Swine Fever (OIE) (7–10). ASFV is a large and complex double-stranded DNA virus with icosahedral morphology (5, 6, 11). Although it was generally considered that there is only one serotype of ASF virus, the classification of ASFV isolates in eight different serogroups based on a hemadsorption inhibition assay (HAI) (12). However, genetic characterization of all the ASF virus isolates known so far has demonstrated 24 geographically related genotypes with numerous subgroups (1, 7, 10). ASFV was first reported in China in August 2018; analysis showed that the causative strain belonged to the p72 genotype II and CD2v serogroup 8 (13, 14).

Due to the presence of seropositive animals to subacute or chronic forms of ASF, there is always a need for an accurate serological diagnosis. Serological assays are the most commonly used diagnostic tests due to their simplicity, comparatively low cost, and their necessitating few specialized pieces of apparatus or facilities. Since there is no vaccine against ASF, the presence of ASFV antibodies always indicates current or historic infection (7, 15). Also, 2–10% of animals recover from the acute form may act as persistent viral shedding sources (7). Studies have shown that the infectious virus genome was detected in tissues (retropharyngeal and submandibular lymph nodes, bone marrow, and tonsil) but was not detected in whole blood from the recovered animals (16). In addition, there were reported variant strains in China, with relatively weak virulence and atypical clinical symptoms (17, 18). Since the antibody IgG appears 7–10 days post-infection and persists for months and even lifetime (7, 15). Therefore, a sensitive and reliable serological diagnostic assay is required, so laboratories can effectively and quickly detect ASFV infection. Corresponding to this, identifying potential antigenic ASFV protein targets that suit to develop a diagnostic assay is very important, of which the p30, p72, and p54 are the best targets (19–25).

The major capsid protein p72 is used to establish numerous ELISA-based serological assays (24, 25). Among them, the p72 protein is mostly used in research. It has good immunogenicity, strong conservation, and high expression. The blocking-ELISA for ASFV antibody detection depends on the use of monoclonal antibodies against p72 (Ingenasa-Ingezim PPA COMPAC K3; Ingenasa, Madrid, Spain) (26, 27), but the detection time upon using p30 protein as the antigen can be earlier than that of p72 protein (20). The p54 protein in different regions has a certain variation in the amino acid sequence, which is easy to cause false-negative results, so it is usually not used as a detection antigen for ASF (20). Compared with the p54 and p72 proteins, the p30 protein is produced earlier and can neutralize the virus before or after the virus adsorption to the cell. The p30 protein is abundantly expressed early in cells and has excellent antigenicity

(20); it is also an important target for early diagnosis of the virus (28–30). Therefore, p30 protein can be used as an antigen to develop the early detection antibody method of ASFV infection.

In the current study, monoclonal antibodies (mAbs) against recombinant protein p30 were generated and their characterizations were investigated. Due to the high specificity of blocking ELISA, a blocking ELISA based on p30 mAb was developed. The established blocking ELISA showed high diagnostic sensitivity and specificity for ASFV antibody detection, providing a new tool for ASFV antibody detection.

MATERIALS AND METHODS

Production of Recombinant p30 in *Escherichia coli*

The ASFV CP204L (582 bp) gene sequence from positive samples during the surveillance was used for the preparation of p30 recombinant protein fragments. His-tagged full-length CP204L constructs were cloned into the pET-30a vector, and recombinant proteins were expressed in *E. coli*, as described previously (31, 32). CP204L was amplified by PCR using a forward primer 5′-GGCCATGGCTATGGATTTTATTTTAAATAT-3′ and a reverse primer 5′-CCGCTCGAGTTTTTTTTTTTAAAAGTTTA-3′. The primers were designed based on African swine fever virus isolate Pig/HLJ/2018 (accession. no. MK333180.1) (16, 17). The single underline is the sequence of the restriction sites of NcoI and XhoI. Briefly, polymerase chain reaction (PCR) amplified CP204 gene (582 bp) and pET-30a vector were digested with NcoI and XhoI (TakaRa, TakaRa Biotechnology Co., Ltd., Dalian, China) restriction enzymes and accordingly ligated with T4 DNA ligase. Recombinant genes were then transformed to Transetta (DE3) *E. coli* competent cells (TransGen Biotech Co., Ltd., Beijing, China) and incubated overnight at 37°C in an agar plate containing kanamycin. Subsequently, perfection of the correct insert was checked by PCR and positive samples were confirmed by DNA sequencing (Sangon Biotech Co., Ltd., Shanghai, China).

Expression and Purification of Recombinant ASFV-P30 Protein

Expression of the p30 protein was facilitated by adding 1 mM isopropyl-β-D-1-thiogalactoside (IPTG), and successful expression was examined by sodium dodecyl sulfate-polyacrylamide gel electrophoresis (SDS-PAGE) analysis of cell lysates. To purify p30 recombinant protein, bacterial cells were harvested by centrifugation, resuspended in pre-cold PBS (50 ml/liter of bacterial culture) (Dalian Meilun Biotechnology Co., Ltd., Dalian, China), and lysed by high-pressure crushing. After centrifugation at 12,000 rpm for 30 min, supernatants were collected and filtered through a 0.22-μm filter and purified using a Ni-NTA resin-based column. The protein sample p30 was taken for analysis by SDS-PAGE; anti-His mAb (Proteintech Group, Inc., Rosemont, IL, USA) and ASFV-positive serum were used as primary antibodies for Western blot verification.

mAb Production

As previously described (33, 34), 4–6-week-old BALB/C mice were immunized with 100 μg/mouse of purified p30 protein mixed with an equal volume of incomplete Freund's adjuvant (Sigma-Aldrich (Shanghai) Trading Co. Ltd., Shanghai, China). Mice were immunized intraperitoneally three times with 2 weeks between each immunization. The mice were euthanized 3 days after the final immunization, after which splenocytes were collected and fused with SP2/0 myeloma cells. After fusion, cells were cultured in 96-well plates (Corning Incorporated Co., Ltd., Kennebunk, ME, USA) in HAT selection media. Cell supernatants were assayed 10 days post cell fusion, and wells with confluent hybridomas were initially screened by indirect ELISA using p30 recombinant protein as a coating antigen. Then, the positive culture supernatants were screened for p30-specific antibodies by immunofluorescence assay (IFA) on PMA cells infected with ASFV which was isolation during the surveillance. Hybridoma clones that produced p30-specific antibodies were subcloned into single-cell clones (monoclones).

Indirect ELISA

Purified recombinant p30 protein constructs were coated on flat-bottom polystyrene plates (1 μg/ml; 100 μl/well) in carbonated coating buffer (pH 9.6) and incubated overnight at 4°C. The plate was washed five times with PBST (0.05% Tween in PBS, v/v), and the plate was blocked with 5% skimmed milk in PBS, for 1 h at 37 °C. After washing the plates as above, 50 μl undiluted hybridoma supernatants was added. Positive serum from mice immunized with p54 recombinant protein and negative serum from unimmunized mice, diluted 1:10,000, were also included in duplicate as a control. The plate was incubated for 30 min at 37°C, and a washing step was repeated. Thereafter, horseradish peroxidase (HRP) conjugated goat anti-mouse IgG (Proteintech Group, Inc., Rosemont, IL, USA) diluted 1:10,000 was added and incubated for 30 min at 37°C. Following washing five times, reaction was developed by adding a chromogenic substrate solution (TMB) (Beyotime Biotechnology Co., Ltd., Shanghai, China) for 10 min and stopped with Stop Solution for TMB Substrate (Beyotime Biotechnology Co., Ltd., Shanghai, China). The plates were read at 630 nm.

IFA

IFA tests on ASFV-infected cells were conducted on porcine alveolar macrophage (PAM) cells infected with ASFV (The virus was isolated and produced by PAM cells, and the virus $TCID_{50}$ was measured by the Reed–Muench method. The virus was stored at −80°C. The virus was isolated and stored in the Animal Biosafety Level 3 Laboratory of Huazhong Agricultural University.). PAM cells were collected from 20 to 30-day-old pigs, and the cells were plated on 96-well plates in 10% FBS (Gibco, Thermo Scientific, USA) RPMI 1640 medium (Gibco, Thermo Scientific, Waltham, MA, USA) at 37°C with 5% CO_2 and infected with ASFV at an MOI of 0.1. At 36 hpi, cell monolayers were fixed with 4% paraformaldehyde in PBS for 30 min at room temperature. The above operations are carried out in the Animal Biosafety Level 3 Laboratory of Huazhong Agricultural University. Cells were incubated with anti-p30 mAb

followed by incubation with FITC conjugated goat anti-mouse IgG (ABclonal Technology Co., Ltd., Wuhan, China). Nuclei were stained with DAPI, and the plates were examined using the fluorescence microscope (EVOS FL Auto, Thermo Fisher Scientific, USA).

Serum Standard and Testing Samples

The serum samples were used for blocking ELISA development and validation. One hundred and eighty-six serum samples were analyzed with the established blocking ELISA, including 88 negative sera and 98 ASFV-positive sera. These 88 samples were collected before the outbreak of ASFV in China and were confirmed to be negative by the commercial ASFV antibody detection kit (INgezim PPA COMPAC, Ingenasa, Madrid, Spain). All the 98 ASFV-positive samples used in this study were from clinically infected pigs, and their positivity was determined by the commercial ASFV antibody detection kit (INgezim PPA COMPAC, Ingenasa, Madrid, Spain). ASFV-positive and -negative sera were kindly gifted by the National African Swine Fever Reference Laboratory of the China Animal Health and Epidemiology Center.

Procedure for ASFV Indirect ELISA and Blocking ELISA

The purified p30 mAb was labeled with horseradish peroxidase (HRP) (Shandong Galaxy Bio-Tech Co., Ltd., Jining, China) to establish a blocking ELISA antibody detection method. Purified recombinant p30 protein constructs were coated on flat-bottom polystyrene plates (0.5 μg/ml; 100 μl/well) in carbonated coating buffer (pH 9.6) and incubated overnight at 4°C. The plate was washed five times with PBST (0.05% Tween in PBS, v/v), and the plate was blocked with 2% skimmed milk in PBS, for 1 h at 37°C. After washing, 100 μl of the diluted control and testing sera was added and incubated at 37°C for 30 min, and a washing step was repeated. All control and testing sera samples were diluted 1:1 in dilution buffer (0.01% Tween 20 in 1× PBS). Next, 100 μl of biotinylated anti-p30 mAb (HPR-anti-p30 mAb; 1 μg/ml) was added into each well, and the plate was incubated at 37°C for another 30 min. Following extensive washing, reaction was developed by adding chromogenic substrate solution (TMB) (Beyotime Biotechnology Co., Ltd., Shanghai, China) for 10 min and stopped with Stop Solution for TMB Substrate (Beyotime Biotechnology Co., Ltd., Shanghai, China). The plates were read at 630 nm, and the raw data were transformed to an Excel sheet and consequently the percent of inhibition (PI value) of each test sample was calculated using the formula: PI (%) = [(OD_{630} value of negative controls − OD_{630} value of sample)/OD_{630} value of negative controls] × 100%, as described by Wang et al. (35).

Cut-Off Value, Diagnostic Sensitivity, and Specificity Determination

To calculate the optimal cutoff value, and associated diagnostic sensitivity and specificity, serum samples from individual pigs of known ASFV-positive and -negative testing sample were tested by blocking ELISA. Receiver operating characteristic (ROC) analysis and degree of agreement (kappa value) were analyzed using SPSS software for windows, version 26.0 (IBM,

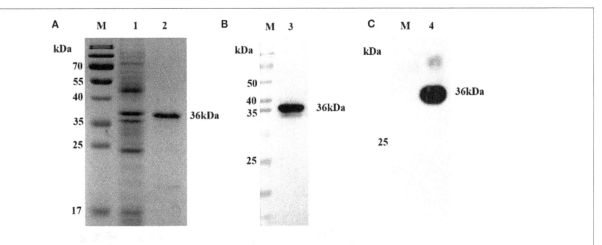

FIGURE 1 | Analysis of p30 protein. **(A)** SDS-PAGE analysis of recombinant p30 protein. The recombinant protein can be seen at 36 kD (Black). **(B)** Western blot analysis of recombinant p30 protein with anti-His tag antibody. The recombinant protein can be seen at 36 kD (Black). It can be seen that the recombinant protein can react specifically with anti-His mAb. **(C)** Western blot analysis of recombinant p30 protein with ASFV positive serum. The recombinant protein can be seen at 36 kD (Black). It can be seen that the recombinant protein can react specifically with ASFV positive serum; M: protein Marker; 1: Negative control; 2, 3, 4: p30 protein.

Armonk, NY, USA). Using the commercial blocking ELISA kit as a standard evaluating method, the sensitivity and specificity of the established ELISA were calculated by the web-based MedCalc statistical software [https://www.medcalc.org/calc/diagnostic test.php (accessed on 7 June 2021)].

Assessment of Blocking ELISA Specificity and Repeatability

To confirm the specificity, the developed blocking ELISA was used to detect six polyclonal anti-sera against other swine viruses (PCV2, PCV3, CSFV, PRV, PRRSV, O-FMDV).

The repeatability of blocking ELISA was assessed by running 10 control sera (three positive control, three medium-positive control, and four negative control). The within-run assay precision was calculated using a standard serum tested on three plates in one run, and the between-run precision was calculated from a standard serum tested in three different runs. Means, standard deviations, and percent coefficient of variation (% CV) were calculated using SPSS software for windows, version 26.0.

Detection Antibody in ASFV-Infected Pig Sera, ASFV Positive Standard Serum

ASFV-infected pig sera were collected at different time-points (0, 5, 10, 15, and 20 Dpi) from experimentally infected pigs. Five sera were collected at each stage. The ASFV-infected pig sera were donated by Harbin Veterinary Research Institute. The ASFV-positive standard serum (no. 202101) and the ASFV-positive standard serum against CD2v-negative (no. 202101) (swine sera infected with ASFV delete the CD2v gene) were purchased from the China Veterinary Drug Administration. The ASFV-positive standard serum and the ASFV-positive standard serum against CD2v-negative at different dilutions were titrated with twofold dilutions from 1:4 to 1:1,024. All collected serum samples were tested by the p30 mAb-based blocking ELISA.

RESULTS

Antigen Preparation

The synthetic DNA fragment of the CP204L gene from ASFV-positive DNA was cloned and expressed in *E. coli* as a His-tagged recombinant protein. The p30 protein was expressed at a high level but formed inclusion bodies. Coomassie blue staining showed a sharp band at the predicted size of the purity His-tagged p30 (~36 kDa) in sodium dodecyl sulfate–polyacrylamide gel electrophoresis (SDS-PAGE) (**Figure 1A**). The identity of the recombinant protein was further confirmed by Western blot analysis using an anti-His mAb (**Figure 1B**) and the ASFV-positive serum (**Figure 1C**).

Generation of MAbs Against ASFV p30

To generate anti-p30 mAbs, mice were immunized with recombinant p30 protein. After the fusion process, supernatants from the resulting hybridoma cells were screened by p30 indirect ELISA, Western blot analysis (**Figure 2A**), and IFA using PAMs infected with ASFV (**Figure 2B**). One mAb from each primary clone, mAb 2D6, 6B3, and 10B8, was selected for further characterization. The different mAbs at different dilutions were titrated with 2-fold dilutions from 1:1,000 to 1:1,024,000 (**Figure 2C**). Furthermore, isotypes of mAbs were characterized using the mouse Ig isotyping kit (Southern Biotechnology Associates, Inc., Birmingham, USA) and all were found to be IgG1 with kappa light chain (**Table 1**).

Assessing Potential Uses of p30 Monoclonal Antibodies for Blocking ELISA

To evaluate the potential use of these anti-p30 monoclonal antibodies as a diagnostic reagent for ASFV antibody detection, blocking ELISA based on each monoclonal antibody was investigated. Five positive sera and five negative sera were selected to determine which p30 monoclonal antibody will have a good performance to be applied in blocking ELISA. Each sample

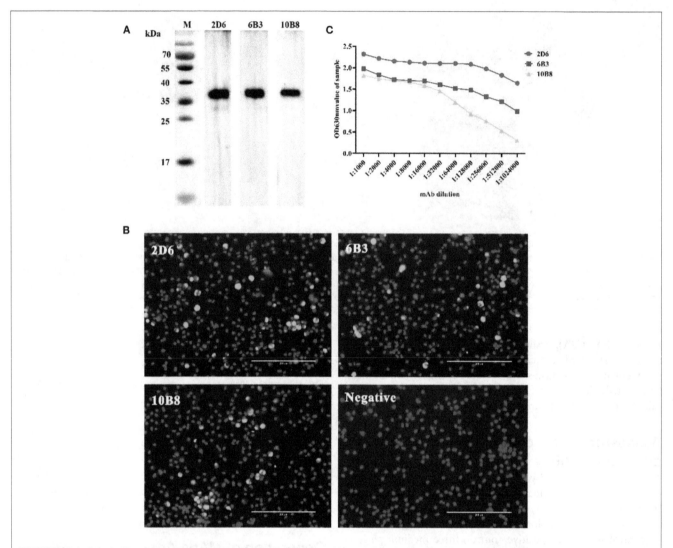

FIGURE 2 | Selection of p30-specific mAb for use in blocking ELISA. **(A)** Western blot analysis anti-p30 mAbs. The three anti-p30 monoclonal antibodies can react specifically with recombinant protein at 36 kD (Black). **(B)** IFA performed on PAMs that were infected with ASFV. Cells were incubated with p30-specific mAbs listed on the top of each panel and stained with FITC-conjugated goat anti-mouse IgG (Green). Cell nucleus was counterstained with DAPI (Blue). Scale bars, 200 μm. **(C)** Different mAbs titer test results. The OD value of mAb-2D6 (Red) at any dilution is higher than mAb-6B3 (Blue) and mAb-10B8 (Green). It is shown that mAb-2D6 has the highest antibody titer.

was tested with the blocking ELISA at a dilution of 1:2, and the percent of inhibition (PI value) of each sample was calculated (**Figure 3**). The result revealed that all test-positive samples were able to block mAb-2D6 by greater than others.

Standardization and Determining the Negative Cut-Off Value for Blocking ELISA

After optimizing the protocol for competitive ELISA, a total of 186 pig serum samples (88 negative samples and 98 positive samples) were tested to assess the performance of the assay. These samples were classified as ASFV seronegative or ASFV seropositive according to their known origin and using a commercial ASFV antibody detection kit (INgezim PPA COMPAC, Ingenasa, Madrid, Spain). All samples were tested in duplicate by the established blocking ELISA, and the percent of inhibition value of each sample was calculated. An ROC curve statistical analysis was performed and allowed us to determine the cutoff value and estimate the diagnostic sensitivity and specificity of the assay (**Figure 4A**). In addition, an interactive dot plot diagram outlined the blocking value of these samples, as shown in **Figure 4B**. An AUC of 1 represents a perfect test, and an AUC above 0.9 indicates high accuracy of the assay. Based on the ROC analysis, the area under the curve (AUC) of the established test was 0.997 (95% confidence interval: 99.2 to 100%). Besides, a diagnostic sensitivity of 97.96% (95% confidence interval: 92.82 to 99.75%) and a specificity of 98.96% (95% confidence interval: 93.83 to 99.97%) were achieved when the cutoff value was set to 38.38%, demonstrating the high accuracy of the assay.

Assessment of Blocking ELISA Specificity and Repeatability

To confirm the specificity, the developed blocking ELISA was used to detect six polyclonal anti-sera against other swine viruses (PCV2, PCV3, CSF, PR, PRRSV, O-FMDV). All sera yielded a negative result in the blocking ELISA with a blocking value much lower than the cutoff value. Thus, non-specific positive swine sera were clearly discriminated from the ASFV-positive sera, suggesting that the established blocking ELISA has a satisfactory analytical specificity.

Reproducibility determines whether an entire experiment or study can be reproduced. In this study, 12 serum samples (eight positive samples and four negative samples) were selected for testing by the developed blocking ELISA while the intra- and inter-assay variations were determined by calculating the coefficient of variation ($CV\%$). The coefficient of variation (CV) <10% was considered to have an adequate repeatability. In this study, an intra-assay CV ranging from 1.09 to 8.56% and an inter-assay CV ranging from 1.21 to 9.92% were observed, indicating that the p30-based blocking ELISA is highly repeatable.

Antibody Response to p30 in ASFV-Infected Pigs

Next, we applied the p30-based blocking ELISA to determine the humoral immune response in ASFV-infected pigs. The ASFV-specific antibody response was determined using blocking ELISA. As shown in **Figure 5**, the antibody response against p30 protein

was detected seroconversion as early as 10 Dpi in two out of five pigs and the p30 response peaked around 20 Dpi.

Analytical Sensitivity of the p30-Based Blocking ELISA

After the assay conditions were optimized, the analytical sensitivity of the p30-based blocking ELISA was evaluated using the ASFV-positive standard serum and the ASFV-positive standard serum against the CD2v-negative one. The maximum dilution of ASFV-positive standard serum detected at different dilutions was 1:512, and the ASFV-positive standard serum against CD2v-negative maximum dilution was 1:64, indicating that the p30-based blocking ELISA is highly sensitive (**Figure 6**).

DISCUSSION

ASFV causes a serious deterioration and incalculable adverse economic impact around the world especially in China which has the largest pig industry (13, 16, 17). Currently, there is no vaccine or other treatments available for ASFV. The principal strategy for control remains early detection, quarantine, and depopulation of affected herds. Cost-effective detection strategies are needed for conducting high-throughput surveillance (2, 7, 24–27). Although the seroconversion time was later than the virus genome-detected time, no significant symptoms were found in the variant strain-infected animals, and the infected pigs underwent intermittent detoxification (18). In addition, in several areas (Africa and Europe), many pigs or wild boar survived infection and presented no clinical signs of ASFV at the time of samplings, without the presence of ASFV attenuated variants (36–38); thus, we need to accurately detect the antibody of the animal to be tested to facilitate the determination of the infection of the pigs. Therefore, a sensitive and reliable serological diagnostic assay is required, so as laboratories can effectively and quickly detect ASFV infection (18, 26).

ELISA is considered a common tool to carry out serological surveillance. Among these ELISA methods, two main types of

TABLE 1 | Identification of subclasses of p30 monoclonal antibodies.

	Monoclonal antibodies		
	2D6	6B3	10B8
Ig subclass	IgG1	IgG1	IgG1
Light chain type	κ	κ	κ

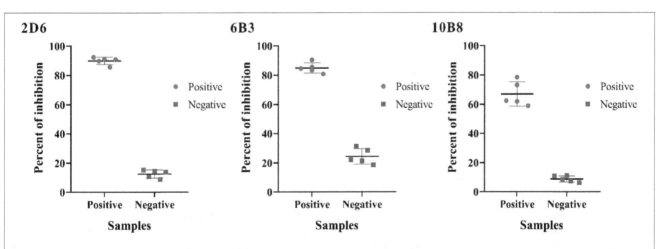

FIGURE 3 | Investigation of p30 monoclonal antibodies on blocking ELISA for ASF detection. The percent of inhibition of five positive samples (Red) and five negative samples (Blue) were determined, and the average percent of inhibition of negative and positive samples was displayed.

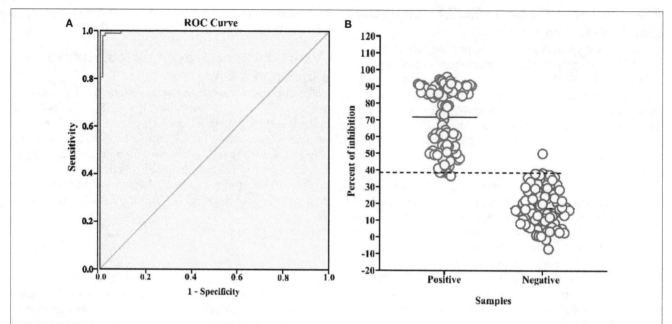

FIGURE 4 | ASFV p30-based blocking ELISA analysis of serum samples. The analysis was performed on known ASFV-negative samples ($n = 88$) and known ASFV-positive samples ($n = 98$). **(A)** ROC analysis of blocking ELISA results while the area under the curve (AUC) of the test was 0.997. **(B)** Interactive dot plot diagram showing the blocking value of serum samples while the cut-off value was set to 38.38%.

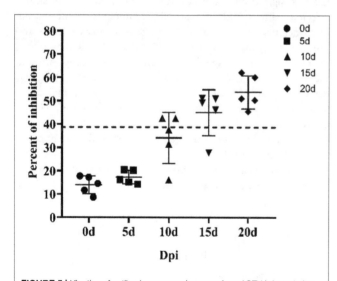

FIGURE 5 | Kinetics of antibody response in serum from ASFV-infected pigs. Serum samples were collected from six pigs infected by ASFV at 0, 5, 10, 15, and 20 days post inoculation. The dashed line represents the cut-off of blocking ELISA.

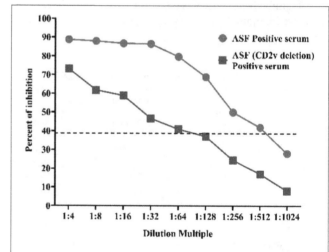

FIGURE 6 | Sensitivity assay. The ASFV-positive standard serum (Red) and the ASFV-positive standard serum against CD2v-negative (Blue) at different dilutions were titrated with 2-fold dilutions from 1:4 to 1:1,024. The dashed line represents the cut-off of blocking ELISA.

ELISAs have been employed in antibody detections. One is indirect ELISA, where coated antigens capture specific antibodies in serum samples directly. The other is blocking or competitive ELISA, where virus-specific antibodies in samples react with antigens to block or compete with the binding of a mAb to the antigens. The specificity of iELISA is generally influenced by high background due to the non-specific reaction of serum antibodies to contaminant antigens in the tests (39). In this study,

we established a blocking ELISA for the detection of antibodies against ASFV in pig serum. The ELISA is a rapid, economical, and sensitive diagnostic method for screening large numbers of sera for antibodies. Additionally, the specificity of this method is supposed to be even higher due to the usage of mAbs. Blocking ELISAs were widely used for a broad range of applications concerning serological diagnosis of various diseases in different animal species (40, 41).

The p30 mAb-based blocking ELISA demonstrated good diagnostic sensitivity of 97.96% and specificity of 98.96%. Based on the selected cutoff value of 38.38%, 1 out of 88 negative sera samples showed false-positive results, with a PI value of 50.01, while 2 out of the 98 positive serum samples showed false-negative results with PI values of 36.59 and 38.03%. It has been reported that intrinsic and external factors, such as autoantibodies, sample quality, and sample storage conditions, can affect the serologic testing (41). Physical and chemical parameters can also affect the test results in the laboratory, such as hemolysis and lipemia (42). In our study, of the two false-negative serum samples and the one false-positive sample, these three serum samples were confirmed as negative by IFA.

The p30 mAb-based blocking ELISA was further validated for detecting seroconversion and monitoring the dynamic of antibody response in experimental pigs infected with ASFV. The blocking ELISA was able to detect seroconversion in two out of five pigs at 10 dpi. It detected an increasing trend of antibody response against p30 protein through the time course of the study (0–20 dpi). The detection of seroconversion at 10 dpi was consistent with the findings in previous studies (23, 43–45), so this detection method can be used as an early detection kit. The maximum dilution of the ASFV-positive standard serum and the ASFV-positive standard serum against the CD2v-negative one at different dilutions were 1:512 and 1:64, respectively, indicating that the p30-based blocking ELISA was highly sensitivity and it can detection for variant strains.

Furthermore, with the emergence of domestic attenuated strains and atypical clinical symptoms, antibody detection methods can be used as an effective means to detect infections. The antibody detection methods can be used to screen ASF antigen–antibody double-negative pigs upon introducing pigs into farm. Due to its simplicity concerning the coating antigen production, easiness to perform, and low cost, the test will be a useful tool for field surveillance and epidemiological studies in swine herd. The non-invasive test for a complete epidemiological investigation in the field is very important, especially ASF. In subsequent studies, an attempt should be made to establish an antibody detection method for oral fluid.

CONCLUSION

This study prepared three monoclonal antibodies against the structural p30 protein of ASFV, and their diagnostic application was investigated. The p30 mAb-based blocking ELISA developed in this study demonstrated a high repeatability with maximized diagnostic sensitivity and specificity in laboratory settings. Through the aforementioned experiments and analysis, we conclude that the newly developed mAb 2D6-based blocking ELISA method offers a promising approach for a rapid and convenient ASFV serodiagnosis. The assay could be a useful tool for field surveillance and epidemiological studies in swine herd.

ETHICS STATEMENT

The animal study was reviewed and approved by the Ethics Committee of the Faculty of Veterinary Medicine of the Huazhong Agricultural University.

AUTHOR CONTRIBUTIONS

XY, XZ, XK, SF, HY, and QH contributed to the conception or design of the work and the acquisition of data. XC, DL, and QX completed the data analysis. LY, QS, and AG drafted the manuscript and revised it critically for important intellectual content. All authors have critically read and edited the manuscript.

ACKNOWLEDGMENTS

We would like to thank the National African Swine Fever Reference Laboratory of the China Animal Health and Epidemiology Center for the ASFV-positive and -negative serum, and the Harbin Veterinary Research Institute for the ASFV-infected pig sera.

REFERENCES

1. Torre A, Bosch J, Iglesias I, Muñoz M, Mur L, Martínez-López B, et al. Assessing the risk of African swine fever introduction into the European Union by Wild Boar. *Transb Emerg Dis.* (2015) 62:272–9. doi: 10.1111/tbed.12129
2. Zakaryan H, Revilla Y. African swine fever virus: current state and future perspectives in vaccine and antiviral research. *Vet Microbiol.* (2016) 185:15–19. doi: 10.1016/j.vetmic.2016.01.016
3. Gaudreault NN, Madden DW, Wilson WC, Trujillo JD, Richt JA. African swine fever virus: an emerging DNA arbovirus. *Front Vet Sci.* (2020) 7:215. doi: 10.3389/fvets.2020.00215
4. Nguyen T, Xuan D, Thi T, Van T, Thi B, Yong J, et al. Molecular profile of African swine fever virus (ASFV) circulating in Vietnam during 2019–2020 outbreaks. *Arch Virol.* (2021) 166:885–90. doi: 10.1007/s00705-020-04936-5
5. Wang N, Zhao D, Wang X, Wang J, Zhang Y, Wang M, et al. Architecture of African swine fever virus and implications for viral assembly. *Science.* (2019) 366:640–4. doi: 10.1126/science.aaz1439
6. Salas ML, Andrés G. African swine fever virus morphogenesis. *Virus Res.* (2013) 173:29–41. doi: 10.1016/j.virusres.2012.09.016
7. Food and Agriculture Organization of Animal Health (FAO), Beltrán-Alcrudo D, FAO Reference Centre, INIA-CISA, Kramer SA, FAO, et al. *African Swine Fever: Detection and Diagnosis.* FAO (2017).
8. OIE. *Global Situation of African Swine Fever.* Report No. 47:2016–2020. Available online at: https://rr-asia.oie.int/en/projects/asf/situational-updates-of-asf-in-asia-and-the-pacific/ (accessed December 15, 2020).
9. OIE. *Global Situation of African Swine Fever.* Report No. 64: February 05 to February 18, 2021. Available online at: https://www.oie.int/en/document/report_64_current_situation_of_asf/ (accessed March 24, 2020).
10. OIE. *Global Control of African Swine Fever: A GF-TADs Initiative (2020–2025).* Available online at: https://www.oie.int/en/global-action-needed-now-to-halt-spread-of-deadly-pig-disease/ (accessed July 17, 2020).
11. Arias M, Jurado C, Gallardo C, Fernández-Pinero J, Sánchez-Vizcaíno JM. Gaps in African swine fever: analysis and priorities. *Transb Emerg Dis.* (2018) 65:235–47. doi: 10.1111/tbed.12695

12. Malogolovkin A, Burmakina G, Titov I, Sereda A, Gogin A, Baryshnikova E, et al. Comparative analysis of African swine fever virus genotypes and serogroups. *Emerg Infect Dis*. (2015) 21:312–5. doi: 10.3201/eid2102.140649

13. Shengqiang G, Jinming L, Xiaoxu F, Fuxiao L, Lin L, Qinghua W, et al. Molecular characterization of African swine fever virus, China, 2018. *Emerg Infect Dis*. (2018) 24:2131–3. doi: 10.3201/eid2411.181274

14. Sánchez-Vizcaíno J, Mur L, Gomez-Villamandos J, Carrasco L. An update on the epidemiology and pathology of African swine fever. *J Comp Pathol*. (2015) 152:9–21. doi: 10.1016/j.jcpa.2014.09.003

15. OIE. Chapter 2.8.1. African swine fever. In: *Manual of Diagnostic Tests and Vaccines for Terrestrial Animals (Mammals, Birds and Bees)*. Paris: World Organisation for Animal Health (2012).

16. Zhao D, Liu R, Zhang X, Li F, Wang J, Zhang J, et al. Replication and virulence in pigs of the first African swine fever virus isolated in China. *Emerg Microbes Infect*. (2019) 8:438–47. doi: 10.1080/22221751.2019.1590128

17. Wen X, He X, Zhang X, Zhang X, Liu L, Guan Y, et al. Genome sequences derived from pig and dried blood pig feed samples provide important insights into the transmission of Africa swine fever virus in China in 2018. *Emerg Microbes Infect*. (2019) 8:303–6. doi: 10.1080/22221751.2019.1565915

18. Gallardo C, Soler A, Nurmoja I, Cano-Gómez C, Cvetkova S, Frant M, et al. Dynamics of African swine fever virus (ASFV) infection in domestic pigs infected with virulent, moderate virulent and attenuated genotype II ASFV European isolates. *Transbound Emerg Dis*. (2021) 68:2826–41. doi: 10.1111/tbed.14222

19. Weldu T, Lulu W, Ghebremedhin T, Yibrah T, Zhenjiang Z, Jiwen Z, et al. Characterization of anti-p54 monoclonal antibodies and their potential use for African swine fever virus diagnosis. *Pathogens*. (2021) 10:178. doi: 10.3390/pathogens10020178

20. Gómez-Puertas P, Rodríguez F, Oviedo J, Brun A, Alonso C, Escribano J. The African swine fever virus proteins p54 and p30 are involved in two distinct steps of virus attachment and both contribute to the antibody-mediated protective immune response. *Virology*. (1998) 243:461–71. doi: 10.1006/viro.1998.9068

21. Rodríguez JM, García-Escudero R, Salas ML, Andrés G. African swine fever virus structural protein p54 is essential for the recruitment of envelope precursors to assembly sites. *J Virol*. (2004) 78:4299–313. doi: 10.1128/JVI.78.8.4299–4313.2004

22. García-Mayoral MF, Rodríguez-Crespo I, Bruix M. Structural models of DYNLL1 with interacting partners: African swine fever virus protein p54 and postsynaptic scaffolding protein gephyrin. *FEBS Lett*. (2011) 585:53–7. doi: 10.1016/j.febslet.2010.11.027

23. Perez-Filgueira DM, Camacho FG, Gallardo C, Resino-Talaván P, Blanco E, Gomez-Casado E, et al. Optimization and validation of recombinant serological tests for African swine fever diagnosis based on detection of the p30 protein produced in Trichoplusia ni larvae. *J Clin Microbiol*. (2006) 44:3114–21. doi: 10.1128/JCM.00406–06

24. Fangfeng Y, Vlad P, Luis G, Jeffrey J, Raymond R, Ying F. Development of a blocking enzyme-linked immunosorbent assay for detection of antibodies against African swine fever virus. *Pathogens*. (2021) 10:760. doi: 10.3390/pathogens10060760

25. Cubillos C, Gómez-Sebastian S, Moreno N, Nuñez MC, Mulumba-Mfumu LK, Quembo CJ, et al. African swine fever virus serodiagnosis: a general review with a focus on the analyses of African serum samples. *Virus Res*. (2013) 173:159–67. doi: 10.1016/j.virusres.2012.10.021

26. Gallardo C, Reis AL, Kalema-Zikusoka G, Malta J, Soler A, Blanco E, et al. Recombinant antigen targets for serodiagnosis of African swine fever. *Clin Vaccine Immunol*. (2009) 16:1012–20. doi: 10.1128/CVI.00408–08

27. Reis AL, Parkhouse RME, Penedos AR, Martins C, Leitão AB. Systematic analysis of longitudinal serological responses of pigs infected experimentally with African swine fever virus. *J Gen Virol*. (2007) 88:2426–34. doi: 10.1099/vir.0.82857–0

28. Ning J, Yunwen O, Zygmunt P, Yongguang Z, Jie Z. Roles of African swine fever virus structural proteins in viral infection. *J Vet Res*. (2017) 61:135–43. doi: 10.1515/jvetres-2017-0017

29. Pamela L, Haru T, Dirk W, Linda D, Dave C. Correlation of cell surface marker expression with African swine fever virus infection. *Vet Microbiol*. (2014) 168:413–19. doi: 10.1016/j.vetmic.2013.12.001

30. Barderas MG, Rodríguez F, Gómez-Puertas P, Avilés M, Beitia F, Alonso C, et al. Antigenic and immunogenic properties of a chimera of two immunodominant African swine fever virus proteins. *Arch Virol*. (2001) 146:1681–91. doi: 10.1007/s007050170056

31. Ann-Maree C, Tatiana AS, David AJ, Philip GB, Rohan TB. An efficient system for high-level expression and easy purification of authentic recombinant proteins. *Prot Sci*. (2004) 13:1331–9. doi: 10.1110/ps.04618904

32. Mallory EH, Maria VM, Ping W, Andre DL, Wei J, Raymond RR. Linear epitopes in African swine fever virus p72 recognized by monoclonal antibodies prepared against baculovirus-expressed antigen. *J Vet Diagn Invest*. (2018) 30:104063871775396. doi: 10.1177/1040638717753966

33. Ying F, Andrew P, Lia H, Eric AN, Raymond RR. Production and characterization of monoclonal antibodies against the nucleocapsid protein of SARS-COV. *Adv Exp Med Biol*. (2006) 581:153–6. doi: 10.1007/978-0-387-33012-9_27

34. Yanhua L, Ali T, Eric JS, Ying F. Identification of porcine reproductive and respiratory syndrome virus ORF1a-encoded non-structural proteins in virus-infected cells. *J Gen Virol*. (2012) 93:829–39. doi: 10.1099/vir.0.039289–0

35. Wang L, Mi S, Gong W, Shi J, Madera R, Ganges L, et al. A neutralizing monoclonal antibody-based competitive ELISA for classical swine fever C-strain post-vaccination monitoring. *BMC Vet Res*. (2020) 16:14. doi: 10.1186/s12917-020-2237-6

36. Atuhaire DK, Afayoa M, Ochwo S, Mwesigwa S, Ojok L. Prevalence of African swine fever virus in apparently healthy domestic pigs in Uganda. *BMC Vet Res*. (2013) 9:263. doi: 10.1186/1746–6148-9-263

37. Patrick BN, Machuka EM, Githae D, Banswe G, Amimo JO, Ongus JR, et al. Evidence for the presence of African swine fever virus in apparently healthy pigs in South-Kivu Province of the Democratic Republic of Congo. *Vet Microbiol*. (2020) 240:108521. doi: 10.1016/j.vetmic.2019.108521

38. Franzoni G, Giudici SD, Loi F, Sanna D, Floris M, Fiori M, et al. African swine fever circulation among free-ranging pigs in Sardinia: data from the eradication program. *Vaccines*. (2020) 8:549. doi: 10.3390/vaccines8030549

39. Sandvik T. Laboratory diagnostic investigations for bovine viral diarrhoea virus infections in cattle. *Vet Microbiol*. (1999) 64:123. doi: 10.1016/S0378–1135(98)00264–8

40. Henriques AM, Fagulha T, Barros SC, Ramos F, Duarte M, Luís T, et al. Development and validation of a blocking ELISA test for the detection of avian influenza antibodies in poultry species. *J Virol Methods*. (2016) 236:47–53. doi: 10.1016/j.jviromet.2016.07.006

41. Isa G, Pfister K, Kaaden OR, Czerny CP. Development of a monoclonal blocking ELISA for the detection of antibodies against Fowlpox virus. *J Vet Med B Infect Dis Vet Public Health*. (2002) 49:21–3. doi: 10.1046/j.1439–0450.2002.0533.x

42. Castro C, Gourley M. Diagnostic testing and interpretation of tests for autoimmunity. *J Allergy Clin Immunol*. (2010) 125:S238–47. doi: 10.1016/j.jaci.2009.09.041

43. Krasowski MD. Educational case: hemolysis and lipemia interference with laboratory testing. *Acad Pathol*. (2019) 6:6. doi: 10.1177/2374289519888754

44. Malmquist WA. Serologic and immunologic studies with African swine fever virus. *Am J Vet Res*. (1963) 24:450–9.

45. Sánchez-Vizcaíno JM, La Dd Omada A, Avilés MM. Editorial: African swine fever. *Front Vet Sci*. (2021) 7:632292. doi: 10.3389/fvets.2020.632292

11

Real-Time Quaking-Induced Conversion Detection of PrP^{Sc} in Fecal Samples from Chronic Wasting Disease Infected White-Tailed Deer using Bank Vole Substrate

*Soyoun Hwang, Justin J. Greenlee and Eric M. Nicholson **

Virus and Prion Research Unit, National Animal Disease Center, United States Department of Agriculture, Agricultural Research Service, Ames, IA, United States

Correspondence:
Eric M. Nicholson
eric.nicholson@ars.usda.gov

Chronic wasting disease (CWD) is a transmissible spongiform encephalopathy (TSE) that is fatal to free-range and captive cervids. CWD has been reported in the United States, Canada, South Korea, Norway, Finland, and Sweden, and the case numbers in both wild and farmed cervids are increasing rapidly. Studies indicate that lateral transmission of cervids likely occurs through the shedding of infectious prions in saliva, feces, urine, and blood into the environment. Therefore, the detection of CWD early in the incubation time is advantageous for disease management. In this study, we adapt real-time quacking-induced conversion (RT-QuIC) assays to detect the seeding activity of CWD prions in feces samples from clinical and preclinical white-tailed deer. By optimizing reaction conditions for temperature as well as the salt and salt concentration, prion seeding activity from both clinical and preclinical animals were detected by RT-QuIC. More specifically, all fecal samples collected from 6 to 30 months post inoculation showed seeding activity under the conditions of study. The combination of a highly sensitive detection tool paired with a sample type that may be collected non-invasively allows a useful tool to support CWD surveillance in wild and captive cervids.

Keywords: CWD, prion disease, RT-QuIC, transmissible spongiform encephalopathy, TSE, feces, white-tailed deer

INTRODUCTION

Chronic wasting disease (CWD) is a form of transmissible spongiform encephalopathy (TSE) or prion disease affecting cervids including deer, elk, reindeer, and moose. Prion diseases result from the misfolding of the cellular prion protein (PrP^C) into a pathogenic form (PrP^{Sc}). Other prion diseases include scrapie in sheep, bovine spongiform encephalopathy (BSE) in cattle, and Creutzfeldt-Jakob disease (CJD), fatal familial insomnia (FFI), Gerstmann-Sträussler-Scheinker syndrome (GSS), and kuru in humans. CWD has been reported across North America including 26 states in the United States and three Canadian provinces. CWD-infected animals have also been reported in South Korea, Norway, Finland, and most recently, Sweden (1–4).

Chronic wasting disease infected cervids have misfolded prion proteins distributed widely, not only in the nervous system but also in lymphoid tissues, muscle, and blood (5–7). These animals are known to shed prions into the environment *via* saliva, urine, blood, and feces. This environmental contamination is often suggested to be the cause for horizontal CWD transmission among captive and free-ranging wild animals. Despite the awareness of potential sources, rising case numbers in wild cervids highlight the lack of effective CWD management strategies. Lacking treatment or vaccination, any management strategy for CWD will be dependent on sensitive and early detection of CWD prions in CWD infected animals. Early detection in a readily accessible sample that can be collected in a non-invasive procedure will afford producers and regulatory entities the opportunity to test prior to shipment as well as upon receipt to reduce the likelihood that an infected animal would be introduced into an otherwise healthy herd. Samples that are shed from animals, particularly early in the incubation period, have low concentrations of detectable prions, which necessitates highly sensitive prion detection methods. Highly sensitive prion detection tools like real-time quaking induced conversion (RT-QuIC) that amplify the prion *in vitro* enabled the detection of prions from early stage of the disease and from various sample types in addition to brain and lymphoid tissues. Several reports have indicated that fecal prions as well as those found in saliva, blood, and urine from cervids could be detected using RT-QuIC, in some cases using preclinical samples (8–14).

In the study, we tested the suitability of bank vole prion protein (BV rPrP) as a substrate for CWD detection in feces samples from clinical and preclinical white-tailed deer. To accomplish this, the reaction conditions were optimized using different enrichment methodologies, different salt concentrations, different temperatures, and different salt ions to amplify fecal prions for improved sensitivity and specificity.

MATERIALS AND METHODS
Source of Fecal Samples
All fecal samples used in this manuscript were collected from white-tailed deer that were experimentally inoculated by the oronasal route with the CWD agent from either a white-tailed deer (deer numbers #1548 and #1553) or an experimentally inoculated raccoon (deer numbers #1542 and #1555). Feces was collected from two non-inoculated, non-CWD exposed deer for use as negative controls (deer numbers #831 and #1801). They are summarized in **Table 1**. All animal experiments were

TABLE 1 | Animal experimental summary of genotype, inoculum, survival period, and enzyme-immunoassay (EIA) in white-tailed deer inoculated oronasally with the agent of chronic wasting disease from white-tailed deer and racoon.

Eartag	Genotype	CWD Inoculum	Months post-incubation (mo.)	[b]EIA O.D.
	96			
1553	GG	WTD	21.4	4.00
1548	GG	WTD	24	4.00
1542	GG	Racoon CWD	34.5	4.00
1555	GG	Racoon CWD	[a]56.7	NT
831	GG	Neg. control	42	[c]0.07
1801	GG	Neg. control	34.1	[c]0.08

NT indicates that samples were not tested.
[a]*This animal has not developed clinical signs at the time of this study.*
[b]*IDEXX HerDCheck CWD Ag test.*
[c]*Values below 0.18 are negative.*

conducted at the National Animal Disease Center under the approval of the Institutional Animal Care and Use Committee (protocol number: ARS-2018-748, date of approval from ethical committee: August 7, 2015). The animal experiments were carried out in accordance with the Guide for the Care and Use of Laboratory Animal (Institute of Laboratory Animal Resources, National Academy of Sciences, Washington DC, USA). Each deer was inoculated oronasally similar to previously described (15) with 1 ml of 10% (wt/vol) brain homogenate from a single animal with clinical signs consistent with prion disease and confirmed positive by immunohistochemistry, enzyme-immunoassay (EIA), and Western blot. Fecal samples were collected at ~6-month intervals until the deer developed clinical signs consistent with CWD. The mean incubation period was 682 days for deer inoculated with the CWD agent from a white-tailed deer. At ~1,700 dpi, the experiment with deer inoculated with the CWD agent from raccoons is ongoing, but deer #1542 was euthanized at 1,035 dpi due to clinical signs consistent with CWD.

Preparation of Cervid Feces Extracts
Cervid feces was prepared as described by Cheng et al. (9). Briefly, 1 g of previously collected fecal pellets was weighed and added into the feces extract buffer (20 mM sodium phosphate (pH 7.1), 130 mM NaCl, 0.05% Tween 20, 1 mM phenylmethylsulfonyl fluoride (PMSF), and 1X complete protease inhibitors (Roche) giving a final concentration of 10% (w/v). Then, the fecal pellets were homogenized in M tubes (GentleMACS M tubes) using a dissociator (GentleMACS, Miltenyi Biotec) for a minute with two to three repeats to ensure complete pellet disruption. The tubes were then placed onto an orbital shaker for 1 h at room temperature. After centrifugation at 18,000 × g for 5 min, supernatants were collected and stored at −80°C for further use.

Sodium Phosphotungstic Acid Precipitation
To each 1 ml volume of 10% (w/v) fecal supernatant, 250 μl of 10% N-lauryl sarcosine was added. Samples were then incubated at 37°C for 30 min at 1,400 rpm in a thermomixer. Using a stock solution of 10% sodium phosphotungstic acid (NaPTA), 170 mM of magnesium chloride (pH 7.4) was added to each sample to give a final concentration of 0.3% NaPTA in the samples. Samples were incubated at 37°C for 2 h with shaking at 400 rpm. Supernatants were removed following centrifugation at 15,800 × g for 30 min. Pellets were washed with wash buffer [10 mM Tris-Cl, pH 7.5, 100 mM NaCl, 0.5% Triton-X 100, 10 mM ethylenediamine tetraacetic acid (EDTA), 0.5% sodium deoxycholate (w/v), and 0.1% sarkosyl (w/v)], and centrifuged again for 15 min at 15,800 g. Pellets were resuspended in 100 μl of Dulbecco's phosphate-buffered saline (DPBS) with 0.05% Sodium dodecyl sulfate (SDS).

PAD-Beads Enrichment
PAD-Beads and all buffers were provided as a kit from (Microsens, London, UK). Standard PAD-Beads enrichment was followed as described by Hwang et al. (16). Briefly, 200 μl of 10% (w/v) fecal samples was mixed with 500 μl of distilled water by gently tapping the tubes, and then 200 μl of capture buffer and

100 μl of beads were added to the tube. The tubes were then shaken for 30 min at room temperature on a rocker. After the incubation, beads were captured on a magnet and the liquid was removed. Then, the samples were washed with wash buffer 1 and wash buffer 2. For elution, 25 μl of elution buffer (0.1 M NaOH, 0.1% Triton X-100) was added to the beads, and the tubes were shaken for 5 min. The tubes were placed on a magnet to capture the beads. While the tubes were on the magnet, the same volume, 25 μl of 0.1 M HCl was added to the tubes to neutralize the NaOH and mixed gently. Finally, the liquid was removed and analyzed by RT-QuIC.

For large scale sample preparation, 1 ml of fecal samples was used instead of 200 μl, and all other buffers were used at five times the previously indicated volume except the elution buffer and HCl neutralization which were both 50 μl.

Recombinant Prion Protein Production and Purification

Escherichia coli [BL21 (λDE3)] was transformed with the pET28a vector containing the bank vole PrP gene (amino acids 23–231; GenBank accession number AF367624), and the recombinant bank vole prion proteins were expressed and purified as described by Vrentas et al. (17). The concentration of pooled protein eluent was measured by UV and calculated from the absorbance at 280 nm using an extinction coefficient of 62,005 $M^{-1}cm^{-1}$ as calculated for the bank vole prion protein (18).

Real-Time Quaking-Induced Conversion Protocol

Real-time quaking-induced conversion reactions were performed as previously described (19–25). The reaction mix was composed of 10 mM phosphate buffer (pH 7.0), either 100, 200, 300, 400, and 500 mM NaCl or 100, 200, 300, 400, and 500 mM sodium iodide (NaI), 0.1 mg/ml recombinant bank vole prion protein, 10 μM thioflavin T (ThT), and 1 mM EDTA tetrasodium salt. Aliquots of the reaction mix (98 μL) were loaded into each well of a black 96-well plate with a clear bottom (Nunc, Thermo Fisher Scientific, USA) and seeded with 2 μL of fecal homogenate dilutions with 0.05% SDS. The plate was then sealed with plate sealer film and incubated at 37, 42, or 48°C in a BMG FLUOstar Omega plate reader with cycles of 1 min shaking (700 rpm double orbital) and 1 min rest for 100 h. ThT fluorescence measurements (excitation 460 nm, emission 480 nm, bottom read, 20 flashes per well, and manual gain 1,400) were taken every 45 min.

All RT-QuIC assays for each dilution of each sample were performed as two repeats of four replicates for a total of eight replicates. ThT fluorescence data are displayed as the average ThT fluorescence of four technical replicates for each time point and, to be considered positive, the ThT fluorescence of at least two replicates out of four reactions must be positive. Positive threshold was calculated as the mean value of non-inoculated control sheep brain homogenates plus 10 SDs, and lag time is defined as the time to reach the positive threshold (20, 26, 27).

RESULTS

Real-Time Quaking-Induced Conversion Detection of PrP^Sc in Non-enriched Fecal Samples From White-Tailed Deer Clinically Affected With CWD

To test whether CWD prions from fecal samples, without enrichment or substrate replacement, could be detected by RT-QuIC using BV rPrP, reactions were seeded with different dilutions of fecal samples collected from clinically affected white-tailed deer at the time of necropsy. Different concentrations of NaCl were tested to find the optimal reaction conditions with BV rPrP and CWD infected deer fecal samples (**Figure 1**). All tested conditions showed an increase in ThT fluorescence typical for the detection of TSE within 30 h except 300 mM NaCl. Using higher salt concentrations (400 and 500 mM NaCl) improved the seeding activity with shorter lag time for assays seeded with feces from positive animal samples while assays seeded with feces from negative control samples remain below the threshold to be considered positive (**Figures 1D,E**).

Real-Time Quaking-Induced Conversion Detection of PrP^Sc in Enriched Fecal Samples by NaPTA Precipitation From White-Tailed Deer Clinically Affected With CWD

To evaluate the efficacy of NaPTA precipitation in detection CWD prions in fecal samples from clinical CWD infected white-tailed deer, reactions containing recombinant BV rPrP were seeded with different dilutions of NaPTA enriched fecal samples. Again, different concentrations of NaCl were tested to find the optimal condition for the detection of PrP^Sc in the fecal samples with RT-QuIC following NaPTA precipitation. Similar to the results observed for non-enriched samples, all tested NaCl concentrations, except 300 mM NaCl, result in fibril seeding based on an observed increase in ThT fluorescence (**Figure 2**). Assays with higher NaCl concentrations (400 and 500 mM) showed shorter lag times with spontaneous conversion with low intensity and extended lag time at 70 h. It is clear that NaPTA precipitation improved the RT-QuIC detection in fecal samples by shortening lag time of seeding activity.

Real-Time Quaking-Induced Conversion Detection of CWD Prions in Fecal Samples of White-Tailed Deer With Clinical Signs of CWD Following PAD-Bead Enrichment

PAD-Beads, a commercially available kit, has been used to successfully enrich brain homogenate samples prior to RT-QuIC (16). To evaluate the efficacy of PAD-Beads enrichment for CWD prion detection from fecal samples, reactions containing BV rPrP were seeded with different dilutions of PAD-Beads eluate in the presence of different NaCl concentrations. Most assays did not show any increase of ThT. However, assays containing 100 mM NaCl showed the increase of ThT fluorescence for the assays seeded with fecal sample of animal #1553 (**Figure 3**). Given the

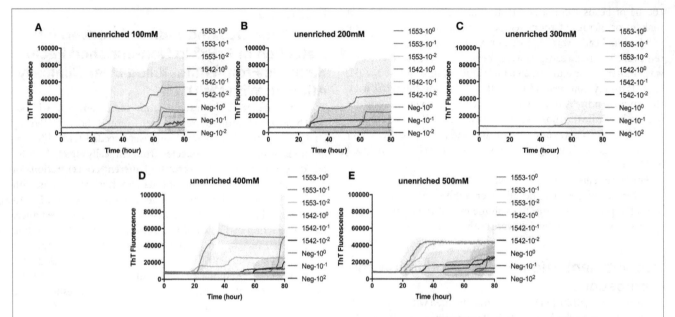

FIGURE 1 | Real-time quacking-induced conversion (RT-QuIC) reactions containing different NaCl concentrations **(A)** 100 mM, **(B)** 200 mM, **(C)** 300 mM, **(D)** 400 mM, and **(E)** 500 mM seeded with fecal dilutions from chronic wasting disease (CWD) infected white-tailed deer brains using BV rPrP as a substrate. RT-QuIC reactions were seeded with 10^0, 10^{-1}, or 10^{-2} dilutions of 10% fecal homogenate. All reactions were seeded with fecal homogenate of white-tailed deer with the addition of 0.001% of SDS. Shown are the average ThT fluorescence readings determined from all replicates (four replicate reactions per each dilution).

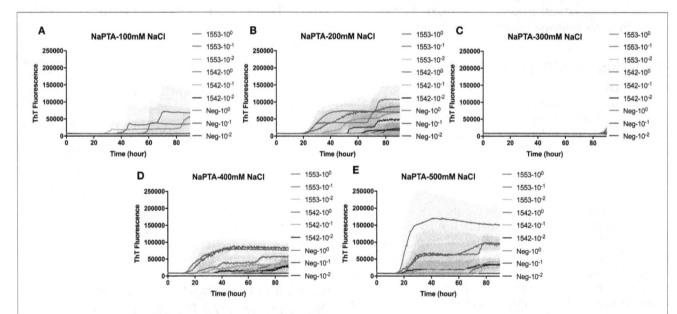

FIGURE 2 | Real-time quacking-induced conversion (RT-QuIC) reactions containing different NaCl concentrations **(A)** 100 mM, **(B)** 200 mM, **(C)** 300 mM, **(D)** 400 mM, and **(E)** 500 mM seeded with sodium phosphotungstic acid (NaPTA) enriched fecal dilutions from CWD infected white-tailed deer brains using BV rPrP as a substrate. RT-QuIC reactions were seeded with 10^0, 10^{-1}, or 10^{-2} dilutions of 10% fecal homogenate. All reactions were seeded with fecal homogenate of white-tailed deer with the addition of 0.001% of SDS. Shown are the average ThT fluorescence readings determined from all replicates (four replicate reactions per each dilution).

presumably lower concentration of PrP^{Sc} in fecal samples relative to brain homogenate, we also assessed a higher starting volume of fecal sample homogenate. The standard PAD-Bead protocol uses 200 µl of 10% fecal homogenates. Therefore, instead of using 200 µl of 10% fecal homogenates (standard protocol), 1 ml of 10% fecal homogenate was used for PAD-Beads enrichment.

All other reagents in the protocol were also increased by five times. At the end, 100 µl of eluate was collected to make the final 1/10 volume of original fecal sample, a volume equivalent to that used in NaPTA enrichment. When assays were seeded with fecal eluate of large scale PAD-Beads enrichment, every assay showed rapid (within 20 h) conversion. However, assays

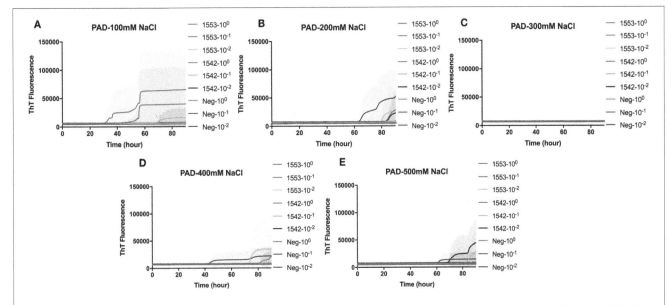

FIGURE 3 | Real-time quacking-induced conversion (RT-QuIC) reactions containing different NaCl concentrations **(A)** 100 mM, **(B)** 200 mM, **(C)** 300 mM, **(D)** 400 mM, and **(E)** 500 mM seeded with PAD-Beads enriched fecal dilutions from CWD infected white-tailed deer brains using BV rPrP as a substrate. RT-QuIC reactions were seeded with 10^0, 10^{-1}, or 10^{-2} dilutions of 10% fecal homogenate. All reactions were seeded with fecal homogenate of white-tailed deer with the addition of 0.001% of SDS. Shown are the average ThT fluorescence readings determined from all replicates (four replicate reactions per each dilution).

seeded the equivalently treated negative control fecal samples showed seeding activity with only a marginally longer lag time. Specifically, assays seeded with negative control in the presence of 400 mM NaCl had a lag time $\sim$5 h longer than from positive animals, and all reactions containing 500 mM NaCl showed the increase of ThT fluorescence in a similar lag time albeit lower intensity (**Figures 4A,B**). ThT fluorescence comparing reactions seeded with unenriched feces, enriched by large scale PAD-Beads, and NaPTA is shown in **Figure 4**. Based on these results, PAD-Bead enrichment was not further pursued for fecal samples, and NaPTA enrichment was used for all further experiments.

Real-Time Quaking-Induced Conversion Detection of CWD Prions in Fecal Samples Collected From White-Tailed Deer in the Preclinical Stage of Prion Disease

To evaluate if RT-QuIC assays can detect prions from fecal samples of preclinical white-tailed deer, fecal samples that were collected at times of routine animal handling were also seeded in RT-QuIC reactions. In total, eight fecal samples from four white tailed deer were collected. Four samples are from animal #1553 and #1548 after 6 and 18 months of inoculation, and another set of four samples received from #1542 and #1555 after 6 and 30 months of inoculation were used to run the assay. All fecal samples were NaPTA enriched and tested for prion detection in RT-QuIC, and assays were measured at 37°C in the presence of 500 mM NaCl (**Figure 5**). However, most assays did not show any increase of ThT fluorescence except the one seeded with #1542 (30 months post inoculation). With low detection under these conditions, assays were repeated at higher temperatures (42 or 48°C) using both 400 mM and 500 mM NaCl (**Figure 6**).

This increased overall conversion as evidenced by increased ThT fluorescence (**Figure 6**). Assays run at 42°C in the presence of 500 mM NaCl showed the increase of ThT fluorescence within 60 h of lag time for most fecal sample collected from biopsy, and the reactions were well-separated from the assay seeded with feces of negative control animal (**Figure 6B**). Assays running at 48°C not only shorten the lag time by $\sim$20 h for most fecal samples but it also shortens the lag time for negative control samples preventing the discrimination of positive samples from negative sample. **Figure 7** shows the lag time for all seeding activity with a cutoff line for time to positive threshold such that positive samples are below the line. In terms of specificity, reactions under 42°C with 500 mM NaCl allowed the best results, and increasing temperature to 48°C improved the conversion efficiency but due to conversion in the negative control samples, the ability to discriminate positive from negative samples was not sufficient for use. It is worth noting that ThT fluorescence intensity from assays seeded with negative samples (**Figure 6**) is lower relative to the assays seeded with positive samples. For example, assays run at 48°C with 500 mM NaCl show higher ThT fluorescence intensity for positive samples compared to the intensity for negative samples.

Sodium Iodide Reduces Lag Time in the Detection of CWD Prions in Fecal Samples Collected From White-Tailed Deer in the Preclinical Stage of Prion Disease

We also tested another salt, NaI, in the reaction mixtures for detecting prions from fecal samples that were collected at times of routine animal handling. Instead of using NaCl, 400 or 500 mM of NaI was added in the RT-QuIC reaction

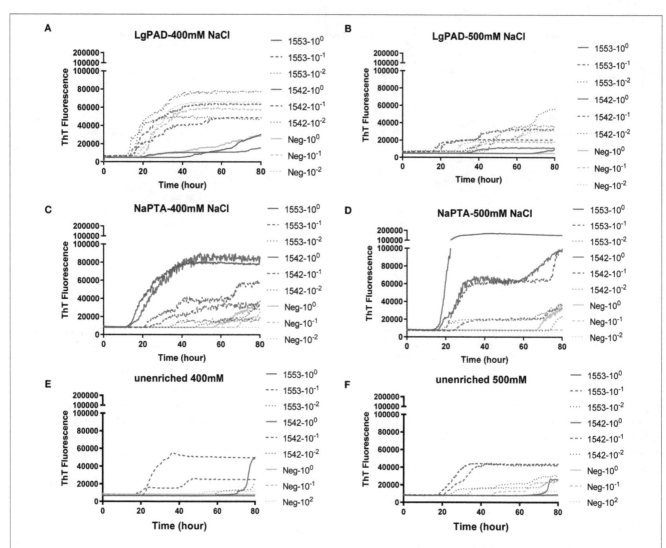

FIGURE 4 | Comparison of RT-QuIC reactions seeded with fecal dilutions from different enrichment. **(A,B)** enriched with PAD-Beads large scale **(C,D)** enriched with NaPTA **(E,F)** non-enriched dilutions. All reactions were seeded with fecal homogenate of white-tailed deer with the addition of 0.001% of SDS. Shown are the average ThT fluorescence readings determined from all replicates (four replicate reactions per each dilution).

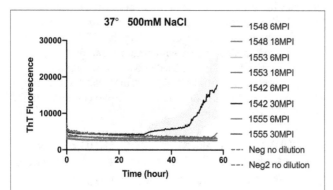

FIGURE 5 | RT-QuIC reactions seeded with biopsy fecal homogenates from preclinical white-tailed deer. RT-QuIC reactions were seeded with 10^{-1} dilution of 10% fecal homogenate. All reaction mixtures contain 500 mM NaCl and measured at 37°C. Shown are the average ThT fluorescence readings determined from all replicates (four replicate reactions per each dilution).

mixtures and they were measured either at 42°C or 48°C. Overall, most reaction assays containing NaI showed a shorter lag time compared to the assays containing NaCl (**Figure 8**). Again, reactions performed at 48°C shorten lag time with NaI but the high temperature stimulated spontaneous reactions for negative control in early lag time. Among the reaction conditions, assays containing 500 mM NaCl measured at 42°C were chosen for optimal conditions to detect prions from biopsy fecal samples when considering both conversion efficiency and specificity. **Figure 9** shows comparison between assays run with 500 mM NaCl or 500 mM NaI. In addition, **Table 2** shows the lag time analysis for the comparison of all the assays containing NaCl and NaI in different temperatures and concentrations. Overall, the replacement of NaCl with NaI allowed us to detect PrP^{Sc} from fecal samples in short lag time but with a reduced separation from the negative control. This is most apparent in **Figure 9** where two inoculated animals at six MPI were no longer differentiated

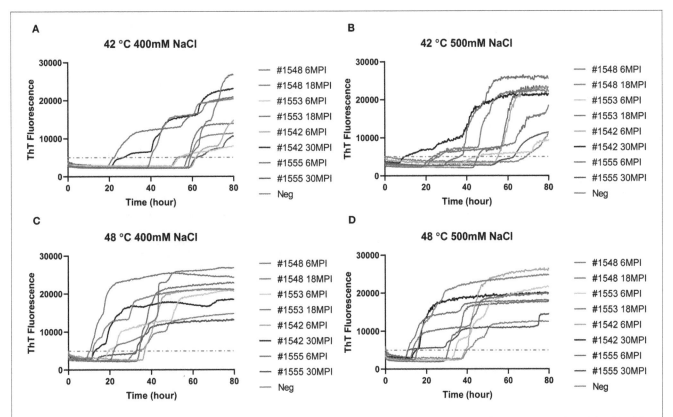

FIGURE 6 | RT-QuIC reactions seeded with biopsy fecal homogenates from preclinical white- tailed deer. Reactions conditions for each sample are followed as **(A)** 400 mM NaCl at 42°C, **(B)** 500 mM at 42°C, **(C)** 400 mM at 48°C, and **(D)** 500 mM at 48°C. Shown are the average ThT fluorescence readings determined from all replicates (four replicate reactions per each dilution).

from negative. This experiment indicates that NaCl is still the better salt choice for fecal samples using bank vole substrate since all fecal samples from inoculated animals exhibited ThT fluorescence indicative of fibril formation in a shorter time relative to the negative control samples.

DISCUSSION

In this study, we have optimized RT-QuIC reaction conditions to enhance the detection of PrP^Sc from fecal homogenates from clinical and preclinical white-tailed deer. Different factors including salt concentrations and temperature were tested with regard to sensitivity and specificity of detection of infectious prions from fecal samples using bank vole recombinant prion protein as the amplification substrate. For fecal samples collected from clinically affected deer, a reaction temperature of 37°C showed prion detection, as previously reported by Henderson and colleagues where they observed less spontaneous reactions by reducing reaction temperature from 42 to 37°C for fecal prion detection in RT-QuIC (8). In the data presented in this study, the assays seeded with fecal samples from clinically affected animals showed prion seeding activity at 37°C even without any enrichment. However, for fecal samples collected from preclinical deer inoculated with CWD, RT-QuIC conditions had to be further optimized to enhance the prion detection. Using high

salt concentration like 500 mM NaCl and increasing temperature from 37 to 42°C enhanced the seeding activity of fecal samples and allowed for discrimination between assays seeded with positive fecal samples and assays seeded with negative controls. We also tested higher temperatures like 48°C for better sensitivity of fecal prions in RT-QuIC. Higher temperatures did shorten the lag time of seeding activity overall, however, assays performed at 48°C also shorten the lag time of assays seeded with negative control, which led to an inability to discriminate positive samples from negative samples. Modified conditions were identified that enhance detection of prions in fecal samples from preclinical animals. Further, it was ultimately determined that for RT-QuIC reactions seeded with fecal samples from preclinical animals, it is desirable to incorporate NaPTA enrichment prior to RT-QuIC for improved detection of seeding activity.

A previously published report that had applied different ions of the Hofmeister series of ions to RT-QuIC reactions showed enhanced sensitivity of seeding activity for assays seeded with ear homogenate from CWD infected deer in the presence of NaI instead of NaCl (28). Here, we compare the seeding activity of fecal samples in the presence of NaI to that of NaCl. As can be seen in **Figure 8**, similar result was observed for fecal samples as was previously reported for ear homogenate such that assays containing NaI had shorter lag times than assays containing NaCl. Assays seeded with negative sample

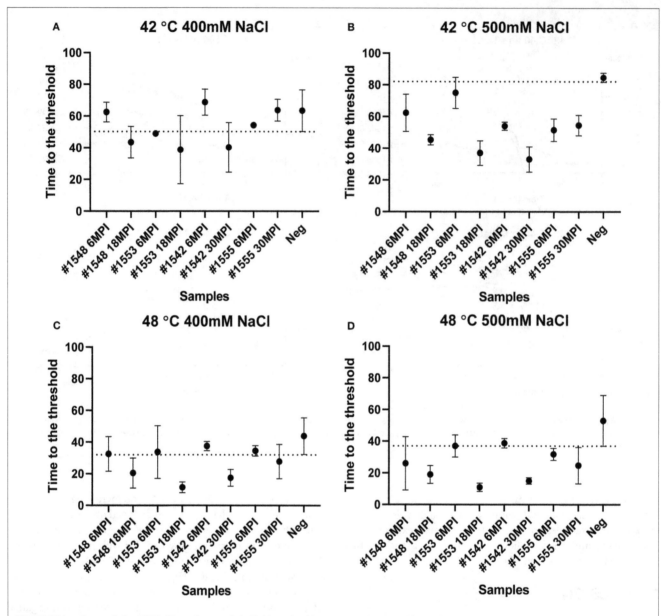

FIGURE 7 | Lag time analysis of RT-QuIC reactions seeded with biopsy fecal homogenates from preclinical white-tailed deer. Reaction conditions for each sample are followed as **(A)** 400 mM NaCl at 42°C, **(B)** 500 mM NaCl at 42°C, **(C)** 400 mM NaCl at 48°C, and **(D)** 500 mM NaCl at 48°C. Circles represent the mean and bars represent SD of four replicate reactions. The horizontal line is the cutoff.

also showed a shortened lag time for unseeded fibril formation under all reaction temperatures complicating discrimination of positive and negative samples. When we compare the results of RT-QuIC with NaI and NaCl, it is clear that NaI could be useful for quick detection with samples that have relatively high amount of prions. However, NaCl, despite the longer lag time, provided 100% sensitivity with better separation of positive assays from negative assays. This is in contrast to the previous report utilizing NaI where assays seeded with ear homogenate from CWD infected deer in the presence of NaI showed higher sensitivity and better specificity for prion detection than NaCl when used in RT-QuIC assays (28).

It is well-documented that fecal samples from cervids infected with CWD contain detectable prions (8–11). RT-QuIC seems practical to detect infectious prions from fecal samples of CWD infected cervids based on our study and previous reports. John and colleagues published a report that had shown RT-QuIC detection of fecal samples obtained from preclinical white-tailed deer. They tested fecal samples collected 20 and 30 months post inoculation, and they were only able to detect PrP^{Sc} from fecal sample collected at 30 months post inoculation possibly due to non-enrichment of the samples (11). Later, Cheng and colleagues showed that fecal prions of CWD infected elk could be detected with a NaPTA enrichment and detection by RT-QuIC

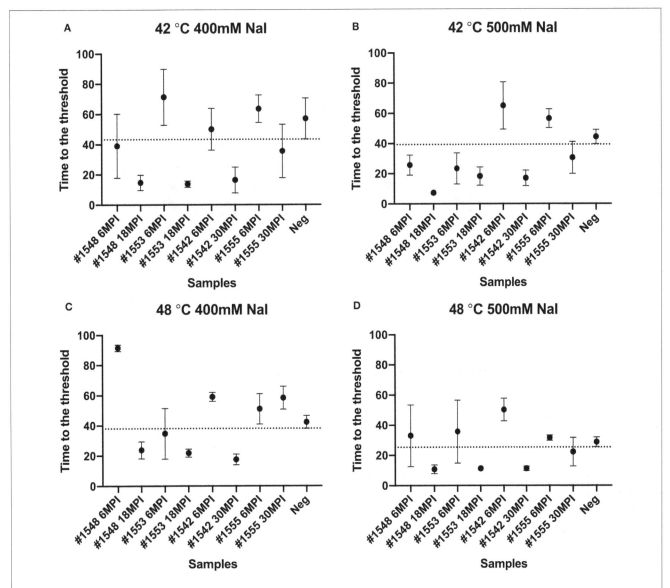

FIGURE 8 | Lag time analysis of RT-QuIC reactions seeded with biopsy fecal homogenates from preclinical white-tailed deer in the presence of NaI. Reactions conditions for each sample are followed as **(A)** 400 mM NaI at 42°C, **(B)** 500 mM NaI at 42°C, **(C)** 400 mM NaI at 48°C, and **(D)** 500 mM NaI at 48 °C. Circles represent the mean and bars represent SD of four replicate reactions. The horizontal line is the cutoff.

using recombinant mouse prion protein (10). Given their choice of substrate and reaction condition, they found it necessary to replace the substrate after 24 h of RT-QuIC reaction in order to see better detection of fecal prions. Henderson and colleagues also published a report indicating that fecal prions could be detected by RT-QuIC using Syrian hamster recombinant prion protein substrate and iron-oxide bead extraction as an enrichment rather than NaPTA precipitation (8). They also evaluated the reaction temperature, 37, 40, or 42°C to reduce the lag time for detection of positive samples and decrease spontaneous fibril formation in negative controls finding 37°C to be optimal for preventing spontaneous reactions while still allowing good sensitivity. In this work, we used recombinant

BV substrate which is generally reported as a universal substrate for detecting various prion diseases from both animals and humans by RT-QuIC (19) to detect CWD prions in fecal samples from white-tailed deer intranasal inoculated with CWD sourced from experimentally passaged through either white-tailed deer or racoon. Like Cheng and colleagues, we applied NaPTA precipitation for enrichment of prions in all fecal samples we collected. We also applied another enrichment methodology PAD-Beads, and has been previously reported for successfully enhanced RT-QuIC assays with brain homogenate of TSE inoculated animals (16). However, when PAD-Beads enrichment was applied for fecal samples, reactions with negative fecal samples were also seeded, which suggested that PAD-Beads may

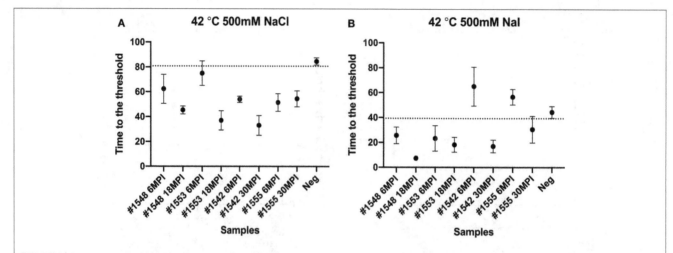

FIGURE 9 | Comparison of lag time analysis of RT-QuIC reactions seeded with biopsy fecal homogenates from preclinical white-tailed deer in the presence of 500 mM NaCl **(A)** or NaI **(B)**. Circles represent the mean and the bars represent SD of four replicate reactions. The horizontal line is the cutoff.

TABLE 2 | Lag time analysis from real-time quacking-induced conversion reactions seeded with preclinical fecal samples in different temperatures, different salt types, and concentrations.

	#1548 6 MPI	#1548 18 MPI	#1553 6 MPI	#1553 18 MPI	#1542 6 MPI	#1542 30 MPI	#1555 6 MPI	#1555 30 MPI	Neg
42°C 400 mM NaI	39.0 ± 21.2	14.7 ± 5.0	71.3 ± 18.5	13.7 ± 2.0	50.0 ± 13.8	16.3 ± 8.5	63.5 ± 9.1	35.5 ± 17.6	57.0 ± 13.6
42°C 500 mM NaI	25.7 ± 6.7	7.25 ± 1.9	23.3 ± 10.3	18.3 ± 6.0	65.0 ± 15.6	17.0 ± 5.1	56.5 ± 6.2	30.5 ± 10.6	44.3 ± 4.7
48°C 400 mM NaI	91.5 ± 2.1	23.8 ± 5.6	34.7 ± 16.8	21.8 ± 2.6	59.0 ± 2.9	17.5 ± 3.5	51.0 ± 10.0	58.3 ± 7.6	42.3 ± 4.3
48°C 500 mM NaI	33.0 ± 20.0	10.8 ± 2.9	35.7 ± 20.8	11.3 ± 1.0	50.3 ± 7.5	11.3 ± 1.5	31.5 ± 1.7	22.3 ± 9.5	28.8 ± 3.2
42°C 400 mM NaCl	62.5 ± 6.2	43.5 ± 9.9	49 ± 1.6	38.7 ± 21.5	68.7 ± 8.2	40.3 ± 15.6	54.3 ± 1.5	63.7 ± 6.9	63.5 ± 13.1
42°C 500 mM NaCl	62.3 ± 11.7	45.3 ± 3.2	75.0 ± 9.9	37.0 ± 7.8	54.0 ± 2.6	33.0 ± 7.9	51.5 ± 7.0	54.5 ± 6.4	84.6 ± 2.9
48°C 400 mM NaCl	32.5 ± 10.9	20.5 ± 9.5	33.8 ± 16.6	11.5 ± 3.4	37.5 ± 2.9	17.5 ± 5.3	34.5 ± 3.3	27.8 ± 10.8	43.9 ± 11.6
48°C 500 mM NaCl	26.0 ± 16.7	19.0 ± 5.6	37.0 ± 6.9	11.0 ± 2.6	38.7 ± 2.9	15.0 ± 2.0	31.7 ± 3.7	24.7 ± 11.4	53.0 ± 16.1

All times were recorded in hours.

not be suitable for fecal sample enrichment coupled with RT-QuIC. Most notable in this work is that by 6 months post-inoculation, prion seeding is identified in both TSE isolates. For the samples included in this study, white-tailed deer CWD showed an incubation time in the 21–24 months range, while CWD passaged through raccoons prior to inoculation in white-tailed deer exhibited an onset of clinical signs in excess of 34 months with one of our samples not showing clinical signs at 56 months post inoculation. This highlights the potential for early clinical detection of TSEs using NaPTA enrichment coupled with RT-QuIC for the detection of CWD. Overall, combination of BV substrate, different salt concentration, and temperature allowed us to detect infectious prions within short lag time with good specificity from clinical or preclinical white-tailed deer.

Altogether, we confirm again that RT-QuIC is a powerful tool to detect infectious fecal prions from CWD infected white-tailed deer. Use of feces is a non-invasive and non-stressing approach to sampling of animals, of particular importance for non-

domesticated animals that may be less tolerant to the handling required for sampling by other means. This is of importance to the management of both wild and farmed cervids and is also of use in experimental settings where repeated sampling of an individual animal would be otherwise difficult. Ultimately, fecal sampling may prove useful in the determination of disease prevalence in a geographic region or within a herd.

ETHICS STATEMENT

The animal study was reviewed and approved by National Animal Disease Center Institutional Animal Care and Use Committee.

AUTHOR CONTRIBUTIONS

SH and EN: conceptualization, methodology, and writing original draft. SH: formal analysis and investigation. EN and JG:

resources. EN: supervision. SH, EN, and JG: writing review and editing. All authors contributed to the article and approved the submitted version.

ACKNOWLEDGMENTS

The authors thank Semakaleng Lebepe-Mazur and Joseph Lesan for providing technical support for this project.

REFERENCES

1. Haley NJ, Hoover EA. Chronic wasting disease of cervids: current knowledge and future perspectives. *Annu Rev Anim Biosci.* (2015) 3:305–25. doi: 10.1146/annurev-animal-022114-111001
2. Benestad SL, Mitchell G, Simmons M, Ytrehus B, Vikoren T. First case of chronic wasting disease in Europe in a Norwegian free-ranging reindeer. *Vet Res.* (2016) 47:88. doi: 10.1186/s13567-016-0375-4
3. Department for Environment FaRA, Agency APH, VSPAT-ID. *Monitoring, Update on Chronic Wasting Disease in Europe* (2018). Available online at: https://assets.publishing.service.gov.uk/government/uploads/system/uploads/attachment_data/file/703368/sa-cwd-norway-20180425.pdf
4. Swedish National Veterinary Institute. *Map of Chronic Wasting Disease (CWD)*, Uppsala (2019).
5. Prusiner SB. Prions. *Proc Natl Acad Sci USA.* (1998) 95:13363–83. doi: 10.1073/pnas.95.23.13363
6. Collinge J. Prion diseases of humans and animals: their causes and molecular basis. *Annu Rev Neurosci.* (2001) 24:519–50. doi: 10.1146/annurev.neuro.24.1.519
7. Caughey B, Chesebro B. Transmissible spongiform encephalopathies and prion protein interconversions. *Adv Virus Res.* (2001) 56:277–311. doi: 10.1016/S0065-3527(01)56031-5
8. Henderson DM, Tennant JM, Haley NJ, Denkers ND, Mathiason CK, Hoover EA. Detection of chronic wasting disease prion seeding activity in deer and elk feces by real-time quaking-induced conversion. *J Gen Virol.* (2017) 98:1953–62. doi: 10.1099/jgv.0.000844
9. Cheng YC, Hannaoui S, John TR, Dudas S, Czub S, Gilch S. Real-time quaking-induced conversion assay for detection of CWD prions in fecal material. *J Vis Exp.* (2017) 127:56373. doi: 10.3791/56373
10. Cheng YC, Hannaoui S, John TR, Dudas S, Czub S, Gilch Early S. Non-invasive detection of chronic wasting disease prions in elk feces by real-time quaking induced conversion. *PLoS ONE.* (2016) 11:e0166187. doi: 10.1371/journal.pone.0166187
11. John TR, Schatzl HM, Gilch S. Early detection of chronic wasting disease prions in urine of pre-symptomatic deer by real-time quaking-induced conversion assay. *Prion.* (2013) 7:253–8. doi: 10.4161/pri.24430
12. Henderson DM, Denkers ND, Hoover CE, Garbino N, Mathiason CK, Hoover EA. Longitudinal detection of prion shedding in saliva and urine by chronic wasting disease-infected deer by real-time quaking-induced conversion. *J Virol.* (2015) 89:9338–47. doi: 10.1128/JVI.01118-15
13. Elder AM, Henderson DM, Nalls AV, Wilham JM, Caughey BW, Hoover EA, et al. *In vitro* detection of prionemia in TSE-infected cervids and hamsters. *PLoS ONE.* (2013) 8:e80203. doi: 10.1371/journal.pone.0080203
14. Atarashi R, Sano K, Satoh K, Nishida N. Real-time quaking-induced conversion: a highly sensitive assay for prion detection. *Prion.* (2011) 5:150–3. doi: 10.4161/pri.5.3.16893
15. Moore SJ, Smith JD, Greenlee MH, Nicholson EM, Richt JA, Greenlee JJ. Comparison of two US sheep scrapie isolates supports identification as separate strains. *Vet Pathol.* (2016) 53:1187–96. doi: 10.1177/0300985816629712
16. Hwang S, Dassanayake RP, Nicholson EM. PAD-beads enrichment enhances detection of PrP(Sc) using real-time quaking-induced conversion. *BMC Res Notes.* (2019) 12:806. doi: 10.1186/s13104-019-4842-7
17. Vrentas CE, Onstot S, Nicholson EM. A comparative analysis of rapid methods for purification and refolding of recombinant bovine prion protein. *Protein Expr Purif.* (2012) 82:380–8. doi: 10.1016/j.pep.2012.02.008
18. Hwang S, Tatum T, Lebepe-Mazur S, Nicholson EM. Preparation of lyophilized recombinant prion protein for TSE diagnosis by RT-QuIC. *BMC Res Notes.* (2018) 11:895. doi: 10.1186/s13104-018-3982-5

19. Orru CD, Groveman BR, Raymond LD, Hughson AG, Nonno R, Zou W, et al. Bank Vole prion protein as an apparently universal substrate for RT-QuIC-based detection and discrimination of prion strains. *PLoS Pathog.* (2015) 11:e1004983. doi: 10.1371/journal.ppat.1004983
20. Dassanayake RP, Orru CD, Hughson AG, Caughey B, Graca T, Zhuang D, et al. Sensitive and specific detection of classical scrapie prions in the brains of goats by real-time quaking-induced conversion. *J Gen Virol.* (2016) 97:803–12. doi: 10.1099/jgv.0.000367
21. Cheng K, Sloan A, Avery KM, Coulthart M, Carpenter M, Knox JD. Exploring physical and chemical factors influencing the properties of recombinant prion protein and the real-time quaking-induced conversion (RT-QuIC) assay. *PLoS ONE.* (2014) 9:e84812. doi: 10.1371/journal.pone.0084812
22. Orru CD, Hughson AG, Groveman BR, Campbell KJ, Anson KJ, Manca M, et al. Factors that improve RT-QuIC detection of prion seeding activity. *Viruses.* (2016) 8:140. doi: 10.3390/v8050140
23. Masujin K, Orru CD, Miyazawa K, Groveman BR, Raymond LD, Hughson AG, et al. Detection of atypical H-type bovine spongiform encephalopathy and discrimination of bovine prion strains by real-time quaking-induced conversion. *J Clin Microbiol.* (2016) 54:676–86. doi: 10.1128/JCM.02731-15
24. Orru CD, Favole A, Corona C, Mazza M, Manca M, Groveman BR, et al. Detection and discrimination of classical and atypical L-type bovine spongiform encephalopathy by real-time quaking-induced conversion. *J Clin Microbiol.* (2015) 53:1115–20. doi: 10.1128/JCM.02906-14
25. Hwang S, Greenlee JJ, Nicholson EM. Use of bovine recombinant prion protein and real-time quaking-induced conversion to detect cattle transmissible mink encephalopathy prions and discriminate classical and atypical L- and H-Type bovine spongiform encephalopathy. *PLoS ONE.* (2017) 12:e0172391. doi: 10.1371/journal.pone.0172391
26. Orru CD, Groveman BR, Hughson AG, Zanusso G, Coulthart MB, Caughey B. Rapid sensitive RT-QuIC detection of human Creutzfeldt-Jakob disease using cerebrospinal fluid. *MBio.* (2015) 6:e02451–14. doi: 10.1128/mBio.02451-14
27. Orru CD, Bongianni M, Tonoli G, Ferrari S, Hughson AG, Groveman BR, et al. A test for Creutzfeldt-Jakob disease using nasal brushings. *N Engl J Med.* (2014) 371:519–29. doi: 10.1056/NEJMoa1315200
28. Metrick MA II, do Carmo Ferreira N, Saijo E, Hughson AG, Kraus A, Orru C, et al. Million-fold sensitivity enhancement in proteopathic seed amplification assays for biospecimens by Hofmeister ion comparisons. *Proc Natl Acad Sci USA.* (2019) 116:23029–39. doi: 10.1073/pnas.1909322116

12

Immunofluorescence Targeting PBP2a Protein: A New Potential Methicillin Resistance Screening Test

Serenella Silvestri[1]*†, Elisa Rampacci[1], Valentina Stefanetti[1], Michele Trotta[2], Caterina Fani[2], Lucia Levorato[3], Chiara Brachelente[1‡] and Fabrizio Passamonti[1‡]

[1] Department of Veterinary Medicine, University of Perugia, Perugia, Italy, [2] CDVet Laboratorio Analisi Veterinarie, Rome, Italy, [3] Department of Medicine and Surgery, University of Perugia, Perugia, Italy

*Correspondence:
Serenella Silvestri
silvestri.serenell@gmail.com

The indiscriminate use of first-line drugs contributed to the spread of resistant bacteria, a major concern for both human and veterinary medicine. Methicillin resistance is acquired through the *mecA* gene, which encodes for the PBP2a protein and lends the resistance to β-lactams. Verifying the correspondence between gene harboring and protein expression and accelerating methicillin resistance diagnosis is critical to improve the management of antimicrobial administration and to reduce the spread of drug resistances. We tested the applicability of immunofluorescence targeting PBP2a protein to identify a new potential methicillin resistance screening test, ancillary to conventional culture methods. We collected 26 clinical *Staphylococcus pseudintermedius* (SP) isolates: 25 from canine pyoderma and 1 from dermatitis in a dog owner. SP is one of the most important etiological agents in canine pyoderma and can harbor the *mecA* gene. We performed PCR for *mecA* gene detection, broth microdilution (BMD) for phenotypic methicillin resistance, and immunofluorescence targeting PBP2a protein. Compared to the PCR as the gold standard, immunofluorescence showed an apparent prevalence of 34.6% vs. a true prevalence of 53.8%, with 100% specificity, 64.3% sensitivity, and 80.8% diagnostic accuracy. PBP2a expression showed isolate-dependent variability: in some isolates, most of the bacterial cells showed an intense and clearly membranous pattern, while in others only a few of them could be detected. Performing the assay in duplicate improved the diagnostic accuracy. Since the *mecA* gene is shared among the members of the *Staphylococcus* genus, the test can be applied to identify methicillin resistance independently from the staphylococcal species, both in human and animal samples. Being a rapid and easy method and providing the unique possibility to study the expression of PBP2a by directly visualizing the morphology, it could represent a new interesting tool for both research and diagnostics. To accelerate methicillin resistance diagnosis, it would be worth further testing of its performance on cytological samples.

Keywords: *Staphylococcus pseudintermedius*, methicillin resistance, fluorescent antibody technique, penicillin-binding protein 2a, antimicrobial drug resistance, pyoderma, dogs, humans

INTRODUCTION

The indiscriminate use of first-line drugs has sparked off the development of resistance mechanisms to antimicrobials by bacteria over time. This is a growing problem afflicting both human and veterinary medicine, so that, in 2019 the World Health Organization (WHO) included the antimicrobial-resistance in the list of the ten major threats to human health (1, 2). The spreading worldwide of methicillin resistance in *Staphylococcus aureus* (SA) is a particular health concern, that poses serious problems in the choice of the proper therapy (2, 3). Methicillin resistance is due to the acquisition and expression of the *mecA* gene. It is located on a mobile element called staphylococcal cassette chromosome *mec* (SCC*mec*) (4) and can be easily transferred between staphylococcal species (5).

Staphylococcus pseudintermedius (SP) is a normal colonizer of the dog skin, which often acts as an opportunistic pathogen, and is one of the most important pyogenic agents in canine pyoderma. Failure in identifying/resolving the primary cause of pyoderma, inappropriate therapy, antimicrobial resistance, or lack of owner's compliance can lead to infection recurrence or persistence and repeated therapy (6, 7).

Similarly to SA, SP can acquire resistance to β-lactams, the most used antimicrobial drugs, through the *mecA* gene. The gene encodes for penicillin-binding protein 2a (PBP2a), resulting in an altered cell wall composition and lower affinity for β-lactams (4, 8).

In SA, a strain-dependent variability in methicillin/oxacillin resistance level is reported (4, 9). Additionally, despite the detection of the *mecA* gene, some isolates were found susceptible to oxacillin (OXA). This status was defined as the "pre-methicillin-resistant" phenotype (10, 11). These previous findings suggest that the *mecA* gene harboring could not correspond to the protein expression. Indeed, Rohde et al. underlined the importance of verifying the congruity between gene presence and the expression of the related protein (12). In experimental conditions, they demonstrated that an immunofluorescence test can be successfully employed for this purpose, suggesting its use as a rapid screening test for susceptibility. To the best of our knowledge, similar studies have never been conducted on clinical isolates of SP.

Additionally, SP isolates harboring the *mecA* gene are often resistant to other classes of antimicrobial agents, showing a "multi-drug resistant" (MDR) phenotype, which increases the effort of establishing an adequate targeted therapy (7, 13–15). SP also has a zoonotic potential and people in close contact with dogs (e.g., pet owners, veterinarians) are at maximum risk for infection, especially if they have a compromised immune system (6, 7, 16).

In such a context, speeding up the detection of methicillin resistance is a key factor to avoid choosing an inappropriate antimicrobial agent that would affect both the disease resolution and the further development of resistances (13, 17–19).

Our study aimed firstly to test the possibility to use a commercially available antibody targeting PBP2a protein in methicillin-resistant *Staphylococcus aureus* (MRSA), never validated in immunofluorescence or tested in methicillin-resistant *Staphylococcus pseudintermedius* (MRSP). Secondly, to evaluate the performance of immunofluorescence targeting PBP2a protein on clinical SP isolates from canine pyoderma. We compared those findings with the minimum inhibitory concentration (MIC) of OXA obtained by broth microdilution (BMD) and with PCR for the *mecA* gene, to investigate the agreement between the methods, as well as the matching between *mecA* gene harboring and PBP2a protein expression. Finally, we sought to explore the potentiality of this technique as a rapid screening test ancillary to conventional culture methods.

MATERIALS AND METHODS

Bacteria Isolation and Antimicrobial Susceptibility Testing

Twenty-six SP isolates, previously included in a larger study on susceptibility testing methods comparison (20), were used in this study: 25 were isolated from canine pyoderma and 1 from a dermatitis sample of a dog owner. Only one isolate per subject was collected. Bacteria were isolated in clinical microbiology laboratories of Central Italy during routine work throughout 2019. Identification of the isolates was performed to the species level both by PCR-restriction fragment length polymorphism approach (RFLP), based on the detection of the MboI restriction site on *pta* locus (21), and by the Vitek-2 system (bioMérieux Inc., Durham, NC), using the most up-to-date GP ID cards, as previously described (20). Before testing, all isolates were cultured from −20°C storage onto Mannitol Salt Agar plates supplemented with 5% v/v Egg Yolk Emulsion and sub-cultured on cation-adjusted Mueller-Hinton agar (CAMHA). The MICs of OXA for the selected isolates, which is the recommended method to phenotypically predict methicillin resistance in SP, were investigated by BMD as previously described (20). Additionally, the MICs for amoxicillin/clavulanate, cephalothin, gentamicin, enrofloxacin, clindamycin, trimethoprim/sulfamethoxazole, doxycycline, and mupirocin were also determined (20). Bacteria resistant to at least three antimicrobial classes were classified as MDR (22). A methicillin-resistant SP isolate, from which the *mecA* gene was sequenced, was used as a positive control in PCR and immunofluorescence assay.

PCR-Based Identification of *mecA* Gene

PCR for the *mecA* gene is the gold standard method for the detection of methicillin resistance (23). DNA from pure SP cultures was extracted by boiling. Bacterial colonies were resuspended in 500 μL of ultrapure molecular biology-grade water and subjected to boiling at 100°C. The suspension was cooled on ice and centrifuged at 14,000 rpm for 10 min. The supernatants were collected for conventional PCR analyses. Single PCR amplifications were performed in 25-μL reaction mixtures using Recombinant Taq DNA polymerase (Takara, Dalian, China) according to the manufacturer's instructions. The chromosomic *mecA* gene was amplified using 0.4 μM of primer f-AAAATCGATGGTAAAGGTTGGC and r-AGTTCTGCAGTACCGGATTTGC (Sigma–Genosys, Milan, Italy) (24). All PCR were performed in the GeneAmp PCR System 2400 thermocycler (Applied Biosystems, Foster City, CA), according to the following amplification conditions: initial denaturation at 94°C for 5 min, followed by 40 cycles of amplification at 94°C for 30 s, annealing at 55°C for 30 s, extension at 72°C for 1 min, and a final extension step at 72°C for 5 min. Positive control, from which the *mecA* gene was previously sequenced, a negative control (negative sample), as well as a negative reaction mix control (containing the reagents and water instead of DNA), were included in each run. The presence and size of the amplified products were confirmed by electrophoresis on 1.5% agarose gel.

Immunofluorescence

For bacteria fixation, a modified protocol was used (12). Briefly, all isolates were fixed adding 3 volumes of 4% formaldehyde in Tris-buffered saline (TBS) buffer. After 1 h incubation at 4°C, bacteria were washed 3 times through centrifugation and resuspension in TBS buffer. Finally, bacteria were suspended in a 1:1 ethanol/TBS solution and used directly. Bacteria solution could be also stored at −20°C before use. Ten μl of each bacteria solution were pipetted on a glass slide and dried for 3 min at 52°C on a hot plate. Slides were stored in the dark until used.

To permeabilize bacteria, slides were incubated with a lysozyme solution (213 μg/ml in TRIS buffer 50 mM, pH 7; Lysozyme, 8259.1, Carl Roth, Karlsruhe, Germany) for 30 min at room temperature (RT) in a humidified chamber and rinsed in TBS buffer. Slides were blocked with blocking buffer (2% bovine serum albumin in TBS buffer; bovine serum albumin solution, A7034, Sigma-Aldrich, Saint Louis, MO) for 10 min at RT. Since the *mecA* gene is shared by the *Staphylococcus* genus (5, 25), we used a specific anti-PBP2a primary antibody validated for application in ELISA and WB to detect MRSA (130-10073, RayBiotech, Peachtree Corners, GA), thus testing its applicability in immunofluorescence and in the detection of MRSP. Slides were incubated overnight at 4°C in a humidified chamber with the rabbit primary antibody diluted 1:200 in blocking buffer. Slides were rinsed in TBS and incubated with a biotinylated goat anti-rabbit secondary antibody (BA-1000, Vector Laboratories, Burlingame, CA) diluted 1:200 in TBS for 1 h at RT. After rinsing in TBS buffer, samples were incubated in a dark humidified chamber with the Alexa Fluor® 488 streptavidin conjugate (S-32354, Life Technologies, Paisley, UK) diluted 1:200 in blocking buffer for 1 h at RT. Finally, the rinsed slides were incubated in the dark with 4′, 6-diamidino-2-phenylindole, dilactate (DAPI; D3571, Invitrogen, Eugene, OR) diluted 1:1000 in TBS buffer for 5 min at RT. After carefully rinsing in TBS, slides were coverslipped with ProLong™ Gold antifade mountant (P36930, TermoFisher Scientific, Rockford, USA). As a positive control for the immunofluorescence assay, we used the isolate used for PCR validation, which resulted as methicillin-resistant also by BMD. The same isolate was used as a negative control, omitting the primary antibody. To verify the specificity of the antibody, we selected one of the isolates confirmed for being methicillin-sensitive both by PCR and BMD as additional negative control (**Table 1**).

TABLE 1 | Results of methicillin resistance investigation in the SP isolates and their MDR status.

Isolate	MIC*	Category	PCR	IF**	MDR
Pos ctr	>32	R	+	+	+
Neg ctr	≤0.125	S	−	−	−
SP01	≤0.125	S	−	−	−
SP02	≤0.125	S	−	−	−
SP03	≤0.125	S	−	−	−
SP04	>32	R	+	+	+
SP05	>32	R	+	+	+
SP06	>32	R	+	+	+
SP07	>32	R	+	+	+
SP08	≤0.125	S	−	−	−
SP09	8	R	+	+	+
SP10	≤0.125	S	−	−	−
SP11	1	R	−	−	+
SP12	>32	R	+	+	+
SP13	>32	R	+	−	+
SP14	1	R	+	−	−
SP15	0.25	S	−	−	−
SP16	≤0.125	S	−	−	−
SP17	>32	R	+	+	+
SP18	≤0.125	S	−	−	−
SP19	>32	R	+	−	+
SP20	≤0.125	S	−	−	−
SP21	>32	R	+	+	+
SP22	0.5	R	+	−	−
SP23	1	R	+	−	ND
SP24	≤0.125	S	−	−	−

R, resistant; S, sensitive; ND, not determined; SP24, human isolate.
*Results of BMD were previously published (15).
**The immunofluorescence (IF) results after 2 replicates are shown.

We performed two technical replicates of the immunofluorescence assay. Except for the positive and negative controls, all the slides were blindly evaluated for PBP2a expression by one operator to avoid inter-operator variability. When at least one of the immunofluorescence assays was positive, we considered the PBP2a expressed. Samples were evaluated using a fluorescent microscope Olympus BX51 equipped with the camera Nikon mod.DS-Qi2Mc. NIS-ELEMENTS D software was used for image analysis.

Statistical Analysis

For descriptive statistics data are shown as absolute and relative frequencies. To evaluate the inter-method agreement, we calculated both the categorical agreement and Cohen's kappa. The categorical agreement is represented by the proportion of the isolates producing the same category result (methicillin-sensitive or -resistant) as compared to the reference method. Major error (ME) was reported when the reference test returned a sensitive result, while the method under evaluation returned resistant. Conversely, a very major error (VME) indicates that the reference test returned a resistant result but the method under evaluation returned sensitive (26). Unweighted Cohen's kappa with 95% confidence interval ($CI_{95\%}$) based on bootstrap (10,000 replicates) was calculated and interpreted as previously described (27). Finally, referring to PCR as the gold standard, the sensitivity, specificity, positive predictive value (PPV), negative predictive value (NPV), likelihood ratio for a positive test, likelihood ratio for a negative test, and diagnostic accuracy of the immunofluorescence assay were also calculated according to previous literature (28, 29). Statistical analyses were performed using the software R (R version 4.0.3) (30).

RESULTS

We examined 25 SP isolates from canine pyoderma and 1 from a dermatitis sample of a dog owner (**Table 1**). Based on MIC determination, 57.7% (15/26) of the samples were resistant to OXA and 52% (13/25; one case not determined) were MDR. The majority of MDR SP were OXA resistant (92.3%, 12/13; **Figure 1**).

Based on the results of PCR, 14/26 (53.8%) SP isolates harbored the *mecA* gene, and, with only one exception, results of MIC evaluation and PCR were in agreement. Specifically, the isolate SP11 was classified as resistant to OXA with a MIC of 1 mg/L, but PCR did not detect the *mecA* gene for this SP. Consequently, one ME was produced and the categorical agreement between the two methods was 96.1% (25/26).

Overall, a clear division between OXA MICs was found between *mecA*-positive and -negative isolates. The majority of *mecA*-positive SP (10/14, 71.4%) showed an OXA MIC > 32 mg/L while, except for SP11, all *mecA*-negative isolates had an OXA MIC ≤ 0.25 mg/L (11/12, 91.6%;

Supplementary Figure 1A). A low level of resistance to OXA was found also for the isolates SP14 and SP21, but, in these cases, PCR detected the *mecA* gene (**Table 1**).

In the immunofluorescence assay, the PBP2a expression has a clear membranous pattern with isolate-dependent variability: while in some isolates the expression was evident in most of the bacteria on the slide, in others PBP2a was expressed by a minor proportion of SP, sometimes making the detection challenging (**Figure 2** and **Supplementary Table 1**). The agreement between the two immunofluorescence replicates was almost perfect ($k = 0.82$, $CI_{95\%} = 0.52–1.00$), since only for 2/26 (7.7%) isolates the results disagreed. In both cases, the positive bacteria identified on the slides were scarce. However, when at least one of the two replicates showed detectable PBP2a protein, the isolate was classified as positive. Overall, 9/26 isolates resulted positive (**Table 1**), with an apparent prevalence of 34.6% vs. a true prevalence of 53.8% (based on PCR results; **Table 2**). Indeed, although the agreement with PCR was substantial ($k = 0.62$, $CI_{95\%} = 0.34–0.91$), in 5/26 (19.2%) isolates PBP2a was not detected while PCR demonstrated *mecA* gene harboring (**Figure 3**). The isolate SP11, where PCR and MIC showed opposite results, was correctly classified as negative for PBP2a expression through both immunofluorescence replicates. Consequently, the categorical agreement with PCR for the *mecA* gene was 80.8% (21/26), while with OXA MIC was 76.9% (20/26). Particularly, in 3/5 (60%) cases in which PBP2a expression was not evident by immunofluorescence, the MICs ranged between 0.5 and 1 mg/L (**Supplementary Figure 1B**), while when it was ≥8 mg/L PBP2a expression was generally detected (9/11, 81.8%).

Since no false-positive results were obtained, both the specificity and the positive predictive value (PPV) reached 100%,

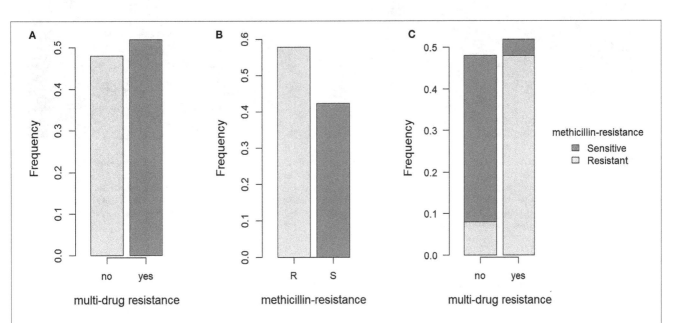

FIGURE 1 | Methicillin resistance and multi-drug resistance in SP isolates. **(A)** Proportions of multidrug-resistant (MDR) SP and not MDR SP. R, resistant; S, sensitive. **(B)** Proportions of methicillin-resistant SP (MRSP) and methicillin-sensitive SP (MSSP). **(C)** Proportions of MRSP and MSSP in MDR SP and not MDR SP.

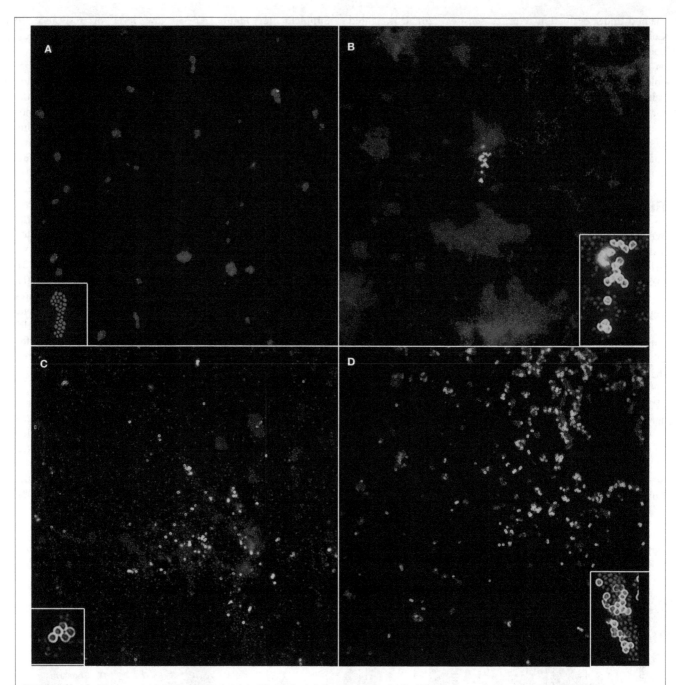

FIGURE 2 | Immunofluorescence targeting PBP2a protein in SP, showing isolate-dependent variability in PBP2a expression level. **(A)** Negative control. Insert: a cluster of SP whose cell walls stained negative and only the nucleoid can be seen (blue). **(B)** A cluster of SP clearly expressing PBP2a protein (green) is shown; the majority of SP does not express the protein. Insert: a magnification of cell walls staining positive, with a well-defined membranous pattern. **(C)** Several SP, both in clusters and sparse, stained positive, while a large proportion of them is negative. Insert: bacteria with cell wall expression of PBP2a protein. **(D)** Most of the SP showed positive cell walls. Insert: a cluster of bacteria where most of them have distinct positivity of the cell walls, together with other negative bacteria where only the nucleoid is stained. Blue: DAPI; Green: Alexa Fluor® 488.

while the sensitivity and the negative predictive value (NPV) were lower. Overall, the diagnostic accuracy of the method was 80.8% (CI$_{95\%}$ = 60.6–93.4%; **Table 2**).

Finally, in our case series, all the SP isolates showing positivity by immunofluorescence were MDR bacteria.

DISCUSSION

Pyoderma is a common skin problem in the canine species and frequently leads to antimicrobial use in clinical practice (7). Since the spreading of resistant bacteria is growing and therapeutic

TABLE 2 | Measures of diagnostic test accuracy.

Measure	Estimate	$CI_{95\%}$
Apparent prevalence	34.6%	17.2–55.7%
True prevalence	53.8%	33.4–73.4%
Sensitivity	64.3%	35.1–87.2%
Specificity	100%	64.0–100%
Positive predictive value	100%	55.5–100%
Negative predictive value	70.6%	44.0–89.7%
Likelyhood ratio for positive test	inf	NA
Likelyhood ratio for negative test	0.357	0.177–0.721
Diagnostic accuracy	80.8%	60.6–93.4%

$CI_{95\%}$, 95% confidence interval.
inf, infinity; NA, non applicable.

options are limited, antimicrobial management optimization is crucial (1, 2, 31). SP, one of the most important etiological agents involved in canine pyoderma (32), can harbor the *mecA* gene that, coding for the PBP2a protein, mediates the methicillin resistance (4).

We tested a new technique potentially applicable in diagnostics as a rapid screening test to detect PBP2a expression. This would help to identify methicillin-resistant staphylococci, providing the clinician with an initial guide for starting the therapy while waiting for antimicrobial susceptibility test results.

Comparing the immunofluorescence assay to PCR for the *mecA* gene, the gold standard for identification of MRSP, the agreement was substantial, but in 19.2% of cases it failed to detect MRSP. Given the specificity of the antibody chosen, we had no false-positive results and the specificity was 100%. However, the sensitivity of the assay was much lower, being equal to 64.3%. Often, the lack of detection of methicillin resistance involved the isolates with low MICs (0.5–1 mg/L). This could be due to the lower sensitivity of immunofluorescence compared to PCR. Additionally, an isolate-dependent variability in PBP2a expression level was observed in our study. When the positive bacteria on the slide are a few, they could be missed, resulting in false-negative results. In our case series, in 2 methicillin-resistant SP isolates, one of the replicates failed to detect the expression of the PBP2a protein. Hence, repeating the assay in duplicate can improve the diagnostic accuracy. Additionally, *mecA* gene expression can be induced by OXA and cefoxitin stimulation (23, 33), but the isolates used in our study for immunofluorescence were not previously exposed to antimicrobials, in order to mimic diagnostic conditions. As a result, the PBP2a protein could have a lower or no expression in some isolates, affecting the general sensitivity of the method. Finally, the sample size we used was relatively limited, hence the lacking of PBP2a detection in a few samples might be overweighed. Testing the method on a larger number of samples might help obtain a more precise evaluation of its performance.

Whit one exception, the results of MIC and PCR overlapped in all cases. The mechanism of OXA resistance, in this case, remains to be determined. Notably, immunofluorescence classification of this isolate was in agreement with PCR, which is why the

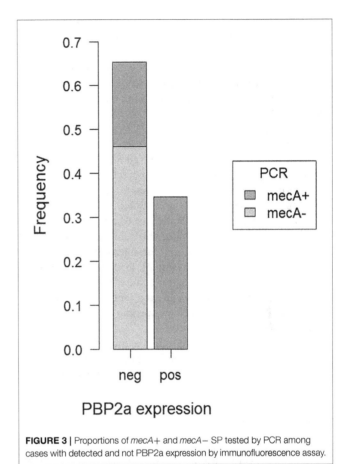

FIGURE 3 | Proportions of *mecA+* and *mecA–* SP tested by PCR among cases with detected and not PBP2a expression by immunofluorescence assay.

categorical agreement with BMD was lower compared to those with PCR.

Despite its limitations, immunofluorescence has several advantages. In our study, the diagnostic accuracy reached 80.8%, showing high reliability when methicillin-resistant SP are identified (PPV = 100%; NPV = 70.6%). In agreement with previous studies reporting a high prevalence of MDR among MRSP (14, 34), in our case series, all of the isolates expressing PBP2a protein were also MDR. Accordingly, the detection of PBP2a expression could help suspect MDR. Results of immunofluorescence targeting PBP2a protein can be rapidly obtained, especially if the primary antibody incubation time is shortened. The method might also be easily applied on cytological samples with the potential to get the results within the same day, so it would be worth testing it in this application. As a further development, a modified method could be employed in immunohistochemistry, allowing the study of the resistant bacteria directly on tissue samples and representing a new interesting tool for both research and diagnostics. However, the suitability of the selected antibody in immunohistochemistry has to be determined. Moreover, since the *mecA* gene is shared by several staphylococci, including SA (5, 25), the methicillin resistance could be detected independently from the staphylococcal species isolated in both human and animal hosts.

To the best of the author's knowledge, two commercially available kits can be used for the rapid detection of PBP2a protein on cultured colonies. The Alere PBP2a Culture Colony Test is a sensitive and specific immunochromatographic assay to test isolates. Although the test itself is very simple and rapid, the colonies should be cultured for at least 24 h and the highest sensitivity is reached when bacteria are harvested from the edges of the cefoxitin zone of growth inhibition (23, 25). The other is the PBP2a latex agglutination test, whose sensitivity and specificity are almost comparable to PCR (35, 36). However, it is technically more complicated and needs additional equipment (3). Being performed on isolates, these commercial tests strictly depend on the timing of bacteria growth. Compared to those tests, the immunofluorescence assay has a lower sensitivity but a corresponding specificity. It is a simple technique and can be carried on in pathology laboratories that routinely perform immunocytochemistry or immunohistochemistry (ICC/IHC) and are equipped with a fluorescent microscope. It is rapid and, if applied on cytological samples, it might be carried out independently from bacteriological culture. Finally, it provides the unparalleled possibility to study the expression of PBP2a by directly visualizing the morphology, opening new possibilities for research purposes.

In conclusion, we demonstrated that immunofluorescence can be successfully used to detect the PBP2a protein in SP isolates, hence methicillin-resistant bacteria. When compared to the gold standard method (PCR for *mecA* gene), immunofluorescence targeting PBP2a protein showed good diagnostic accuracy, with 100% specificity, although the sensitivity is lower. It is a rapid and easy method that can represent a new interesting tool for both research and diagnostics. It would be worth testing its performance on cytological samples to further accelerate the diagnosis of methicillin resistance in SP.

AUTHOR CONTRIBUTIONS

SS: conceptualization, design, investigation, first draft writing, data acquisition, data analysis, visualization, and software. ER: conceptualization, design, investigation, first draft sections writing, data acquisition, data analysis, and software. VS: conceptualization, investigation, data acquisition, and software. MT and LL: investigation, data acquisition, and software. CF: funding acquisition, resources, and supervision. CB: conceptualization, design, resources, and supervision. FP: conceptualization, funding acquisition, resources, and supervision. All authors contributed to the manuscript's critical revision and editing and approved the submitted version.

REFERENCES

1. World Health Organization (WHO) I. Ten *Treats to Global Health in 2019*. (2019). Available online at: https://www.who.int/news-room/spotlight/ten-threats-to-global-health-in-2019
2. Yarbrough M, Lainhart W, Burnham C-A. Epidemiology, clinical characteristics, antimicrobial susceptibility profiles of human clinical isolates of Staphylococcus intermedius group. *J Clin Microbiol*. (2018) 56:e01788–17. doi: 10.1128/JCM.01788-17
3. Yamada K, Wanchun J, Ohkura T, Murai A, Hayakawa R, Kinoshita K, et al. Detection of methicillin-resistant *Staphylococcus aureus* using a specific anti-PBP2a chicken IgY antibody. *Jpn J Infect Dis*. (2013) 66:103–8. doi: 10.7883/yoken.66.103
4. Ballhausen B, Kriegeskorte A, Schleimer N, Peters G, Becker K. The mecA homolog mecC confers resistance against β-lactams in *Staphylococcus aureus* irrespective of the genetic strain background. *Antimicrob Agents Chemother*. (2014) 58:3791–8. doi: 10.1128/AAC.02731-13
5. Somayaji R, Priyantha MAR, Rubin JE, Church D. Human infections due to *Staphylococcus pseudintermedius*, an emerging zoonosis of canine origin: report of 24 cases. *Diagn Microbiol Infect Dis*. (2016) 85:471–6. doi: 10.1016/j.diagmicrobio.2016.05.008
6. Bajwa J. Canine superficial pyoderma and therapeutic considerations. *Diagnostic Dermatology*. (2016) 52:204–6.
7. Loeffler A, Lloyd D. What has changed in canine pyoderma. A narrative review. *Vet J*. (2018) 235:73–82. doi: 10.1016/j.tvjl.2018.04.002
8. Priyantha R, Gaunt MC, Rubin JE. Antimicrobial susceptibility of *Staphylococcus pseudintermedius* colonizing healthy dogs in Saskatoon, Canada. *Can Vet J La Rev Vet Can*. (2016) 57:65–9.
9. Pardos de la Gandara M, Borges V, Chung M, Milheiriço C, Gomes JP, de Lencastre H, et al. Genetic determinants of high-level oxacillin resistance in methicillin-resistant *Staphylococcus aureus*. *Antimicrob Agents Chemother*. (2018) 62:e00206–18. doi: 10.1128/AAC.01096-18
10. Kuwahara-Arai K, Kondo N, Hori S, Tateda-Suzuki E, Hiramatsu K. Suppression of methicillin resistance in a mecA-containing pre-methicillin-resistant Staphylococcus aureus strain is caused by the mecI-mediated repression of PBP 2 production. *Antimicrob Agents Chemother*. (1996) 40:2680–5. doi: 10.1128/AAC.40.12.2680

11. Oliveira DC, de Lencastre H. Methicillin-resistance in *Staphylococcus aureus* is not affected by the overexpression in trans of the mecA gene repressor: a surprising observation. Van Melderen L, editor. *PLoS ONE*. (2011) 6:e23287. doi: 10.1371/journal.pone.0023287
12. Rohde A, Hammerl JA, Al Dahouk S. Rapid screening for antibiotic resistance elements on the RNA transcript, protein and enzymatic activity level. *Ann Clin Microbiol Antimicrob*. (2016) 15:55. doi: 10.1186/s12941-016-0167-8
13. Perreten V, Kadlec K, Schwarz S, Andrsson UG, Finn M, Greko C, et al. Clonal spread of methicillin-resistant *Staphylococcus pseudintermedius* in Europe and North America: an international multicentre study. *J Antimicrob Chemother*. (2010) 65:1145–54. doi: 10.1093/jac/dkq078
14. Stefanetti V, Bietta A, Pascucci L, Marenzoni ML, Coletti M, Franciosini MP, et al. Investigation of the antibiotic resistance and biofilm formation of *Staphylococcus pseudintermedius* strains isolated from canine pyoderma. *Vet Ital*. (2017) 53:289–96. doi: 10.12834/VetIt.465.2275.6
15. Ventrella G, Moodley A, Grandolfo E, Parisi A, Corrente M, Buonavoglia D, et al. Frequency, antimicrobial susceptibility and clonal distribution of methicillin-resistant *Staphylococcus pseudintermedius* in canine clinical samples submitted to a veterinary diagnostic laboratory in Italy: A 3-year retrospective investigation. *Vet Microbiol*. (2017) 211:103–6. doi: 10.1016/j.vetmic.2017.09.015
16. Phumthanakorn N, Schwendener S, Donà V, Chanchaithong P, Perreten V, Prapasarakul N. Genomic insights into methicillin-resistant *Staphylococcus pseudintermedius* isolates from dogs and humans of the same sequence types reveals diversity in prophages and pathogenicity islands. *PLoS ONE*. (2021) 16:e0254382. doi: 10.1371/journal.pone.0254382
17. Epstein CR, Yam WC, Peiris JSM, Epstein RJ. Methicillin-resistant commensal staphylococci in healthy dogs as a potential zoonotic reservoir for community-acquired antibiotic resistance. *Infect Genet Evol*. (2009) 9:283–5. doi: 10.1016/j.meegid.2008.11.003
18. Vanderhaeghen W, Van De Velde E, Crombé F, Polis I, Hermans K, Haesebrouck F, et al. Screening for methicillin-resistant staphylococci in dogs admitted to a veterinary teaching hospital. *Res Vet Sci*. (2012) 93:133–6. doi: 10.1016/j.rvsc.2011.06.017
19. Kjellman EE, Slettemeås JS, Small H, Sunde M. Methicillin-resistant *Staphylococcus pseudintermedius* (MRSP) from healthy dogs in Norway -

occurrence, genotypes and comparison to clinical MRSP. *Microbiologyopen.* (2015) 4:857–66. doi: 10.1002/mbo3.258

20. Rampacci E, Trotta M, Fani C, Silvestri S, Stefanetti V, Brachelente C, et al. Comparative performances of Vitek-2, disk diffusion, and broth microdilution for antimicrobial susceptibility testing of canine *Staphylococcus pseudintermedius*. *J Clin Microbiol.* (2021) 59:e0034921. doi: 10.1128/JCM.00349-21

21. Bannoehr J, Franco A, Iurescia M, Battisti A, Fitzgerald JR. Molecular diagnostic identification of *Staphylococcus pseudintermedius*. *J Clin Microbiol.* (2009) 47:469–71. doi: 10.1128/JCM.01915-08

22. Magiorakos A-P, Srinivasan A, Carey R, Carmeli Y, Falagas M, Giske C, et al. Multidrug-resistant, extensively drug-resistant and pandrug-resistant bacteria: an international expert proposal for interim standard definitions for acquired resistance. *Clin Microbiol Infect.* (2012) 18:268–81. doi: 10.1111/j.1469-0691.2011.03570.x

23. Wu M, Burnham C, Westblade L, Dien Bard J, Lawhon S, Wallace M, et al. Evaluation of oxacillin and cefoxitin disk and MIC breakpoints for prediction of methicillin resistance in human and veterinary isolates of Staphylococcus intermedius Group. Richter SS, editor. *J Clin Microbiol.* (2016) 54:535–42. doi: 10.1128/JCM.02864-15

24. Strommenger B, Kettlitz C, Werner G, Witte W. Multiplex PCR assay for simultaneous detection of nine clinically relevant antibiotic resistance genes in *Staphylococcus aureus*. *J Clin Microbiol.* (2003) 41:4089–94. doi: 10.1128/JCM.41.9.4089-4094.2003

25. Arnold A, Burnham C-A, Ford B, Lawhon S, McAllister S, Lonsway D, et al. Evaluation of an immunochromatographic assay for rapid detection of penicillin-binding protein 2a in human and animal Staphylococcus intermedius Group, *Staphylococcus lugdunensis*, and *Staphylococcus schleiferi* clinical isolates. *J Clin Microbiol.* (2016) 54:745–8. doi: 10.1128/JCM.02869-15

26. Humphries, Romney M Ambler J, Mitchell SL, Castanheira M, Dingle T, Hindler JA, et al. CLSI methods development and standardization working group best practices for evaluation of antimicrobial susceptibility tests. *J Clin Microbiol.* (2018) 56:e01934-17. doi: 10.1128/JCM.01934-17

27. Landis JR, Koch GG. The measurement of observer agreement for categorical data. *Biometrics.* (1977) 33:159–74. doi: 10.2307/25 29310

28. Šimundić A-M. Measures of diagnostic accuracy: basic definitions. *EJIFCC.* (2009) 19:203–11.

29. Shim SR, Kim S-J, Lee J. Diagnostic test accuracy: application and practice using R software. *Epidemiol Health.* (2019) 41:e2019007. doi: 10.4178/epih.e2019007

30. R Core Team. *R: A Language and Environment for Statistical Computing.* Vienna: R Foundation for Statistical Computing (2020).

31. Committee for Medicinal Products for Veterinary Use I. *Reflection Paper on Meticillin-Resistant Staphylococcus pseudintermedius.* London: European Medicine Agency (2010).

32. Miller W, Griffin C, Campbell K. *Muller&Kirk's Small Animal Dermatology. 7th ed.* Saint Louis, MI: Elsevier (2013).

33. Dupieux C, Bouchiat C, Larsen A, Pichon B, Holmes M, Teale C, et al. Detection of mecC-positive *Staphylococcus aureus*: what to expect from immunological tests targeting PBP2a? *J Clin Microbiol.* (2017) 55:1961–3. doi: 10.1128/JCM.00068-17

34. Little SV, Bryan LK, Hillhouse AE, Cohen ND, Lawhon SD. Characterization of agr Groups of *Staphylococcus pseudintermedius* Isolates from Dogs in Texas. D'Orazio SEF, editor. *mSphere.* (2019) 4:e00033-19. doi: 10.1128/mSphere.00033-19

35. Cavassini M, Wenger A, Jaton K, Blanc DS, Bille J. Evaluation of MRSA-Screen, a simple anti-PBP 2a slide latex agglutination kit, for rapid detection of methicillin resistance in *Staphylococcus aureus*. *J Clin Microbiol.* (1999) 37:1591–4. doi: 10.1128/JCM.37.5.1591-1594.1999

36. Sakoulas G, Gold HS, Venkataraman L, Degirolami PC, Eliopoulos GM, Qian Q. Methicillin-resistant *Staphylococcus aureus*: Comparison of susceptibility testing methods and analysis of mecA-positive susceptible strains. *J Clin Microbiol.* (2001) 39:3946–51. doi: 10.1128/JCM.39.11.3946-3951. 2001

13

New Diagnostic Assays for Differential Diagnosis between the Two Distinct Lineages of Bovine Influenza D Viruses and Human Influenza C Viruses

Faten A. Okda[1,2]*, Elizabeth Griffith[3], Ahmed Sakr[4], Eric Nelson[5] and Richard Webby[1]*

[1] Department of Infectious Diseases, St. Jude Children's Research Hospital, Memphis, TN, United States, [2] Veterinary Division, National Research Center, Cairo, Egypt, [3] Department of Chemical and Therapeutic, St. Jude Children's Research Hospital, Memphis, TN, United States, [4] Department of Business Administration and Management, Dakota State University, Madison, SD, United States, [5] Veterinary & Biomedical Sciences Department, Animal Disease Research and Diagnostic Laboratory, South Dakota State University, Brookings, SD, United States

*Correspondence:
Faten A. Okda
faten.okda@stjude.org;
faten.okda@jacks.sdstate.edu
Richard Webby
richard.webby@stjude.org

Influenza D virus (IDV), a novel orthomyxovirus, is currently emerging in cattle worldwide. It shares >50% sequence similarity with the human influenza C virus (HICV). Two clades of IDV are currently co-circulating in cattle herds in the U.S. New assays specific for each lineage are needed for accurate surveillance. Also, differential diagnosis between zoonotic human influenza C virus and the two clades of IDV are important to assess the zoonotic potential of IDV. We developed an enzyme-linked immunosorbent assay (ELISA) based on two different epitopes HEF and NP and four peptides, and fluorescent focus neutralization assay to differentiate between IDV bovine and swine clades. Calf sera were obtained, and bovine samples underwent surveillance. Our results highlight the importance of position 215 with 212 in determining the heterogeneity between the two lineages. We needed IFA and FFN for tissue culture–based analysis and a BSL2 facility for analyzing virus interactions. Unfortunately, these are not available in many veterinary centers. Hence, our second aim was to develop an iELISA using specific epitopes to detect two lineages of IDVs simultaneously. Epitope-iELISA accurately detects neutralizing and non-neutralizing antibodies against the IDV in non-BSL2 laboratories and veterinary clinics and is cost-effective and sensitive. To differentiate between IDVs and HICVs, whole antigen blocking, polypeptides, and single-peptide ELISAs were developed. A panel of ferret sera against both viruses was used. Results suggested that both IDV and ICV had a common ancestor, and IDV poses a zoonotic risk to individuals with prior or current exposure to cattle. IDV peptides IANAGVK (286–292 aa), KTDSGR (423–428 aa), and RTLTPAT (448–455 aa) could differentiate between the two viruses, whereas peptide AESSVNPGAKPQV (203–215 aa) detected the presence of IDV in human sera but could not deny that it could be ICV, because the only two conserved influenza C peptides shared 52% sequence similarity with IDV and cross-reacted with IDV. However, blocking ELISAs differentiated between the two viruses. Diagnostic tools and assays to differentiate between ICV and IDV are required for serological and epidemiological analysis to clarify the complexity and evolution and eliminate misdiagnosis between ICV and IDV in human samples.

Keywords: influenza D viruses, influenza C viruses, differential diagnosis, peptide ELISAs, blocking ELISA, diagnostic assay

INTRODUCTION

Influenza viruses (IVs) are a public health threat, as they are associated with a high rate of morbidity and mortality every year (1). Although both influenza A viruses (IAVs) and influenza B viruses (IBVs) cause annual epidemics in human populations, IAVs have been associated with several pandemics in past decades due to their wide host range and cross-species transmission (2, 3). As the host range of IBVs and influenza C viruses (ICVs) is limited, their mutational capacity is also limited, so they do not cause pandemics (1). IDV is a novel IV detected in cattle and swine and is antigenically and biologically distinct from the human ICV [2]. Several studies suggest that bovine species is the natural host reservoir, and IDV is possibly involved in the bovine respiratory disease complex (4).

Serological studies show the presence of IDV in beef cattle at least since 2004 (5). Bovine species are the main reservoir for IDV. However, young weaned and immunologically naive calves are very susceptible to IDV, as there is a reduction in maternal antibodies from birth to 6 months (6). IDV seroprevalence is ~62% in cattle, alone or with other respiratory viruses, that could influence the severity of respiratory syndrome disease in cattle (7). Moreover, serological studies on small ruminants in different US states report that 13.5 and 13.3% of sheep and goat farms, respectively, have IDV exposure (8). Calves weaned and co-mingled play a critical role in circulation and transmission of IDV, and neonatal calves acquire maternal immunity against IDV within the first 24 h through colostrum. However, this declines within 6 months (9, 10), as the passively acquired IgG has a half-life of 21.2–35.9 days (11). Enzyme-linked immunosorbent

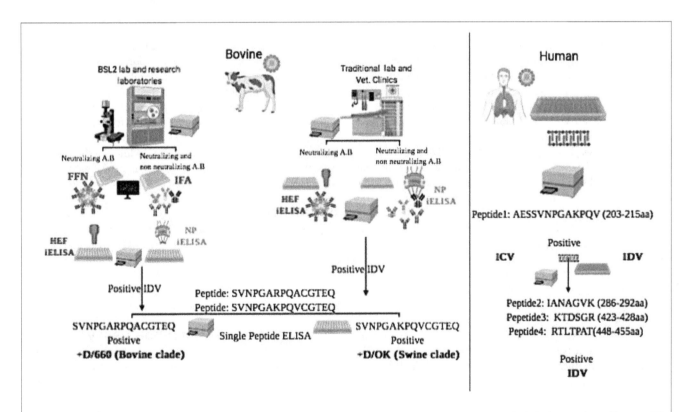

Graphical Abstract | Graphical Abstract represents schematic flowchart for differential diagnosis between the two clades of IDV in bovine samples and between IDV and HICV in human samples using new diagnostic assays:
*NP-iELISA and HEF-iELISA for detection of IDV in non-BSL2 laboratories in bovine samples.
*Immunofluorescence and neutralization assays for detection of IDV in bovine samples.
*Peptide ELISA for differentiation between the swine and bovine lineage of IDV in bovine samples.
*Blocking ELISA and a panel of peptide ELISAs for differentiation between IDV and human ICV in human samples.

assays (ELISAs) and virus neutralization assays are considered accurate and rapid serological and diagnostic assays in veterinary and human medicine (12).

Common diagnostic tests for IVs include direct detection of virus attachment to sialic acid–linked receptors on red blood cells by the hemagglutinin assay (HA), or by detecting virus-specific neutralizing antibodies that inhibit virus binding to RBCs by using hemagglutination inhibition (HI), an agar gel precipitation test (AGP), or the micro-neutralization (MN) assay, an ELISA-based virus neutralization test (13, 14). Both the HA and HI are commonly used, but different IVs show variations in the avidity to RBCs (15). In a recent study, several IVs showed low binding to RBCs, and low avidity of some recent IVs has caused major issues due to inconsistent HI tests, especially for evidence relating to antigenic drift or determining changes related to the IV vaccine (16). Also, the HI test is labor intensive and requires many standardizations (17). Disadvantages of the agar gel precipitation test are low sensitivity and high time consumption (18, 19). The MN assay is considered more sensitive than the HI or agar gel precipitation tests, but it requires further standardization for routine evaluation of vaccine efficacy (20). HI requires reference sera specific for each virus for each test performed (14). HI can detect antibodies that can block the binding of viral hemagglutinin to receptors on RBCs, However, the MN test is a tissue culture–based assay to identify functional antibodies for hemagglutinin to prevent infection of cells (13, 21).

Reverse-transcription PCR detects viral nucleic acids and is commonly used to diagnose IDV (4). It is a highly sensitive assay for virus identification, but has low efficacy in large-scale surveillance, due to early clearance of viral nucleic acids (22). Given that two lineages of IDV are not cross-reacted using the HI test but they showed low or no HI titer to each other (4), an accurate ELISA test based on conserved antigen specificity for IDV, along with a fluorescence-based neutralization assay, is required for effective IDV surveillance. Moreover, new diagnostic assays specific for each IDV lineage are needed to obtain critical information about viral evolution and vaccine efficacy (12). Highly conserved proteins in the genus of IVs include nucleoproteins (NPs), with only 20–30% of intergenic homologies (4). Therefore, we aimed to develop a highly sensitive and specific ELISA based on two different epitopes NP and HEF for serological studies and four different peptides to differentiate between the two circulating lineages of IDV. We also planned to optimize a quick and accurate fluorescent focus neutralization (FFN) assay using a high-avidity-binding polyclonal antibody specific for the whole viral antigen.

Influenza D virus (IDV) can cause respiratory disease in pigs and cattle and is closely related to human ICV (23). IDV shares 50% amino acid sequence identity with ICV, lacks the neuraminidase gene, and has seven genes instead of eight seen in IAV and IBV (4). Based on the National Center for Biotechnology Information analysis, Sequence similarity between ICV and IDV is as follows: PB2 gene, 58.5%; PB1 gene, 66.7%; P3 gene: 57.29%; HEF gene: 55.7%; NP gene: 51.4%; NS gene: 47.5%; and P42 gene; 52.4% (**Table 3** and **Figure 5**). ICV infection is characterized by mild clinical respiratory illness with a low frequency of infection, commonly in young and elderly individuals (24). IDV can infect

ferrets, but has not transmitted from human to humans to date (4, 5). ICV has a global distribution in children (25), and is reported in pigs (26), dogs (27), and camels (28). In contrast, IDV has been reported in swine (23), cattle (4), goat (8), and equine (29) species. IDV has shown serological reactivity with plasma collected from human exposed to cattle (30). In 2017, IDV was detected in rectal swabs, raising the concern that it could replicate in the intestinal tract as IAV and IBV do (31). ICV lacks an open channel due to a salt bridge interaction. However, IDV has an open channel that can accommodate a diverse range of glycans, which can contribute to broad cell tropism. Some genetic and antigenic IDV lineages do not reassort with ICV or IDV or cross-react with antibodies against some human ICVs (32). In our study, we optimized IDV and ICV blocking and peptide ELISAs with known antibody panels specific to each virus, which can be used to detect and distinguish between ICVs and IDVs in human serum samples.

MATERIALS AND METHODS

Cell Culture and Virus Production
Madin-Darby canine kidney (MDCK) cells were cultured in DMEM supplemented with 10% fetal bovine serum (FBS) and 1% penicillin and streptomycin. Influenza D/bovine/Oklahoma/660/2013 (D/660 or bovine clade) and D/swine/ Oklahoma/1334/2011 (D/OK or swine clade) were previously isolated from bovine or swine showing symptoms of respiratory disease (23). Influenza C/Human/Johannesburg-1/1966 were obtained from St. Jude Children Research Hospital. Viruses were propagated by infecting confluent MDCK cells at a multiplicity of infection of 0.01, and then incubated at 33°C with ~5% CO_2 for 5 days, using virus growth/maintenance media and DMEM with 0.1 μg/mL TPCK-treated trypsin. After 5 days, infected cell cultures were frozen and thawed thrice, and the supernatant was centrifuged at 500 × g for 15 min at 4 degree to remove cellular debris. Virus titer was determined by using MDCK cells according to the Reed and Meunch method (33).

Serum Samples
Approximately 500 randomly selected bovine serum samples were collected (South Dakota State Animal Disease Research and Veterinary Diagnostic Laboratory) mostly 6-month-old calves. Sample from 1 year to 2 years old bovine, bovine sera from different seasons, and ferret sera (from previous experiments) were supplied by St. Jude Children's Research Hospital.

Hemagglutination Inhibition Assay
The HI assay was run in bovine serum samples as per World Health Organization standard manual (5). Samples were pre-treated with receptor-destroying enzyme (Denka 261 Seiken, Chuo-ku, Tokyo, Japan). The HI assay was performed using 1% turkey RBCs (Lampire Biological Laboratories, PA, USA). Serial 2-fold dilutions of serum samples were tested in duplicate. Titers were expressed as reciprocal of the highest serum dilution of serum yielding complete hemagglutination. All samples were assayed in three separate experiments, and mean antibody titers were calculated.

Indirect Immunofluorescence Assay

All bovine samples were tested by immunofluorescence analysis (IFA) developed and previously optimized (12) and classified as positive or negative.

Preparation of Antigens Used for ELISA
Bacterial Expression and Purification of the IDV Nucleocapsid Protein (NP)

A full-length IDV NP gene sequence of the IDV strain D/bovine/Ok/660/2013 (GenBank: KF425663.1) was previously synthesized and used (12). Purified proteins were run on a western blot (WB) using anti-rabbit IDV polyclonal antisera previously generated in our laboratories.

Bacterial and Mammalian Expression and Purification of IDV Hemagglutinin Esterase

A recombinant plasmid with the synthetic truncated sequence of the region from 400 to 1,665 of the HE sequence of the IDV strain D/bovine/Ok/660/2013 (GenBank: KF425662.1) with the addition of a 3′ 6 × -His tag by GeneArt® Gene Synthesis (GeneScript, Piscataway, NJ, USA) was subcloned in the Pet28 system for bacterial expression as reported previously (34). Plasmid DNA of the HEF-truncated sequence (60-400) and the mutation at amino acid site 212 were linearized by digestion with restriction enzymes BamH1 and Xho1 and then cloned into the pcDNA3.1 mammalian expression vector.

Whole-Virus Antigen

Sucrose-purified/ultraviolet-inactivated IDV strain D/660, C/OK, and HICV strains were used as a whole virus purified control antigen for IFA, WB, and ELISA. Trypsin-treated cleavage viruses were used as a control for HE cross-reactivity.

Preparation of Antibody Panels

The panel of antibodies included ferret α-C/VICTORIA/1/2011, ferret α-Johannesburg-1/1966, ferret α-D/OK/1334/2011, and ferret α-D/OK/660/2013, which were generated at St. Jude Children's Research Hospital (5). Experimental bovine α-D/OK/660/2013 and Experimental D/bovine/Mississippi/C00046N/2014 and D/bovine/Mississippi/C00013N/2014 were kindly provided by Dr. Xiufeng Wan and Dr. Lucas Ferguson, Mississippi State University. Convalescence-positive bovine D, rabbit α-D/OK/1334/2011, rabbit Dα-D/OK/660/2013, and negative control were prepared in South Dakota State University.

Peptide Design to Determine Heterogeneity Between the Two Lineages of IDV in Antibody Recognition

We designed four different peptide covers for amino acids K212 and R212 in both lineages. Four peptides were synthesized by Genscript. Four different peptides, SVNPGARPQACGTEQ (206-220aa), SVNPGAKPQACGTEQ (206-220aa), SVNPGAKPQVCGTEQ (206-220aa), and SVNPGARPQVCGTEQ (206-220aa), covering the region of position 212, were used. In the D/OK lineage, the K is in position 212 and the V in position 215, whereas in the D/660 lineage only R is in position 212 and A in position 215.

Preparation of Polypeptides and Single Peptides to Differentiate Between ICV and IDV

Based on the alignment between the HEF of ICV and IDV, we selected four different conserved peptides for each virus that were different in amino acid sequences. Amino acid sequences ranged from 7 to 16 amino acids (**Figure 5**). A combination of equal concentration of each peptide was used as a polypeptide antigen. For optimization, a panel of antibodies specific for ICV and IDV was used. The ICV sequence was used as antigen (which did not include the influenza D sequence) to reflect the antigenicity of ICV. Then, using the ICV sequence as antigen and IDV sequence as negative control, synthetic peptides were purchased (GenScript). Peptides were chosen based on conserved amino acid differences in the HEF protein. RTDKSNSAFPRSAD (74–87 aa), in which its conserved but like IDV 58%. GSRKESGGGVTKES (484–497 aa). We did not find conserved peptides specific to ICV, and they did not share any amino acids with IDV. For IDV, we found four conserved peptides different from those in ICV: AESSVNPGAKPQV (203–215 aa), IANAGVK (286–292 aa), KTDSGR (423–428 aa), and RTLTPAT (448–455 aa) (**Figures 4A, 5**).

Cross-Reactivity Between the Two IDV Lineages

Rabbit polyclonal primary antibodies (IgG) against IDV D/660 and D/OK were used as controls to study the cross-reactivity between clades D/660 and D/OK, which are antigenically different. Monoclonal antibodies generated in our laboratories against D/660 were also used. Cross-reactivity between the two lineages was evaluated by WB and IFA of the mammalian expression system of the HE protein.

Western Blot

WB was performed using sucrose-purified viruses and recombinant NP and HE proteins. First, 50 μg of protein was resolved by SDS-PAGE in 7% acrylamide gels and transferred to nitrocellulose membranes. After blocking blots with 5% non-fat dry milk in TBS-Tween 20 (0.1%; TBS-T 20) solution for 2 hr at RT, they were probed with hyperimmune polyclonal antibodies, monoclonal antibodies, and selected bovine antibodies diluted overnight in 5% non-fat dry milk TBS-T 20 were incubated at 4°C. Blots were washed thrice with TBS-T 20 for 10 min at RT and incubated with a goat anti-bovine IgG-HRP (Jackson ImmunoResearch Laboratories, INC, USA) conjugate secondary antibody for bovine sera, a goat anti-rabbit IgG-HRP conjugate secondary antibody for rabbit-polysera, and a goat anti-mouse IgM-HRP conjugate secondary antibody for mAbs for 2 h at RT. Commercial anti-HIS antibody (Invitrogen, Carlsbad, CA) at 1:10,000 was used as primary antibody to confirm expression of the recombinant protein. FBS was used as a negative control. Blots were washed thrice with TBS-T 20 for 10 min, and bands were visualized by staining with 4-chloro-1-naphthol (ThermoFisher, Grand Island, NY).

Assay Development and Validation

Positive bovine samples from HI, IFA, and WB were collected to prepare strong positive bovine sera specific for IDV and used for assay development.

Indirect ELISA Development and Optimization

Ultraviolet radiation–inactivated, sucrose purified viruses, NP and HE recombinant proteins expressed in *E. coli* were used in indirect ELISA (iELISA). Polysorb microtiter plates (Immunolon Polysorb, 96 well, Thermo Scientific, Waltham, MA) were coated with the appropriate antigen, 50 ng/well of ultraviolet radiation–inactivated sucrose-purified whole virus antigen, HE, 100 ng/well; and NP, 25 ng/well (35). Optimal assay conditions (concentration of antigen, serum, anti-bovine biotinylated antibodies, and secondary antibody dilutions) were determined by a checkerboard titration, which gave the highest signal-to-noise ratio. In addition, FBS was used as negative control and a single lot of pooled convalescent IDV serum positive by IFA, HI, and WB was used to establish quality control standards that gave high and low optical density (high OD = 2.0–2.5, low OD = 0.5–1.0, and negative OD = <0.2). The ELISA was performed as previously reported (12, 34).

Blocking ELISA Antigen

Using ICV protein as the antigen to generate antibodies, we performed two rounds of purification for the anti-serum: affinity purification using ICV to obtain antibodies that recognize ICV, and perform cross-absorption using IDV to remove the portion of the antibody that could also recognize IDV; hence, the portion left would recognize ICV but not IDV. Blocking ELISA was performed as described previously (34).

Blocking Polypeptide ELISA

A combination of equal concentration of each peptide was used as a polypeptide antigen. For optimization, a panel of antibodies specific for ICV and IDV were used to block each alternatively.

Fluorescent Focus Neutralization Test

An IDV virus neutralization assay using an FFN format was developed and evaluated using specific, highly neutralized bovine serum samples as described previously (12).

Seroconversion of IDV in Experimentally Infected Calves

Calf sera for the study was provided by the Department of Basic Sciences, College of Veterinary Medicine, Mississippi State University, and Mississippi State, Mississippi, USA.

Measurement of Statistical Testing Agreement and Correlation

Multiple-comparison inter-rater agreement (kappa measure of association) and Pearson's correlation tests were calculated for all four tests (HI, iELISA [iELISA], FFN, and IFA), using the IBM SPSS version 20 software (SPSS Inc., Chicago, IL).

3D Structure for the ICV, PIC1, PIC2, IDV, PID1, PID2, PID3, and PID4

Are done sing the Phyre2 web portal for protein modeling, prediction and analysis using Kelley LA et al. Nature Protocols 10, 845-858 (2015). In intensive mode it was able to generate a theoretical model covering this region. The images were generated in Pymol (The PyMOL Molecular Graphics System, Version 2.3.5 Schrödinger, LLC).

Alignment Between the Selective IDV Peptides Represented in USA Selected Strain and the Non-american IDV Strains

Multiple-sequence alignment of the influenza D virus HEF protein including the four different peptides in comparison to ICV. The HEF protein (NCBI Reference Sequence: NC_036618.1) used in this study were blasted using the NCBI Influenza Virus Resource and the sequences with 97% or more were aligned using muscle v3.8.31, and the aligned sequences of representative viruses at each peptide site are shown along with the consensus sequence (**Figure 4**, **Supplementary Materials 1**, **3**). Alignment between the NP protein of the two clades of IDV to the non-American strains are shown in **Supplementary Material 2**.

RESULTS

HI Assay

All randomly collected serum samples from different states were tested by HI, using D/660 after RDE treatment. About 317 samples were positive from 400 cows and bulls, and 100 serum samples were negative from 7- to 8-month old young cattle and calves. However, the HI test using D/OK showed only 166 positive cases from 400 cows and bulls and 100 serum samples negative out of 100. Remaining samples with known HI titers were from St. Jude Children's Research Hospital.

Expression of Recombinant IDV-NP and IDV-HE Antigens by the Bacterial System

Protein yield by the IPTG-induced *E. coli* culture was approximately 25 mg IDV-NP/liter of 2XYT medium, with a purity of >95%. Purity of the recombinant protein was assessed by SDS-PAGE, and the expected band of 64 kDa for NP and 65 kDa for HE migrated in Coomassie brilliant blue staining. Specificity of recombinant proteins was confirmed by WB, using convalescent IDV-positive serum, FBS as negative control, and anti-His mAb and anti-rabbit-IDV polysera (**Figure 1A**).

Immunofluorescence Assay

About 166 of 400 field samples tested by the IFA were classified as positive and 100 of 100 as negative. The IDV-positive control serum showed clear cytoplasmic fluorescence starting at a 1:40 dilution, whereas the IDV-negative serum did not (**Figure 1B**). We developed an accurate and sensitive IFA specific for both lineages of IDV (**Figure 1B**) by using control-positive and control-negative serum samples evaluated by WB to avoid non-specific binding (**Figure 1A**).

Western Blot

WB was done for three purposes. First, WB was used to investigate some selective serum samples against the whole virus, NP, and HE, using the anti-bovine HRP antibody to confirm seroconversion status (**Figure 1A**). Second, WB was used to map the monoclonal antibody generated in our laboratory. To map the mAb of isotype IgM, sucrose-purified whole virus D/660 and D/OK were treated with trypsin for 1 h at a concentration of 10 µg/ml before running the gel. Non-treated viruses were used

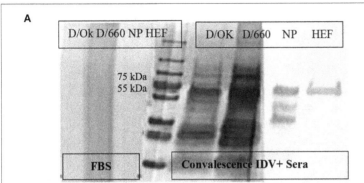

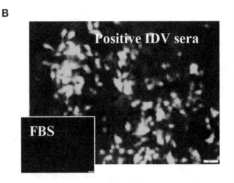

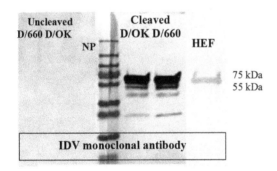

FIGURE 1 | Specificity of recombinant proteins vs. that for the whole virus at the IDV convalescent stage. **(A)** Specificity of recombinant proteins vs. that for the whole virus at the IDV convalescent stage. **(B)** IFA of IDV-infected MDCK cells using positive and negative bovine serum samples and anti-bovine fluorescein isothiocyanate (FITC) including positive convalescent bovine anti-IDV sera showing strong fluorescent staining of virus-infected cells and Negative serum sample showing no specific fluorescent staining. **(C)** Mapping of the IDV mAb.

as a control along with NP and HE proteins. Our mAb cross-reacted with the HE recombinant protein and did not cross-react with NP. It also cross-reacted with both D/660 and D/OK under trypsin treatment and did not react with the whole virus (**Figure 1C**) compared to non-cleaved virus with anti-rabbit sera. To map whether IDV produced mAbs that could be used in competitive ELISA, we used WB. We blotted the whole virus of both IDV clades in two forms: cleaved or not cleaved by trypsin. Our IDV-mAb did not recognize the non-cleaved whole virus but reacted strongly with the cleaved version (**Figure 1C**). Blotting this mAb with the two recombinant NP and HE bacterial expressed proteins showed no recognition with NP but a strong signal with HEF (**Figure 1C**).

Indirect ELISA

Receiver operating characteristic analysis of the indirect ELISA with the IFA was used to determine sensitivity and specificity values and cutoffs. Optimal cutoff values and corresponding sensitivity and specificity of NP- and HEF-based tests are shown in **Figures 2A,B**, respectively. Receiver operating characteristic analysis for the NP-iELISA showed 94.4% sensitivity and

91.9% specificity with a cutoff of 0.357. Receiver operating characteristic analysis for the HEF-iELISA showed an estimated sensitivity and specificity of 96.6 and 96.2%, respectively, with a cutoff of 0.321. We detected 332 positive samples out of 350 expected positive samples and 120 negative samples from 150 archived samples (1984–1999), since IDV did not circulate before 2003 (5). We found an ∼90% preliminary prevalence of IDV in dairy cattle and 4–7% prevalence in healthy 7-month-old calves. We optimized and validated the HEF- iELISA, and our results showed high specificity and sensitivity (**Figure 2B**) as well as high correlation with the two neutralizing tests HI and FFN. These results not only confirm the specificity of HI and FFN directed toward protective antibodies against HEF, but also indicate that neutralizing tissue culture-based assays that require BSL2 facilities and a highly prepared lab to perform ELISA to determine neutralizing antibodies can be easily performed in a traditional lab, clinical lab, and veterinary clinics (**Table 1**). Based on the blast and alignment analysis, both Np and HEF ElISA developed here can be used for the non-American IDV strains (**Figure 5** and **Supplementary Material 2**).

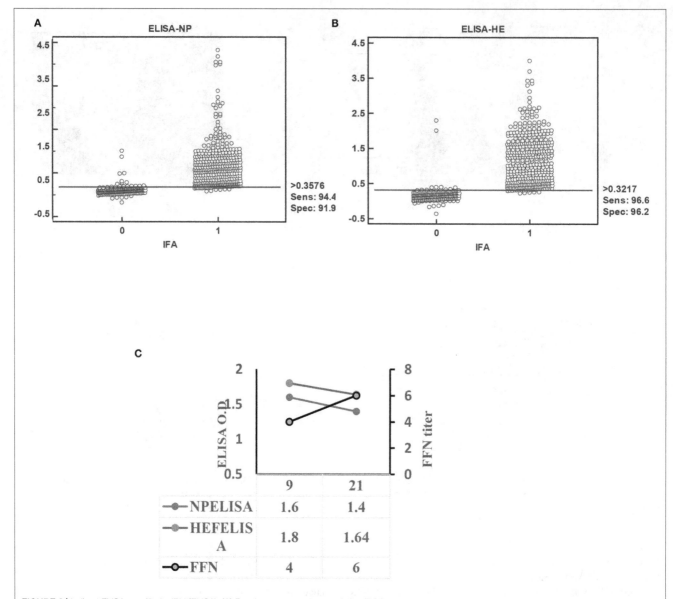

FIGURE 2 | Indirect ELISA specific for IDV (iELISA). **(A)** Receiver operator characteristics (ROC) and diagnostic sensitivity and specificity of IDV-NP. **(B)** ROC analysis and diagnostic sensitivity and specificity of IDV-HE (MedCalc version 11.1.1.0, MedCalc software, Mariakerke, Belgium) In each panel, dot plot on the left and right denote negative and positive testing populations, respectively. The horizontal line bisecting the dot plots denotes the cutoff value for optimal diagnostic sensitivity and specificity. **(C)** Seroconversion of IDV in infected calves using ELISA-based NP, HE, and FFN in calves experimentally infected with IDV.

Seroconversion of Influenza D Virus in Experimentally Infected Calves

Calf sera showed seropositivity at day 9 post infection with Np and HEF-iELISA, with high titers of neutralization seen with FFN at 21 DPI (**Figure 2C**).

FFN

The FFN assay was initially run by using well-recognized positive convalescent serum samples by WB, IFA, HI, and ELISA. Essentially, the 100 negative samples showed serum FFN endpoint titers of <1:20 and included calves 6–7 months old. Of the 350 positive sample set of cows and bulls, 349 had endpoint

titers from 1:80 to 1:1280. We optimized and developed FFN by using high-throughput methods specific for IDVs.

Statistical Correlation Among HI, FFN, and HEF-iELISA

Pearson's correlation test among all diagnostic platforms showed high correlation values among assays. There was a good correlation between HI results after transformation to log 2: FFN value was 0.732 between HEF-iELISA and FFN-log 2 was 0.556, and that of iELISA based on HEF and HI log 2 was 0.532 (**Table 1**). The HI results using both clades D/660 and D/OK were different in seropositive status but the FFN results were able to

TABLE 1 | Pearson correlation coefficients for diagnostic assays between HI results after log-2 transformation and FFN.

	Total no. 450	HEF-iELISA	NP-iELISA	FFN (Log)	HI Log	IFA Log
ELISA-HE	Correlation coefficient		0.517	0.548	0.522	0.556
	Significance level P		<0.0001	<0.0001	<0.0001	<0.0001
ELISA-NP	Correlation coefficient	0.517		0.484	0.435	0.512
	Significance level P	<0.0001		<0.0001	<0.0001	<0.0001
FFN (Log)	Correlation coefficient	0.548	0.484		0.581	0.705
	Significance level P	<0.0001	<0.0001		<0.0001	<0.0001
Hi_Log	Correlation coefficient	0.522	0.435	0.581		0.732
	Significance level P	<0.0001	<0.0001	<0.0001		<0.0001
IFA_log	Correlation coefficient	0.556	0.512	0.705	0.732	
	Significance level P	<0.0001	<0.0001	<0.0001	<0.0001	

Correlation coefficient values were 0.581 between HI and FFN, 0.548 between HI and HEF-iELISA, and 0.522 between iELISA based on HEF and FFN-log2.

cover both. Our IFA, iELISAs and FFN tests specific for IDV will detect both the protective and non-protective antibodies against the two IDV antigenically different clades that co-circulating in the U.S. Indirect HE ELISA and FNN showed a high correlation with HI results, which confirm that the HI test can be replaced by HEF- iELISA and FFN. The HI results from clades D/660 and D/OK revealed differences in seropositive status, but FFN results were consistent.

Cross-Reactivity Between the Two Lineages of IDV

Cross-reactivity between IDV-D/660 and IDV-D/OK was determined using rabbit antisera specific for both IDV lineages generated in our laboratories. We used WB with different epitopes from whole-virus D/660, D/OK, trypsin and no trypsin treated D/660, trypsin and no trypsin treated D/OK, and recombinant N and HE proteins against rabbit antisera specific for both lineages alternatively. **Figure 3A** shows that both anti-rabbit sera reacted with both viruses treated or not treated with trypsin, demonstrating cross-reactivity between the two clades when using our rabbit antisera. Therefore, our rabbit antisera will serve as an accurate tool for general diagnosis of IDV in the US. Moreover, to investigate whether the amino acid 212, located in the apex of the HE receptor binding domain, has a critical role in antibody recognition, we introduced a deletion mutation in this region and cloned the mutant in the PcDNA3.1 mammalian expression vector and then transfected MDCK cells with the construct. Transfected cells were stained by both rabbit polyclonal antisera specific to the two IDV clades and cross-reacted with mutant HEF. The mutation introduced by deleting the amino acid site 212 of the HE protein and transfection in MDCK cells using lipofectamine 3000 did not affect the antigenic recognition of the epitope against mAb and rabbit antisera for both lineages using IFA (**Figure 3B**).

Peptide ELISA to Assess the Heterogeneity of Recognition Between the Two Lineages

Despite the genetic differences between the two lineages, mutation in position 212 did not show differences in the recognition of antibodies. Therefore, we investigated the

importance of K, R, A, and V amino acids in the heterogeneity of the IDV-circulated lineage and found that positions 215 play an important role in heterogeneity (**Figure 3**). We treated both sucrose-purified viruses with TPCK-treated trypsin to cleave the HE protein and used both rabbit polyclonal antisera against both clades alternatively (**Figure 3A**). Both cleaved and non-cleaved viruses reacted to both rabbit antisera. Also, both polyclonal antisera specific to both clades reacted with the D/OK HE recombinant protein. Therefore, we developed peptide ELISA using a panel of four different peptides. Each peptide had 14 amino acids covering the region from positions 206 to 220 (**Figure 3C**). Both positions 212 and 215 are important for the heterogeneity between the two lineages (**Figure 3**, graphical abstract and **Table 2**). Peptide ELISA with the anti-IDV ferret serum was positive with D/OK and D/660 m in position 215 (A to V), with no cross reaction with D/660. The list of peptides and recognition of both D/OK and D/660 antibodies are given in (**Figure 3C** and **Table 2**). These results highlight the importance of position 215 with 212 in the zoonotic importance of IDV. Using the peptides ELISA with anti-IDV from ferret showed only positive with the D/OK lineage and D/660 mutant in position 215 (A to V).

Structural Representation of the Haemagglutinin Esterase Fusion Glycoprotein From the Influenza C Virus and the Influenza D Virus

Structural representation of the haemagglutinin esterase fusion glycoprotein from the influenza C virus in green [PDB:1FLC (32, 36)] and the influenza D virus in blue [PDB:5E64 (32)]. ICV peptide one (PIC1) is found in esterase domain one and has the sequence RTDKSNSAFPRSAD. ICV peptide two (PIC2) is found in fusion domain two and has the sequence GSRKESGGGVTKES (**Figure 4A**). IDV peptide one (PID1) is found in the receptor domain and has the sequence AESSVNPGAKPQVCGT. IDV peptide two (PID2) is also found in the receptor domain and has the sequence IANAGVK. IDV peptide three (PID3) is found in the fusion domain and has the sequence KTDSGR. An enzymatic cleavage site was noted adjacent to IDV peptide three. IDV peptide four (PID4) falls within a 17 amino acid region not represented in structural data. Its location is highlighted with a

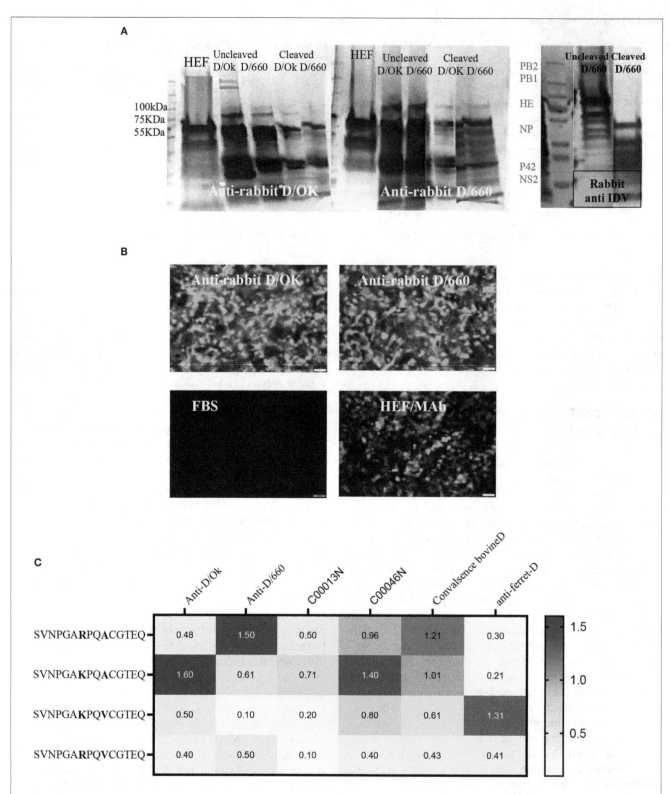

FIGURE 3 | Cross-reactivity between two IDV different clades of D/660 and C/OK. **(A)** Cross-reactivity between the two IDV different clades of D/660 and C/OK using specific polyclonal rabbit anti-IDV sera against each clade and using polyclonal rabbit anti-IDV/D/660 and polyclonal rabbit anti-IDV/C/OK sera against cleaved and non-cleaved viruses. **(B)** Cross reactivity of the mutant HE protein at the site 212 amino acid. MDCK cells were stained with both IDV lineages of anti-rabbit-sera and mAb after transfection in MDCK cells. **(C)** List of peptides used and recognition of both D/OK and D/660 antibodies.

TABLE 2 | Summary for the representative assays in this study compared to the shaded standard assay used for influenza viruses.

Epitope	Sequence	Assay	Analyte	BSL2	Sample/host	Application	Limitation
IDV/OK/or IDV/660	Whole virus	FFN	IgG/IgM	Yes	Bovine serum	IDV antibodies	BSL2/expensive
IDV/OK/or IDV/660	Whole virus	IFA	Poly	Yes	Bovine serum	IDV antibodies	BSL2/expensive
IDV-NP	40-600 AA	Indirect ELISA	IgG	No	Bovine serum	IDV antibodies	Very specific
IDV-HEF	60-400 AA	Indirect ELISA	IgG	No	Bovine serum	IDV antibodies	Very specific
IDV/OK/Whole-Viral-Ag	Sucrose purified virus	Indirect ELISA	IgG	No	Bovine serum	IDV/OK (swine clade) antibodies	Very specific
IDV/660/Whole-Viral-Ag	Sucrose purified virus	Indirect ELISA	IgG	No	Bovine serum	IDV/660 (Bovine clade) antibodies	Very specific
IDV peptide	SVNPGA**R**PQ**A**CGTEQ (206-220aa)	Indirect ELISA	IgG	No	Bovine serum	IDV/660 (Bovine clade) antibodies	Not cheap
IDV peptide	SVNPGA**K**PQ**A**CGTEQ (206-220aa)	Indirect ELISA	IgG	No	Bovine serum	IDV/OK (swine clade) antibodies	Not cheap
IDV peptide	SVNPGA**R**PQ**V**CGTEQ (206-220aa)	Indirect ELISA	IgG	No	Bovine serum	IDV/660 (Bovine clade) antibodies	Not cheap
IDV peptide	SVNPGA**K**PQ**V**CGTEQ (206-220aa)	Indirect ELISA	IgG	No	Bovine serum	IDV/OK (swine clade) antibodies	Not cheap
HICV/Whole-Viral-Ag	Sucrose purified virus	Indirect ELISA	IgG	No	Human serum	HICV antibodies	Very specific
IDV/OK/Whole-Viral-Ag	Sucrose purified virus	Blocking ELISA	IgG	No	Human serum	IDV antibodies	Very specific
HICV/Whole-Viral-Ag	Sucrose purified virus	Blocking ELISA	IgG	No	Human serum	HICV antibodies	Very specific
Peptide 1 IDV (PID1)	AESSVNPGAKPQV (203–215 aa)	Indirect ELISA	IgG	No	Human serum	IDV antibodies	Not cheap
Peptide 2 IDV (PID2)	IANAGVK (286–292 aa)	Indirect ELISA	IgG	No	Human serum	IDV antibodies	Not cheap
Peptide 3 IDV (PID3)	KTDSGR (423–428 aa)	Indirect ELISA	IgG	No	Human serum	IDV antibodies	Not cheap
Peptide 4 IDV (PID4)	RTLTPAT (448–455 aa)	Indirect ELISA	IgG	No	Human serum	IDV antibodies	Not cheap
Peptide 1 ICV (PIC1)	RTDKSNSAFPRSAD (74–87 aa)	Indirect ELISA	IgG	No	Human serum	HICV antibodies	Not cheap
Peptide 2 ICV (PIC2)	GSRKESGGGVTKES (484–497 aa)	Indirect ELISA	IgG	No	Human serum	HICV antibodies	Not cheap
IDV-Polypeptide	Equal concentration of P1D1 to PID4	Blocking ELISA	IgG	No	Human serum	IDV antibodies	Not cheap
ICV-Polypeptide	Equal concentration of (P1D1-2)	Blocking ELISA	IgG	No	Human serum	HICV antibodies	Not cheap
HI test	IDV/OK, IDV/660, HICV	HI	Poly	Yes	Human/bovine	Based on the virus	Time/less sensitivity
Microneutralization assay	IDV/OK, IDV/660, HICV	ELISA based tissue culture immunoperoxidase	poly	Yes	Human/bovine	Based on the virus	Time consumed
Reverse-transcription PCR	IDV/OK, IDV/660	PCR	Nucleic acid	Yes	Swap	Number of cycles	Expensive

dashed circle. IDV peptide four has the sequence RTLTPAT and occupies the fusion domain (**Figure 4A**).

Blocking Polypeptide ELISA and Single-Peptide ELISA to Differentiate Between ICV and IDV

On the basis of the alignment between the HEF of ICV and IDV, we selected four different conserved peptides for each virus that have different amino acid sequences. The amino acid sequences had seven to 16 amino acids. A combination of equal concentration of each peptide was used as a polypeptide antigen. For optimization, a panel of antibodies specific for ICV and IDV were used (**Figure 4B**). To establish a serological test to differentiate between two closely related viruses, we developed peptides, blocking polypeptides, and blocking whole antigen ELISAs. Our IDV blocking and peptide 2–4 ELISAs can be used to detect and distinguish between ICV and IDV. IDV was more conserved and had three different peptides that did

not cross-react with ICV, whereas the only two conserved ICV peptides were positive for IDV (**Figure 4B**). This indicates that ICV can cross-react with IDV and vice versa.

Representation of the IDV HEF Protein and Peptides Among Non-american IVD

Representation of the IDV HEF protein including the four IDV peptides of the strain in our study. The IDV Peptides showed more similarities to the European strains than of the Asian. The two clades IDV virus led sequence are cataloged with other virus sequences from the blast then an alignment using Bio edit program has been done. As part of this process, we compared the ICV sequence with the other virus sequences and looks for differences among them to visually represent how genetically different the Peptides are from each virus strain to other (**Figure 5** and **Supplementary Materials 1**, **3**). PID1 showed a 100% similar to (D/bovine/Guangdong/SQ/

TABLE 3 | IDV similarities to ICV IDV shares 50% amino acid sequence identity with ICV, lacks the neuraminidase gene, and has seven genes instead of eight seen in IAV and IBV (4).

IDV gene	Similarities to ICV
PB2	58.5%
PB1	66.7%
P3	57.29%
HEF	55.7%
NP	51.4%
NS	47.5%
P42	52.4%

Sequence similarity between ICV and IDV is as follows: PB2 gene, 58.5%; PB1 gene, 66.7%; P3 gene, 57.29%; HEF gene, 55.7%; NP gene, 51.4%; NS gene, 47.5%; and P42 gene, 52.4%.

2018), (D/swine/Guangdong/LX-2/2018), (D/bovine/Guangdong/YC/2017), (D/bovine/Shandong/Y125/2014), (D/bovine/Shandong/Y217/2014), (D/bovine/Guangdong/SQ/2018) (D/bovine/France/5920/2014), (D/bovine/Italy/108524/2018), (D/swine/Italy/173287-4/2016), (D/swine/Italy/268344-2/2015), (D/bovine/Italy/46484/2015) and (D/swine/Italy/254578/2015) (**Figure 5** and **Supplementary Material 3**), while PID2 showed 100 % similarities to (D/bovine/Guangdong/SQ/2018), (D/swine/Guangdong/LX-2/2018), (D/bovine/Guangdong/YC/2017), (D/bovine/Shandong/Y125/2014), (D/bovine/Shandong/Y217/2014), (D/bovine/Guangdong/SQ/2018), and (D/swine/Italy/354017/2015) (**Figure 5** and **Supplementary Material 3**). PID3 showed 100 % similarities with (D/bovine/Quebec/3E-H/2018), (D/bovine/Quebec/3M-B/2020), (D/bovine/Mexico/S56/2015), (D/bovine/France/5920/2014), (D/bovine/France/2986/2012), (D/bovine/Italy/108524/2018), (D/swine/Italy/173287-4/2016), (D/bovine/Italy/46484/2015), (D/swine/Italy/254578/2015), (D/swine/Italy/354017/2015), (D/bovine/Italy/28300/2019), (D/bovine/Italy/28145/2019), (D/bovine/Italy/19RS176-11/2018), (D/swine/Italy/199724-3/2015), and (D/bovine/Italy/1/2014),while it showed 90% to (D/bovine/Yamagata/1/2019).

PID 4 showed 100% similarities to all the European and Eurasian strains except a 90 % to (D/bovine/Italy/108524/2018). (**Figure 5** and **Supplementary Materials 1, 3**).

DISCUSSION

Although the HI test is commonly used for IVs, it cannot be used to detect the antibodies against the two genetic lineages IDV, D/OK-like virus (swine clade) and D/660-like virus (bovine clade), which are antigenically distinct (37). Therefore, each lineage requires a specific standard test. For better diagnosis of IDV, our aim was to develop general, sensitive antibody-based tissue culture assays that can detect both lineages of IDV. Neutralization assays (e.g., MN) cannot detect cross-reactive antibodies in the highly conserved stem region of different IVs, especially in the elderly (38). Also, they identify protective antibodies against specific epitopes, but not non-neutralizing antibodies produced by the immune system against

other epitopes (e.g., PB1, PB2, M, and other IV proteins), which can reflect the serostatus of the animal but are missing in MN or HI tests. There are different formats of the MN assay worldwide, such as a 2-day ELISA protocol (39), a 3-day HA protocol, and a 7-day HA protocol (18). Because time is critical for sero-epidemiology and early diagnosis, an accurate and shorter protocol of 2 days is optimal (12).

Our proposed diagnostic assays can be a sensitive and accurate diagnostic tool for high-throughput surveillance and detection of both D/OK-like and D/660-like IDVs co-circulating in the same herds in both research and clinical labs. We needed IFA and FFN for tissue culture–based analysis for analyzing virus interactions. The IFA is the gold standard of infectious disease serology, rapid, accurate, highly sensitive and highly specific technique that can be used for viral identification (40, 41). IFA has been used efficiently for the management and surveillance of several IVs (42, 43). However, the IFA assay is very expensive to use in surveillance and cannot differentiate between neutralizing and non-neutralizing antibodies (12). FFN is a neutralization test based on high avidity binding of rabbit polyclonal antisera prepared in our lab against IDV as a detection antibody. The FFN assay can detect neutralizing antibodies against both IDV clusters, using either type of IDV as the virus indicator. The biggest advantage of FFN over iELISA is that iELISA requires species-specific enzyme-conjugated antibodies but FFN does not (34). Furthermore, FFN detects only neutralizing antibodies (35), so it can be used for further optimization by using milk and colostrum samples from cow herds that experienced an acute IDV outbreak. Serum samples can be used to quantify maternal and acquired immunity transferred to calves (44). Unfortunately, IFA and FFN require BSL2 facilities that are not available in many veterinary centers. Hence, our second aim was to develop an iELISA using specific epitopes to detect two lineages of IDVs simultaneously.

Epitope-iELISA accurately detects neutralizing and non-neutralizing antibodies against the IDV in non-BSL2 laboratories and veterinary clinics (12) and is cost-effective and sensitive (12, 22). The IDV NP is considered a genus-specific antigen that can distinguish among different genera of IVs. NP is responsible for the loss of cross-recognition of viral antigens between different IVs (4). NP is a conserved domain with 94% similarities between IDV swine and bovine clades (**Supplementary Material 2**). Therefore, it represents the best epitope target for general seroprevalence of IDV in clinical labs and veterinary clinics. We established two separate and optimized iELISAs based on NP and HEF. The HEF epitope is specific for ICV and IDV but not IAV and IBV (32). The sensitivity and specificity of our NP- iELISA were very good (**Figure 2A**), However, the specificity was higher than the sensitivity, which may be related to fewer negative samples than positive samples in our study. Therefore, further analysis of known negative samples are next steps in optimizing the test. NP-iELISA can detect antibodies that target common viral proteins (34) and can be effective for large-scale surveillance of IDV in herds. The HEF protein of IDV recognizes and binds the specific receptor, and consequently mediates viral entrance and virus infection (23). Our HEF- iELISA showed high sensitivity and specificity

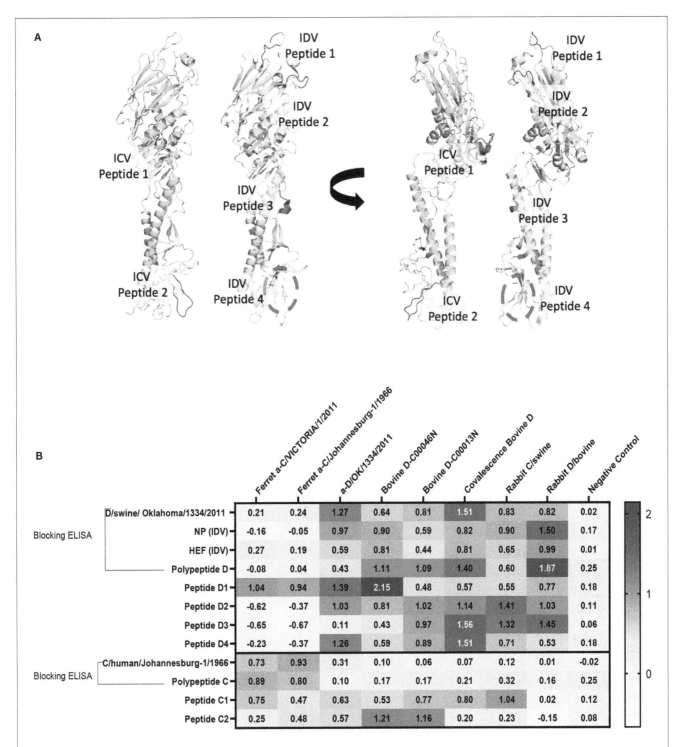

FIGURE 4 | Differentiation between IDV and ICV. **(A)** Structural representation of the haemagglutinin esterase fusion glycoprotein from the influenza C virus in green (PDB:1FLC) and the influenza D virus in blue (PDB:5E64). Peptides of interest are represented in red. ICV peptide one is found in esterase domain one and has the sequence RTDKSNSAFPRSAD. ICV peptide two is found in fusion domain two and has the sequence GSRKESGGGVTKES. IDV peptide one is found in the receptor domain and has the sequence AESSVNPGAKPQVCGT. IDV peptide two is also found in the receptor domain and has the sequence IANAGVK. IDV peptide three is found in the fusion domain and has the sequence KTDSGR. An enzymatic cleavage site was noted adjacent to IDV peptide three. IDV peptide four falls within a 17 amino acid region not represented in structural data. Its location is highlighted with a dashed circle. IDV peptide four has the sequence RTLTPAT and occupies the fusion domain. **(B)** NP, HEF, and IDV antigens were blocked by anti-ICV antibodies. ICV was blocked by anti-IDV antibodies. Compared to blocking ELISA, polypeptides and single peptide ELISA had higher sensitivity and specificity of peptides to differentiate between IDV and ICV.

(**Figure 2B**). Furthermore, comparison of seroprevalence of 6- to 7-month-old calves and adult cattle revealed a significant increase of 10% in 8-month-old calves compared to 89% in adult cattle (8). Our results highlight the high spread rate of IDV among cattle in the US, in contrast to a study reporting a spread rate of 11.3% in calves and 66.5% in adult cows (9). The variation seen between calves and adult cows could be due to passive immunity against IDV transferred from positive adult cattle to calves, which may aid temporary protection (9). Calf sera showed seropositivity at 9 days post infection and high titers of neutralization by FFN at 21 days post infection (**Figure 2C**).

The above assays can determine whether the status of tested samples is positive or negative against IDV in general but cannot determine the specific lineage (graphical abstract). Therefore, our third aim was to develop another diagnostic assay to differentiate between the two IDV lineages. The IDV/D/660 clade has a K replacing R of the D/OK clade at position 212. HI results and molecular models of the two clades revealed that amino acid 212 plays an important role in IDV antigenicity and antibody recognition (37). For understanding the two IDVs lineages at the molecular level, we developed an assay to serologically differentiate between the two viral clades. First, we tested cross-reactivity between the two clades using our rabbit polyclonal

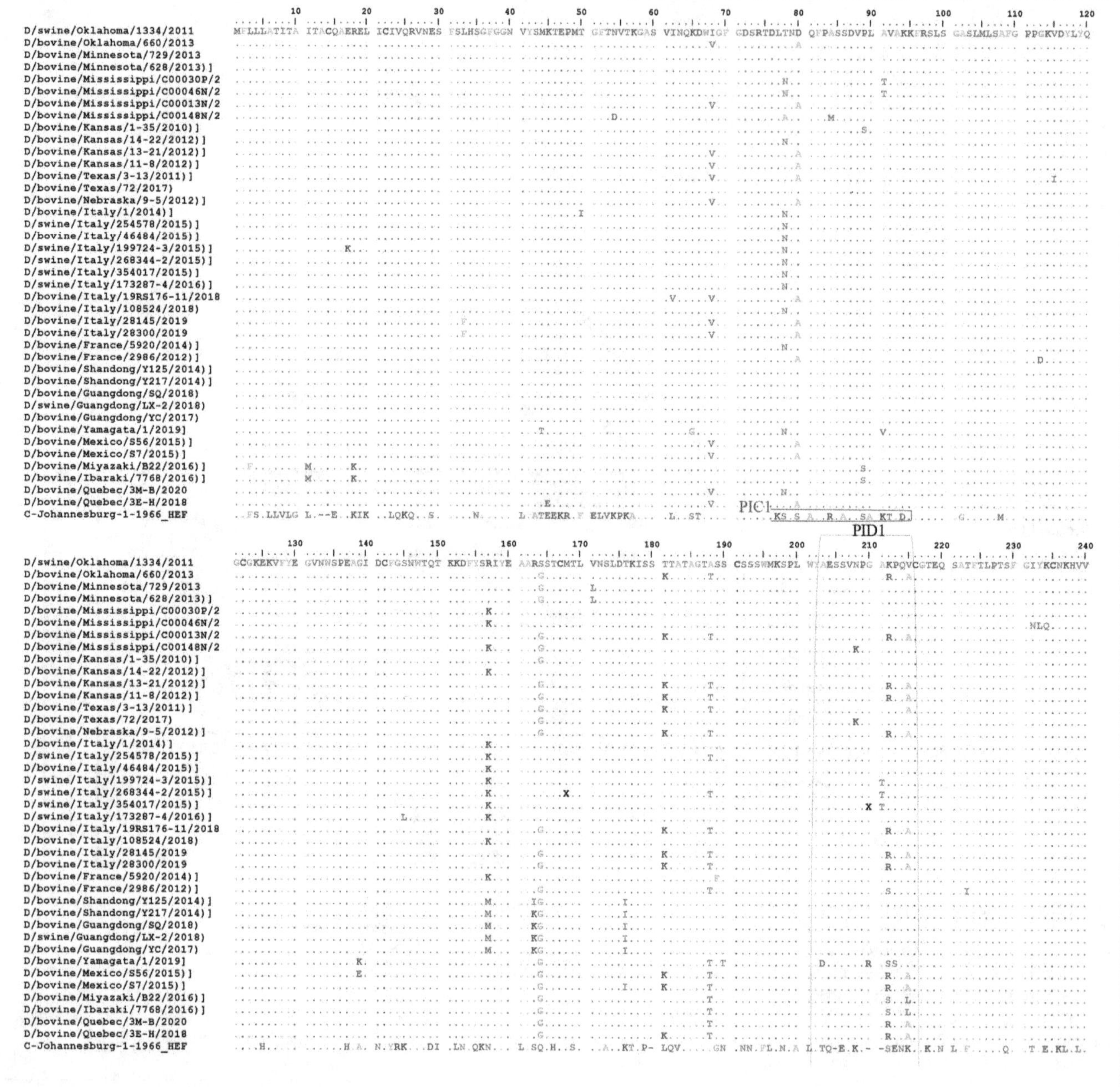

FIGURE 5 | Continued

antisera against both D/OK and D/660. A strong cross-reactivity was found when using the alternative rabbit polyclonal antisera (**Figures 3A,B**). A deletional mutation at the amino acid site 212 in only the HEF protein did not affect antigenic recognition of the epitope against mAb and rabbit antisera for both lineages (**Figure 3B**), which suggested that the amino acid 212 region alone does not cause a difference in HI titers between the two clades. Another region such as V115I or D372G in the esterase domain (37) may also play a critical role in antigenic differences in recognizing the receptor.

Peptide ELISA with anti-IDV antibodies from ferret were only positive with the synthetized peptide with a mutation in position 215 (A to V) in both the swine lineage D/OK and the bovine lineage D/660 (**Figure 3C**). This indicates that IDV is a zoonotic hazard, and more samples of individual coworkers handling swine and bovine lineages need to be screened. Our results from peptide ELISA can be an important tool to differentiate between the zoonotic ability of both lineages and determine drifts in HEF protein between swine and bovine lineages after transmission.

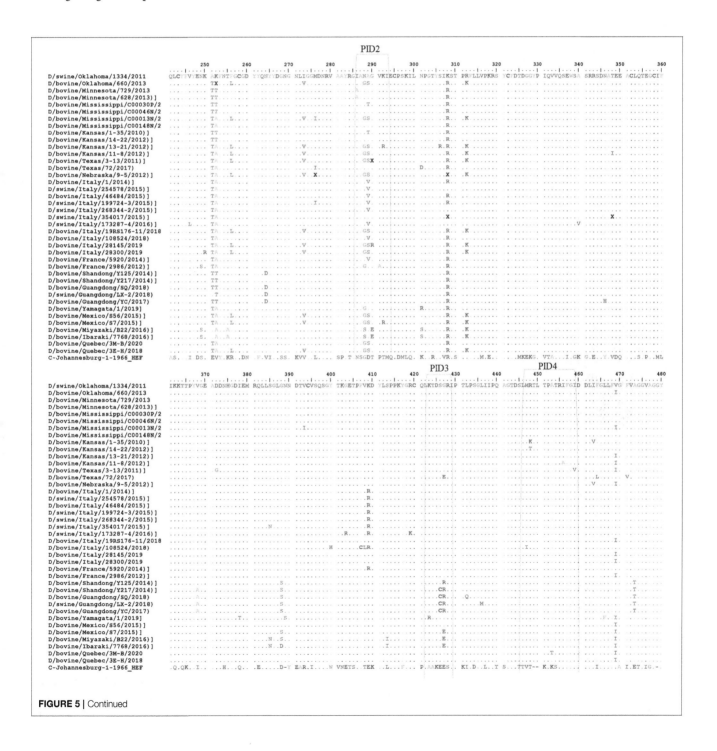

FIGURE 5 | Continued

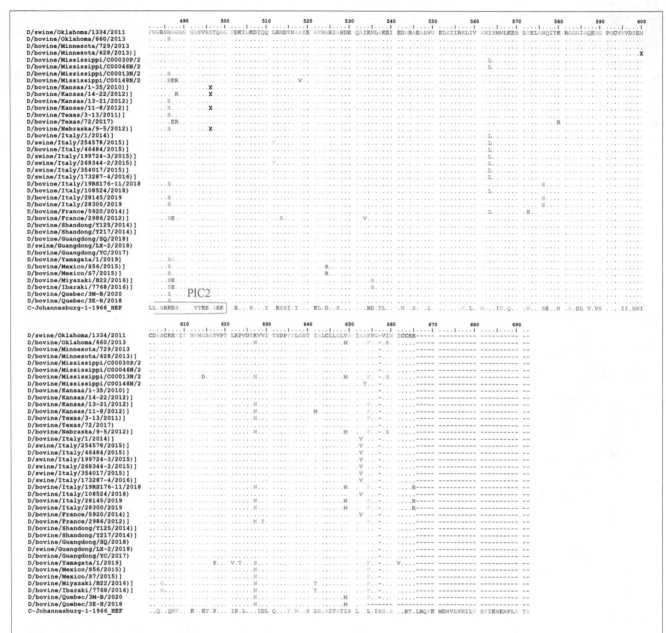

FIGURE 5 | Alignment between the selective IDV peptides represented in USA and the non-American IDV strains. Representation of the IDV HEF protein including the four IDV peptides of the strain in our study. Multiple-sequence alignment of the influenza D virus HEF protein and four different peptides in comparison to ICV. The HEF protein used in this study were blasted using the NCBI Influenza Virus Resource and the sequences with 97% or more were aligned using muscle v3.8.31, and the aligned sequences of representative viruses at each peptide site are shown along with the consensus sequence. Dots represent identical residues, PID1, PID2, PID3, and PID4 are outlined, and the location of the fusion peptide is shown.

To date, viral zoonotic diseases maintain to cause pandemic in human (45). Although the zoonotic potential of IDV remains unclear, it can efficiently replicate and transmit in ferrets which considered a good model for human IVs (46). In contrast to a recent study in Scotland showing that no evidence of seroprevalence of IDV but a seroprevalence of ICV in human respiratory samples (47), another study revealed high seroprevalence of IDV in sera from humans exposed to calves, indicating the zoonotic potential of IDV (30).

Importantly, the frequent mutations in IVs necessitate measures to prepare for the potential threat to human and public health. Therefore, it is critical to develop diagnostic tools and assays to differentiate between ICV and IDV due to their similar genomic structures. Such accurate assays are required for serological and epidemiological analysis to clarify the complexity and evolution and eliminate misdiagnosis between ICV and IDV. Here, we developed a new diagnostic and serological-based assay, which will serve as an excellent tool for veterinarians and researchers in

IDV surveillance and vaccine evaluation, along with diagnostic assays to serologically differentiate between ICV and IDV (**Figure 4** and **Table 2**). Our results agree with those from a previous study showing that IDV clusters most closely with and is derived from human ICV (48), which indicates that ICV can cross-react with IDV and vice versa (**Figure 4B**). Blocking ELISAs and IDV peptides IANAGVK (286–292 aa), KTDSGR (423–428 aa), and RTLTPAT (448–455 aa). Our blocking ELISA, PID3 and PID4 will be an excellent approach to differentiate between IDV and ICV in human samples in USA and Europe based on the alignment and blast results from the NCBI and Uniport (**Figure 5, Supplementary Materials 1, 3**).

In conclusion, our study and the assays we have developed will play key roles in seroprevalence studies, surveillance, diagnosis of IDV, and vaccine evaluation (graphical abstract and **Table 2**). Also, our new diagnostic tests will play a critical role in vaccine evaluation. The indirect HE ELISA and FNN showed the possible replacement of the HI test by HE based iELISA and FFN. Our IDV tissue culture–based assays IFA and FFN are important for research labs and vaccine evaluation, and our NP-iELISA and/or HEF-iELISA can be used in clinical laboratories lacking BSL2 facilities. Peptide-iELISA of the two IDV lineages highlighted the importance of position 215 with 212 in the zoonotic importance of IDV and the heterogeneity between the two lineages. Blocking ELISAs and IDV peptides IANAGVK (286-292aa), KTDSGR (423-428aa), and RTLTPAT (448-455aa) will be a great tool to differentiate between IDV and ICV in human samples. The two IDV's lineage peptides-iELISA highlighted the importance of position 215 with 212 in the zoonotic importance of IDV and the heterogeneity between the two lineages.

AUTHOR CONTRIBUTIONS

FO: conceptualization, writing, and visualization. AS and FO: methodology, software, validation, and formal analysis. EN and RW: investigation, supervision, project administration, and funding acquisition. RW: resources. FO and RW: data curation. AS and FO: writing, review, and editing. All authors contributed to the article and approved the submitted version.

ACKNOWLEDGMENTS

We are grateful for the technical assistance from Julie Nelson and Aaron Singrey. We thank Dr. Dr. Xiufeng Wan and Dr. Lucas Ferguson, Mississippi State University for providing experimental samples, and we thank Dr. Webby's group in St. Jude Children Research hospital for the laboratory trainings and the funding supported by from National Institutes of Health and South Dakota State University board of education. We thank Vani Shanker, PhD, ELS, for editing the manuscript. Also, the authors would like to thank Maria Smith for helping in the technical process.

REFERENCES

1. Kumar B, Asha K, Khanna M, Ronsard L, Meseko CA, Sanicas M. The emerging influenza virus threat: status and new prospects for its therapy and control. *Arch Virol.* (2018) 163:831–44. doi: 10.1007/s00705-018-3708-y

2. Khanna M, Saxena L, Gupta A, Kumar B, Rajput R. Influenza pandemics of 1918 and 2009: a comparative account. *Future Virol.* (2013) 8:335–42. doi: 10.2217/fvl.13.18

3. Khanna M, Kumar B, Gupta A, Kumar P. Pandemic influenza A H1N1 2009 virus: lessons from the past and implications for the future. *Indian J Virol.* (2012) 23:12–7. doi: 10.1007/s13337-012-0066-3

4. Hause BM, Collin EA, Liu R, Huang B, Sheng Z, Lu W, et al. Characterization of a novel influenza virus in cattle and Swine: proposal for a new genus in the *Orthomyxoviridae* family. *MBio.* (2014) 5:e00031-14. doi: 10.1128/mBio.00031-14

5. Eckard LE. Assessment of the zoonotic potential of a novel bovine influenza virus. Ph.D. Thesis, The University of Tennessee Health Science Center, Memphis, TN. doi: 10.21007/etd.cghs.2016.0405

6. Cox NJ, Neumann G, Donis RO, Kawaoka Y. Orthomyxoviruses: influenza. In: Topley WWC, Wilson, editors. *Topley & Wilson's Microbiology and Microbial Infections.* John Wiley & Sons, Ltd (2010). doi: 10.1002/9780470688618.taw0238

7. Ng TFF, Kondov NO, Deng X, van Eenennaam A, Neibergs HL, Delwart E. A metagenomics and case-control study to identify viruses associated with bovine respiratory disease. *J Virol.* (2015) 89:5340–49. doi: 10.1128/JVI.00064-15

8. Quast M, Sreenivasan C, Sexton G, Nedland H, Singrey A, Fawcett L, et al. Serological evidence for the presence of influenza D virus in small ruminants. *Vet Microbiol.* (2015) 180:281–5. doi: 10.1016/j.vetmic.2015.09.005

9. Ferguson L, Eckard L, Epperson WB, Long L-P, Smith D, Huston C, et al. Influenza D virus infection in mississippi beef cattle. *Virology.* (2015) 486:28–34. doi: 10.1016/j.virol.2015.08.030

10. Quigley JD, Kost CJ, Wolfe TM. Absorption of protein and IgG in calves fed a colostrum supplement or replacer. *J Dairy Sci.* (2002) 85:1243–8. doi: 10.3168/jds.s0022-0302(02)74188-x

11. Fulton RW, Ridpath JF, Confer AW, Saliki JT, Burge LJ, Payton ME. Bovine viral diarrhoea virus antigenic diversity: impact on disease and vaccination programmes. *Biologicals.* (2003) 31:89–95. doi: 10.1016/s1045-1056(03)00021-6

12. Okda FA. *Surveillance of Emerging Livestock Viruses.* (2017). Available online at: https://openprairie.sdstate.edu/etd/1180/ (accessed November 21, 2020).

13. Julkunen I, Pyhälä R, Hovi T. Enzyme immunoassay, complement fixation and hemagglutination inhibition tests in the diagnosis of influenza A and B virus infections. Purified hemagglutinin in subtype-specific diagnosis. *J Virol Methods.* (1985) 10:75–84. doi: 10.1016/0166-0934(85)90091-6

14. Petric M, Comanor L, Petti CA. Role of the laboratory in diagnosis of influenza during seasonal epidemics and potential pandemics. *J Infect Dis.* (2006) 194:S98–110. doi: 10.1086/507554

15. Nycholat CM, McBride R, Ekiert DC, Xu R, Rangarajan J, Peng W, et al. Recognition of sialylated poly-N-acetyllactosamine chains on N- and O-linked glycans by human and avian influenza A virus hemagglutinins. *Angew Chemie Int Ed.* (2012) 51:4860–3. doi: 10.1002/anie.201200596

16. Gulati S, Smith DF, Cummings RD, Couch RB, Griesemer SB, St. George K, et al. Human H3N2 influenza viruses isolated from 1968 to 2012 show varying preference for receptor substructures with no apparent consequences for disease or spread. *PLoS ONE.* (2013) 8:e66325. doi: 10.1371/journal.pone.0066325

17. Prince HE, Leber AL. Comparison of complement fixation and hemagglutination inhibition assays for detecting antibody responses following influenza virus vaccination. *Clin Diagn Lab Immunol.* (2003) 10:481–2. doi: 10.1128/cdli.10.3.481-482.2003

18. Meulemans G, Carlier MC, Gonze M, Petit P. Comparison of hemagglutination-inhibition, agar gel precipitin, and enzyme-linked immunosorbent assay for measuring antibodies against influenza viruses in chickens. *Avian Dis.* (1987) 31:560. doi: 10.2307/1590740

19. Snyder DB, Marquardt WW, Yancey FS, Savage PK. An enzyme-linked immunosorbent assay for the detection of antibody against avian influenza virus. *Avian Dis.* (1985) 29:136. doi: 10.2307/1590702

20. Verschoor CP, Singh P, Russell ML, Bowdish DME, Brewer A, Cyr L, et al. Microneutralization assay titres correlate with protection against seasonal influenza H1N1 and H3N2 in children. *PLoS ONE.* (2015) 10:e0131531. doi: 10.1371/journal.pone.0131531

21. Lambrecht B, Steensels M, Van Borm S, Meulemans G, van den Berg T. Development of an M2e-specific enzyme-linked immunosorbent assay for differentiating infected from vaccinated animals. *Avian Dis.* (2007) 51:221-6. doi: 10.1637/7589-040206r.1

22. Chomel JJ, Thouvenot D, Onno M, Kaiser C, Gourreau JM, Aymard M. Rapid diagnosis of influenza infection of NP antigen using an immunocapture ELISA test. *J Virol Methods.* (1989) 25:81-91. doi: 10.1016/0166-0934(89)90102-x

23. Hause BM, Ducatez M, Collin EA, Ran Z, Liu R, Sheng Z, et al. Isolation of a novel swine influenza virus from Oklahoma in 2011 which is distantly related to human influenza C viruses. *PLoS Pathog.* (2013) 9:e1003176. doi: 10.1371/journal.ppat.1003176

24. Crescenzo-Chaigne B, Barbezange C, Van Der Werf S. Non coding extremities of the seven influenza virus type C vRNA segments: effect on transcription and replication by the type C and type a polymerase complexes. *Virol J.* (2008) 5:132. doi: 10.1186/1743-422X-5-132

25. Homma M, Ohyama S, Katagiri S. Age distribution of the antibody to type C influenza virus. *Microbiol Immunol.* (1982) 26:639-42. doi: 10.1111/mim.1982.26.7.639

26. Yuanji G, Fengen J, Ping W. Isolation of influenza C virus from pigs and experimental infection of pigs with influenza C virus. *J Gen Virol.* (1983) 64:177-82. doi: 10.1099/0022-1317-64-1-177

27. Ohwada K, Kitame F, Sugawara K, Nishimura H, Nakamura K, Homma M. Distribution of the antibody to influenza c virus in dogs and pigs in yamagata prefecture, Japan. *Microbiol Immunol.* (1987) 31:1173-80. doi: 10.1111/j.1348-0421.1987.tb01351.x

28. Salem E, Cook EAJ, Lbacha HA, Oliva J, Awoume F, Aplogan GL, et al. Serologic evidence for influenza c and d virus among ruminants and Camelids, Africa, 1991-2015. *Emerg Infect Dis.* (2017) 23:1556-9. doi: 10.3201/eid2309.170342

29. Nedland H, Wollman J, Sreenivasan C, Quast M, Singrey A, Fawcett L, et al. Serological evidence for the co-circulation of two lineages of influenza D viruses in equine populations of the Midwest United States. *Zoonoses Public Health.* (2018) 65:e148-54. doi: 10.1111/zph.12423

30. White SK, Ma W, McDaniel CJ, Gray GC, Lednicky JA. Serologic evidence of exposure to influenza D virus among persons with occupational contact with cattle. *J Clin Virol.* (2016) 81:31-3. doi: 10.1016/j.jcv.2016.05.017

31. Zhai SL, Zhang H, Chen SN, Zhou X, Lin T, Liu R, et al. Influenza D virus in animal species in Guangdong Province, Southern China. *Emerg Infect Dis.* (2017) 23:1392-6. doi: 10.3201/eid2308.170059

32. Song H, Qi J, Khedri Z, Diaz S, Yu H, Chen X, et al. An open receptor-binding cavity of hemagglutinin-esterase-fusion glycoprotein from newly-identified influenza D virus: basis for its broad cell tropism. *PLoS Pathog.* (2016) 12:e1005411. doi: 10.1371/journal.ppat.1005411

33. Reed LJ, Muench H. A simple method of estimating fifty per cent endpoints12. *Am J Epidemiol.* (1938) 27:493-7. doi: 10.1093/oxfordjournals.aje.a118408

34. Okda F, Liu X, Singrey A, Clement T, Nelson J, Christopher-Hennings J, et al. Development of an indirect ELISA, blocking ELISA, fluorescent microsphere immunoassay and fluorescent focus neutralization assay for serologic evaluation of exposure to North American strains of porcine epidemic diarrhea virus. *BMC Vet Res.* (2015) 11:180. doi: 10.1186/s12917-015-0500-z

35. Okda F, Lawson S, Liu X, Singrey A, Clement T, Hain K, et al. Development of monoclonal antibodies and serological assays including indirect ELISA and fluorescent microsphere immunoassays for diagnosis of porcine deltacoronavirus. *BMC Vet Res.* (2016) 12:95. doi: 10.1186/s12917-016-0716-6

36. Rosenthal PB, Zhang X, Formanowski F, Fitz W, Wong C-H, Meier-Ewert H, et al. Structure of the haemagglutinin-esterase-fusion glycoprotein of influenza C virus. *Nature.* (1998) 396:92-96. doi: 10.1038/23974

37. Collin EA, Sheng Z, Lang Y, Ma W, Hause BM, Li F. Cocirculation of two distinct genetic and antigenic lineages of proposed influenza D virus in cattle. *J Virol.* (2015) 89:1036-42. doi: 10.1128/JVI.02718-14

38. Sui J, Hwang WC, Perez S, Wei G, Aird D, Chen L, et al. Structural and functional bases for broad-spectrum neutralization of avian and human influenza A viruses. *Nat Struct Mol Biol.* (2009) 16:265-73. doi: 10.1038/nsmb.1566

39. Li OTW, Barr I, Leung CYH, Chen H, Guan Y, Peiris JSM, et al. Reliable universal RT-PCR assays for studying influenza polymerase subunit gene sequences from all 16 haemagglutinin subtypes. *J Virol Methods.* (2007) 142:218-22. doi: 10.1016/j.jviromet.2007.01.015

40. Anestad G, Breivik N, Thoresen T. Rapid diagnosis of respiratory syncytial virus and influenza A virus infections by immunofluorescence: experience with a simplified procedure for the preparation of cell smears from nasopharyngeal secretions. *Acta Pathol Microbiol Immunol Scand Sect B Microbiol.* (1983) 91:267-71. doi: 10.1111/j.1699-0463.1983.tb00045.x

41. Fauvel M, Ozanne G. Immunofluorescence assay for human immunodeficiency virus antibody: investigation of cell fixation for virus inactivation and antigen preservation. *J Clin Microbiol.* (1989) 27:1810-3. doi: 10.1128/JCM.27.8.1810-1813.1989

42. Daisy JA, Lief FS, Friedman HM. Rapid diagnosis of influenza A infection by direct immunofluorescence of nasopharyngeal aspirates in adults. *J Clin Microbiol.* (1979) 9:688-92.

43. Anestad G, Maagaard O. Rapid diagnosis of equine influenza. *Vet Rec.* (1990) 126:550-1.

44. Clement T, Singrey A, Lawson S, Okda F, Nelson J, Diel D, et al. Measurement of neutralizing antibodies against porcine epidemic diarrhea virus in sow serum, colostrum, and milk samples and in piglet serum samples after feedback. *J Swine Heal Prod.* (2016) 24:147-53.

45. Gupta S, Elkhenany H, Kumar P, Okda FA. Animals in the COVID-19 era: between being a source, victims, or maybe our hope to overcome it! *Int J Coronaviruses.* (2020) 1:12-25. doi: 10.14302/issn.2692-1537.ijcv-20-3481

46. Maines TR, Chen LM, Matsuoka Y, Chen H, Rowe T, Ortin J, et al. Lack of transmission of H5N1 avian-human reassortant influenza viruses in a ferret model. *Proc Natl Acad Sci USA.* (2006) 103:12121-6. doi: 10.1073/pnas.0605134103

47. Smith DB, Gaunt ER, Digard P, Templeton K, Simmonds P. Detection of influenza C virus but not influenza D virus in Scottish respiratory samples. *J Clin Virol.* (2016) 74:50-3. doi: 10.1016/j.jcv.2015.11.036

48. Ishida H, Murakami S, Kamiki H, Matsugo H, Takenaka-Uema A, Horimoto T. Establishment of a reverse genetics system for influenza D virus. *J Virol.* (2020) 94:e01767-19. doi: 10.1128/JVI.01767-19

14

Design of a High-Throughput Real-Time PCR System for Detection of Bovine Respiratory and Enteric Pathogens

Nicole B. Goecke [1,2]*, Bodil H. Nielsen [3], Mette B. Petersen [4] and Lars E. Larsen [2]

[1] Centre for Diagnostics, Technical University of Denmark, Lyngby, Denmark, [2] Department of Veterinary and Animal Sciences, University of Copenhagen, Copenhagen, Denmark, [3] Department of Animal Science, Aarhus University, Aarhus, Denmark, [4] Department of Veterinary Clinical Sciences, University of Copenhagen, Copenhagen, Denmark

Correspondence:
Nicole B. Goecke
nbgo@sund.ku.dk

Bovine respiratory and enteric diseases have a profound negative impact on animal, health, welfare, and productivity. A vast number of viruses and bacteria are associated with the diseases. Pathogen detection using real-time PCR (rtPCR) assays performed on traditional rtPCR platforms are costly and time consuming and by that limit the use of diagnostics in bovine medicine. To diminish these limitations, we have developed a high-throughput rtPCR system (BioMark HD; Fluidigm) for simultaneous detection of the 11 most important respiratory and enteric viral and bacterial pathogens. The sensitivity and specificity of the rtPCR assays on the high-throughput platform was comparable with that of the traditional rtPCR platform. Pools consisting of positive and negative individual field samples were tested in the high-throughput rtPCR system in order to investigate the effect of an individual sample in a pool. The pool tests showed that irrespective of the size of the pool, a high-range positive individual sample had a high influence on the cycle quantification value of the pool compared with the influence of a low-range positive individual sample. To validate the test on field samples, 2,393 nasal swab and 2,379 fecal samples were tested on the high-throughput rtPCR system as pools in order to determine the occurrence of the 11 pathogens in 100 Danish herds (83 dairy and 17 veal herds). In the dairy calves, *Pasteurella multocida* (38.4%), rotavirus A (27.4%), *Mycoplasma* spp. (26.2%), and *Trueperella pyogenes* (25.5%) were the most prevalent pathogens, while *P. multocida* (71.4%), *Mycoplasma* spp. (58.9%), *Mannheimia haemolytica* (53.6%), and *Mycoplasma bovis* (42.9%) were the most often detected pathogens in the veal calves. The established high-throughput system provides new possibilities for analysis of bovine samples, since the system enables testing of multiple samples for the presence of different pathogens in the same analysis test even with reduced costs and turnover time.

Keywords: high-throughput, real-time PCR, viruses, bacteria, bovine pathogens, prevalence

INTRODUCTION

Bovine respiratory and enteric diseases have a profound negative impact on animal, health, welfare, and productivity. The two major calf disease syndromes are bovine respiratory disease (BRD) and bovine enteric disease (BED) which are multifactorial diseases associated with presence of a range of pathogens, environmental factors, stress conditions, and health and immunological status of the animal. Bovine respiratory disease and BED can have substantive economic consequence due to reduced productivity, increased mortality, and/or morbidity, as well as decreased animal welfare and increased use of antibiotics (1–3).

Bovine respiratory disease is most severe in calves between 2 weeks and 6 months of age. A wide range of viruses and bacteria are involved in BRD, including bovine adenovirus, bovine coronavirus (BCoV), bovine herpesvirus 1 (BHV1), bovine parainfluenza virus type 3, bovine respiratory syncytial virus (BRSV), bovine viral diarrhea virus (BVDV), *Mannheimia haemolytica*, *Pasteurella multocida*, *Histophilus somni*, and *Mycoplasma bovis* (4–6). The viruses BHV1 and BVDV have been eradicated in several countries, including Denmark (7). In addition to the abovementioned viruses, influenza D virus (IDV), bovine rhinitis A virus, and bovine torovirus (BToV) have recently been shown to be involved in BRD (8–10). Furthermore, the bacterium *Trueperella pyogenes* has also been associated with BRD (6). Development of severe respiratory signs often involves a primary viral infection followed by a secondary bacterial infection (1, 11, 12). The progression of BRD is believed to be related to suppression of the immune system, allowing for inflammation and damage of the respiratory tissue, which in severe cases can lead to pneumonia or even death (13).

Bovine enteric disease is often associated with diarrhea, which is one of the most economically costly disorders in the calves industry due to weight loss and deaths of young animals (3). Multiple viruses, bacteria, and parasites have been identified as the causative agents of diarrhea. The most important infectious agents are BCoV, rotavirus A (RVA), BVDV, *Escherichia coli* F5 (K99+), *Salmonella* spp., *Clostridium perfringens*, *Cryptosporidium parvum*, and *Eimeria* spp. Several of these pathogens are associated with diarrhea within a particular age group (14–17). Furthermore, viruses such as bovine norovirus, bovine enterovirus, rotavirus B and C, BToV, and nebovirus have also been shown to be potential diarrhea-causing pathogens (14, 18–21). Each of these pathogens can cause disease individually, but mixed infections are also commonly seen, which often lead to more severe disease (14, 22).

Since a vast number of viral and bacterial pathogens are involved in both BRD and BED, it is essential to have a highly specific and sensitive diagnostic method for rapid identification of the causative pathogens. A variety of laboratory tests, including culture and molecular methods, have been described and these methods all have their benefits and limitations in regard to sensitivity, specificity, predictive values, speed, and costs (23). During recent years, a range of multiplex real-time PCR (rtPCR) tests targeting pathogens involved in BRD and/or BED have been developed (24–28). The multiplex rtPCR test allows for simultaneous analysis of three–five pathogens in a single sample. However, the number of available targets that can be tested in one run is limited because multiplex rtPfoCR is based on traditional rtPCR platforms, which have a limited number of detection channels. A general disadvantage of the common used tests is the high costs. Therefore, pooling of individual samples can be beneficial and cost effective especially as it requires no additional equipment or materials (29). Pooling can be favorable in screening and surveillance programs, and if information at the individual sample level is required, subsequent individual tests can be performed if the pooled sample is positive.

In order to diminish the limitations of the traditional rtPCR platforms, we previously have established high-throughput rtPCR systems for detection and screening of respiratory and enteric viral and bacterial porcine pathogens (30, 31) and for detection and differentiation of influenza A viruses circulating in Danish pigs (32). The high-throughput rtPCR platform BioMark HD (Fluidigm, South San Francisco, CA) and the dynamic array (DA) integrated fluidic circuit (IFC) nanofluidic chip have been utilized. Different DA IFC chips exist which can combine either 48 samples with 48 assays (48.48DA), 96 samples with 96 assays (96.96DA), 192 samples with 24 assays (192.24DA), or 24 samples with 192 assays (24.192DA), resulting in 2,304, 9,216 or 4,608 individual reactions, respectively. The rtPCR reactions are carried out in the DA IFC chip, which contains microfluidic networks that automatically combine the samples and rtPCR reagents in the reaction chambers. Furthermore, the high-throughput platform has also been used as a screening and detection tool for tick-borne and food- and water-borne pathogens (33, 34).

In the present paper, we describe the design, optimization, validation, and use of a similar high-throughput rtPCR system consisting of 11 rtPCR assays targeting 11 respiratory and enteric viral and bacterial bovine pathogens known to be involved in BRD and BED. The purpose of the high-throughput rtPCR system was to develop a system that can function as a rapid screening and detection tool suitable for the detection of disease-causing pathogen(s) within calf herds. Furthermore, pools consisting of different numbers of positive and negative individual field samples were tested in order to investigate the effect of the individual samples in a pool. Lastly, the occurrence of the 11 respiratory and enteric viral and bacterial pathogens in Danish calves was evaluated by using the developed high-throughput rtPCR system.

MATERIALS AND METHODS
Samples and Sampling
Known positive samples (controls) were used for optimization and initial validation of the high-throughput rtPCR system and the associated rtPCR assays. The positive controls consisted of pure bacterial cultures, cell culture lysates (viruses), and synthesized plasmids coding for the specific PCR targets. Initially, the positive controls were tested by culturing and/or by established and validated PCR assays and/or sequencing. The positive controls were obtained from the routine diagnostic laboratory at the Centre for Diagnostics, Technical University

of Denmark (DTU). Furthermore, field samples (nasal swab and fecal samples) collected from Danish calves were used for validation of the high-throughput rtPCR system. Nasal swab samples were collected by inserting a sterile cotton swab (Technical University of Denmark, Lyngby, Denmark) approximately 8–10 cm into one nostril and turning the swab around for a few seconds. No prior cleaning of the nostril was performed. Immediately after, the swabs were placed and stored in 1.5 ml phosphate-buffered saline (PBS). Fecal samples were collected from each calf by gathering the feces in a 10-ml tube when the calf was expelling feces from the rectum. If the calf did not defecated spontaneously, a finger was inserted into the rectum and defecation was stimulated by gentle manipulation of the intestinal wall. The samples were kept refrigerated (approximately 5°C) for up to 48 h prior to shipment, and they were sent in a box containing freezer packs to the Centre for Diagnostics, DTU, where the samples were stored at −80°C until nucleic acid extraction. Prior to extraction, a 10% dilution in PBS was made for each of the individual fecal samples by weighing 0.1 g of the feces and adding PBS. The nasal swab samples were vortexed to transfer the biological material to PBS. The nasal swab and fecal samples were analyzed as individual samples and/or as pools. Before the nucleic acid extraction, the samples were pooled based on herd and age group with five to 10 samples per pool. The 10% feces dilutions were pooled with equal volume (μl) of each individual sample. The nasal swab samples were also pooled with equal volume (μl) of each individual sample. For the samples, which were analyzed both individually and in a pool, the sample material used for both analyses originated from the same original sample for the nasal swab samples. For the feces samples, the sample material used came from the same 10% dilution of the original sample.

For the field study, 4,772 field samples (2,393 nasal swab and 2,379 fecal samples) were collected from 100 Danish, intensive, commercial herds (83 dairy and 17 veal herds). The veal herds were rosé veal producers that produce meat from calves fed on a diet without restriction of iron intake. The rosé veal calves are slaughtered when they are between 8 and 12 months old. Sampling was done in the winter period from September to April in 2018 and 2019. The samples were collected from three age groups in the dairy herds (0–10 days, 3 weeks, 3 months) and two age groups in the veal herds (2 weeks after arrival and at 3 months of age). In the first and second age groups, calves were primarily kept in single pens. In the two oldest age groups, calves were kept indoor in groups. Feeding regimes differed according to local management. Typically, the calves were milk fed for 8–12 weeks. In 14 cases, it was not possible to obtain a fecal sample, as the calf did not defecate and the rectum was empty. Therefore, the number of fecal samples differed from the number of nasal swab samples.

Nucleic Acid Extraction

RNA and DNA were extracted from the nasal swab samples using the extraction robot QIAcube HT (QIAGEN, Hilden, Germany) and the Cador Pathogen 96 QIAcube HT kit (QIAGEN) using the manufacturer's instructions. Before

nucleic acid extraction, nasal swab samples were prepared by centrifuging 400 μl of each individual sample or pool for 5 min at 9,000×g at room temperature (15–25°C), and 200 μl of the supernatant was subsequently used for extraction. Positive and negative (nuclease-free water; Amresco, Cleveland, OH) controls were included in each extraction. The nucleic acids were stored at −80°C until further analysis.

RNA and DNA were extracted from 10% fecal dilutions of the individual samples or from pools consisting of the 10% fecal dilutions using the extraction robot QIAcube HT (QIAGEN) and the Cador Pathogen 96 QIAcube HT kit (QIAGEN). Prior to nucleic acid extraction, one 5-mm steel bead was added to each sample or pool and the samples or pools were homogenized in a TissueLyser II (QIAGEN) for 20 s at 15 Hz. The homogenate was centrifuged for 90 s at 6,700×g, and 200 μl of the supernatant was used for extraction. Positive and negative (nuclease-free water; Amresco) controls were included in each extraction. The nucleic acid extractions were stored at −80°C until further analysis.

Primer and Probe Design

Eleven rtPCR assays targeting respiratory and enteric viral and bacterial pathogens were established (**Table 1**). The primer and probe sequences were copied either from previously published assays or designed in this study. Some of the published primer and probe sequences were modified to improve the specificity or to adapt to the selected PCR conditions. New primer and probe sequences were designed based on alignments containing sequences of the target gene for the selected pathogens. The sequences were retrieved from GenBank (35) and aligned using CLC Main Workbench version 8.0 (QIAGEN). The specificity of the oligonucleotides were tested *in silico* using nucleotide BLAST search (36), and the melting temperature and basic properties were approximated using OligoCalc (37). The oligonucleotides were purchased from Eurofins Genomics (Ebersberg, Germany).

Traditional rtPCR Platform

Initially, the sensitivity and specificity of the rtPCR assays were validated on the Rotor-Gene Q rtPCR platform (QIAGEN) using 10-fold serial dilutions of the positive controls. For the rtPCR assays targeting RNA viruses, AgPath-ID one-step RT-PCR reagents kit (Applied Biosystems, Foster City, CA) was used with a final reaction volume of 15 μl. The PCR mix consisted of 7.5 μl RT-PCR buffer (2×), 0.45 μl of each primer (10 μM), 0.45 μl probe (10 μM), 0.6 μl RT-PCR enzyme mix (25×), 3.55 μl nuclease-free water, and 2 μl RNA. The PCR reactions were run at the following thermal cycling conditions: 45°C for 20 min, 95°C for 10 min, followed by 45 cycles of 94°C for 15 s, and 60°C for 45 s.

For the rtPCR assays targeting DNA viruses and bacteria, JumpStart Taq ready mix (Sigma-Aldrich, St. Louis, MO) was used with a final reaction volume of 25 μl. The PCR mix contained 12.5 μl JumpStart Taq ready mix (2×), 0.75 μl of each primer (10 μM), 0.2 μl probe (30 μM), 3.5 μl MgCl$_2$ (25 mM),

TABLE 1 | Viruses and bacteria, assay names, and primer and probe sequences used for detection of viruses and bacteria.

Pathogen	Target gene	Name	Sequence (5'-3')	Length (bp)	Reference
BRSV	F	BRSV-F-485F	AAGGGTCAAACATCTGCTTAACTAG	85	Hakhverdyan et al. (66)
		BRSV-F-569R	TCTGCCTGWGGGAAAAAAG		
		BRSV F Taqman-546	FAM-AGAGCCTGCATTRTCACAATACCACCCA-BHQ1		
BCoV	M	BCoV-F	GTTGGTGGAGTTTCAACCCAG	90	F, R, and P (modified): Decaro et al. (65)
		BCoV-R	GGTAGTCCTCAATTATCGGCC		
		BCoV-P	FAM-CATCCTTCCCTTCATATCTATACACATC-BHQ1		
E. coli F5		E. coli F5-F	GAGGTCAATGGTAATCGTACATC	117	This study
		E. coli F5-R	CGCTAGGCAGTCAYTACTGC		
		E. coli F5-P	FAM-GATCTTGGGCAGGCTGCTATTAGTGGT-BHQ1		
H. somni	16S rRNA	HS-F	GAAGATACTGACGCTCGAGT	115	F and P: this study; R: Angen et al. (64)
		HS-R	TTCGGGCACCAAGTRTTCA		
		HS-P	FAM-TCCCCAAATCGACATCGTTTACAGCGTG-BHQ1		
IDV	PB1	IDV-F	GCTGTTTGCAAGTTGATGGG	136	Hause et al. (50)
		IDV-R	TGAAAGCAGGTAACTCCAAGG		
		IDV-P	FAM-TTCAGGCAAGCACCCGTAGGATT-BHQ1		
M. haemolytica	sodA	M. hae-F	GCCGTTGTTTCAACCGCTAAC	100	This study
		M. hae-R	CGTGTTCCCAAACGTCTAAGAC		
		M. hae-P	FAM-TCGGATAGCCTGAAACGCCTGCCAC-BHQ1		
M. bovis	oppD	PMB996-F	TCAAGGAACCCCACCAGAT	71	Sachse et al. (68)
		PMB1066-R	AGGCAAAGTCATTTCTAGGTGCAA		
		Mbovis1016	FAM-TGGCAAACTTACCTATCGGTGACCCT-TAMRA		
Mycoplasma spp.	16S rRNA	Mycoplasma-F	GATCCTGGCTCAGGATGAAC	103	This study
		Mycoplasma-R	CGTTGAGTACGTGTTACTCAC		
		Mycoplasma-P	FAM-GGCTGTGTGCCTAATACATGCATGTCG-BHQ1		
P. multocida	kmt1	PM-ny-F	GACTACCGACAAGCCCACTC	125	F and R: this study; P: Goecke et al. (30)
		PM-ny-R	CTATCCGCTATTTACCCAGTGG		
		PM-P	FAM-GTGCGAATGAACCGATTGCCGCG- BHQ1		
RVA	NSP3	Rota A-F	ACCATCTACACATGACCCTC	84	F and P: Pang et al. (67); R: this study
		Rota A-ny-R	CACATAACGCCCCTATAGCC		
		Rota A-P	FAM-ATGAGCACAATAGTTAAAAGCTAACACTGTCAA-TAMRA		
T. pyogenes	plo-Pyolysin	T. pyogenes-F	CATCAACAATCCCACGAAGAG	98	F (modified) and R: Kishimoto et al. (25); P: this study
		T. pyogenes-R	TTGCAGCATGGTCAGGATAC		
		T. pyogenes-P	FAM-CCGTGACTCAAGGACTGAACGGCCT-BHQ1		

4.3 μl nuclease-free water, and 3 μl DNA. The PCR reactions were tested at the following thermal cycle conditions: 94°C for 2 min, followed by 40 cycles of 94°C for 15 s, and 60°C for 60 s.

Data, including quantification cycle (Cq) values and amplification curves, obtained from the abovementioned PCR reactions were analyzed using Rotor-Gene series software version 2.3.1 (QIAGEN) with the following parameter adjustments: dynamic tube normalization, on; noise slope correction, on; ignore first cycle; outlier removal, 10%; and Cq fixed, 0.01. All reactions, samples, and positive and negative (nuclease-free water; Amresco) controls were run in duplicates. For each of the rtPCR assays, a standard curve was constructed from the Cq values. The amplification efficiency was calculated based on the slope of the standard curve, as previously described (38).

Reverse Transcription and Preamplification Prior to High-Throughput rtPCR

For RNA targets, one-tube combined reverse-transcription and preamplifications were performed in a final volume of 15 μl using AgPath-ID one-step RT-PCR reagents kit (Applied Biosystems); 7.5 μl RT-PCR buffer (2×), 0.75 μl of 200 nM primer mix (containing the different sets of primers (20 μM each) listed in **Table 1**), 0.6 μl random hexamer (50 μM), 0.6 μl RT-PCR enzyme mix (25×), 2.55 nuclease-free water, and 3 μl RNA were mixed. The PCR was performed on a T3 Thermocycler (Biometra, Fredensborg, Denmark) with the following thermal cycle conditions: 45°C for 20 min, 95°C for 10 min, followed by 24 cycles at 94°C for 15 s, and 60°C for 45 s. The preamplified complementary DNA (cDNA) was stored at −20°C.

For DNA targets, preamplification were performed using TaqMan PreAmp master mix (Applied Biosystems) in a final volume of 10 μl containing 5 μl master mix, 2.5 μl of 200 nM primer mix [containing the different sets of primers (20 μM each) listed in **Table 1**], and 2.5 μl DNA. Preamplification was performed on a T3 Thermocycler (Biometra) with the following thermal cycle conditions: 95°C for 10 min, followed by 14 cycles at 95°C for 15 s, and 60°C for 4 min. The preamplified DNA was stored at −20°C until testing.

High-Throughput rtPCR

For the rtPCR analysis, the high-throughput rtPCR platform BioMark HD (Fluidigm) and the BioMark 192.24 DA IFC chip (Fluidigm) were used. For each sample, a 4-μl sample mix containing 2 μl TaqMan gene expression master mix (2×) (Applied Biosystems), 0.2 μl sample loading reagent (20×) (Fluidigm), and 1.8 μl preamplified sample was prepared. For each assay, a 4-μl assay mix containing 2 μl assay loading reagent (2×) (Fluidigm) and 2 μl primer-probe stock (final concentration: 16 μM primers and 5 μM probe) was prepared. Three-microliter sample mix and 3 μl assay mix were loaded into the respective inlets of the 192.24 DA IFC chip. The 192.24.DA IFC chip was placed in the IFC controller RX (Fluidigm) for loading and mixing for approximately 30 min and then subject to thermal cycling in the high-throughput rtPCR instrument BioMark HD (Fluidigm) with the following cycle conditions: 50°C for 2 min, 95°C for 10 min, followed by 40 cycles of 95°C for 15 s and 60°C for 60 s. Samples were tested in single reactions, and the assays were performed in duplicates. In each 192.24 DA IFC chip run, positive and negative (nuclease-free water; Amresco) PCR and extraction controls were included. Data, including Cq values and amplification curves, obtained on the BioMark system, were analyzed using the Fluidigm Real-Time PCR Analysis software version 4.5.2 (Fluidigm).

Assessment of the Sensitivity, Specificity and Application of the rtPCR Assays

Initially, the rtPCR assays were validated on the Rotor-Gene Q (QAGEN) and BioMark HD (192.24 DA IFC) (Fluidigm) platforms by running 10-fold serial dilutions for each of the positive controls in duplicates in order to analyze the sensitivity and amplification efficiency on the two platforms. For each of the rtPCR assays, a standard curve was constructed from the Cq values. The amplification efficiency was calculated based on the slope of the standard, curve as previously described (38).

To assess the specificity of the rtPCR assays on the high-throughput rtPCR platform (BioMark HD; Fluidigm), the positive controls were initially tested, followed by testing of 32 field samples (19 nasal swab and 13 fecal samples). Six field samples positive for either *E. coli* F5 or *M. haemolytica* were selected for Sanger sequencing in order to verify the specificity of the rtPCR assays. Prior to sequencing, the selected samples were PCR amplified on the Rotor-Gene Q platform (QIAGEN), and the PCR products were purified using the High Pure PCR Product Purification kit (Roche, Basel, Switzerland) according to the manufacturer's instructions. The samples were sequenced at LGC Genomics GmbH (Berlin, Germany). The obtained sequences were assembled and analyzed using CLC Main Workbench version 8.0 (QIAGEN). The analyzed sequences

were aligned to published sequences using the database NCBI BLAST (36).

To evaluate the repeatability of the rtPCR assays on the high-throughput rtPCR platform (BioMark HD; Fluidigm), the positive controls were tested on 13 separated 192.24 DA IFC chip runs and the outcomes were compared along the chip runs.

The application of the high-throughput rtPCR platform (BioMark HD; Fludigm) and 192.24 DA IFC chip was validated by testing 4,772 field samples, which were pooled in 980 pools (491 pools of nasal swab and 489 pools of fecal samples).

Assessment of Test of Pooled Samples Contra Test of Individual Samples

In order to compare test of pooled samples with test of individual samples, a pilot study was performed. Three different setups were made for five selected assays (*Mycoplasma* spp., *M. bovis*, *H. somni*, *T. pyogenes*, and RVA) using field samples selected based on the results obtained in the high-throughput rtPCR analysis.

In the first and second setup, the effect of increasing the number of positive samples and decreasing the number of negative samples within a pool was tested. In the first setup, the pools consisted of 10 samples with a varying number of positive and negative samples. The pools were made with the following distribution of positive and negative samples; 1:9, 2:8, 3:7, 4:6, 5:5, 6:4, 7:3, 8:2, and 9:1 (number of positive samples:number of negative samples). Similarly, the second setup tested pools consisting of five samples instead of 10 samples. In the third setup, the effect of increasing the number of negative samples within a pool containing one positive sample was tested. Here, the pools consisted of one positive sample and an increasing number of negative samples with the following structure 1:1, 1:2, 1:3, 1:4, 1:5, 1:6, 1:7, and 1:8 (number of positive samples:number of negative samples). The constructed pools from the three setups were analyzed on the high-throughput rtPCR system, as described above.

RESULTS

Sensitivity and Amplification Efficiency of the rtPCR Assays

To evaluate the sensitivity and amplification efficiency of the rtPCR assays, 10-fold serial dilutions of the positive controls were tested on the Rotor-Gene Q (QIAGEN) and BioMark HD (Fluidigm) platforms. Standard curves were constructed using mean Cq values from duplicate 10-fold serial dilutions, in which the efficiency was calculated for each of the rtPCR assays (**Table 2**).

The sensitivity of the rtPCR assays was in the range of 3–7 $\log_{10}$, and the results were identical or differed by one $\log_{10}$ between the two platforms (**Table 2**). Similarly, the dynamic range of the rtPCR assays was either identical or differed by one $\log_{10}$. Furthermore, the amplification efficiency of the rtPCR assays was comparable for the Rotor-Gene Q (QIAGEN) and the BioMark HD (Fluidigm) platforms and was 78–103% and 79–118%, respectively. For some of the rtPCR assays (*H. somni*, *T. pyogenes*), the undiluted and the first diluted sample were excluded from the calculation of efficiency of the BioMark HD (Fluidigm) platform because the Cq was too low. This exclusion resulted in a shorter dynamic range for these rtPCR assays when run on the BioMark HD (Fluidigm) platform compared with the Rotor-Gene Q (QIAGEN) run.

The Cq values obtained by the BioMark HD (Fluidigm) platform were allocated into three categories; high-range positive (Cq value ≤13), mid-range positive (Cq value 14–20), and low-range positive (Cq value ≥21).

Test of the Specificity of the rtPCR Assays

Initially, the specificity of the rtPCR assays was tested on the BioMark HD (Fluidigm) platform and the 192.24 DA IFC chip by testing the positive controls for each pathogen in all assays. For each rtPCR assay, the specificity was assessed based on the Cq value and the corresponding amplification curve obtained from the respective positive control. Positive results were obtained in the rtPCR assay specific for the correct positive control sample only—that is, no cross-reaction to any of the other positive control samples was detected (**Figure 1**). Furthermore, 32 field samples (nasal swab and fecal samples) were tested on the high-throughput system in order to investigate the performance on field samples (**Table 3**). Six of these field samples, which tested positive for either E. coli F5 or M. haemolytica, were selected for Sanger sequencing (**Table 4**). The obtained sequences were aligned to previously published sequences using the database NCBI BLAST (36). Eight sequences showed 100% identity to the two field samples positive for E. coli F5 (samples 2 and 4). For three out of four M. haemolytica-positive field samples, 89 sequences showed 100% identity to these (samples 15, 19, and 20), while for the last field sample (sample 21), the 89 sequences showed 98.7–99.0% identity. The accession numbers of the published sequences which showed the highest identity to the sequences obtained in this study are listed in **Table 4**.

Test of Repeatability of the rtPCR Assays on the High-Throughput rtPCR Platform

The repeatability of the rtPCR assays on the high-throughput rtPCR platform (BioMark HD) was evaluated by testing the positive controls in 13 separate chip runs. The mean Cq value and standard deviation (SD) were calculated for each of the positive controls, and the SD was found to be between ±0.35 and 1.00 for all the positive control samples (**Table 5**).

Comparative Testing of Pooled and Individual Samples

The results of the three different pool setups are shown for each pathogen in **Supplementary Tables 1A–E**. In general, the results from the first and second setup showed that irrespective of the size of the pool, an individual sample with a high-range positive Cq value had a higher influence on the Cq value of the pool compared with the influence of an individual sample with a low-range positive Cq value.

TABLE 2 | Sensitivity and amplification efficiency of rtPCR assays on the Rotor-Gene Q and BioMark platforms.

Dilution	BRSV		BCoV		E. coli F5		H. somni		IDV		M. haemolytica		M. bovis		Mycoplasma spp.		P. multocida		RVA		T. pyogenes	
	Rotor-gene	BioMark gene	Rotor-gene	BioMark gene	Rotor-gene	BioMark gene	Rotor-gene	BioMark gene	Rotor-gene	BioMark gene	Rotor-gene	BioMark gene	Rotor-gene	BioMark gene	Rotor-gene	BioMark gene	Rotor-gene	BioMark gene	Rotor-gene	BioMark gene	Rotor-gene	BioMark gene
10	12.7	NA	18.6	12.6	12.6	3.3	9.0	(3.3)	23.6	11.0	11.0	(2.5)	12.6	(2.5)	13.0	(3.4)	10.9	(3.5)	18.4	6.3	(11)	(2.5)
10^{-1}	15.5	13.0	22.0	16.5	15.5	7.7	11.4	(3.7)	26.5	14.3	14.1	2.8	15.9	3.3	15.9	3.9	13.8	3.9	21.6	8.9	12.8	(2.5)
10^{-2}	18.6	18.8	25.4	19.5	19.6	13.0	14.5	2.5	30.1	17.4	17.7	5.8	19.1	6.0	19.5	7.6	17.7	6.7	25.4	12.4	15.5	2.5
10^{-3}	22.4	21.0	28.6	21.4	23.6	15.8	17.6	6.2	34.1	21.4	21.1	9.3	22.6	9.1	22.9	10.9	21.1	10.3	28.1	15.7	19.4	6.0
10^{-4}	25.4	25.4	32.3	24.7	28.6	17.6	20.9	9.0	–	–	24.6	12.4	26.2	12.8	26.3	15.0	24.6	14.1	32.0	18.5	23.6	9.9
10^{-5}	28.2	27.9	35.4	–	(33.1)	20.9	24.5	12.6	–	–	28.0	16.0	29.5	15.9	29.9	17.3	27.8	16.7	34.9	23.7	27.0	13.3
10^{-6}	32.3	–	–	–	(37.8)	23.9	28.7	16.8	–	–	31.1	19.0	33.3	18.7	32.9	19.9	31.0	19.8	–	26.0	30.3	17.4
10^{-7}	(34.4)	–	–	–	–	–	32.2	19.3	–	–	–	22.2	–	21.2	36.3	–	–	(24.6)	–	–	33.2	–
10^{-8}	–	–	–	–	–	–	–	–	–	–	–	–	–	(23.7)	–	–	–	–	–	–	–	–
Efficiency	1.03	0.79	0.98	1.18	0.78	1.02	0.99	0.97	0.92	1.03	0.97	1.01	0.95	1.09	0.98	1.09	0.97	1.03	0.99	0.99	0.92	0.83

Numbers: Cq values. "–" negative sample; NA, sample was not analyzed. Number in parentheses is not included in the efficiency calculation.

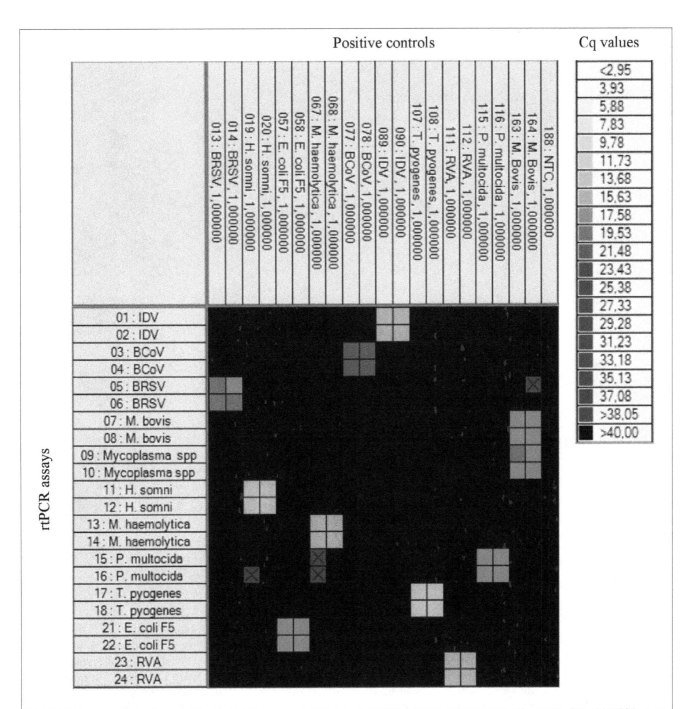

FIGURE 1 | Heat map showing the specificity of the rtPCR assays on the high-throughput rtPCR system by testing known positive controls. To the left: rtPCR assays (**Table 1**). At the top: the positive controls and a no-template control (NTC). Each square corresponds to a single rtPCR reaction. Cq values for each reaction are indicated by color; the corresponding color scale is presented in the legend on the right. A black square is considered a negative result. A black X is shown if the amplification curve deviates too much from an ideal amplification curve.

For all five pathogens in the first setup, there was a decrease in the Cq value of the first pool (1:9) to the last pool (9:1), meaning that the pool became increasingly positive. However, the degree of decrease was varied between the different pathogens. For *Mycoplasma* spp., *H. somni*, and RVA there was a decrease of 5.3–6.4 Cq values, while for *M. bovis* and *T. pyogenes*, the decrease in Cq was 1.6 and 0.3, respectively. In the second setup, the Cq value of the pool decreased (became more positive) with increasing numbers of positive samples for four of the pathogens. For *H. somni*, the Cq values for two of the pools (3:2 and 4:1)

TABLE 3 | Feces and nasal swab samples analyzed on the high-throughput rtPCR system.

Sample	Material	BRSV	BCoV	M. bovis	Mycoplasma spp.	M. haemolytica	H. somni	IDV	P. multocida	RVA	E. coli F5
1	Feces		–	–	–					–	29.0
2	Feces		–	–	–					17.0	22.4
3	Feces		–	–	–					6.5	–
4	Feces		–	–	–					–	21.5
5	Feces		–	–	–					–	27.6
6	Feces		–	–	–					–	–
7	Feces		–	–	–					–	–
8	Feces		–	–	–					–	–
9	Feces		–	–	–					–	–
10	Feces		19.0	–	–					–	–
11	Feces		–	–	–					–	–
12	Feces		–	–	–					–	–
13	Feces		–	–	–					–	–
14	Nasal swab	–	–	–	24.0	–	–	–	–		
15	Nasal swab	–	–	–	23.4	22.4	–	–	17.2		
16	Nasal swab	–	–	–	–	–	–	–	–		
17	Nasal swab	–	–	–	–	–	–	–	–		
18	Nasal swab	–	–	–	–	–	–	–	–		
19	Nasal swab	–	–	17.4	13.1	15.0	–	–	18.3		
20	Nasal swab	–	–	15.9	15.5	18.1	–	–	17.5		
21	Nasal swab	–	–	–	15.2	16.8	18.6	–	21.0		
22	Nasal swab	–	26.2	16.5	12.8	13.8	–	–	18.9		
23	Nasal swab	–	–	25.9	11.3	14.7	19.5	–	19.9		
24	Nasal swab	–	–	–	NA	–	20.0	–	18.2		
25	Nasal swab	–	–	–	NA	17.2	–	–	18.6		
26	Nasal swab	–	–	–	NA	20.7	14.1	–	19.7		
27	Nasal swab	–	–	–	NA	–	20.5	–	17.7		
28	Nasal swab	–	–	–	NA	–	–	–	21.3		
29	Nasal swab	–	–	–	NA	–	–	–	–		
30	Nasal swab	–	–	–	NA	22.5	19.1	–	–		
31	Nasal swab	–	–	–	NA	21.3	23.2	–	–		
32	Nasal swab	–	–	–	NA	20.66	–	–	27.4		

Numbers: Cq values. "–" negative result; NA, sample was not analyzed. Gray cell: analysis not relevant.

were 17.0 and 17.1, respectively, and therefore a decrease in the Cq value of the pool was not observed. In the third setup, in which an increasing number of negative individual samples were added to a pool containing one positive sample, the pool became less positive (higher Cq value) as the number of negative samples increased. For all of the five pathogens, the pool was only made to dilution 1:8 due to a limited amount of available negative samples. For the RVA pool, the Cq value increased from 8.8 (pool 1:1) to 16.4 (pool 1:8), which was more than expected in relation to a 10-fold dilution in theory should increase the Cq value with a value of 3.3. The positive sample in the RVA pool had a high-range positive Cq value (8.3) compared with the positive samples in the *Mycoplasma* spp., *M. bovis*, *H. somni*, and *T. pyogenes* pools, which had a Cq value between 16.4 and 17.9.

Occurrences of Respiratory and Enteric Pathogens in Danish Calves

The occurrence of the different pathogens in Danish calves was evaluated by testing 980 pools of nasal swab and feces samples on the high-throughput rtPCR system. The samples were collected from dairy and veal calves at different ages from 100 Danish herds (83 dairy and 17 veal herds). In total, 491 nasal swab pools and 489 feces pools were analyzed and the overall occurrence of each pathogen was calculated (**Figure 2**; **Table 6**). Furthermore, the occurrence of each pathogen in each age group on the herd level was calculated as the number of herds with at least one positive pool divided by the total number of herds (**Table 7**).

Overall Pathogen Occurrence

In general, the overall occurrence of the respiratory pathogens in the different age groups showed that the bacterial pathogens were more frequent than the viruses both in the dairy and veal calves (**Table 6**). In the dairy calves, *P. multocida* (38.4%), *Mycoplasma* spp. (26.2%), *T. pyogenes* (25.5%), and *M. haemolytica* (17.5%) were found to be the most prevalent pathogens across all age groups followed by *H. somni* (6.9%) and *M. bovis* (4.4%). For the bacterial pathogens, the highest occurrences were found in the oldest age group except for *T. pyogenes*, which was most

TABLE 4 | Samples sequenced by Sanger sequencing.

Sample	Pathogen	BLAST results — accession no.
2	E. coli F5	MH916617, KR870316, KR606337, KP054295, JX987524, GU951525, FJ864678, M35282 (100% identity)
4	E. coli F5	MH916617, KR870316, KR606337, KP054295, JX987524, GU951525, FJ864678, M35282 (100% identity)
15	M. haemolytica	CP017484-17552, CP026857-58, CP029638, LS483299, CP023043-44, CP023046-47, CP006957, CP004752-53, CP011098-99, CP006619, CP005972-74, CP005383, AY702551, AY702512 (100% identity)
19	M. haemolytica	CP017484-17552, CP026857-58, CP029638, LS483299, CP023043-44, CP023046-47, CP006957, CP004752-53, CP011098-99, CP006619, CP005972-74, CP005383, AY702551, AY702512 (100% identity)
20	M. haemolytica	CP017484-17552, CP026857-58, CP029638, LS483299, CP023043-44, CP023046-47, CP006957, CP004752-53, CP011098-99, CP006619, CP005972-74, CP005383, AY702551, AY702512 (100% identity)
21	M. haemolytica	CP017484-17552, CP026857-58, CP029638, LS483299, CP023043-44, CP023046-47, CP006957, CP004752-53, CP011098-99, CP006619, CP005972-74, CP005383, AY702551, AY702512 (98.96%—98.73% identity)

Comparison of percentage identity with already published sequences.

TABLE 5 | Test of repeatability of the rtPCR assays on the high-throughput rtPCR platform.

Positive control	No. of repeats	Mean Cq value	Standard deviation (±)
BRSV	13	21.7	1.00
BCoV	13	21.0	0.92
E. coli F5	13	13.7	0.97
H. somni	13	16.5	0.48
IDV	13	19.0	0.83
M. haemolytica	13	16.2	0.44
M. bovis	13	18.8	0.70
Mycoplasma spp.	13	20.2	0.60
P. multocida	13	14.0	0.35
RVA	13	16.3	0.76
T. pyogenes	13	12.5	0.46

frequent in the middle age group. The viral pathogens BCoV and BRSV were present at a very low level (2.3 and 0.7%, respectively), while none of the pools from the dairy calves tested positive for IDV. In the veal calves, more than 50% of the pools were positive for Mycoplasma spp., M. haemolytica, or P. multocida, and the occurrence increased with age. Also, M. bovis (42.9%) was frequently detected, while H. somni (26.8%) and T. pyogenes (23.2%) were less frequently detected. For the viral pathogens, BCoV was the virus with the highest overall occurrence (17.9%) followed by IDV (7.1%), while BRSV was not detected in any pools from the veal calves. Bovine coronavirus was most frequently detected in the youngest age group (24.1%), while IDV was most frequently detected in the oldest age group (11.1%).

The enteric pathogens generally had lower occurrence than the respiratory pathogens. Rotavirus A was the most frequently detected enteric pathogen both in the dairy (27.4%) and veal (10.9%) calves with the highest occurrence in the youngest age groups (17.9%–33.9%). Bovine coronavirus was observed in all age groups and was most prevalent in the veal calves (12.7%). E. coli F5 was only detected in the youngest age group in dairy calves (1.8%), and M. bovis was only

detected in a single pool in the 3-month age group in dairy calves (0.2%).

Occurrence of Pathogens at the Herd Level

The occurrence of the pathogens at the herd level in the different age groups is shown in **Table 7**. At the overall herd level, the majority of the dairy herds had at least one nasal swab pool testing positive for P. multocida (67 herds, 80.7%), Mycoplasma spp. (53 herds, 63.9%), T. pyogenes (51 herds, 61.5%), or M. haemolytica (45 herds, 54.2%). Seventeen herds (20.5%) were positive for H. somni and 13 herds (15.7%) for M. bovis, while BCoV and BRSV were detected in six (7.2%) and two (2.4%) of the dairy herds, respectively. Influenza D virus was not detected in any of the dairy herds. Six dairy herds (7.2%) had at least one feces pool positive for E. coli F5 and one herd (1.2%) tested positive for M. bovis. Rotavirus A and BCoV were detected in 55 (66.3%) and six (7.2%) herds, respectively.

In the veal herds, the majority of the herds had at least one nasal swab pool testing positive for P. multocida (16 herds, 94.1%), Mycoplasma spp. (16 herds, 94.1%), M. haemolytica (16 herds, 94.1%), or M. bovis (13 herds, 76.5%). H. somni was detected in eight herds (47.0%) and T. pyogenes in seven herds (41.2%). The viruses BCoV and IDV were found in six (35.3%) and four veal herds (23.5%), respectively, while none of the veal herds tested positive for BRSV. Considering the feces pools from veal herds, none of the herds tested positive for E. coli F5, Mycoplasma spp., or M. bovis, while six herds (35.3%) were positive for BCoV, and RVA was detected in five herds (29.4%).

DISCUSSION

The validation of the high-throughput rtPCR system revealed that it was possible simultaneously to test for 11 respiratory and enteric pathogens, including four viruses and seven bacteria known to be associated with BRD and/or BED. The sensitivity and specificity of the rtPCR assays were evaluated using positive controls tested both on the high-throughput BioMark HD and the Rotor-Gene Q platforms. These analyses revealed that all assays had an acceptable PCR efficiency, and only minor differences in the dynamic range and efficiency were

TABLE 6 | The occurrence of respiratory and enteric pathogens by age group and in total.

| | Number of positive nasal swab pools | | | | | | | Number of positive feces pools | | | | | | |
| | Dairy calves | | | | Veal calves | | | Dairy calves | | | | Veal calves | | |
Pathogens	0–10 days N = 168 (%)	~3 weeks N = 154 (%)	~3 months N = 113 (%)	Overall N = 435 (%)	~2 weeks N = 29 (%)	~3 months N = 27 (%)	Overall N = 56 (%)	0–10 days N = 168 (%)	~3 weeks N = 154 (%)	~3 months N = 112 (%)	Overall N = 434 (%)	~2 weeks N = 28 (%)	~3 months N = 27 (%)	Overall N = 55 (%)
BRSV	0 (0)	1 (0.7)	2 (1.8)	3 (0.7)	0 (0)	0 (0)	0 (0)							
BCoV	0 (0)	8 (5.2)	2 (1.8)	10 (2.3)	7 (24.1)	3 (11.1)	10 (17.9)	1 (0.6)	2 (1.3)	4 (3.6)	7 (1.6)	4 (14.3)	3 (11.1)	7 (12.7)
IDV	0 (0)	0 (0)	0 (0)	0 (0)	1 (3.5)	3 (11.1)	4 (7.1)	0 (0)	0 (0)	1 (0.9)	1 (0.2)	0 (0)	0 (0)	0 (0)
M. bovis	0 (0)	10 (6.5)	9 (8.0)	19 (4.4)	16 (55.2)	8 (29.6)	24 (42.9)							
Mycoplasma spp.	16 (9.5)	54 (34.4)	45 (39.8)	114 (26.2)	16 (55.2)	17 (63.0)	33 (58.9)							
M. haemolytica	5 (3.0)	23 (14.9)	48 (42.5)	76 (17.5)	10 (34.5)	20 (74.1)	30 (53.6)							
H. somni	3 (1.8)	8 (5.2)	19 (16.8)	30 (6.9)	2 (6.9)	13 (48.2)	15 (26.8)							
P. multocida	22 (13.1)	68 (44.2)	77 (68.1)	167 (38.4)	17 (58.6)	23 (85.2)	40 (71.4)							
T. pyogenes	27 (16.1)	62 (40.3)	22 (19.5)	111 (25.5)	6 (20.7)	7 (25.0)	13 (23.2)							
E. coli F5								8 (4.8)	0 (0)	0 (0)	8 (1.8)	0 (0)	0 (0)	0 (0)
RVA								57 (33.9)	51 (33.1)	11 (9.8)	119 (27.4)	5 (17.9)	1 (3.7)	6 (10.9)

Number of positive pools, followed by prevalence (%) in parentheses.
N, number of analyzed pools; %, percent of positive pools. Gray cell: analysis not relevant.

seen between the two platforms. In general, the Cq values obtained on the BioMark HD platform were lower than those of the traditional rtPCR platform. This discrepancy in values is probably due to the preamplification of the samples in the high-throughput setup (39). Preamplification of samples is often required due to the small reaction volumes in the BioMark system, and this step is also recommended from the supplier and other studies using this platform for pathogen detection (30, 33, 40). An important aspect to consider when using the BioMark HD platform is the risk of false-negative results that can occur for very positive samples, since this preamplification will lower the Cq value of the sample even more. Furthermore, the rtPCR assays will also have a lower cutoff value in the BioMark platform than in the Rotor-Gene Q platform, which also was the case in our study.

The high-throughput rtPCR system can easily be expanded to include more targets since the assay capacity of the 192.24 DA IFC chip used in this study was 24 assays, and thereby an even wider detection system could be developed. However, the added primer-probe sets should be optimized to the temperature conditions selected for the PCR. If more than 24 targets are included, one of the other available DA IFC chips, 48.48 or 96.96, should be utilized. The change in chip format will, however, result in fewer samples that can be analyzed in one run since the choice of chip depends on the application. The high-throughput rtPCR system designed in this study was developed in the frame of a project in which several thousand samples collected from Danish calves were analyzed and, therefore, the 192.24 DA IFC chip was chosen.

The occurrence of pathogens in the field was based on test of pools of pathogen, since it is a much cheaper way of analyzing a large number of animals. One important consideration in the test of pools is to decide on the number of samples to be included in each pool. The schism is to find a balance between the wish to test as many animals as possible and the impact of the number of samples on the sensitivity of the test. Pool size can be theoretically and mathematically calculated (41, 42); however, in real life, this number can be different since pooling of samples have to consider different parameters, such as age and gender. In the present study, both pools consisting of five and 10 individual field samples were examined with the purpose of determining if an acceptable correlation between the results for the individual samples and the pools could be established. Traditionally, when testing pools of samples, it is assumed that each individual sample has the same probability of being positive. However, this is often an erroneous and unrealistic assumption. There exists different pool testing procedures and concluding which one is the best is not an easy task, since parameters such as assay accuracy, availability of risk factor information, prevalence levels, and risk probability distributions all play a role in determining which procedure is best (29, 41, 42). The field samples tested in this study displayed varying Cq values, making it difficult to construct a fully controlled setup. However, the test of pooled samples contra test of individual samples showed that a high-range positive individual sample had a greater influence on the Cq value of the pool than a low-range positive individual sample had, which was observed in all three pool setups. The degree of

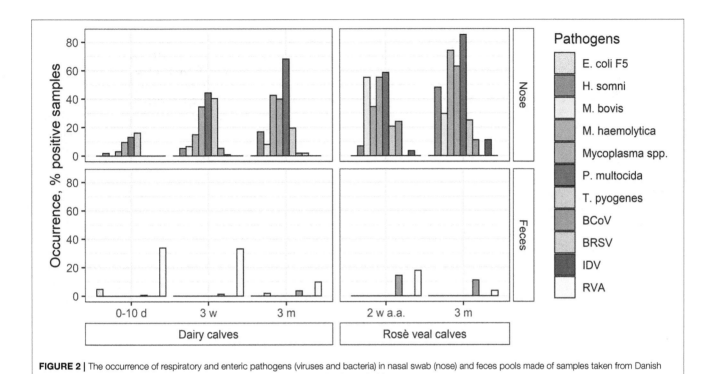

FIGURE 2 | The occurrence of respiratory and enteric pathogens (viruses and bacteria) in nasal swab (nose) and feces pools made of samples taken from Danish dairy and rosé veal calves at different ages (d, day; w, week; m, month; a.a., after arrival) in percentage.

decrease in the pool's Cq value was affected by either the addition of one or few high-range positive individual sample(s) or by the addition of several mid-range positive individual samples. Whereas the addition of low-range positive individual samples did not noticeably change the Cq value of the pool. This was observed both for the bacteria (*Mycoplasma* spp., *M. bovis*, *H. somni*, *T. pyogenes*) and the virus (RVA) in pools consisting of five and 10 individual samples, respectively. Testing pools consisting of a large number of samples can be economically advantageous since it minimize the number of pools. A potential limitation of using larger pools in a group of animals with low occurrence of a given pathogen is the risk of diluting the few positive samples to an extent, that it will no longer be detectable in the rtPCR analysis. However, this study was not able to show how many negative samples were needed to dilute a positive sample so that it was no longer detectable—but again, this depends on the Cq value of the positive sample. Larger pools can nevertheless be preferable in prevalence and screening studies where the purpose often is to test a large number of animals, which also was the case in this study. Since one positive sample in a pool in most cases will lead to a positive test result, the calculation of the occurrence/prevalence of pathogens may be overestimated if it is based on test of pools compared with test of individual animals given the same number of tests performed in each herd.

The high-throughput rtPCR system designed in this study was used to analyze pools of nasal swab and feces field samples in order to determine the occurrence of selected pathogens in Danish calves. The samples were taken from dairy (heifer) and veal (bull) calves at different age groups, and the analysis showed that bacteria were found to be more prevalent than

viruses in the nasal swab pools, while it was opposite in the feces pools. The most prevalent respiratory pathogens found in nasal swab pools from the dairy calves were *Mycoplasma* spp., *M. haemolytica*, *P. multocida*, and *T. pyogenes* (17.5–38.4%), while the other pathogens were observed more sporadically (0–6.9%). All pathogens except for BRSV and *T. pyogenes* were found to be more widespread in the veal calves than in the dairy calves. This was not surprising in that most veal herds commingle with calves from several different sources. Analysis of the occurrence of the pathogens at the herd level revealed that *Mycoplasma* spp., *M. haemolytica*, and *P. multocida* were present in more than 50% of all herds (54.2–94.1%) no matter the herd type. The role of *P. multocida* in the development of pneumonia in calves has been widely discussed, while some studies have reported *P. multocida* as being an opportunistic pathogen, others have found strong indications for *P. multocida* having a pathogenic role (11, 43, 44). Tegtmeier et al. (45) showed that *P. multocida*, *H. somni*, *M. haemolytica*, and *T. pyogenes* are among the most common bacteria associated with severe calf pneumonia in Denmark (45). These findings are supported by a newer study, which found *P. multocida*, *H. somni*, and *M. haemolytica* to be more prevalent in sick cattle than in healthy cattle. Interestingly, >50% of the healthy cattle was found to harbor these bacteria in the lower airways (46), although not showing any symptoms of disease. Benchmarking the laboratory data with information on clinical signs, herd management, housing, and biosecurity may explain why some cattle harboring bacterial pathogens in their lower airways remained healthy, while others developed bronchopneumonia. These analyses are outside the scope of the present study that focused on the

TABLE 7 | The occurrence of respiratory and enteric pathogens at herd level by age group.

Pathogens	Number of positive nasal swab pools							Number of positive feces pools						
	Dairy calves				Veal calves			Dairy calves				Veal calves		
	0–10 days N = 83 (%)	~3 weeks N = 83 (%)	~3 months N = 83 (%)	Overall^	~2 weeks N = 16 (%)	~3 months N = 17 (%)	Overall^	0–10 days N = 83 (%)	~3 weeks N = 83 (%)	~3 months N = 82* (%)	Overall^	~2 weeks N = 16* (%)	~3 months N = 17 (%)	Overall^
BRSV	0 (0)	1 (1.2)	2 (2.4)	2 (2.4)	0 (0)	0 (0)	0 (0)							
BCoV	0 (0)	5 (6.0)	2 (2.4)	6 (7.2)	5 (31.3)	3 (17.7)	6 (35.3)	1 (1.2)	1 (1.2)	4 (4.9)	6 (7.2)	4 (25.0)	3 (17.7)	6 (35.3)
IDV	0 (0)	0 (0)	0 (0)	0 (0)	1 (6.3)	3 (17.7)	4 (23.5)	0 (0)	0 (0)	1 (1.2)	1 (1.2)	0 (0)	0 (0)	0 (0)
M. bovis	0 (0)	7 (8.4)	8 (9.6)	13 (15.7)	12 (75.0)	6 (35.3)	13 (76.5)				0 (0)			0 (0)
Mycoplasma spp.	12 (14.5)	38 (45.8)	37 (44.6)	53 (63.9)	13 (81.3)	13 (76.5)	16 (94.1)							
M. haemolytica	5 (6.0)	17 (20.5)	40 (48.2)	45 (54.2)	8 (50.0)	15 (88.2)	16 (94.1)							
H. somni	3 (3.6)	7 (8.4)	14 (16.9)	17 (20.5)	1 (6.3)	8 (47.1)	8 (47.1)							
P. multocida	19 (22.9)	43 (51.8)	61 (73.5)	67 (80.7)	14 (87.5)	15 (88.2)	16 (94.1)							
T. pyogenes	23 (27.7)	44 (53.0)	22 (26.5)	51 (61.5)	5 (31.3)	5 (29.4)	7 (41.2)							
E. coli F5								6 (7.2)	0 (0)	0 (0)	6 (7.2)	0 (0)	0 (0)	0 (0)
RVA								37 (44.6)	40 (48.2)	11 (13.4)	55 (66.3)	4 (25.0)	1 (5.9)	5 (29.4)

Number of herds with at least one positive pool in the age group, followed by prevalence (%) in parentheses.

N, number of analyzed pools; %, percent of positive pools. Gray cell: analysis not relevant.

^ Across all age groups in the herd.

* In one herd, we obtained no fecal samples.

establishment and validation of a sensitive and specific system for the detection of pathogens in calves. Nevertheless, the findings in the present study can substantiate that *P. multocida*, *H. somni*, *M. haemolytica*, and *T. pyogenes* are present in Danish cattle herds.

In many countries, *M. bovis* is regarded as one of the major causes of respiratory disease in cattle (47). This is supported in the present study, in which the bacterium was detected in 76.5% of the veal herds. Interestingly, this finding is different from older Danish studies, in which *M. bovis* either was not detected in the examined herds or only detected with low occurrence (11, 48, 49). Influenza D virus was detected in four of the veal herds (23.5%), and this is the first time IDV has been found in Danish calves. The virus was isolated for the first time in 2011 in the USA (50), and it has subsequently been detected in cattle from multiple geographic areas across Asia, Europe, and the USA (25, 51–55). In Denmark, BRSV and BCoV have previously been found to be the most common viral agents in relation to calf pneumonia (56). However, BRSV was only detected in very few of the herds (2.4%), while BCoV was found to be more prevalent especially in the veal herds (35.3%). The reason for the low occurrence of the viruses found in the study herds is probably that the herds included in the present study were not tested based on a history of severe respiratory clinical disease which is often the hallmark of especially BRSV.

For the enteric pathogens, RVA was clearly the most prevalent pathogen in the dairy calves (27.4%), while other pathogens were only sporadically detected (0%−1.8%). In the veal calves, RVA (10.9%) and BCoV (12.7%) were the only pathogens detected. Rotavirus A was primary detected in calves below 3 weeks of age, which also was expected since RVA is known to be pathogenic only in young calves (57). Bovine corona virus is also considered an important neonatal calf diarrhea pathogen (58); however, the highest occurrence was detected in veal calves. In contrast, a study from Argentina found BCoV to be most prevalent in the dairy herds (12.1%) compared with veal herds (4.3%) (59). The reason for this discrepancy is probably that only calves with diarrhea was included in the Argentinian study. Another important neonatal diarrhea-causing pathogen is *E. coli* F5, which is known to cause diarrhea within the first 4 days of life (60). In the present study, this pathogen was only detected in the group of 0–10-day-old calves and with a low occurrence (4.8%). This occurrence is similar to the prevalence reported in the Netherlands (2.6%), New Zealand (3.3%), Scotland, and northern England (7.5%) (61–63).

In summary, the developed high-throughput rtPCR system showed good sensitivity and specificity, and the use of it provides new possibilities for more intensive monitoring of bovine respiratory and enteric viral and bacterial pathogens in dairy and veal herds. Furthermore, the system enables testing of multiple samples for the presence of different pathogens in the same setup even with reduced cost and turnover time. Combining the results from continuous monitoring of pathogens with information on clinical signs, productivity, health status, and medicine consumption, the high-throughput rtPCR system presents a new and innovative tool for routine diagnostics, and this even at a lower cost than the traditional diagnostic methods.

ETHICS STATEMENT

Ethical review and approval was not required for the animal study because the samples used in the present study were taken from field animals by veterinarians. The samples were taken and submitted to Centre for Diagnostics, Technical University of Denmark, as if it was a routine submission.

AUTHOR CONTRIBUTIONS

LL, BN, MP, and NG contributed to the experimental design of the study. The design of the rtPCR assays used in the present study was done by NG. rtPCR analyses were conducted and interpreted by NG. The manuscript was drafted by NG. LL contributed to the manuscript preparation, while all authors participated in proofreading of the manuscript. All authors read and approved the final manuscript.

ACKNOWLEDGMENTS

The authors would like to thank Anne Marie Michelsen, Nina Dam Otten, Stine Lindgren, Masja Feline Reipurth Søndergaard, Henrik Hjul Møller, Franziska Helene Skaarup Pedersen, Thomas Damm Poulsen, Jesper Kjærgård Davidsen, Sofie Jeppesen, Maëva Durand, Lucie Jeanne Marie Dupont, Anaëlle Bouqueau, Alicia Fokje Klompmaker, Maria Brydensholt, Sascha Coes, Jensine Wilm, Mette Gerdes Wilson, Emma Madsen, Helge Kromann, and Henrik Læssøe Martin for collection of the samples. Thanks to the herd owners and their staff for their help and cooperation. Thanks to Nina Dam Grønnegaard, Jonathan Rahlff Rogersen, and Sari Mia Dose for their work with the samples in the laboratory. Thanks to Martin Bjerring for organizing the results.

REFERENCES

1. Hodgson PD, Aich P, Manuja A, Hokamp K, Roche FM, Brinkman FSL, et al. Effect of stress on viral-bacterial synergy in bovine respiratory disease: Novel mechanisms to regulate inflammation. *Comp Funct Genomics.* (2005) 6:244–50. doi: 10.1002/cfg.474
2. Gorden PJ, Plummer P. Control, management, and prevention of bovine respiratory disease in dairy calves and cows. *Vet Clin North Am Food Anim. Pract.* (2010) 26:243–59. doi: 10.1016/j.cvfa.2010.03.004
3. Cho Y, il, Yoon KJ. An overview of calf diarrhea - infectious etiology, diagnosis, and intervention. *J Vet Sci.* (2014) 15:1–17. doi: 10.4142/jvs.2014.15.1.1
4. Ellis JA. Update on viral pathogenesis in BRD. *Anim Health Res Rev.* (2009) 10:149–53. doi: 10.1017/S146625230999020X
5. Fulton RW. Bovine respiratory disease research (1983-2009). *Anim Health Res Rev.* (2009) 10:131–9. doi: 10.1017/S146625230999017X
6. Griffin D, Chengappa MM, Kuszak J, McVey DS. Bacterial pathogens of the bovine respiratory disease complex. *Vet Clin North Am Food Anim Pract.* (2010) 26:381–94. doi: 10.1016/j.cvfa.2010.04.004
7. Pansri P, Katholm J, Krogh KM, Aagaard AK, Schmidt LMB, Kudirkiene E, et al. Evaluation of novel multiplex qPCR assays for diagnosis of pathogens associated with the bovine respiratory disease complex. *Vet J.* (2020) 256:105425. doi: 10.1016/j.tvjl.2020.105425
8. Ito T, Okada N, Okawa M, Fukuyama S, ichi, Shimizu M. Detection and characterization of bovine torovirus from the respiratory tract in Japanese cattle. *Vet Microbiol.* (2009) 136:366–71. doi: 10.1016/j.vetmic.2008.11.014
9. Ng TFF, Kondov NO, Deng X, Van Eenennaam A, Neibergs HL, Delwart E. A metagenomics and case-control study to identify viruses associated with bovine respiratory disease. *J. Virol.* (2015) 89:5340–9. doi: 10.1128/JVI.00064-15
10. Ferguson L, Olivier AK, Genova S, Epperson WB, Smith DR, Schneider L, et al. Pathogenesis of influenza D virus in cattle. *J Virol.* (2016) 90:5636–42. doi: 10.1128/JVI.03122-15
11. Angen Ø, Thomsen J, Larsen LE, Larsen J, Kokotovic B, Heegaard PMH, et al. Respiratory disease in calves: microbiological investigations on trans-tracheally aspirated bronchoalveolar fluid and acute phase protein response. *Vet Microbiol.* (2009) 137:165–71. doi: 10.1016/j.vetmic.2008.12.024
12. Sudaryatma PE, Nakamura K, Mekata H, Sekiguchi S, Kubo M, Kobayashi I, et al. Bovine respiratory syncytial virus infection enhances Pasteurella multocida adherence on respiratory epithelial cells. *Vet Microbiol.* (2018) 220:33–8. doi: 10.1016/j.vetmic.2018.04.031

13. Srikumaran S, Kelling CL, Ambagala A. Immune evasion by pathogens of bovine respiratory disease complex. *Anim Heal Res Rev.* (1996) 8:215–29. doi: 10.1017/S1466252307001326
14. Cho Y, Il, H.an JI, Wang C, Cooper V, Schwartz K. Engelken T, et al. Case-control study of microbiological etiology associated with calf diarrhea. *Vet Microbiol.* (2013) 166:375–85. doi: 10.1016/j.vetmic.2013.07.001
15. Enemark HL, Dahl J, Dehn Enemark. J. M. Eimeriosis in danish dairy calves—correlation between species, oocyst excretion and diarrhoea. *Parasitol Res.* (2013) 112:169–76. doi: 10.1007/s00436-013-3441-0
16. Delafosse A, Chartier C, Dupuy MC, Dumoulin M, Pors I, Paraud C. Cryptosporidium parvum infection and associated risk factors in dairy calves in western France. *Prev Vet Med.* (2015) 118:406–12. doi: 10.1016/j.prevetmed.2015.01.005
17. Ngeleka M, Godson D, Vanier G, Desmarais G, Wojnarowicz C, Sayi S, et al. Frequency of Escherichia coli virotypes in calf diarrhea and intestinal morphologic changes associated with these virotypes or other diarrheagenic pathogens. *J Vet Diagnostic Investig.* (2019) 31:611–5. doi: 10.1177/1040638719857783
18. Chang KO, Parwani AV, Smith D, Saif LJ. Detection of group B rotaviruses in fecal samples from diarrheic calves and adult cows and characterization of their VP7 genes. *J Clin Microbiol.* (1997) 35:2107–10. doi: 10.1128/JCM.35.8.2107-2110.1997
19. Hoet AE, Nielsen PR, Hasoksuz M, Thomas C, Wittum TE, Saif LJ. Detection of bovine torovirus and other enteric pathogens in feces from diarrhea cases in cattle. *J Vet Diagnostic Investig.* (2003) 15:205–12. doi: 10.1177/104063870301500301
20. Mawatari T, Taneichi A, Kawagoe T, Hosokawa M, Togashi K, Tsunemitsu H. Detection of a bovine group C rotavirus from adult cows with diarrhea and reduced milk production. *J Vet Med Sci.* (2004) 66:887–90. doi: 10.1292/jvms.66.887
21. Zhu L, Xing Z, Gai X, Li S, San Z, Wang X. Identification of a novel enterovirus e isolates HY12 from cattle with severe respiratory and enteric diseases. *PLoS ONE.* (2014) 9:e97730. doi: 10.1371/journal.pone.0097730
22. Izzo MM, Kirkland PD, Mohler VL, Perkins NR, Gunn AA, House JK. Prevalence of major enteric pathogens in Australian dairy calves with diarrhoea. *Aust Vet J.* (2011) 89:167–73. doi: 10.1111/j.1751-0813.2011.00692.x
23. Fulton RW, Confer AW. Laboratory test descriptions for bovine respiratory disease diagnosis and their strengths and weaknesses: Gold standards for diagnosis, do they exist? *Can Vet J.* (2012) 53:754–61.

24. Tsuchiaka S, Masuda T, Sugimura S, Kobayashi S, Komatsu N, Nagai M, et al. Development of a novel detection system for microbes from bovine diarrhea by real-time PCR. *J Vet Med Sci.* (2016) 78:383–9. doi: 10.1292/jvms.15-0552

25. Kishimoto M, Tsuchiaka S, Rahpaya SS, Hasebe A, Otsu K, Sugimura S, et al. Development of a one-run real-time PCR detection system for pathogens associated with bovine respiratory disease complex. *J Vet Med Sci.* (2017) 79:517–23. doi: 10.1292/jvms.16-0489

26. Wisselink HJ, Cornelissen JBWJ, van der Wal FJ, Kooi EA, Koene MG, et al. Evaluation of a multiplex real-time PCR for detection of four bacterial agents commonly associated with bovine respiratory disease in bronchoalveolar lavage fluid. *BMC Vet Res.* (2017) 13:1–10. doi: 10.1186/s12917-017-1141-1

27. Loy JD, Leger L, Workman AM, Clawson ML, Bulut E, Wang B. Development of a multiplex real-time PCR assay using two thermocycling platforms for detection of major bacterial pathogens associated with bovine respiratory disease complex from clinical samples. *J Vet Diagnostic Investig.* (2018) 30:837–47. doi: 10.1177/1040638718800170

28. Goto Y, Yaegashi G, Fukunari K, Suzuki T. Design of a multiplex quantitative reverse transcription-PCR system to simultaneously detect 16 pathogens associated with bovine respiratory and enteric diseases. *J Appl Microbiol.* (2020) 129:832–47. doi: 10.1111/jam.14685

29. Muñoz-Zanzi CA, Johnson WO, Thurmond MC, Hietala SK. Pooled-sample testing as a herd-screening tool for detection of bovine viral diarrhea virus persistently infected cattle. *J Vet Diagnostic Investig.* (2000) 12:195–203. doi: 10.1177/104063870001200301

30. Goecke NB, Hjulsager CK, Krog JS, Skovgaard K, Larsen LE. Development of a high-throughput real-time PCR system for detection of enzootic pathogens in pigs. *J Vet Diagnostic Investig.* (2020) 1:51–64. doi: 10.1177/1040638719890863

31. Goecke NB, Kobber,ø M, Kusk TK, Hjulsager CK, Pedersen KS, Kristensen CS, et al. Objective pathogen monitoring in nursery and finisher pigs by monthly laboratory diagnostic testing. *Porc Heal Manag.* (2020) 6:1–14. doi: 10.1186/s40813-020-00161-3

32. Goecke NB, Krog JS, Hjulsager CK, Skovgaard K, Harder TC, Breum SØ, et al. Subtyping of swine influenza viruses using a high-throughput real-time PCR platform. *Front Cell Infect Microbiol.* (2018) 8:165. doi: 10.3389/fcimb.2018.00165

33. Ishii S, Segawa T, Okabe S. Simultaneous quantification of multiple food- and waterborne pathogens by use of microfluidic quantitative PCR. *Appl Environ Microbiol.* (2013) 79:2891–8. doi: 10.1128/AEM.00205-13

34. Michelet L, Delannoy S, Devillers E, Umhang G, Aspan A, Juremalm M, et al. High-throughput screening of tick-borne pathogens in Europe. *Front Cell Infect Microbiol.* (2014) 4:1–13. doi: 10.3389/fcimb.2014.00103

35. NCBI Resource Coordinators Database Resources of the National Center for Biotechnology Information. *Nucleic Acids Res.* (2017) 45:D12–7. doi: 10.1093/nar/gkw1071

36. Altschul SF, Gish W, Miller W, Myers EW, Lipman DJ. Basic local alignment search tool. *J Mol Biol.* (1990) 215:403–10. doi: 10.1016/S0022-2836(05)80360-2

37. Kibbe WA. OligoCalc: an online oligonucleotide properties calculator. *Nucleic Acids Res.* (2007) 35:W43–46. doi: 10.1093/nar/gkm234

38. Bustin SA, Benes V, Garson JA, Hellemans J, Huggett J, Kubista M, et al. The MIQE guidelines:minimum information for publication of quantitative real-time PCR experiments. *Clin Chem.* (2009) 55:611–22. doi: 10.1373/clinchem.2008.112797

39. Korenková V, Scott J, Novosadov,á V, Jindrichov,á M, Langerov,á L. Švec D, et al. Pre-amplification in the context of high-throughput qPCR gene expression experiment. *BMC Mol Biol.* (2015) 16:5–15. doi: 10.1186/s12867-015-0033-9

40. Spurgeon SL, Jones RC, Ramakrishnan R. High throughput gene expression measurement with real time PCR in a microfluidic dynamic array. *PLoS ONE.* (2008) 3:e1662. doi: 10.1371/journal.pone.0001662

41. Bilder CR, Tebbs JM. Pooled-testing procedures for screening high volume clinical specimens in heterogeneous populations. *Stat Med.* (2012) 31:3261–8. doi: 10.1002/sim.5334

42. Nguyen NT, Bish EK, Aprahamian H. Sequential prevalence estimation with pooling and continuous test outcomes. *Stat Med.* (2018) 37:2391–426. doi: 10.1002/sim.7657

43. Autio T, Pohjanvirta T, Holopainen R, Rikula U, Pentikäinen J, Huovilainen A, et al. Etiology of respiratory disease in non-vaccinated, non-medicated calves in rearing herds. *Vet Microbiol.* (2007) 119:256–65. doi: 10.1016/j.vetmic.2006.10.001

44. Nikunen S, Härtel H, Orro T, Neuvonen E, Tanskanen R, Kivel,ä SL, et al. Association of bovine respiratory disease with clinical status and acute phase proteins in calves. *Comp Immunol Microbiol Infect Dis.* (2007) 30:143–51. doi: 10.1016/j.cimid.2006.11.004

45. Tegtmeier C, Uttenthal A, Friis N, Jensen N, Jensen H. Pathological and microbiological studies on pneumonic lungs from danish calves. *J Vet Med.* (1999) 46:693–700. doi: 10.1046/j.1439-0450.1999.00301.x

46. Timsit E, Hallewell J, Booker C, Tison N, Amat S, Alexander TW. Prevalence and antimicrobial susceptibility of Mannheimia haemolytica, Pasteurella multocida, and Histophilus somni isolated from the lower respiratory tract of healthy feedlot cattle and those diagnosed with bovine respiratory disease. *Vet Microbiol.* (2017) 208:118–25. doi: 10.1016/j.vetmic.2017.07.013

47. Nicholas RAJ, Ayling RD. Mycoplasma bovis: disease, diagnosis, and control. *Res Vet Sci.* (2003) 74:105–12. doi: 10.1016/S0034-5288(02)00155-8

48. Friis N, Krogh H. Isolation of mycoplasmas from Danish cattle. *Nord Vet Med.* (1983) 35:74–81.

49. Feenstra A, Madsen EB, Friis NF, Meyling A, Ahrens P. A field study of mycoplasma bovis infection in cattle. *J Vet Med Ser B.* (1991) 38:195–202. doi: 10.1111/j.1439-0450.1991.tb00861.x

50. Hause BM, Ducatez M, Collin EA, Ran Z, Liu R, Sheng Z, et al. Isolation of a novel swine influenza virus from oklahoma in 2011 which is distantly related to human influenza C viruses. *PLoS Pathog.* (2013) 9:e1003176. doi: 10.1371/journal.ppat.1003176

51. Jiang WM, Wang SC, Peng C, Yu JM, Zhuang QY, Hou GY, et al. Identification of a potential novel type of influenza virus in Bovine in China. *Virus Genes.* (2014) 49:493–6. doi: 10.1007/s11262-014-1107-3

52. Ducatez MF, Pelletier C, Meyer G. Influenza d virus in cattle, France, 2011–2014. *Emerg Infect Dis.* (2015) 21:368–71. doi: 10.3201/eid2102.141449

53. Ferguson L, Eckard L, Epperson WB, Long LP, Smith D, Huston C, et al. Influenza D virus infection in Mississippi beef cattle. *Virology.* (2015) 486:28–34. doi: 10.1016/j.virol.2015.08.030

54. Chiapponi C, Faccini S, De Mattia A, Baioni L, Barbieri I, Rosignoli C, et al. Detection of influenza D virus among swine and cattle, Italy. *Emerg Infect Dis.* (2016) 22:352–4. doi: 10.3201/eid2202.151439

55. Flynn O, Gallagher C, Mooney J, Irvine C, Ducatez M, Hause B, et al. Influenza D virus in cattle, Ireland. *Emerg Infect Dis.* (2018) 24:389–91. doi: 10.3201/eid2402.170759

56. Larsen LE, Tjørnehøj K, Viuff B, Jensen NE, Uttenthal Å. Diagnosis of enzootic pneumonia in Danish cattle: reverse transcription-polymerase chain reaction assay for detection of bovine respiratory syncytial virus in naturally and experimentally infected cattle. *J Vet Diagnostic Investig.* (1999) 11:416–22. doi: 10.1177/104063879901100505

57. Dhama K, Chauhan RS, Mahendran M, Malik SVS. Rotavirus diarrhea in bovines and other domestic animals. *Vet Res Commun.* (2009) 33:1–23. doi: 10.1007/s11259-008-9070-x

58. Mebus CA, Stair EL, Rhodes MB, Twiehaus MJ. Neonatal calf diarrhea: propagation, attenuation, and characteristics of a coronavirus-like agent. *Am J Vet Res.* (1973) 34:145–50.

59. Bok M, Miño S, Rodriguez D, Badaracco A, Nuñes I, Souza SP, et al. Molecular and antigenic characterization of bovine Coronavirus circulating in Argentinean cattle during 1994–2010. *Vet Microbiol.* (2015) 181:221–9. doi: 10.1016/j.vetmic.2015.10.017

60. Foster DM, Smith GW. Pathophysiology of diarrhea in calves. *Vet Clin North Am Food Anim Pract.* (2009) 25:13–36. doi: 10.1016/j.cvfa.2008.10.013

61. Sherwood D, Snodgrass D, Lawson G. Prevalence of enterotoxigenic Escherichia coli in calves in Scotland and northern England. *Vet Rec.* (1983) 113:208–12. doi: 10.1136/vr.113.10.208

62. Bartels CJM, Holzhauer M, Jorritsma R, Swart WAJM, Lam TJGM. Prevalence, prediction and risk factors of enteropathogens in normal and non-normal faeces of young Dutch dairy calves. *Prev Vet Med.* (2010) 93:162–9. doi: 10.1016/j.prevetmed.2009.09.020

63. Al Mawly J, Grinberg A, Prattley D, Moffat J, French N. Prevalence of endemic enteropathogens of calves in New Zealand dairy farms. *N Z Vet J.* (2015) 63:147–52. doi: 10.1080/00480169.2014.966168

64. Angen Ø, Ahrens P, Tegtmeier C. Development of a PCR test for identification of Haemophilus somnus in pure and mixed cultures. *Vet Microbiol.* (1998) 63:39–48. doi: 10.1016/S0378-1135(98)00222-3

65. Decaro N, Elia G, Campolo M, Desario C, Mari V, Radogna A, et al. Detection of bovine coronavirus using a TaqMan-based real-time RT-PCR assay. *J Virol Methods.* (2008) 151:167–71. doi: 10.1016/j.jviromet.2008.05.016

66. Hakhverdyan M, Hägglund S, Larsen LE, Belák S. Evaluation of a single-tube fluorogenic RT-PCR assay for detection of bovine respiratory syncytial virus in clinical samples. *J Virol Methods.* (2005) 123:195–202. doi: 10.1016/j.jviromet.2004.09.016

67. Pang XL, Lee B, Boroumand N, Leblanc B, Preiksaitis JK, Ip CCY. Increased detection of rotavirus using a real time reverse transcription-polymerase chain reaction (RT-PCR) assay in stool specimens from children with diarrhea. *J Med Virol.* (2004) 72:496–501. doi: 10.1002/jmv.20009

68. Sachse K, Salam HSH, Diller R, Schubert E, Hoffmann B, Hotzel H. Use of a novel real-time PCR technique to monitor and quantitate Mycoplasma bovis infection in cattle herds with mastitis and respiratory disease. *Vet J.* (2010) 186:299–303. doi: 10.1016/j.tvjl.2009.10.008

15

Estimating Clinically Relevant Cut-Off Values for a High-Throughput Quantitative Real-Time PCR Detecting Bacterial Respiratory Pathogens in Cattle

Alicia F. Klompmaker[1†], Maria Brydensholt[1†], Anne Marie Michelsen[1], Matthew J. Denwood[1], Carsten T. Kirkeby[1], Lars Erik Larsen[1], Nicole B. Goecke[1,2], Nina D. Otten[1] and Liza R. Nielsen[1*]

[1] Department of Veterinary and Animal Sciences, Faculty of Health and Medical Sciences, University of Copenhagen, Copenhagen, Denmark, [2] Centre for Diagnostics, Technical University of Denmark, Kongens Lyngby, Denmark

*Correspondence:
Liza R. Nielsen
liza@sund.ku.dk

[†] These authors have contributed equally to this work and share first authorship

Bovine respiratory disease (BRD) results from interactions between pathogens, environmental stressors, and host factors. Obtaining a diagnosis of the causal pathogens is challenging but the use of high-throughput real-time PCR (rtPCR) may help target preventive and therapeutic interventions. The aim of this study was to improve the interpretation of rtPCR results by analysing their associations with clinical observations. The objective was to develop and illustrate a field-data driven statistical method to guide the selection of relevant quantification cycle cut-off values for pathogens associated with BRD for the high-throughput rtPCR system "Fluidigm BioMark HD" based on nasal swabs from calves. We used data from 36 herds enrolled in a Danish field study where 340 calves within pre-determined age-groups were subject to clinical examination and nasal swabs up to four times. The samples were analysed with the rtPCR system. Each of the 1,025 observation units were classified as sick with BRD or healthy, based on clinical scores. The optimal rtPCR results to predict BRD were investigated for *Pasteurella multocida*, *Mycoplasma bovis*, *Histophilus somni*, *Mannheimia haemolytica*, and *Trueperella pyogenes* by interpreting scatterplots and results of mixed effects logistic regression models. The clinically relevant rtPCR cut-off suggested for *P. multocida* and *M. bovis* was ≤ 21.3. For *H. somni* it was ≤ 17.4, while no cut-off could be determined for *M. haemolytica* and *T. pyogenes*. The demonstrated approach can provide objective support in the choice of clinically relevant cut-offs. However, for robust performance of the regression model sufficient amounts of suitable data are required.

Keywords: bovine respiratory disease, calf, diagnostics, nasal swab, rtPCR, clinically relevant cut-off

INTRODUCTION

Bovine respiratory disease (BRD) is a multifactorial disease which involves multiple stressors, environmental and host factors, and various infectious agents. The disease is a common health problem and a cause of mortality and welfare issues in calves between 1 and 6 months old (1, 2). Furthermore, BRD is associated with economic losses due to direct costs of treatment and lost calves, but also because of long-term impacts on animal performance e.g., reduced weight gain and thereby age at first calving (3). Costs of treatment for respiratory disease in feedlot cattle in the United States were estimated to ∼€20 per case (4), while a Dutch study estimated annual losses per dairy heifer to €31 on average (5). Respiratory disease among calves is also associated with high levels of antimicrobial use. In the year 2015, antibiotics registered for respiratory disease covered 71% of the total amount of antibiotics prescribed for Danish calves (6).

Obtaining a timely and accurate diagnosis of BRD is challenging (7) due to the uncertainty of whether pathogens recovered from the sample are in fact the cause of the respiratory disease or simply a part of the microbiota. Ante-mortem diagnosis of respiratory disease is typically based on clinical examinations (8), where the most common clinical signs are fever, coughing, nasal- and ocular discharge, depression, increased respiratory rate and laboured breathing (9). Clinical respiratory scoring systems to detect calves with respiratory disease have been developed and scientifically validated with moderate sensitivity and relatively high specificity (10). However, the clinically sick animal will rarely display signs which are specific for a single aetiology (7). Diagnostic laboratory testing is therefore necessary for identification of the pathogens associated with BRD (11), allowing correct treatment and prevention to be initiated. A new high-throughput real-time PCR (rtPCR) detection system using the BioMark HD platform (Fluidigm, South San Francisco, USA) established at the Centre for Diagnostics, Technical University of Denmark can detect genetic material from multiple bovine viruses and bacteria in the same setup while running numerous samples at once.

We used this new high-throughput rtPCR system for detection of nine respiratory agents. In this manuscript, we report on analysis of five of these for which we had a presumably sufficient sample of test-positive samples, namely *Mycoplasma bovis* (*M. bovis*), *Histophilus somni* (*H. somni*), *Mannheimia haemolytica* (*M. haemolytica*), *Pasteurella multocida* (*P. multocida*), and *Trueperella pyogenes* (*T. pyogenes*) in nasal swabs. Several studies in the veterinary and human medical field have shown that clinical presentation and disease severity can be related to (semi-)quantitative PCR results representing the pathogenic load (12–14). On the other hand, several pathogens associated with BRD can also be found in clinically healthy animals showing that merely detecting the pathogen is not sufficient for making a diagnosis (15). To the authors' knowledge, clinically relevant rtPCR cut-off values have not yet been defined for bovine respiratory pathogens. Therefore, there is a need to determine cut-offs for which the test result is associated with respiratory disease and not just presence of the pathogen, thereby improving the interpretation of molecular diagnostics, to assist veterinarians and farmers in making more objective and accurate interventions. The study objective was to develop and provide proof-of-concept of a new data-driven statistical approach, providing evidence to suggest field-relevant rtPCR quantification cycle (Cq) cut-off values, and to test this model on common bovine pathogens associated with respiratory disease tested by the high-throughput rtPCR system (Fluidigm). The study was based on data from a Danish field study providing systematically collected clinical recordings paired with rtPCR results from nasal swab samples.

MATERIALS AND METHODS

Herd and Calf Selection

The data used in this study were collected between September 2018 and March 2020. A total of 36 cattle herds including nine veal herds and 27 dairy herds participated. In Denmark, a veal herd is a rosé veal calf producing unit, where mainly bull calves purchased from dairy herds are slaughtered as veal (8–12 months) or young bulls (>12 months) (16). Selection criteria for veal herds were the use of electronic disease registration and regular dairy calf suppliers. Qualifying herds were selected by convenience to ensure wide geographical coverage in Denmark. For each of the nine selected veal herds, the three dairy farms supplying the highest number of calves on a regular basis were asked to participate. For all 36 herds, participation was voluntary.

At the beginning of the study period for each herd, up to 12 calves between 0 and 10 days old were randomly selected (this age group is referred to as "Age 1w"). On most farms, 12 calves were not yet available for sampling at the first herd visit, so follow-up visits were necessary to increase the number of animals. The lack of calves at initial visits also meant that it was not always possible to select calves at random, but necessary to include all available calves. The selected cohorts of calves were subsequently examined at 3 weeks of age ("Age 3w"), 2 weeks after introduction to the veal herds ("Age 2wai"), and at 3 months of age ("Age 3m"), resulting in four age groups. A total of 340 individual calves were sampled up to four times resulting in 1,025 observation units. In this study, an observation unit refers to a calf in a particular age group.

Clinical Examination and Sample Collection

A clinical examination protocol was developed prior to herd visits, and the participating veterinary researchers underwent a joint training session aiming to harmonise their scoring. Clinical examinations were primarily performed by two veterinarians, and data were registered onsite and synchronised with an online platform and project database. Clinical measures relevant to the study presented in this paper included rectal temperature and coughing as well as nasal and ocular discharge. Each calf was also subject to nasal swab collection using 15 cm unguarded polyester-tipped swabs. A swab was guided into one naris, rotated against the mucosal wall, and withdrawn. The tip of the swab was placed in an Eppendorf tube containing PBS and stored at ∼5°C for a maximum of 4 days until sample preparation and extraction.

Sample Analysis

The nasal swab samples were analysed at the Centre for Diagnostics, Technical University of Denmark. Samples were vortexed, after which bacterial DNA were extracted using the extraction robot QIAcube HT (QIAGEN, Hilden, Germany) and the Cador Pathogen 96 QIAcube HT kit (QIAGEN) according to the manufacturer's instructions. The extracted samples were pre-amplified (DNA-targets) as described by Goecke et al. (17). This pre-amplification step prior to the rtPCR, results in distinctly lower Cq values compared to other rtPCR systems. The primer and probe sequences used were either from previously published assays or designed for the project (17). For the high-throughput rtPCR amplification, the BioMark HD (Fluidigm) and the BioMark 192.24 Dynamic Array (DA) Integrated Fluidic Circuit (IFC) chip (Fluidigm) were used. This platform automatically combines 192 pre-amplified samples with 24 assays, thus enabling 4,608 individual rtPCR reactions simultaneously. The chip was placed in the RX IFC controller (Fluidigm) for loading and mixing. After 30 min, the chip was transferred to and run on the rtPCR BioMark HD platform. Known positive and negative control samples were included in each run, and if the Cq values of the positive controls were not within two Cq values of the pre-determined value, the DA IFC chip was run again. The output data, including the Cq values and amplification curves, obtained from the BioMark HD system were analysed using the Fluidigm Real-Time PCR Analysis software 4.1.3 (Fluidigm).

Respiratory Clinical Status

The calves were classified as either sick with respiratory disease or not, using a clinical scoring system. Calves classified as not having respiratory disease are referred to as healthy for the purpose of this study. The scoring system was adapted from two existing scoring systems for BRD (11, 18). The clinical score was based on the four clinical signs: coughing, rectal temperature, nasal discharge, and ocular discharge, where both unilateral and bilateral discharge were considered on equal terms. For each sign, points were given depending on the severity, and the total of these points for each sign equalled the clinical score for the calf. For all signs, a score of zero was given if the sign was not present, or in the case of rectal temperature, if the temperature was $<39°$ C. For nasal discharge, serous discharge equalled one point while mucopurulent discharge equalled four points. For ocular discharge, serous discharge equalled one point while mucopurulent discharge equalled two points. In addition, one point was added to the total score if a calf had both nasal and ocular discharge of any severity. For rectal temperature, 39–39.3°C equalled one point while a temperature $\geq 39.4°$C equalled two points. Finally, at least one spontaneous cough equalled three points. A calf with a clinical score equal to or greater than five points was classified as sick with respiratory disease.

Statistical Analyses

Statistical analyses were conducted using the statistical software R (19). All data were extracted from the SQL database located at Aarhus University into an Excel spreadsheet pairing clinical registrations and rtPCR Cq values for each observation unit. The pathogens for which attempts were made to find a clinically relevant Cq value were *M. bovis, H. somni, M. haemolytica, P. multocida,* and *T. pyogenes.*

Scatterplots depicting the clinical score for each observation unit plotted against Cq values were created for each of the five tested pathogens. The scatterplots were visually inspected to attempt to identify a plausible Cq cut-off value for each pathogen by considering the distribution of Cq values for observation units defined as either sick with respiratory disease or not. To aid the

visualisation of a cut-off, data points were displayed as black dots if the observation units were classified as sick with respiratory disease, or grey triangles if not. Nasal swab samples in which the pathogen in question was not found were given the Cq value 32 (referred to as test-negative), as no samples with a Cq value (referred to as test-positive) reached this value. Both positive and negative test-results were included in the scatter plots.

The following procedure was used to determine the "optimal cut-off value," i.e., the cut-off value leading to the test-result interpretation with the highest predictive value for respiratory disease being present in the calves. First, an interval of Cq values in which to search for optimal cut-off values was specified for each pathogen. The interval was based on the observed distribution of Cq values and excluded the extreme ends of the distribution with sparse data. Each of the potential cut-off values for rtPCR Cq within this interval were then evaluated based on the predictive ability to determine the observation units' respiratory health status using a mixed-effects logistic regression model fit using the lme4 package (20) within R (19). The outcome variable "sick with respiratory disease" was dichotomised into yes or no, with yes referring to observation units with a clinical score equal to or above five, and no referring to observation units with a clinical score below five. The main explanatory variable of interest was the rtPCR results dichotomised according to the threshold being tested. The explanatory variable "Age Group" had four levels as explained above. Data hierarchies (e.g., data with a nested or clustered structure) were adjusted for in the mixed-effects model at herd- and age-group level by including them as a combined random effect factor ("Group ID"). The model was re-fit using each potential value of rtPCR threshold. Predicted probability plots were then created for each pathogen based on the predictive ability of each mixed-effects model.

RESULTS

Descriptive Analyses

A total of 1,025 observations were available from 340 calves. In each of the nine veal herds between 14 and 36 individual calves were sampled. In the 27 dairy herds between three and 33 individual calves were sampled in each herd. In total, 417 (40.7%) observation units were scored as being sick with respiratory disease (Age 1w: 17.5%, Age 3w: 9.4%, Age 2wai: 29.3%, Age 3m: 43.9%). Hence, the prevalence of BRD was generally higher in older than younger calves. This was taken into account in the model results reported below.

Of these, 296 (71%) were positive (had DNA-material detected as defined by Cq < 32) for at least one of the five investigated respiratory pathogens, and 121 (29%) were test-negative. The median clinical score and mean age of the sick observation units were seven points and 57 days (SD 35.7), respectively. The remaining 608 (59.3%) observation units had a clinical score below five and were per definition scored as not being sick with respiratory disease. In 362 (59.5%) of these 608 observation units none of the pathogens were detected, while in 246 (40.5%) observation units, DNA from at least one pathogen was detected. The median clinical score and mean age for the observation

Estimating Clinically Relevant Cut-Off Values for a High-Throughput Quantitative Real-Time PCR Detecting...

141

units classified as healthy were two points and 29 days (SD 31.5), respectively.

The data for the five investigated pathogens are summarised in **Table 1**. Generally, the minimum and maximum Cq values for these pathogens did not differ meaningfully. For observation units, which had measurable Cq values for *M. bovis*, *H. somni*, *M. haemolytica*, and *P. multocida*, ~60–70% were classified as sick with respiratory disease. However, only 36.6% of the observation units with Cq values < 32 for *T. pyogenes* were classified as sick. The mean age for observation units positive for *T. pyogenes* was lower for both healthy and sick calves, compared to the other four pathogens. *H. somni* was the pathogen detected the fewest times as the only pathogen detected in a sample. The pathogens were most often found in combination with *P. multocida*.

Real-Time PCR Cut-Off Analyses
P. multocida
Based on the scatterplot in **Figure 1**, it was not possible to visually estimate a clinically relevant cut-off for *P. multocida*, because it did not show any clear association between clinical score and the rtPCR results. The interval chosen for the mixed-effects model for *P. multocida* was 14–25 and the results are given in **Table 2**. Dichotomised rtPCR results based on a cut-off of Cq ≤ 21.3 was found to be significantly associated with being scored as sick with respiratory disease ($p = 0.026$). The proportion of observation units with *P. multocida* Cq values ≤ 21.3 being classified as sick with respiratory disease was 0.61, whereas it was 0.36 for observation units with Cq values > 21.3. In **Figure 2**, the predicted probability plot illustrates that the probability of being classified as sick with respiratory disease within each age-group for samples with *P. multocida* Cq ≤ 21.3 was slightly higher than when the Cq was >21.3, and the difference was largest in the 3w age-group.

M. bovis
By visual inspection of the scatterplot in **Figure 1**, the cut-off for *M. bovis* was tentatively placed at Cq value 21. Mixed-effects models for *M. bovis* were run over the interval of Cq 15–26 and the results are shown in **Table 2**. Dichotomised rtPCR results based on a cut-off of ≤ 21.3 was significantly associated with a clinical score indicating respiratory disease ($p = 0.042$). The overall proportion of observation units being classified as sick with respiratory disease with Cq values ≤ 21.3 was 0.72, whereas it was 0.39 for observation units with *M. bovis* Cq values > 21.3. **Figure 2** illustrates that the predicted probability of being classified as sick with respiratory disease within each age-group for samples with *M. bovis* Cq ≤ 21.3 was generally higher than when the Cq was >21.3. However, there were no observation units with Cq values ≤ 21.3 in the 1w age-group.

H. somni
The visual inspection of **Figure 1** placed the Cq cut-off for *H. somni* at Cq 20. For *H. somni,* the mixed-effects model was run over the interval of Cq 15–25, and the results are seen in **Table 2**. Dichotomised rtPCR based on a cut-off at Cq ≤ 17.4 was significantly associated with a clinical score indicating respiratory disease ($p = 0.002$). The proportion of observation units being classified as sick with respiratory disease with *H. somni* Cq values ≤ 17.4 was 0.86, whereas it was 0.40 for observation units with Cq values > 17.4. **Figure 2** illustrates that the predicted probability of being classified as sick with respiratory disease within each age-group for samples with *H. somni* ≤ 17.4 was generally markedly higher than when the Cq was >17.4. However, few observations were available with Cq values ≤ 17.4 in the 1w and 3w age-groups.

TABLE 1 | Summary of the pathogens [*M. bovis* (MB), *H. somni* (HS), *M. haemolytica* (MH), *P. multocida* (PM), and *T. pyogenes* (TP)] with the percentage of the observation units, in which the respective pathogen was detected, which were classified as sick and the minimum and maximum Cq value for both healthy (H) and sick (S) observation units.

| | | Cq value | | | | | | | | | |
| | | Min | | Max | | Median score | | Mean age | | # detected as the only pathogen | | |
Pathogen	Scored as sick (%)	H	S	H	S	H	S	H	S	H	S	In combination with (%)
MB	64.8	13.1	12.8	27.5	27.8	4	7	44.5	55.0	17	19	PM (56) MH (37)
HS	69.4	15.6	11.9	24.8	25.1	4	7	75.8	85.8	3	7	PM (68) MH (47)
MH	60.0	10.5	11.1	26.7	24.4	3	7	65.0	74.9	23	17	PM (56) MB (30)
PM	61.0	12.5	12.9	25.2	26.6	3	7	61.1	70.9	51	76	MH (30) MB (25)
TP	36.6	13.8	17.8	26.3	25.1	2	7	23.5	47.6	66	22	PM (31) MH (19)

The median clinical score and mean age for the healthy (H) and sick (S) observation units and the number of healthy (H) and sick (S) observation units where the pathogen was detected as the only pathogen. Finally, the pathogens which the respective pathogen was most often found in combination with are shown.

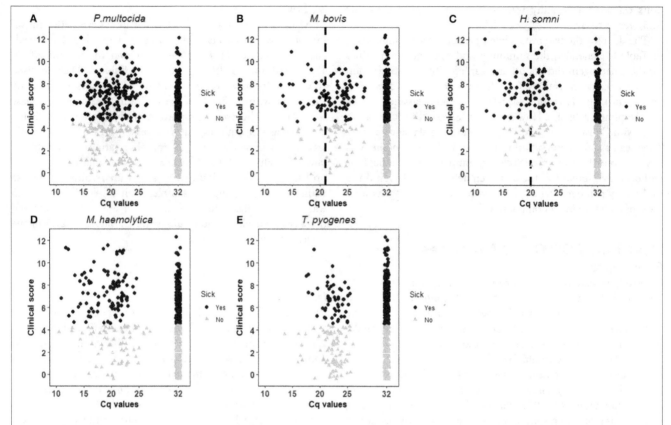

FIGURE 1 | Distribution of respiratory clinical score against Cq values for *P. multocida* **(A)**, *M. bovis* **(B)**, *H. somni* **(C)**, *M. haemolytica* **(D)** and *T. pyogenes* **(E)**, and additionally grouped by respiratory disease classification with black dots indicating an observation unit sick with respiratory disease and grey triangles indicating a healthy. The vertical dotted lines in **(B,C)** represent the visually estimated clinically relevant Cq values.

M. haemolytica and *T. pyogenes*

A visual cut-off could not be placed for neither *M. haemolytica* nor *T. pyogenes*, based on **Figure 1** because no clear associations between clinical score and Cq values were found. The interval chosen for the mixed-effects model was 14–26 for *M. haemolytica* and 20–26 for *T. pyogenes*. As shown in the results in **Table 2**, none of the potential cut-offs were found to yield a dichotomised rtPCR result with a significant association with being classified as sick vs. healthy for these pathogens with the available data.

DISCUSSION

This study shows that it is possible to suggest clinically relevant cut-off values with statistically significant associations with clinical scores indicating respiratory disease for the three pathogens *P. multocida*, *M. bovis*, and *H. somni*. A cut-off of Cq ≤ 17.4 was found for *H. somni*, accompanied by the highest probability of being scored as sick with respiratory disease.

Meaningful cut-off values could not be determined for *M. haemolytica* and *T. pyogenes* in this study. For *M. haemolytica*, this might be explained by the assay used for the rtPCR in this study, which did not distinguish between different serotypes. Several serotypes of *M. haemolytica* exist, for instance serotype A1, which is associated with clinical disease, and

serotype A2, which occurs as a commensal (21). Basing the statistical calculations also on commensal serotypes complicates determining clinically relevant Cq cut-off values. For further investigations, it would be relevant to only test samples for the pathogenic serotypes of *M. haemolytica*.

For *T. pyogenes*, 36.6% of the observation units test-positive (Cq value < 32) for this bacterium were scored as sick with respiratory disease, whereas this was more than 60% for the other four pathogens. Furthermore, in most of the observation units positive for *T. pyogenes*, it was found as the only pathogen. These findings suggest that the majority of the *T. pyogenes* detected in this study were a part of the commensal nasal microbiota, as supported by published literature (22), making it difficult to determine a clinically relevant Cq cut-off for that pathogen.

One thing to consider when using the high-throughput rtPCR platform BioMark is the risk of false negative results, which can occur if a sample is very positive. This results from the additional pre-amplification step that may lead to saturation due to the very high level of templates. In such cases, it will be necessary to dilute the sample and re-test it in the BioMark platform. In general, the optimal range of measurable Cq values in the high-throughput rtPCR platform is ~8–10 cycles lower compared to regular rtPCR cyclers (23) and therefore, the cutoff value will also be lower for rtPCR assays in the high-throughput setup.

TABLE 2 | Results of the mixed-effects model for analysis of variables associated with respiratory disease in calves including analysis of the best rtPCR Cq cut-off differentiating between sick and healthy calves for *P. multocida, M. bovis, H. somni, M. haemolytica* and *T. pyogenes.*

Pathogen	Variables	Estimate	SE	p	σ²	SD
P. multocida	Fixed effects					
	Intercept	−1.33	0.19	***		
	Cq > 21.3	0	–	–		
	Cq ≤ 21.3	0.44	0.2	*		
	Age 1w	0	–	–		
	Age 3w	−0.30	0.29	–		
	Age 2wai	1.66	0.32	***		
	Age 3m	1.85	0.28	***		
	Random effect					
	Group ID				0.34	0.58
M. bovis	Fixed effects					
	Intercept	−1.31	0.19	***		
	Cq > 21.3	0	–	–		
	Cq ≤ 21.3	0.77	0.38	*		
	Age 1w	0	–	–		
	Age 3w	−0.29	0.28	–		
	Age 2wai	1.63	0.31	***		
	Age 3m	1.96	0.27	***		
	Random effect					
	Group ID				0.32	0.56
H. somni	Fixed effects					
	Intercept	−1.33	0.18	***		
	Cq > 17.4	0	–	–		
	Cq ≤ 17.4	2.38	0.75	**		
	Age 1w	0	–	–		
	Age 3w	−0.34	0.28	–		
	Age 2wai	1.75	0.30	***		
	Age 3m	1.95	0.27	***		
	Random effect					
	Group ID				0.30	0.54
M. haemolytica	Fixed effects					
	Intercept	−1.31	0.18	***		
	Cq > 22.2	0	–	–		
	Cq ≤ 22.2	0.37	0.23	–		
	Age 1w	0	–	–		
	Age 3w	−0.28	0.28	–		
	Age 2wai	1.67	0.31	***		
	Age 3m	1.88	0.27	***		
	Random effect					
	Group ID				0.31	0.56
T. pyogenes	Fixed effects					
	Intercept	−1.29	0.19	***		
	Cq > 23.7	0	–	–		
	Cq ≤ 23.7	−0.18	0.24	–		
	Age 1w	0	–	–		
	Age 3w	−0.26	0.29	–		
	Age 2wai	1.78	0.31	***		
	Age 3m	1.98	0.27	***		
	Random effect					
	Group ID				0.33	0.58

The estimates describe the log-transformed fixed effects of Cq cut-off and age and standard error (SE) and p-value (p) are provided for the estimates. Variance (σ²) and standard deviation (SD) are provided for the random effect, GroupID (*p-value < 0.05, **p-value < 0.01, ***p-value < 0.001).

It was not possible to investigate combinations of pathogens using the optimisation and modelling approach, which would have required a larger dataset with a higher sample size of the different pathogen combinations. Thus, the clinically relevant Cq cut-offs were calculated without accounting for the central interactions between the respiratory pathogens. BRD often has a polymicrobial aetiology and it is likely that the presence of some pathogens influence the presence and/or growth of others (24), thereby affecting the Cq values. In addition, other pathogens than those investigated in the current study are associated with BRD, for instance bovine respiratory syncytial virus, bovine coronavirus, influenza D virus, and bovine parainfluenzavirus type 3. However, result on the viruses were not included in the statistical analyses as there were either very few positive samples, or because it was not yet possible to test for the pathogen using the high-throughput rtPCR system (Fluidigm) as it was set up for this project. To exploit the full potential of the rtPCR system it would be necessary to determine possible cut-off Cq values for the remaining important respiratory infectious agents. As many of the pathogens involved in BRD are also commensals, their mere presence may not be indicative of disease. Establishing clinically relevant Cq cut-offs would make it possible to differentiate between harmless commensals and disease-causing pathogens under different conditions. Furthermore, repeated testing in the same herd would enable improved understanding of the effect of changing pathogen occurrence in age groups or barn sections over time.

Due to the inclusion of multiple factors, the mixed-effects model was valued as the most precise method to indicate relevant cut-offs. However, as evident from the scatterplots, the correlation between Cq values and clinical scores was not very clear. Hence, the level of noise in the data affected the performance of the regression model and the robustness of the model results. This limitation could be levitated by access to larger datasets with more test-positive samples combined with stringent clinical scoring of the calves. Another method frequently used for test comparison and test performance studies in the literature, receiver operating characteristic (ROC) curves, used by e.g., Loy et al. (25), would likely have encountered similar data noise issues.

Another limitation in this study was that the same calves were included as individual observations up to four times (equal to four age groups). However, using the mixed-effects model, a random factor combining herd- and age-group was included. This factor includes herd differences, but also differences between age groups within the herds, such as calf and colostrum management, housing environment etc., all of which could impact disease as well as the calves' ability to overcome disease.

The course of a disease is dynamic and the pathogens which initiate BRD in a calf are not necessarily the same in the later stages or at post-mortem (24). Thomas et al. (15) described varying carriage rates of *H. somni, P. multocida,* and *M. haemolytica* in healthy beef calves. It showed that not all calves became colonised with the bacteria even though they were placed in the same environment. Furthermore, the carriage rates decreased over time which can be explained by the calves getting immunologically more mature and thereby better at clearing

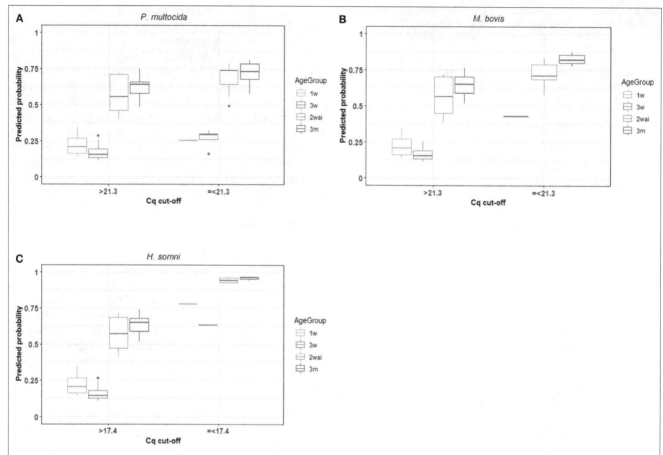

FIGURE 2 | The model predicted probability of calves being classified as sick with respiratory disease using the Cq cut-offs providing the highest predictive value of the Fluidigm rt-PCR for detection of *P. multocida* **(A)**, *M. bovis* **(B)** and *H. somni* **(C)** in each age group of calves in 27 dairy and nine veal herds (1w, 1 week old; 3w, 3 weeks old; 2wai, 2 weeks after introduction to veal herds; and 3m, 3 months old).

pathogens (15). In the present study, 29% of the observation units which were scored as sick with respiratory disease did not have any respiratory pathogens detected in their nasal swabs. Likewise, in 40.5% of the observation units classified as not sick with respiratory disease, respiratory agents able to act as primary pathogens were detected. While one reason for this could be the detection of commensals, another explanation could be that visits to the same calves, in which samples were taken and clinical assessments were performed were carried out with intervals of at least 2 weeks. Therefore, disease course in individual calves could not be followed over time but should rather be considered as snapshots. This may have led to misclassification of BRD status in some observation units. It is thereby possible that a calf presenting with a low clinical score, but a high microbial load (low Cq value) could present with more severe clinical sign in the days following assessment and sampling. Another explanation for this opposing result could be rtPCR detecting DNA material from non-viable organisms still present in the respiratory tract (15).

BRD is a problem at group level as calves are housed together and sometimes mixed from different herds (26). Therefore, it would be interesting to investigate the potential of the rtPCR

system to be used at group level and determine relevant cut-off values for group level testing. In groups, calves are usually in different stages of infection at any given time. Therefore, testing groups might be more representative of which pathogens are associated with disease than individual animal testing, as the latter may be more affected by the mentioned snapshots. Again, repeated testing of groups of calves over time would allow for improved understanding of the effect of changing pathogen profiles. It should be emphasised that treatment decisions cannot be made solely based on the results of this test, but should always be made together with clinical evaluations of the calves.

In conclusion, this study demonstrated how the selection of clinically relevant rtPCR Cq cut-offs could be guided by use of a mixed-effects logistic regression model for three well-known BRD-pathogens. A Cq cut-off of ≤ 21.3 was identified for *P. multocida* and *M. bovis*, while a cut-off of ≤ 17.4 was identified for *H. somni*. Further investigations are warranted to define cut-off values for all relevant respiratory pathogens in bovine calves to make more relevant diagnoses and thereby improve treatment and prevention of BRD.

ETHICS STATEMENT

Ethical review and approval was not required for the animal study because before the initiation of this research project, the Animal Experiment Council under the Danish Veterinary and Food Administration was contacted for ethical approval. It was stated by the council that due to the observational and diagnostic nature of the research further approval was not needed. Written informed consent was obtained from the herd owners for the participation of their animals in this study and allowing the researchers access to data from their herds for research purposes. All procedures in the code for conduct of responsible conduct of research at the University of Copenhagen were adhered to.

AUTHOR CONTRIBUTIONS

The study was conceived by LN, LL, AM, AK, and MB. AK and MB analysed data and wrote the manuscript. AM, NO, AK, and MB were responsible for data collection. NG was responsible for sample analysis. MD and CK were responsible for the specification of the mixed-effects logistic regression model and statistical supervision. LN, LL, and AM supervised the study and contributed with major revision of the manuscript. All authors contributed to the article and approved the submitted version.

ACKNOWLEDGMENTS

The authors would like to thank Bodil Højlund Nielsen from Department of Animal Science, Aarhus University, for the help with data extraction and Henrik Læssøe Martin from SEGES Dairy and Beef Research Centre for help with guidance in the field and with the development of the clinical scoring system.

REFERENCES

1. Brscic M, Leruste H, Heutinck LFM, Bokkers EAM, Wolthuis-Fillerup M, Stockhofe N, et al. Prevalence of respiratory disorders in veal calves and potential risk factors. *J Dairy Sci*. (2012) 95:2753–64. doi: 10.3168/jds.2011-4699

2. Svensson C, Linder A, Olsson SO. Mortality in Swedish dairy calves and replacement heifers. *J Dairy Sci*. (2006) 89:4769–77. doi: 10.3168/jds.S0022-0302(06)72526-7

3. Virtala A-MK, Mechor GD, Gröhn YT, Erb HN. The effect of calfhood diseases on growth of female dairy calves during the first 3 months of life in New York State. *J Dairy Sci*. (1996) 79:1040–9. doi: 10.3168/jds.S0022-0302(96)76457-3

4. USDA–APHIS–VS. *National Animal Health Monitoring System Beef Feedlot Study 2011. Types Costs of Respiratory Disease Treatments in U.S. Feedlots. Info Sheet*. (2013) Available online at: https://www.aphis.usda.gov/aphis/ourfocus/animalhealth/monitoring-and-surveillance/nahms/NAHMS_Feedlot_Studies (accessed February 15, 2021).

5. Van der Fels-Klerx HJ, Sorensen JT, Jalvingh AW, Huirne RBM. An economic model to calculate farm-specific losses due to bovine respiratory disease in dairy heifers. *Prev Vet Med*. (2001) 51:75–94. doi: 10.1016/S0167-5877(01)00208-2

6. Jensen VF, Svensmark B, Larsen G, Pedersen K, Toft N, Jorsal E, et al. Diagnostiske undersøgelser af luftvejsinfektioner og antibiotikabehandling af kalve. *Dansk Veterinaertidsskrift*. (2018) 6:28–35. Available online at: https://backend.orbit.dtu.dk/ws/portalfiles/portal/161803810/DVT_2018_laboratorieUS_og_antibiotika_til_svin.pdf (accessed May 13, 2021).

7. Fulton RW, Confer AW. Laboratory test descriptions for bovine respiratory disease diagnosis and their strengths and weaknesses: gold standards for diagnosis, do they exist? *Can Vet J*. (2012) 53:754–61.

8. Buczinski S, Forté G, Francoz D, Bélanger AM. Comparison of thoracic auscultation, clinical score, and ultrasonography as indicators of bovine respiratory disease in preweaned dairy calves. *J Vet Intern Med*. (2014) 28:234–42. doi: 10.1111/jvim.12251

9. Griffin D, Chengappa MM, Kuszak J, McVey DS. Bacterial pathogens of the bovine respiratory disease complex. *Vet Clin North Am Food Anim Pract*. (2010) 26:381–94. doi: 10.1016/j.cvfa.2010.04.004

10. Love WJ, Lehenbauer TW, Van Eenennaam AL, Drake CM, Kass PH, Farver TB, et al. Sensitivity and specificity of on-farm scoring systems and nasal culture to detect bovine respiratory disease complex in preweaned dairy calves. *J Vet Diagnostic Investig*. (2016) 28:119–28. doi: 10.1177/1040638715626204

11. Love WJ, Lehenbauer TW, Kass PH, Van Eenennaam AL, Aly SS. Development of a novel clinical scoring system for on-farm diagnosis of bovine respiratory disease in pre-weaned dairy calves. *PeerJ*. (2014) 2:1–25. doi: 10.7717/peerj.238

12. Best N, Zanandrez L, Gwozdz J, Klien E, Buller N, Suter R, et al. Assessment of a rtPCR for the detection of virulent and benign Dichelobacter nodosus, the causative agent of ovine footrot, in Australia. *BMC Vet Res*. (2018) 14:1–12. doi: 10.1186/s12917-018-1575-0

13. Dormond L, Jaton K, de Vallière S, Genton B, Greub G. Malaria real-time PCR: correlation with clinical presentation. *New Microbe New Infect*. (2015) 5:10–12. doi: 10.1016/j.nmni.2015.02.004

14. Trang NV, Choisy M, Nakagomi T, Chinh NTM, Doan YH, Yamashiro T, et al. Determination of cut-off cycle threshold values in routine RT-PCR assays to assist differential diagnosis of norovirus in children hospitalized for acute gastroenteritis. *Epidemiol Infect*. (2015) 143:3292–9. doi: 10.1017/S095026881500059X

15. Thomas AC, Bailey M, Lee MRF, Mead A, Morales-Aza B, Reynolds R, et al. Insights into Pasteurellaceae carriage dynamics in the nasal passages of healthy beef calves. *Sci Rep*. (2019) 9:1–14. doi: 10.1038/s41598-019-48007-5

16. Fertner M, Toft N, Martin HL, Boklund A. A register-based study of the antimicrobial usage in Danish veal calves and young bulls. *Prev Vet Med*. (2016) 131:41–7. doi: 10.1016/j.prevetmed.2016. 07.004

17. Goecke NB, Hjulsager CK, Krog JS, Skovgaard K, Larsen LE. Development of a high-throughput real-time PCR system for detection of enzootic pathogens in pigs. *J Vet Diagnostic Investig*. (2020) 32:51–64. doi: 10.1177/1040638719890863

18. McGuirk SM. Disease management of dairy calves and heifers. *Vet Clin North Am Food Anim Pract*. (2008) 24:139–53. doi: 10.1016/j.cvfa.2007. 10.003

19. R Core Team. *R: A Language and Environment for Statistical Computing*. (2020) Available online at: https://www.r-project.org/ (accessed February 15, 2021).

20. Bates D, Mächler M, Bolker B, Walker S. Fitting linear mixed-effects models using {lme4}. *J Stat Softw*. (2015) 67:1–48. doi: 10.18637/jss.v067.i01

21. Cozens D, Sutherland E, Lauder M, Taylor G, Berry CC. Pathogenic *Mannheimia haemolytica* invades differentiated bovine airway epithelial cells. *Infect Immun*. (2019) 87:1–20. doi: 10.1128/IAI.00078-19

22. Jost BH, Billington SJ. Arcanobacterium pyogenes: molecular pathogenesis of an animal opportunist. *Antonie Van Leeuwenhoek*. (2005) 88:87–102. doi: 10.1007/s10482-005-2316-5

23. Korenková V, Scott J, Novosadová V, Jindrichová M, Langerová L, Švec D, et al. Pre-amplification in the context of high-throughput qPCR gene expression experiment. *BMC Mol Biol*. (2015) 16:5. doi: 10.1186/s12867-015-0033-9

24. Taylor JD, Fulton RW, Lehenbauer TW, Step DL, Confer AW. The epidemiology of bovine respiratory disease: what is the evidence for predisposing factors? *Can Vet J.* (2010) 50:1095–1102.

25. Loy JD, Leger L, Workman AM, Clawson ML, Bulut E, Wang B. Development of a multiplex real-time PCR assay using two thermocycling platforms for detection of major bacterial pathogens associated with bovine respiratory disease complex from clinical samples. *J Vet Diagn Inv.* (2018) 30:837–47. doi: 10.1177/1040638718800170

26. Sanderson MW, Dargatz DA, Wagner BA. Risk factors for initial respiratory disease in United States' feedlots based on producer-collected daily morbidity counts. *Can Vet J.* (2008) 49:373–8.

16

Development of an Online Tool for *Pasteurella multocida* Genotyping and Genotypes of *Pasteurella multocida* from Different Hosts

Zhong Peng[1†], Junyang Liu[2], Wan Liang[1,3], Fei Wang[1], Li Wang[2], Xueying Wang[1], Lin Hua[1], Huanchun Chen[1], Brenda A. Wilson[4*], Jia Wang[2*] and Bin Wu[1*†]

[1] State Key Laboratory of Agricultural Microbiology, The Cooperative Innovation Center for Sustainable Pig Production, College of Animal Science and Veterinary Medicine, Huazhong Agricultural University, Wuhan, China, [2] Hubei Key Laboratory of Agricultural Bioinformatics, College of Informatics, Huazhong Agricultural University, Wuhan, China, [3] Key Laboratory of Prevention and Control Agents for Animal Bacteriosis (Ministry of Agriculture and Rural Affairs), Animal Husbandry and Veterinary Institute, Hubei Academy of Agricultural Sciences, Wuhan, China, [4] Department of Microbiology, School of Molecular and Cellular Biology, University of Illinois at Urbana-Champaign, Urbana, IL, United States

*Correspondence:
Brenda A. Wilson
wilson7@illinois.edu
Jia Wang
wang.jia@mail.hzau.edu.cn
Bin Wu
wub@mail.hzua.edu.cn

Pasteurella multocida is a versatile zoonotic pathogen. Multiple systems have been applied to type *P. multocida* from different diseases in different hosts. Recently, we found that assigning *P. multocida* strains by combining their capsular, lipopolysaccharide, and MLST genotypes (marked as capsular: lipopolysaccharide: MLST genotype) could help address the biological characteristics of *P. multocida* circulation in different hosts. However, there is still lack of a rapid and efficient tool to diagnose *P. multocida* according to this system. Here, we developed an intelligent genotyping platform PmGT for *P. multocida* strains according to their whole genome sequences using the web 2.0 technologies. By using PmGT, we determined capsular genotypes, LPS genotypes, and MLST genotypes as well as the main virulence factor genes (VFGs) of *P. multocida* isolates from different host species based on their whole genome sequences published on NCBI. The results revealed a closer association between the genotypes and pasteurellosis rather than between genotypes and host species. With the advent of high-quality, inexpensive DNA sequencing, PmGT represents a more efficient tool for *P. multocida* diagnosis in both epidemiological studies and clinical settings.

Keywords: *Pasteurella multocida*, genotyping, whole genome sequence, PmGT, genotypes

INTRODUCTION

Rapid and accurate diagnosis of sources of infections is critical for both medical and veterinary activities, and it is important for improved understanding of disease mechanisms and measures to control the illness (1). Microbial typing is an important link for the diagnosis of pathogens associated with diseases. The most widely used typing methods consist of serological typing systems and PCR-based molecular typing methods (2, 3). The establishment of discriminatory typing systems help in the understanding and control of pathogens, especially those with multiple serovars and/or genotypes from different environmental or host sources. Whole genome sequencing combined with the high-end computational technology is such an emerging approach for microbial diagnosis (4). Using the whole genome sequencing technologies, it is possible to determine the causative agent of infectious diseases rapidly and accurately, including newly emerged ones (5, 6). However, interpretation of the sequencing results to formulate a definitive diagnosis still requires technical experts with computational and bioinformatics skills. Therefore, a practical, automated platform that combines whole genome sequencing with computational technologies to provide diagnostic outcomes would be beneficial in advancing the field.

Pasteurella multocida is an important zoonotic pathogen and it can colonize and cause infections in a wide range of domestic and wild animals including food producing animals (e.g., poultry, pigs, beef, sheep) and companion animals (e.g., cats and dogs) as well as in humans (7–9). Animal diseases associated with P. multocida such as fowl cholera in poultry and other birds, progressive atrophic rhinitis and pneumonic pasteurellosis in pigs, haemorrhagic septicaemia and respiratory diseases in cattle and buffalos, leporine atrophic rhinitis and pneumonic pasteurellosis, are of great economic significance in agriculture (9). In humans, opportunistic infections of soft tissue, including wound dermonecrosis, respiratory disease with chronic pulmonary, urinary tract infection and bacteremic meningitis have also been reported (9). Most of these infections are associated with animal biting, scratching, kissing, and/or licking (10–12). In this regard, P. multocida represents a risk to public health. P. multocida strains from different hosts are serologically classified into five serogroups (A, B, D, E, F) (13–15) and/or 16 serovars (serovars 1 to 16) (16), according to their capsular and lipopolysaccharide (LPS) antigens, respectively. However, these two traditional serological typing methods require high-quantity antisera that are challenging to prepare, particularly for clinical use, such those methods are no longer widely used for large-scale epidemiological studies (7, 17).

In 2001, a multiplex PCR-based method was established to type the five serogroups into five capsular genotypes (A, B, D, E, F) (18), and in 2015, another multiplex PCR-based method was also developed to classified the 16 serovars into eight LPS genotypes (L1~L8) (19). In 2004 and 2010, two multilocus sequencing typing systems were also developed to genotype P. multocida strains (https://pubmlst.org/pmultocida/) from multiple mammalian hosts and birds, respectively (20, 21). In 2017, a virulence genotyping system based on the detection of different virulence factor gene (VFG) profiles was also reported for distinguishing P. multocida strains from different hosts (22). Compared to the traditional serological typing methods, these molecular DNA-based typing systems are indeed highly effective and accurate, and they are now widely used to determine the epidemiological and genetic characteristics of clinical isolates (23–27).

Despite of more than 135 years of research, differences on the molecular biological characteristics of P. multocida prevalence in different host species remain to be addressed. For example, P. multocida type A strains have been recovered from avian species, pigs, bovine species, and many other host species (8, 9), but little is known about differences on those type A isolates from different hosts. Recently, we developed a system to assign P. multocida strains from different host species by combining their capsular, LPS, and MLST genotypes (marked as capsular genotype: LPS genotype: MLST genotype), as well as determine the VFG profiles, which contributes to address the molecular biological characteristics of P. multocida prevalence in different host species (7, 23, 27). However, this strategy requires bioinformatics experts for data analysis and interpretation. Here, we report the development of an automated platform to type P. multocida strains from multiple hosts that combines the use of whole genome sequencing.

MATERIALS AND METHODS

Bacterial Strains and Nucleotide Sequences

P. multocida strains used in this study include one isolate of bovine origin (strain HB01), one isolate of avian origin (strain HB02), and 50 isolates of porcine origin (strains HB03, HN04, HN05, HN06, HN07, HNA01~HNA22, HND01~HND21, HNF01 and HNF02) (**Supplementary Table S1**). All of these strains are from our laboratory collection, for which we have previously sequenced their whole genome sequences (27–30).

Nucleotide sequences specific for the determination of P. multocida strains (KMT1, 460 bp), and their the five capsular genotypes (A, 1044 bp; B, 760 bp; D, 657 bp; E, 511 bp; F, 851 bp); as well as their eight LPS genotypes (L1, 1307 bp; L2, 810 bp; L3, 474 bp; L4, 550 bp; L5, 1175 bp; L6, 668 bp; L7, 931 bp; L8, 255 bp) were extracted from the genome sequences of the different P. multocida strains according to the positions documented in previous publications (18, 19) and were deposited in GenBank under accession numbers MT570166, MN938443~MN938455 (**Supplementary Text 1**).

The nucleotide sequences of 23 types of virulence genes commonly detected in P. multocida epidemiological studies, including those encoding fimbriae and other adhesins (ptfA, fimA, hsf-1, hsf-2, pfhA, and tadD), toxin (toxA), iron acquisition proteins (exbB, exbD, tonB, hgbA, hgbB, fur, and tbpA), sialidases (nanB and nanH), hyaluronidase (pmHAS), outer membrane proteins (OMPs) (ompA, ompH, oma87, and plpB), and superoxide dismutase (sodA and sodC), were amplified from the genomic DNA of P. multocida HN06 and HB01 by PCR assays using the protocols documented elsewhere (23, 31). These nucleotide sequences were deposited in GenBank under accession numbers MT570167~ MT570189 (**Supplementary Text 1**).

The publicly available whole genome sequences of 262 P. multocida strains from bovine species [n = 106; including those recovered bovine haemorrhagic septicaemia cases (32)], avian species (n = 39), porcine species (n = 66), leporine species (n = 20), ovine species (n = 6), humans (n = 13), canines (n = 3), murine species (n = 2), horses (n = 2), cats (n = 2), alpacas (n = 2) and 1 synthetic DNA sequence in NCBI genome database were downloaded for use (**Supplementary Table S1**).

System Implementation

The PmGT platform was integrated on a CentOS server, mainly providing two kinds of online services: genotyping tool, and data query and display. To establish the genotyping online service, we first used Apache (https://www.apache.org) as the web

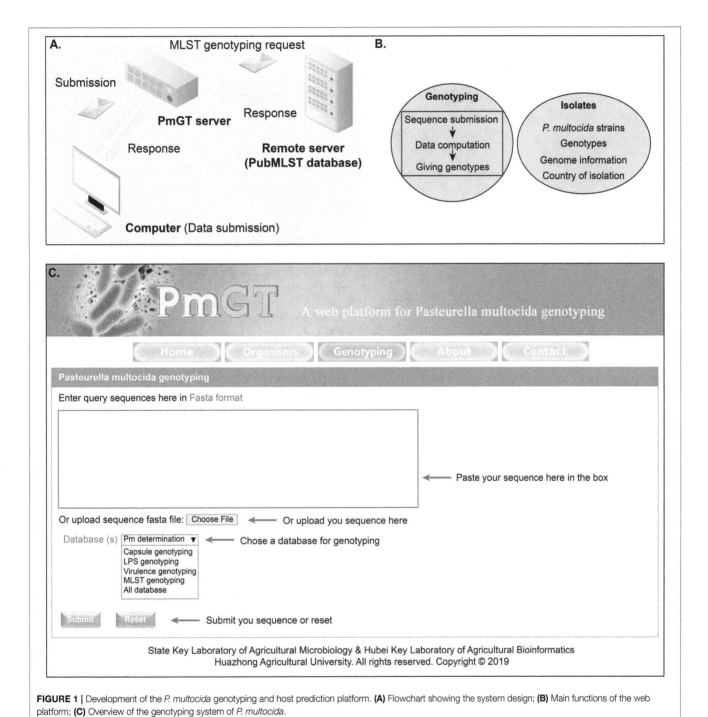

FIGURE 1 | Development of the *P. multocida* genotyping and host prediction platform. **(A)** Flowchart showing the system design; **(B)** Main functions of the web platform; **(C)** Overview of the genotyping system of *P. multocida*.

container. Then, we downloaded the BLAST package (ftp://ftp. ncbi.nlm.nih.gov/blast/executables/LATEST/) from NCBI, which was thereafter installed and configured on the web container. PHP was used as the server-side language and the browser-side script used jQuery, which is a fast, small, and feature-rich JavaScript library. The view pages were constructed with Hypertext Markup Language (HTML) and Cascading Style Sheets (CSS). For the target strain, the format of the sequence was first verified by the web user interface and then the

sequence data was uploaded to the server through the PHP program which subsequently called the localized BLAST to align the uploaded sequence with the reference database. The nucleotide sequences specific for the determination of *P. multocida* strains, capsular genotypes, LPS genotypes, and the 23 types of virulence factor genes (VFGs) were packaged and used as the reference database for sequence alignment. Finally, the result was returned and displayed in the web page. In addition, if the user selected the option of "MLST

TABLE 1 | Genotypes of 52 *Pasteurella multocida* strains determined via the PmGT Platform.

Strain	Capsular genotype	LPS genotype	MLST genotype (Sequence type)	GenBank accession numbers
HB01	A	L3	ST1	CP006976
HB02	A	L1	ST128	LYOX00000000
HB03	A	L3	ST3	CP003328
HN04	B	L2	ST44	PPVE00000000
HN05	D	L6	ST11	PPVF00000000
HN06	D	L6	ST11	CP003313
HN07	F	L3	ST12	CP007040
HNA01	A	L3	ST133	PPVG00000000
HNA02	A	L6	ST10	PPVH00000000
HNA03	A	L3	ST3	PPVI00000000
HNA04	A	L6	ST10	PPVJ00000000
HNA05	A	L6	ST10	PPVK00000000
HNA06	A	L6	ST10	PPVL00000000
HNA07	A	L6	ST10	PPVM00000000
HNA08	A	L3	ST3	PPVN00000000
HNA09	A	L3	ST3	PPVO00000000
HNA10	A	L6	ST10	PPVP00000000
HNA11	A	L6	ST10	PPVQ00000000
HNA12	A	L6	ST10	PPVR00000000
HNA13	A	L3	ST3	PPVS00000000
HNA14	A	L3	ST3	PPVT00000000
HNA15	A	L3	ST3	PPVU00000000
HNA16	A	L6	ST10	PPVV00000000
HNA17	A	L3	ST3	PPVW00000000
HNA18	A	L3	ST3	PPVX00000000
HNA19	A	L3	ST3	PPVY00000000
HNA20	A	L3	ST3	PPVZ00000000
HNA21	A	L6	ST10	PPWA00000000
HNA22	A	L6	ST10	PPWB00000000
HND01	D	L6	ST11	PPWC00000000
HND02	D	L6	ST134	PPWD00000000
HND03	D	L6	ST11	PPWE00000000
HND04	D	L6	ST11	PPWF00000000
HND05	D	L6	ST11	PPWG00000000
HND06	D	L6	ST11	PPWH00000000
HND07	D	L6	ST11	PPWI00000000
HND08	D	L6	ST11	PPWJ00000000
HND09	D	L6	ST11	PPWK00000000
HND10	D	L6	ST11	PPWL00000000
HND11	D	L6	ST11	PPWN00000000
HND12	D	L6	ST134	PPWM00000000
HND13	D	L6	ST134	PPWO00000000
HND14	D	L6	ST11	PPWP00000000
HND15	D	L6	ST11	PPWQ00000000
HND16	D	L6	ST11	PPWR00000000
HND17	D	L6	ST11	PPWS00000000
HND18	D	L6	ST11	PPWT00000000
HND19	D	L6	ST11	PPWU00000000
HND20	D	L6	ST11	PPWV00000000
HND21	D	L6	ST11	PPWW00000000
HNF01	F	L3	ST12	PPWX00000000
HNF02	F	L3	ST12	PPWY00000000

genotyping," the http request function "curl_setopt" in PHP was used to request PubMLST's RESTful interface (http://rest.pubmlst.org/db/pubmlst_Pmultocida_seqdef/sequence) and the function "curl_exec" was used to catch the response which thereafter was parsed to the result and displayed in the genotyping page.

PCR Detection of Capsular Genotypes, LPS Genotypes, MLST Genotypes, and Virulence Genes of *P. multocida* Strains From Pigs

Capsular genotypes and LPS genotypes of *P. multocida* strains from our laboratory collection were determined using multiplex PCR-based assays, as documented elsewhere (18, 19). Profiles of 23 types of virulence genes mentioned above were determined by PCR assays, as described previously (23). Sequence types (STs) were determined according to the protocols described in *Pasteurella multocida* MLST database (https://pubmlst.org/organisms/pasteurella-multocida/multi-host).

Data Availability

Nucleotide sequences specific for *P. multocida* and its capsular genotypes, LPS genotypes, as well as VFGs were publicly available in GenBank under accession numbers MN938443-MN938455 and MT570167~MT570189. The typing system developed in the present study is available at: http://vetinfo.hzau.edu.cn/PmGT.

RESULTS

Development and Implementation of PmGT

The general process for genotyping is summarized as: when a query sequence is submitted via the web user interface, this sequence will be then submitted to the CentOS server via HTTP protocol. Thereafter, the sequence is evaluated by the PHP program, and the passed sequence will be BLASTed against the genotype database to yield a result, which will be returned to the webpage through the PHP program (**Figures 1A,B**). Through the above procedures, the genotyping module of PmGT (http://vetinfo.hzau.edu.cn/PmGT) was developed (**Figure 1**).

Currently, PmGT provides the above services includes five menus: (1) the "Home" page gives a brief introduction of *P. multocida* etiological characteristics to help the users understand the bacterium; (2) the "Isolates" page displays the genotypes of *P. multocida* strains based on their whole genome sequences that are publicly available in NCBI; this page also provides the link for the users to download the genomes of these *P. multocida* strains from NCBI; (3) the "Genotyping" page enables the users to determine whether a putative isolate is a *P. multocida* and genotype *P. multocida* strains by using the whole genome sequence assembled from the sequencing reads (**Figure 1C**); (4) the "About" page summarizes the guidelines for the use of this web tool; (5) the "Contact" page provides the contact information of the developers.

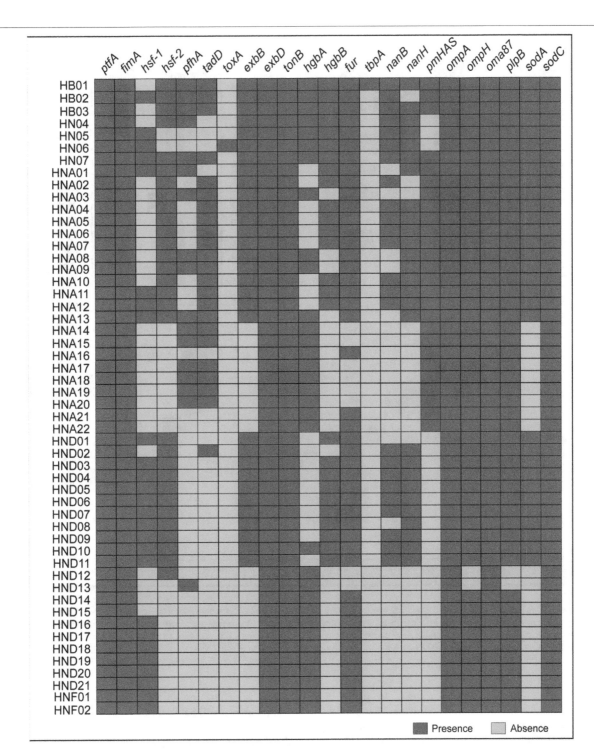

FIGURE 2 | Heatmap showing the distribution of the 23 types of virulence genes (VFGs) among the 52 *P. multocida* strains from pigs. Boxes in red indicate a VFG is presence in the strain while boxes in green represent a VFG is missing in the strain.

PmGT Shows the Same Accuracy With PCR Methods in Genotyping *P. multocida* Strains

To test the accuracy of PmGT, we used two methods to type 52 *P. multocida* isolates (HB01, HB02, HB03, HN04, HN05,

HN06, HN07, HNA01~HNA22, HND01~HND21, HNF01, and HNF02) from our laboratory collection (27). First, we submitted their whole genome sequences to PmGT for genotyping. As a comparison, we also determined the capsular genotypes, LPS genotypes, sequence types, as well as the profile of the

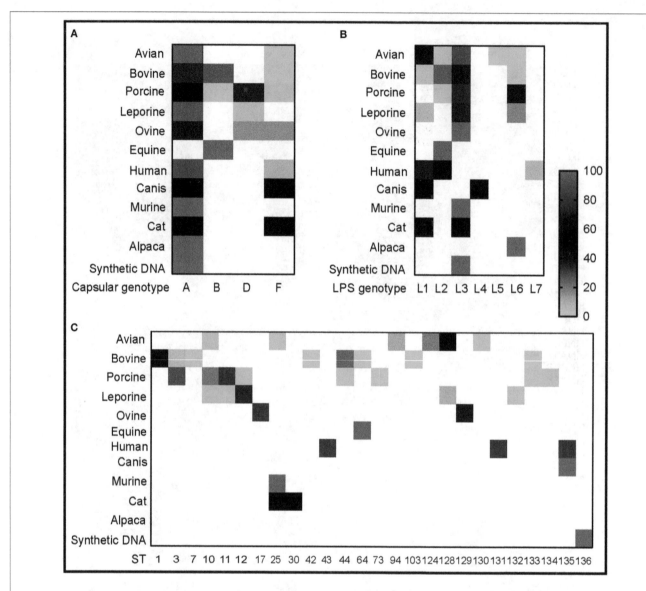

FIGURE 3 | Heatmap revealing the association between capsular/LPS/MLST genotypes and *P. multocida* strains from different host species determined by PmGT. **(A)** Heatmap revealing the association between capsular genotypes and *P. multocida* strains from different host species; **(B)** Heatmap revealing the association between LPS genotypes and *P. multocida* strains from different host species; **(C)** Heatmap revealing the association between MLST genotypes and *P. multocida* strains from different host species. Percentages of sequences typed are shown with different colors displayed at right corner.

abovementioned 23-kinds of virulence genes by using PCR assays. All these 52 strains were genotyped by PmGT and through this online genotyping platform (**Table 1**). Genotyping by PCR assays confirmed these capsular, LPS, and MLST genotypes. PCR results of capsular and LPS genotypes are provided in **Supplementary Figures S1, S2**.

Determination of the 23 types of virulence genes for each of the 52 strains by using this online system revealed that several genes (*ptfA*, *fimA*, *oma87*, and *sodC*) were broadly presented in the genome sequences genotyped (**Figure 2**). However, several genes (*hsf-1*, *hsf-2*, *pfhA*, and *tadD)* were heterogeneously distributed, and in particularly, none of the 52 sequences genotyped carried the *toxA* or *tbpA* genes

(**Figure 2**). These results were also confirmed by PCR assays (**Supplementary Table S1**).

Genotypes of *P. multocida* From Different Hosts

To understand the genotypes of *P. multocida* strains circulation in different host species, the 262 whole genome sequences of *P. multocida* strains were genotyped by PmGT. The results revealed that *P. multocida* isolates from different hosts displayed a certain preference for "capsular/LPS/MLST genotypes" (**Figure 3**). For example, most of the porcine strains were determined as capsular genotypes A (52%) and D (39%), LPS genotypes L3 (36%) and L6 (61%), sequence types ST3 (29%), ST11 (22%), and ST10 (34%),

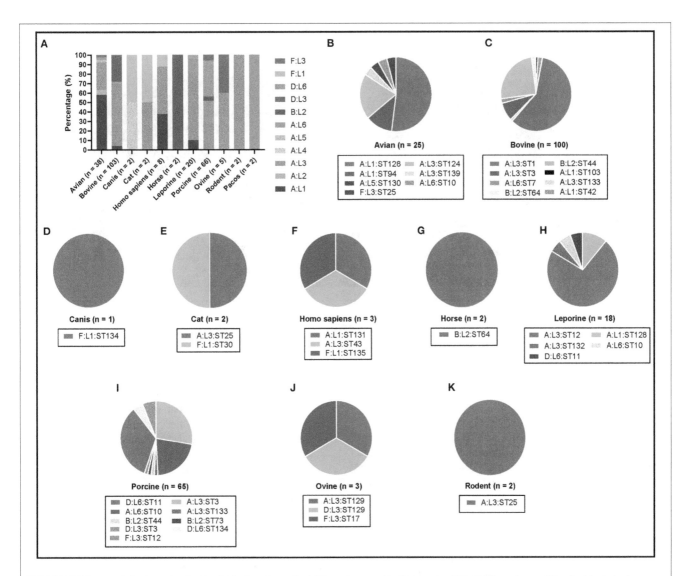

FIGURE 4 | Column and pie charts showing the distribution of capsular: LPS genotypes and/or the capsular: LPS: MLST genotypes of *P. multocida* strains from different host species determined by PmGT by using the whole genome sequences. **(A)** Column chart showing the distribution of capsular: LPS genotypes of *P. multocida* strains from different host species; **(B–K)** Pie charts showing the distribution of capsular: LPS: MLST genotypes of *P. multocida* strains from avian species, bovine species, canis, cats, humans, horses, leporine species, pigs, ovine species, and rodents, respectively.

respectively; while most of the genotyped bovine strains were determined as capsular genotypes A (72%) and B (28%), LPS genotypes L3 (67%) and L2 (27%), and sequence types ST1 (59%) and ST44 (25%), respectively (**Figure 3**). When combining the capsular genotypes and the LPS genotypes, it revealed that most of the genotyped avian *P. multocida* were typed as A:L1 and A:L3, while most of the genotyped bovine *P. multocida* were typed as A:L3 and B:L2; the genotyped porcine *P. multocida* mainly belonged to D:L6, A:L3, and A:L6; while the genotyped leporine *P. multocida* mainly belonged to A:L3; most of the genotyped human *P. multocida* were typed as A:L3 and A:L1 (**Figure 4A**). If the capsular genotypes, LPS genotypes, and MLST genotypes were combined, most of the genotyped avian *P. multocida* were typed as A:L1:ST128, while most of the genotyped bovine *P. multocida* were typed as A:L3:ST1 and B:L2:ST44; the genotyped

porcine *P. multocida* mainly belonged to D:L6:ST11, A:L3:ST3, and A:L6:ST10; while the genotyped leporine *P. multocida* mainly belonged to A:L3:ST12 (**Figure 4**).

Virulence genotyping using the system developed herein revealed that the presence of multiple VFGs, including *ptfA*, *fimA*, *hsf-2*, *exbB*, *exbD*, *tonB*, *hgbA*, *hgbB*, *fur*, *nanB*, *nanH*, *ompA*, *ompH*, *oma87*, *plpB*, *sodA*, and *sodC*, was a broad characteristic of *P. multocida* strains from multiple host species (**Figure 5**). However, several VFGs were only determined in the genome sequences of *P. multocida* from certain hosts. For example, *toxA*, a gene encoding a dermonecrotic toxin, was found only in strains from pig, sheep, and alpacas, while *tbpA*, a transferrin binding protein coding gene, was found only in strains from cattle, sheep, and alpacas (**Figure 5**).

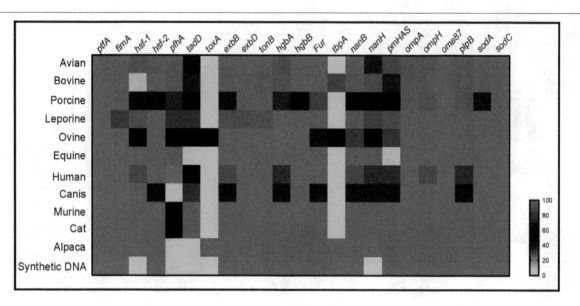

FIGURE 5 | Heatmap revealing the association between virulence genes and *P. multocida* strains from different host species.

DISCUSSION

P. multocida is the causative agent of multiple diseases with a wide spectrum of host species, including humans and other primates (7–9). In addition, *P. multocida* isolates recovered from different hosts with different diseases can be classified in many different serovars/genotypes according to different typing systems (7, 9). Relying on only one or two typing systems is difficult to address the characteristics of *P. multocida* isolates from different host species and/or their association with different diseases. For example, *P. multocida* isolates from different host species might have the same capsular genotypes but possess different LPS genotypes and/or MLST genotypes; even those from different host species that share the same capsular, LPS, and MLST genotypes might carry different VFGs (27, 33). Therefore, we have proposed a combined "capsular: LPS: MLST" genotyping system that includes virulence genotyping to discriminate *P. multocida* isolates from different host species and/or those associated with different diseases (7). However, this combined genotyping system is multiplex PCR-based and is laborious and time-consuming.

Advances in bioinformatics and bioinformatical tools enable the application of whole genome sequence data for inclusion of various demographic information for bacterial characterization, such as capsular and LPS genotyping; the presence of adhesins, toxins, or other virulence factors (34). In the present study, we reported the development of a genotyping platform for distinguishing *P. multocida* isolates according to the bacterial whole genome sequences. Validation of the PmGT platform was performed on a collection of *P. multocida* isolates from our laboratory. Results revealed that this genotyping system provides consistent results of

determining the capsular-, LPS-, MLST genotypes, and VFGs, as compared with that obtained using multiplex PCR-based typing systems. Compared to the multiplex PCR-based typing systems (18, 19, 21, 22) and traditional serological typing systems (13, 16), this genotyping system takes less time to yield results and does not require high-quality antisera, which represents a more efficient and cost-saving tool for characterizing *P. multocida* isolates in both epidemiological studies and clinical settings.

By using PmGT, the capsular-, LPS-, MLST genotypes, and VFGs of *P. multocida* strains from different hosts were determined according to the whole genome sequences. These results agree with those of the epidemiological studies (23, 24, 26, 35). For example, *P. multocida* serovars B: 2 and A: 3 strains are frequently associated with bovine haemorrhagic septicaemia and respiratory diseases, respectively (36, 37). It is known that *P. multocida* serogroups A and B are assigned to capsular genotypes A and B by multiplex PCR, respectively (18); while *P. multocida* Heddleston serovars 2 and 3 are assigned to LPS genotypes L2 and L3 by multiplex PCR, respectively (19). That is why the capsular: LPS genotypes of most of the bovine strains were determined as A: L3 and B: L2, respectively. In addition, *P. multocida* strains isolated from bovine haemorrhagic septicaemia are commonly determined as ST122 (38), this sequence type can be reassigned to ST44 by using the multihost MLST database (27). These findings could explain why *P. multocida* strains associated with bovine haemorrhagic septicaemia were typed as capsular: LPS: MLST genotype B: L2: ST44. Similar findings were also observed in *P. multocida* strains from the other host species. In particularly, most of the *P. multocida* strains from pigs were determined as capsular: LPS: MLST genotypes D: L6:

ST11, A: L3: ST3, and A: L6: ST10. These results are also in agreement with the results of our previously epidemiological study (23), suggesting that these three genotypes, particularly genotype D/L6/ST11, are likely to be strongly associated with swine respiratory diseases. However, during our test we also found the capsular-, LPS-, and/or MLST-genotypes of several strains could not be determined by PmGT according to the whole genome sequences. After check the data we put forward several reasons to explain this result: (1) most of these non-typeable genomes are sequenced and assembled using the second-generation sequencing technologies and the quality of these genomes are not high, some of the genes used for capsular/LPS/MLST genotyping fell within the gaps between genome contigs in the assemblies (7); (2) the genome sequences might be those of the capsular nontypeable strains reported (23, 39); (3) several strains belong to novel sequence types and the current *Pasteurella multocida* MLST database do not include these sequence types.

In conclusion, we developed an online platform for *P. multocida* genotyping (PmGT platform), which combines whole genome sequence analysis tools with web 2.0 technologies. By using this system, we determined the genotypes of *P. multocida* isolates from different host species. Overall, this system represents a more convenient tool for *P. multocida* diagnosis in both epidemiological studies and clinical settings. More importantly, our study provides an example to develop rapid and efficient tools for bacterial diagnosis by using their whole genome sequences in the coming age of artificial intelligence.

AUTHOR CONTRIBUTIONS

ZP, BWi, JW, and BWu contributed to conception and design of the study. ZP, JL, WL, FW, LW, XW, and LH performed the experiments. ZP, JL, LW, and JW performed the statistical analysis. ZP wrote the first draft of the manuscript. ZP, HC, BWi, JW, and BWu revised the manuscript. All authors contributed to manuscript revision, read, and approved the submitted version.

ACKNOWLEDGMENTS

We sincerely acknowledge Huazhong Agricultural University College of Informatics for providing the CentOS server and the PubMLST database for the RESTful port for connection.

SUPPLEMENTARY MATERIAL

Supplementary Text 1 | Nucleotide sequences and their GenBank accession numbers for the construction of a comparative database for *P. multocida* genotyping.

Supplementary Figure S1 | PCR results of capsular genotypes of tested *P. multocida* strains in the present study.

Supplementary Figure S2 | PCR results of LPS genotypes of tested *P. multocida* strains in the present study.

Supplementary Table S1 | *Pasteurella multocida* genome sequences used in the present study.

REFERENCES

1. Kessel M. Why microbial diagnostics need more than money. *Nat Biotechnol.* (2015) 33:898–900. doi: 10.1038/nbt.3328
2. Peng Z, Ling L, Stratton CW, Li C, Polage CR, Wu B, et al. Advances in the diagnosis and treatment of Clostridium difficile infections. *Emerg Microbes Infect.* (2018) 7:15. doi: 10.1038/s41426-017-0019-4
3. Schmitz JE, Tang YW. The GenMark ePlex((R)): another weapon in the syndromic arsenal for infection diagnosis. *Future Microbiol.* (2018) 13:1697–708. doi: 10.2217/fmb-2018-0258
4. Lecuit M, Eloit M. The diagnosis of infectious diseases by whole genome next generation sequencing: a new era is opening. *Front Cell Infect Microbiol.* (2014) 4:25. doi: 10.3389/fcimb.2014.00025
5. Zhang YZ, Holmes EC. A genomic perspective on the origin and emergence of SARS-CoV-2. *Cell.* (2020) 181:223–7. doi: 10.1016/j.cell.2020.03.035
6. Török ME, Peacock SJ. Rapid whole-genome sequencing of bacterial pathogens in the clinical microbiology laboratory–pipe dream or reality? *J Antimicrob Chemother.* (2012) 67:2307–8. doi: 10.1093/jac/d ks247
7. Peng Z, Wang X, Zhou R, Chen H, Wilson BA, Wu B. *Pasteurella multocida*: genotypes and genomics. *Microbiol Mol Biol Rev.* (2019) 83:e00014–9. doi: 10.1128/MMBR.00014-19
8. Wilkie IW, Harper M, Boyce JD, Adler B. *Pasteurella multocida*: diseases and pathogenesis. *Curr Top Microbiol Immunol.* (2012) 361:1–22. doi: 10.1007/82_2012_216
9. Wilson BA, Ho M. *Pasteurella multocida*: from zoonosis to cellular microbiology. *Clin Microbiol Rev.* (2013) 26:631–55. doi: 10.1128/CMR.00024-13
10. Ryan JM, Feder HM Jr. Dog licks baby Baby gets *Pasteurella multocida* meningitis. *Lancet.* (2019) 393:e41. doi: 10.1016/S0140-6736(19)30953-5
11. Dryden MS, Dalgliesh D. *Pasteurella multocida* from a dog causing Ludwig's angina. *Lancet.* (1996) 347:123. doi: 10.1016/S0140-6736(96)90250-0
12. Godey B, Morandi X, Bourdinière J, Heurtin C. Beware of dogs licking ears. *Lancet.* (1999) 354:1267–8. doi: 10.1016/S0140-6736(99)04197-5
13. Carter GR. Studies on *Pasteurella multocida*. I A hemagglutination test for the identification of serological types. *Am J Vet Res.* (1955) 16:481–4.
14. Carter GR. A new serological type of *Pasteurella multocida* from Central Africa. *Veterinary Record.* (1961) 73:1052.
15. Rimler RB, Rhoades KR. Serogroup F. A new capsule serogroup of *Pasteurella multocida*. *J Clin Microbiol.* (1987) 25:615–8. doi: 10.1128/jcm.25.4.615-618.1987
16. Heddleston KL, Gallagher JE, Rebers PA. Fowl cholera: gel diffusion precipitin test for serotyping Pasteurella multocida from avian species. *Avian Dis.* (1972) 16:925–36. doi: 10.2307/1588773
17. Peng Z, Liang W, Wu B. Molecular typing methods for *Pasteurella multocida*-a review. *Wei Sheng Wu Xue Bao.* (2016) 56:1521–9. doi: 10.13343/j.cnki.wsxb.20160002
18. Townsend KM, Boyce JD, Chung JY, Frost AJ, Adler B. Genetic organization of *Pasteurella multocida* cap loci and development of a multiplex capsular PCR typing system. *J Clin Microbiol.* (2001) 39:924–9. doi: 10.1128/JCM.39.3.924-929.2001
19. Harper M, John M, Turni C, Edmunds M, St Michael F, Adler B, et al. Development of a rapid multiplex PCR assay to genotype *Pasteurella multocida* strains by use of the lipopolysaccharide outer core biosynthesis locus. *J Clin Microbiol.* (2015) 53:477–85. doi: 10.1128/JCM.02824-14
20. Davies RL, MacCorquodale R, Reilly S. Characterisation of bovine strains of *Pasteurella multocida* and comparison with isolates of avian, ovine and porcine origin. *Vet Microbiol.* (2004) 99:145–58. doi: 10.1016/j.vetmic.2003.11.013
21. Subaaharan S, Blackall LL, Blackall PJ. Development of a multi-locus sequence typing scheme for avian isolates of *Pasteurella multocida*. *Vet Microbiol.* (2010) 141:354–61. doi: 10.1016/j.vetmic.2010.01.017
22. Garcia-Alvarez A, Vela AI, San Martin E, Chaves F, Fernandez-Garayzabal JF, Lucas D, et al. Characterization of *Pasteurella multocida* associated with ovine pneumonia using multi-locus sequence typing (MLST) and virulence-

associated gene profile analysis and comparison with porcine isolates. *Vet Microbiol.* (2017) 204:180–7. doi: 10.1016/j.vetmic.2017.04.015

23. Peng Z, Wang H, Liang W, Chen Y, Tang X, Chen H, et al. A capsule/lipopolysaccharide/MLST genotype D/L6/ST11 of *Pasteurella multocida* is likely to be strongly associated with swine respiratory disease in China. *Arch Microbiol.* (2018) 200:107–18. doi: 10.1007/s00203-017-1421-y

24. Li Z, Cheng F, Lan S, Guo J, Liu W, Li X, et al. Investigation of genetic diversity and epidemiological characteristics of *Pasteurella multocida* isolates from poultry in southwest China by population structure, multi-locus sequence typing and virulence-associated gene profile analysis. *J Vet Med Sci.* (2018) 80:921–9. doi: 10.1292/jvms.18-0049

25. Devi LB, Bora DP, Das SK, Sharma RK, Mukherjee S, Hazarika RA. Virulence gene profiling of porcine *Pasteurella multocida* isolates of Assam. *Vet World.* (2018) 11:348–54. doi: 10.14202/vetworld.2018.348-354

26. Massacci FR, Magistrali CF, Cucco L, Curcio L, Bano L, Mangili P, et al. Characterization of *Pasteurella multocida* involved in rabbit infections. *Vet Microbiol.* (2018) 213:66–72. doi: 10.1016/j.vetmic.2017.11.023

27. Peng Z, Liang W, Wang F, Xu Z, Xie Z, Lian Z, et al. Genetic and phylogenetic characteristics of *Pasteurella multocida* isolates from different host species. *Front Microbiol.* (2018) 9:1408. doi: 10.3389/fmicb.2018.01408

28. Peng Z, Liang W, Liu W, Wu B, Tang B, Tan C, et al. Genomic characterization of *Pasteurella multocida* HB01, a serotype A bovine isolate from China. *Gene.* (2016) 581:85–93. doi: 10.1016/j.gene.2016.01.041

29. Liu W, Yang M, Xu Z, Zheng H, Liang W, Zhou R, et al. Complete genome sequence of *Pasteurella multocida* HN06, a toxigenic strain of serogroup D. *J Bacteriol.* (2012) 194:3292–3. doi: 10.1128/JB.00215-12

30. Peng Z, Liang W, Wang Y, Liu W, Zhang H, Yu T, et al. Experimental pathogenicity and complete genome characterization of a pig origin *Pasteurella multocida* serogroup F isolate HN07. *Vet Microbiol.* (2017) 198:23–33. doi: 10.1016/j.vetmic.2016.11.028

31. Khamesipour F, Momtaz H, Azhdary Mamoreh M. Occurrence of virulence factors and antimicrobial resistance in *Pasteurella multocida* strains isolated from slaughter cattle in Iran. *Front Microbiol.* (2014) 5:536. doi: 10.3389/fmicb.2014.00536

32. Moustafa AM, Seemann T, Gladman S, Adler B, Harper M, Boyce JD, et al. Comparative genomic analysis of Asian Haemorrhagic Septicaemia-associated strains of *Pasteurella multocida* identifies more than 90 Haemorrhagic Septicaemia-specific genes. *PLoS One.* (2015) 10:e0130296. doi: 10.1371/journal.pone.0130296

33. Ujvári B, Makrai L, Magyar T. Virulence gene profiling and ompA sequence analysis of *Pasteurella multocida* and their correlation with host species. *Vet Microbiol.* (2019) 233:190–5. doi: 10.1016/j.vetmic.2019.05.005

34. Stoesser N, Sheppard AE, Pankhurst L, De Maio N, Moore CE, Sebra R, et al. Evolutionary history of the global emergence of the escherichia coli epidemic clone ST131. *MBio.* (2016) 7:e02162. doi: 10.1128/mBio.02162-15

35. Ewers C, Lübke-Becker A, Bethe A, Kiebling S, Filter M, Wieler LH. Virulence genotype of *Pasteurella multocida* strains isolated from different hosts with various disease status. *Vet Microbiol.* (2006) 114:304–17. doi: 10.1016/j.vetmic.2005.12.012

36. Shivachandra SB, Viswas KN, Kumar AA. A review of hemorrhagic septicemia in cattle and buffalo. *Anim Health Res Rev.* (2011) 12:67–82. doi: 10.1017/S146625231100003X

37. Welsh RD, Dye LB, Payton ME, Confer AW. Isolation and antimicrobial susceptibilities of bacterial pathogens from bovine pneumonia: 1994–2002. *J Vet Diagn Invest.* (2004) 16:426–31. doi: 10.1177/104063870401600510

38. Hotchkiss EJ, Hodgson JC, Lainson FA, Zadoks RN. Multilocus sequence typing of a global collection of *Pasteurella multocida* isolates from cattle and other host species demonstrates niche association. *BMC Microbiol.* (2011) 11:115. doi: 10.1186/1471-2180-11-115

39. Tang X, Zhao Z, Hu J, Wu B, Cai X, He Q, et al. Isolation, antimicrobial resistance, and virulence genes of *Pasteurella multocida* strains from swine in China. *J Clin Microbiol.* (2009) 47:951–8. doi: 10.1128/JCM.02029-08

17

Detection and Genetic Diversity of Porcine Coronavirus Involved in Diarrhea Outbreaks

Héctor Puente*, Héctor Argüello, Óscar Mencía-Ares, Manuel Gómez-García, Pedro Rubio and Ana Carvajal

Department of Animal Health, Faculty of Veterinary Medicine, Universidad de León, León, Spain

*Correspondence:
Héctor Puente
hpuef@unileon.es

Porcine enteric coronaviruses include some of the most relevant viral pathogens to the swine industry such as porcine epidemic diarrhea virus (PEDV) or porcine transmissible gastroenteritis virus (TGEV) as well as several recently identified virus such as swine enteric coronavirus (SeCoV), porcine deltacoronavirus (PDCoV) or swine enteric alphacoronavirus (SeACoV). The aim of this study is the identification and characterization of enteric coronaviruses on Spanish pig farms between 2017 and 2019. The study was carried out on 106 swine farms with diarrhea outbreaks where a viral etiology was suspected by using two duplex RT-PCRs developed for the detection of porcine enteric coronaviruses. PEDV was the only coronavirus detected in our research (38.7% positive outbreaks, 41 out of 106) and neither TGEV, SeCoV, PDCoV nor SeACoV were detected in any of the samples. The complete S-gene of all the PEDV isolates recovered were obtained and compared to PEDV and SeCoV sequences available in GenBank. The phylogenetic tree showed that only PEDV of the INDEL 2 or G1b genogroup has circulated in Spain between 2017 and 2019. Three different variants were detected, the recombinant PEDV-SeCoV being the most widespread. These results show that PEDV is a relevant cause of enteric disorders in pigs in Spain while new emerging coronavirus have not been detected so far. However, the monitoring of these virus is advisable to curtail their emergence and spread.

Keywords: swine coronavirus, pig, PEDV, S or Spike gene, INDEL strain

INTRODUCTION

Coronaviruses (CoVs) are found in a wide variety of animals including both mammals and birds in which they cause a variety of respiratory, enteric or even hepatic and neurological disorders (1). They belong to the Coronaviridae family which recognizes four genera based on phylogenetic clustering: Alphacoronavirus, Betacoronavirus, Gammacoronavirus, and Deltacoronavirus. The CoVs are enveloped viruses, and their genome is composed of a non-segmented, positive sense and single-stranded RNA with a size of ~30 kb. From the 5′ end to the 3′ end, their genomic structure is made up of at least six open reading frames (ORFs) named ORF1a, ORF1b, spike (S), envelope (E), membrane (M), and nucleocapsid (N). ORF1a and ORF1b encode non-structural polyproteins, whereas S, E, M, and N genes encode the corresponding structural proteins (2).

Two species of the Alphacoronavirus genus, transmissible gastroenteritis virus (TGEV) and the porcine epidemic diarrhea virus (PEDV) have long been recognized as the cause of acute diarrhea outbreaks on swine farms affecting pigs of all ages and causing high mortality in lactating piglets.

The relevance of TGEV on farms is scarce (1), mainly due to the widespread distribution of a respiratory mutant of TGEV, the porcine respiratory coronavirus (PRCV), which partially protects animals against the enteric disease. PEDV was recognized for the first time in Europe and Asia during the seventies and the eighties, respectively (3). In Europe its incidence markedly decreases in the nineties and subsequent years while in Asia PEDV has remained as a major cause of diarrhea outbreaks until now. Moreover, highly pathogenic variants of PEDV have been described in Asia since 2010. This virus emerged in America in 2013–2014 causing substantial economic losses (4). PEDV also re-emerged in Europe soon after its first description in the USA and PEDV outbreaks have been reported in several European countries since 2014 (5–7). Two main PEDV genogroups, named INDEL or G1 and non-INDEL or G2 have been described and differentiated by insertions-deletions in the S1 subunit of the S-gene (8, 9). Non-INDEL isolates have been associated with a higher virulence and better horizontal transmission (10). Both genotypes are reported on infected farms in Asia and America, while in Europe there is no evidence of the presence of the non-INDEL genogroup with the only exception of an Ukrainian isolate (11).

New coronaviruses affecting pigs have been unveiled in recent years. A chimeric virus produced by the recombination of TGEV/PRCV (backbone sequence) with PEDV (S gene), called swine enteric coronavirus (SeCoV), was reported in several European countries including Spain (12–15). A porcine deltacoronavirus (PDCoV) was detected in 2012 in Hong Kong (16) and subsequently on pig farms from the USA, Canada and several Asian countries (17). And finally, a new Alphacoronavirus named swine enteric alphacoronavirus (SeACoV), also known as swine acute diarrhea syndrome coronavirus (SADS-CoV) or porcine enteric alphacoronavirus (PEAV), was identified as the cause of severe diarrhea in neonatal piglets in China (18–22).

The emergence of these new CoVs and re-emergence of PEDV in Europe, immediately after its disruptive appearance in America, requires studies characterizing these CoVs on pig farms so as to allow for an accurate differential diagnosis of viral diarrhea. This study aims at disclosing the current situation of enteric CoVs in Spain, the largest pig producer in Europe, through the identification and characterization of CoVs in diarrhea outbreaks on Spanish pig farms between 2017 and 2019.

MATERIALS AND METHODS

Samples Collection and Preparation

The study was conducted between January 2017 and March 2019 on 106 swine farms (105 from Spain and one from Portugal) with diarrhea outbreaks in which a viral etiology was suspected. The outbreaks affected nursing piglets (<21 days) (28 farms), postweaning-growing pigs (21–70 days) (17 farms), or fattening pigs (>70 days) (61 farms). Location of the farms include 22 provinces in the northeast, center and northwest of Spain (**Figure 1**). Fecal samples were submitted for diagnostic purposes to the Infectious Diseases Unit of the Animal Health Department of the University of León (Spain). From each farm, two to six individual fecal samples were submitted. Individual fecal samples were mixed to prepare one pooled sample per farm.

Pooled samples were diluted 1:2 (v/v) in sterile phosphate buffered saline (PBS), homogenized by vortex mixing and centrifuged for 10 min at 20,000 g. The RNA was extracted from 140 µl of the supernatant using QIAMP Viral RNA Mini Kit (QIAGEN), following the manufacturer's instructions.

Molecular Diagnosis of Porcine Enteric Coronaviruses

Two duplex RT-PCRs were developed for the detection of SeACoV (ORF1ab), TGEV/SeCoV (N gene), PEDV/SeCoV (S gene) and PDCoV (N gene) (**Table 1**). Two conventional RT-PCRs were also developed to confirm SeCoV by excluding a potential PEDV-TGEV co-infection, by detecting the M gene of PEDV and the S gene of TGEV. The RT-PCR was carried out with Verso 1-Step RT-PCR ReddyMix kit (Thermo Scientific). The reaction was conducted under the following conditions: 50°C for 30 min, 95°C for 2 min, 40 cycles at 95°C for 20 s, 50°C for 30 s, and 72°C for 1 min, followed by a final extension step at 72°C for 10 min.

The RT-PCR products were visualized on a 1.5% agarose gel containing RedSafe Nucleic Acid Staining Solution (iNtRON Biotechnology, Inc.). The length of the PCR fragment generated for each CoV is shown in **Table 1**.

PEDV S-gene Sequencing

The S-gene of PEDV positive samples was amplified using four overlapping fragments with the primers described in **Table 1** and the Verso 1-Step RT-PCR ReddyMix kit (Thermo Scientific). The reaction was conducted under the following conditions: 50°C for 30 min, 95°C for 2 min, 45 cycles at 95°C for 20 s, 50°C for 30 s, and 72°C for 2 min, followed by a final extension step at 72°C for 10 min. The RT-PCR products were purified using the GeneMATRIX Basic DNA Purification Kit (EurX). The complete sequences of the S-gene were obtained by using forward and reverse Sanger sequencing. The complete sequence of the S gene of 36 PEDV isolates from different farms can be accessed at the NCBI GenBank with the accession numbers MW251343-MW251378 (**Table 2**). The remaining five PEDV isolates included in this research were previously sequenced by using a RNA virus-specific tailor-made NGS protocol (15).

Phylogenetic Analysis

PEDV and SeCoV genome sequences available in the GenBank database were aligned together with S-gene sequences obtained in this study using CLUSTALW. After the alignment, the evolutionary relationships among sequences were analyzed with a phylogenetic analysis, using the neighbor joining method and the maximum composite likelihood method with MEGAX software (28).

Statistical Analysis

The Fisher exact test was used to compare the frequency of occurrence of PEDV positive outbreaks among age groups and provinces (only those with five or more submitted samples

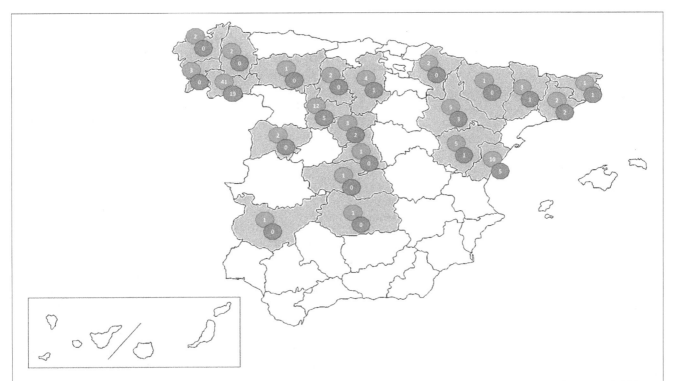

FIGURE 1 | Map showing the distribution of the viral suspected diarrhea outbreaks investigated in this research (shaded area). The number of farms sampled (blue circle) and PEDV positive farms per province (orange circle) are given.

TABLE 1 | Primer sets used for the detection of porcine enteric coronaviruses by multiplex RT-PCR and for the amplification of the S gene of PEDV.

PCR type	Viral agent	Sequence 5' to 3'	Gene target	Product size (bp)	References
Multiplex RT-PCR 1	SeACoV	TTTTGGTTCTTACGGGCTGTT	RNA-dependent	754	(20)
		CAAACTGTACGCTGGTCAACT	RNA polymerase		
	TGEV/SeCoV	GATGGCGACCAGATAGAAGT	Nucleoprotein	612	(23)
		GCAATAGGGTTGCTTGTACC			
Multiplex RT-PCR 2	PEDV/SeCoV	TTCTGAGTCACGAACAGCCA	Spike	651	(24)
		CATATGCAGCCTGCTCTGAA			
	PDCoV	GCTGACACTTCTATTAAAC	Nucleoprotein	497	(25)
		TTGACTGTGATTGAGTAG			
Conventional RT-PCR 1	TGEV	GTGGTTTTGGTYRTAAATGC	Spike	858	(24)
		CACTAACCAACGTGGARCTA			
Conventional RT-PCR 2	PEDV	GGGCGCCTGTATAGAGTTTA	Membrane	412	(23)
		AGACCACCAAGAATGTGTCC			
PEDV S-gene RT-PCR	PEDV	TGCTAGTGCGTAATAATGAC	Spike 1	1,349	(26)
		CGTCAGTGCCATGACCAGTG			(15)
		GGGAAATTGTCATCACCAAG	Spike 2	1,289	(15)
		CTGGGTGAGTAATTGTTTACAACG			(27)
		AGTACTAGGGAGTTGCCTGG	Spike 3	1,216	(15)
		AACCATAACGCTGAGATTGC			
		TTGAACACTGTGGCTCATGC	Spike 4	1,128	(15)
		CATCTTTGACAACTGTGT			(26)

TABLE 2 | List of porcine epidemic diarrhea virus (PEDV) isolates recovered in this study.

Isolate name	Collection date	Country	Province of origin	Accession number
SP-VC2*	12/01/2017	Spain	Valladolid	MN692784
SP-VC3	17/01/2017	Spain	Valladolid	MW251343
SP-VC4	17/01/2017	Spain	Burgos	MW251344
SP-VC16	01/03/2017	Spain	Zaragoza	MW251345
SP-VC18	07/03/2017	Spain	Segovia	MW251346
SP-VC19	07/03/2017	Spain	Segovia	MW251347
SP-VC27	06/06/2017	Spain	Ourense	MW251348
SP-VC29	06/06/2017	Spain	Ourense	MW251349
SP-VC46	11/01/2018	Spain	Valladolid	MW251350
SP-VC51*	02/02/2018	Spain	Ourense	MN692788
SP-VC52	02/02/2018	Spain	Ourense	MW251351
SP-VC53	05/02/2018	Spain	Teruel	MW251352
SP-VT13	14/02/2018	Spain	Valladolid	MW251353
SP-VC54	14/02/2018	Spain	Castellón	MW251354
SP-VC55	15/02/2018	Spain	Girona	MW251355
SP-VC57*	02/03/2018	Spain	Castellón	MN692789
SP-VC61	18/04/2018	Spain	Castellón	MW251356
SP-VC62*	03/05/2018	Spain	Castellón	MN692790
SP-VC63	03/05/2018	Spain	Zaragoza	MW251357
SP-VC66	30/05/2018	Spain	Ourense	MW251358
SP-VC68	20/06/2018	Spain	Zaragoza	MW251359
SP-VC75	05/09/2018	Spain	Castellón	MW251360
SP-VC77	05/09/2018	Spain	Ourense	MW251361
SP-VC81	06/10/2018	Spain	Ourense	MW251362
SP-VC87	07/10/2018	Spain	Lérida	MW251363
SP-VT86	07/11/2018	Spain	Barcelona	MW251364
SP-VT87	29/11/2018	Spain	Valladolid	MW251365
SP-VT108	10/01/2019	Spain	Barcelona	MW251366
SP-VC89	18/01/2019	Spain	Ourense	MW251367
SP-VC90	22/01/2019	Spain	Ourense	MW251368
SP-VC92	24/01/2019	Spain	Ourense	MW251369
SP-VC93	25/01/2019	Spain	Ourense	MW251370
SP-VC94	08/02/2019	Spain	Ourense	MW251371
SP-VC95	12/02/2019	Spain	Ourense	MW251372
SP-VC96	12/02/2019	Spain	Ourense	MW251373
SP-VC97	14/02/2019	Spain	Ourense	MW251374
SP-VC98	19/02/2019	Spain	Ourense	MW251375
SP-VC99	19/02/2019	Spain	Ourense	MW251376
SP-VC100*	28/02/2019	Spain	Ourense	MN692791
SP-VC101	28/02/2019	Spain	Ourense	MW251377
POR-VC102	14/03/2019	Portugal	Coimbra	MW251378

A complete sequence of the S gene was obtained for all PEDV isolates.
*PEDV isolates previously sequenced by de Nova et al. (15).

were included in the analysis). ANOVA test was used to compare the number of investigated outbreaks as well as the percentage of PEDV positive outbreaks among the different trimesters of the year. Epi Info™ was used for data analysis at $\alpha = 0.05$.

RESULTS

Prevalence of Enteric Coronaviruses in Porcine Diarrhea Outbreaks

Neither TGEV, SeCoV, PDCoV nor SeACoV were detected in any of the samples, while PEDV was the only coronavirus detected in 41 out of the 106 investigated outbreaks (38.7%). Most of these outbreaks occurred in fattening pigs (24 positive farms out of 61, 39.3%) or postweaning-growing pigs (nine positive farms out of 17, 52.9%). PEDV was involved to a lesser extent in diarrhea outbreaks affecting nursing piglets (eight positive farms out of 28, 28.6%), although no significant differences in the number of PEDV confirmed outbreaks between age groups arose when compared using the Fisher exact test ($p = 0.094$).

PEDV positive farms were detected throughout the sampled area in northeast, center, and northwest of the country with at least one positive outbreak in 10 out of 22 sampled provinces (**Figure 1**). No significant differences were found in the number of PEDV confirmed outbreaks between provinces ($p = 0.286$).

In addition, it was evidenced that most of the investigated outbreaks occurred during the first trimester of the year ($p = 0.041$) (**Figure 2**). Although most of the PEDV positive outbreaks also occurred during the first 3 months of the year, no significant differences arose when compared using ANOVA test ($p = 0.097$).

Phylogenetic Analysis Based on the Nucleotide and Amino Acid Sequences of PEDV S Gene

The full-length S-gene sequences of all PEDV positive samples (41) were compared to previous and recent sequences of PEDV and SeCoV available in GenBank (**Figure 3**, **Supplementary Data 1**). The phylogenetic tree showed that all PEDV isolates recovered in Spain between 2017 and 2019 were allocated within the INDEL 2 or G1b genogroup together with several recent European PEDV isolates and isolates from the USA and Asia. They clustered in a branch clearly separate from the non-INDEL or G2 genogroup as well as from the original European or Asian PEDV isolates included in the INDEL 1 or G1a genogroup and SeCoV isolates.

Three subgroups or clusters were identified from Spanish PEDV isolates identified as INDEL 2.1, 2.2, and 2.3 (**Figures 3, 4**). The first was formed using two Spanish isolates recovered in 2018 and 2019 together with other Spanish and European PEDV isolates from 2014 to 2016. The INDEL 2.2 cluster included Spanish isolates from 2014 to 2019 and several Asian and American PEDV strains from the same time period. It is worth mentioning that all the isolates identified in this research included in the INDEL 2.2 subgroup correspond to isolates recovered from farms located within the same region and belong to the same pig producing company. Finally, the INDEL 2.3 cluster include recent Spanish isolates from 2017 to 2019 distributed throughout the sampling area together with Hungarian, Slovenian, Dutch, German, and French coetaneous strains. This clade corresponds to a PEDV-SeCoV recombinant

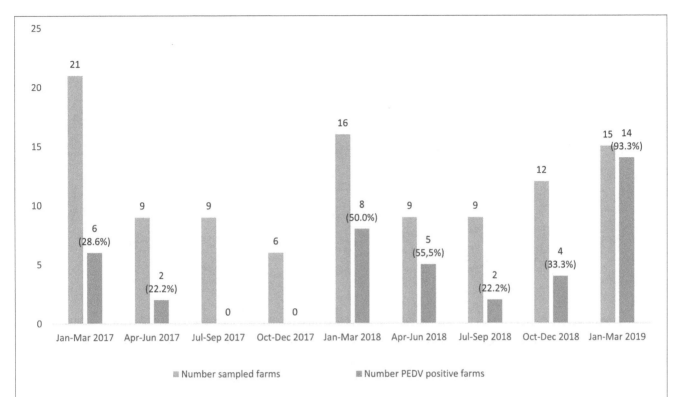

FIGURE 2 | Distribution of the viral suspected diarrhea outbreaks and PEDV positive outbreaks from January, 2017 to March, 2019. The number of sampled farms and PEDV-positive farms is shown above the columns. The percentage of PEDV-positive outbreaks in each trimester studied. The percentage of PEDV-positive outbreaks in each trimester studied is showed.

variant previously described in Hungary and Slovenia (29, 30) as well as in Spain (15).

Three major regions of the S1 gene were further analyzed and characterized at the amino acid level. Compared with three different strains of PEDV (CV777 accession no. AF353511, OH851 accession no. KJ399978 and SLOreBAS-1 accession no. KY019623), four amino acid mutations were found in four out of 41 Spanish PEDV isolates (**Supplementary Data 1**).

DISCUSSION

The recent emergence of several novel porcine enteric coronaviruses such as PDCoV or SeACoV together with the re-emergence of PEDV, a classical coronavirus, and their spread throughout the main pig producing countries over the last years have highlight porcine enteric coronavirus. They have caused significant losses to the pig-farming industry associated to high morbidity acute diarrhea in pigs of all ages and high mortality in neonatal pigs in naive farms. Enteric diseases caused by porcine enteric CoVs are clinically indistinguishable thus making differential diagnosis in the laboratory an essential tool.

A hundred and six viral suspected diarrhea outbreaks were investigated between 2017 and 2019 and confirmed that PEDV was the only enteric coronavirus detected in swine farms in Spain. PEDV was identified in about a 40% of the investigated outbreaks, confirming the re-emergence of PEDV in the Iberian Peninsula

as it has been described in several European countries (31) after its emergence in 2013 in the United States. The difference in the percentage of PEDV positive outbreaks among the different trimesters of the year was near to statistical significance, with most of the PEDV positive outbreaks occurring in winter (68.3%, 28 out of 41 PEDV positive outbreaks), when low temperatures favor the environmental resistance of the virus facilitating its indirect transmission. This results confirms the seasonal distribution of the disease (3, 32). Besides, although no significant differences were shown in the proportion of PEDV outbreaks between age groups, most of the outbreaks were observed among postweaning-growing or fattening pigs. The fact that few PEDV outbreaks were detected in suckling piglets (28.6%, eight PEDV outbreaks out of 28 investigated) could be a consequence of maternal immunity in the sows or high biosecurity level in farrowing facilities. Clearance of maternal antibodies together with the mix of piglets after weaning could explain a higher percentage of positive outbreaks (52.9%, nine PEDV positive outbreaks out of 17 investigated) in postweaning pigs (21–70 days) (1).

Neither TGEV, SeCoV, PDCoV nor SeACoV were detected in any of the investigated diarrhea outbreaks. To our knowledge, this is the first study in Europe actively researching PDCoV or SeACoV on swine farms. While SeACoV has a limited geographic distribution and has only been detected in swine farms in China (18, 19), PDCoV has been reported in the USA, South Korea, Thailand and mainland China (33). Although the

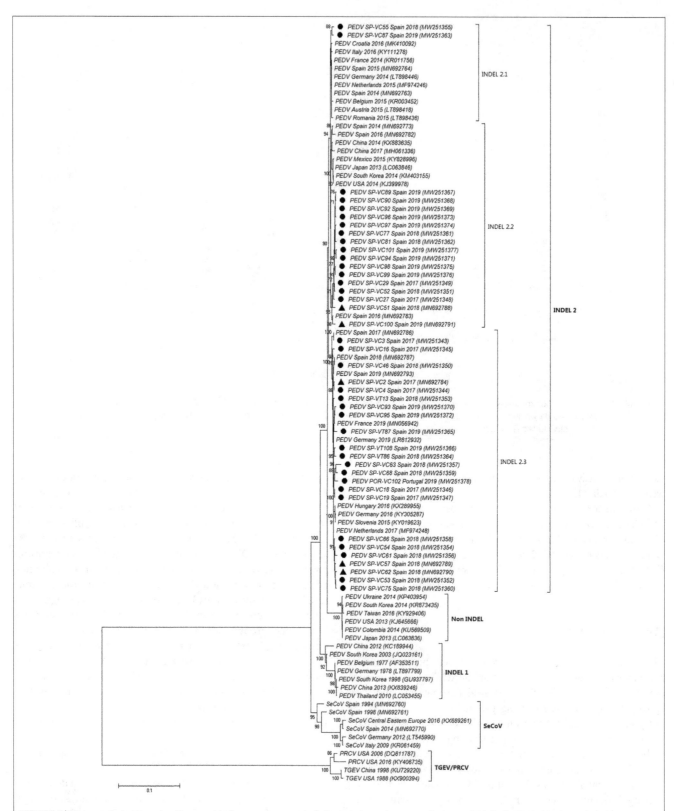

FIGURE 3 | Phylogenetic tree based on the complete S-gene sequences including enteric porcine coronaviruses available in GenBank. Numbers along the tree represent the confidence value for a given internal branch based on 500 Bootstrap replicates (only values >70 are shown). The symbols above the strains highlight the Spanish PEDV isolates of this study. The filled circles identified the isolates sequenced in this research while the filled triangles identified isolates previously sequenced by de Nova et al. (15). GenBank accession number, country and year of the outbreak are also shown below the strains. The genogroups and subgroups referred in the text are included on the right of the tree. Scale bars indicate nucleotide substitutions per site.

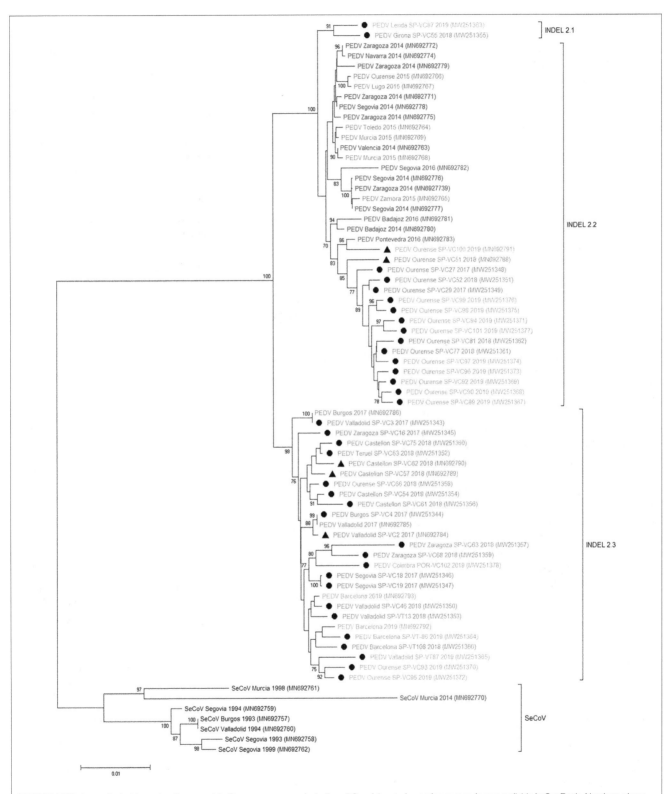

FIGURE 4 | Phylogenetic tree based on the complete S-gene sequences including all Spanish enteric porcine coronaviruses available in GenBank. Numbers along the tree represents the confidence value for a given internal branch based on 500 Bootstrap replicates (only values >70 are shown). The symbols above the strains stand out the Spanish PEDV isolates of this study. The filled circles identified the isolates sequenced in this research and the filled triangles identified the isolates previously sequenced by de Nova et al. (15). GenBank accession number, province and year of the outbreak are also shown below the strains. The genogroups and subgroups referred in the text are included on the right of the tree. Scale bars indicate nucleotide substitutions per site. Black, pre-2000 isolates; Red, 2014 isolates; Gray, 2015 isolates; Purple, 2016 isolates; Yellow, 2017 isolates; Green, 2018 isolates; Blue, 2019 isolates.

country of origin and transmission routes of this virus have not been elucidated, available sequence data suggests that PDCoV identified in South Korea was introduced from the USA (33) indicating its international spread. The ability of porcine CoVs to emerge and re-emerge showed in recent years together with the probable naive status of European pig population for these emerging CoVs allows us to conclude the need of monitoring programmes which allow for a prompt detection and alert to establish strict biosecurity measures which would curtail their spread between countries or continents.

In order to identify PEDV variants currently circulating in Spain, we obtained the complete sequences of the S-gene of all the isolates and compared them to a representative selection of 44 PEDV genome sequences from Europe, Asia and America available in the GenBank (**Figure 3**). Like in other European countries (5–7, 32), only PEDV isolates included in the INDEL 2 or G1b genogroup were identified in Spain between 2017 and 2019. This genogroup has been described as causing a less severe disease than the non-INDEL or G2 genogroup (3, 8) which could explained the limited economic impact of PEDV re-emergence in Europe as compared to its dramatic consequences in the United States or Asia (34).

Phylogenetic analysis allows us to classify recent Spanish PEDV isolates into three clusters with some geographical relationships. The INDEL 2.1 and 2.2 clusters have a limited geographical spread, with the first restricted to two isolates recovered from two farms from Catalonia in the northeast of the country and the second including a number of isolates from farms located in a single province in the northwest and belonging to the same pig-producing company. Nevertheless, the INDEL 2.3 cluster included isolates recovered throughout the country together with recombinant PEDV-SeCoV isolates described in Hungary, Slovenia, Italy, or Spain (14, 15, 29) as well as Dutch, German, and French PEDV recent isolates. These isolates harbor a recombinant fragment of ∼400 nt in the 5′ end of S-gene with PEDV and SeCoV being the major and minor parents, respectively. Since S protein is a key target for PEDV neutralizing antibodies, it has been proposed that this recombination event might provide some advantages (35, 36). Our results confirm this recombinant PEDV-SeCoV variant as the most widespread

in Spain between 2017 and 2019 as previously suggested by de Nova et al. (15) in a research with a limited number of recent PEDV isolates. A similar displacement of other PEDV subgroups by the PEDV-SeCoV cluster has also been reported in Italy (35).

To sum up, this research confirms that PEDV has become endemic in Spain being detected in almost 40% of the viral suspected diarrhea outbreaks between 2017 and 2019 with most of the outbreaks occurring in postweaning-growing or fattening pigs, which limits the severity of the disease. Only the PEDV INDEL 2 or G1b genogroup is circulating and the recombinant PEDV-SeCoV variant is the most widespread strain. In contrast, neither PEDV non-INDEL or G2 genogroup, nor TGEV, SeCoV, PDCoV or SeACoV were detected. The emergence of new virus or variants due to spillover or through mutation or recombination events makes monitoring of porcine enteric CoVs of outmost importance in order to prevent their spread and allow for updated diagnostic tools.

AUTHOR CONTRIBUTIONS

HP, HA, PR, and AC conceived and designed the experiments, analyzed the data, and wrote and revised the manuscript. HP, MG-G, and ÓM-A performed the experiments. All authors contributed to the article and approved the submitted version.

ACKNOWLEDGMENTS

We acknowledge the excellent technique assistance provided by Diana Molina.

SUPPLEMENTARY MATERIAL

Supplementary Data 1 | Comparison of S1 amino acid sequences of PEDV isolates from this study with those of reference strains (GenBank accession nos. AF353511, KJ399978, and KY019623). Amino acid sequence variations in three major epitope regions (aa 220-233, aa 770-776, and aa 784-792) in the S1 genes of 41 Spanish PEDV strains.

REFERENCES

1. Saif LJ, Wang Q, Vlasova AN, Jung K, Xiao S. Coronaviruses. In: Zimmerman JJ, Karriker LA, Ramirez A, Schwartz KJ, Stevenson GW, Zhang J, editors. *Diseases of Swine.* Hoboken: John Wiley and Sons. (2019) p. 488–523. doi: 10.1002/9781119350927.ch31

2. Fehr AR, Perlman S. Coronaviruses: an overview of their replication and pathogenesis. *Methods Mol Biol.* (2015) 1282:1–23. doi: 10.1007/978-1-4939-2438-7_1

3. Carvajal A, Argüello H, Martínez-Lobo FJ, Costillas S, Miranda R, de Nova PJG, et al. Porcine epidemic diarrhoea: new insights into an old disease. *Porc Heal Manag.* (2015) 1:1–8. doi: 10.1186/s40813-015-0007-9

4. Stevenson GW, Hoang H, Schwartz KJ, Burrough ER, Sun D, Madson D, et al. Emergence of Porcine epidemic diarrhea virus in the United States: clinical signs, lesions, and viral genomic sequences. *J Vet Diagnostic Investig.* (2013) 25:649–54. doi: 10.1177/1040638713501675

5. Grasland B, Bigault L, Bernard C, Quenault H, Toulouse O, Fablet C, et al. Complete genome sequence of a porcine epidemic diarrhea S gene indel strain isolated in France in December 2014. *Genome Announc.* (2015) 3:2014–5. doi: 10.1128/genomeA.00535-15

6. Hanke D, Jenckel M, Petrov A, Ritzmann M, Stadler J, Akimkin V, et al. Comparison of porcine epidemic diarrhea viruses from Germany and the United States, 2014. *Emerg Infect Dis.* (2015) 21:493–6. doi: 10.3201/eid2103.141165

7. Theuns S, Conceição-Neto N, Christiaens I, Zeller M, Desmarets LMB, Roukaerts IDM, et al. Complete genome sequence of a porcine epidemic diarrhea virus from a novel outbreak in Belgium, January 2015. *Genome Announc.* (2015) 3:1–2. doi: 10.1128/genomeA.00506-15

8. Vlasova AN, Marthaler D, Wang Q, Culhane MR, Rossow KD, Rovira A, et al. Distinct characteristics and complex evolution of pedv strains, North America, May 2013-February 2014. *Emerg Infect Dis.* (2014) 20:1620–8. doi: 10.3201/eid2010.140491

9. Lee S, Kim Y, Lee C. Isolation and characterization of a Korean porcine

epidemic diarrhea virus strain KNU-141112. *Virus Res.* (2015) 208:215–24. doi: 10.1016/j.virusres.2015.07.010

10. Gallien S, Andraud M, Moro A, Lediguerher G, Morin N, Gauger PC, et al. Better horizontal transmission of a US non-InDel strain compared with a French InDel strain of porcine epidemic diarrhoea virus. *Transbound Emerg Dis.* (2018) 65:1720–32. doi: 10.1111/tbed.12945

11. Dastjerdi A, Carr J, Ellis RJ, Steinbach F, Williamson S. Porcine epidemic diarrhea virus among farmed pigs, Ukraine. *Emerg Infect Dis.* (2015) 21:2235–7. doi: 10.3201/eid2112.150272

12. Akimkin V, Beer M, Blome S, Hanke D, Höper D, Jenckel M, et al. New chimeric porcine coronavirus in Swine Feces, Germany, 2012. *Emerg Infect Dis.* (2016) 22:1314–5. doi: 10.3201/eid2207.160179

13. Belsham GJ, Rasmussen TB, Normann P, Vaclavek P, Strandbygaard B, Bøtner A. Characterization of a novel chimeric swine enteric coronavirus from diseased pigs in Central Eastern Europe in 2016. *Transbound Emerg Dis.* (2016) 63:595–601. doi: 10.1111/tbed.12579

14. Boniotti MB, Papetti A, Lavazza A, Alborali G, Sozzi E, Chiapponi C, et al. Porcine epidemic diarrhea virus and discovery of a recombinant swine enteric coronavirus, Italy. *Emerg Infect Dis.* (2016) 22:83–7. doi: 10.3201/eid2201.150544

15. de Nova PJG, Cortey M, Díaz I, Puente H, Rubio P, Martín M, et al. A retrospective study of porcine epidemic diarrhoea virus (PEDV) reveals the presence of swine enteric coronavirus (SeCoV) since 1993 and the recent introduction of a recombinant PEDV-SeCoV in Spain. *Transbound Emerg Dis.* (2020) 67:2911–22. doi: 10.1111/tbed.13666

16. Woo PCY, Lau SKP, Lam CSF, Lau CCY, Tsang AKL, Lau JHN, et al. Discovery of seven novel mammalian and Avian coronaviruses in the genus Deltacoronavirus supports Bat coronaviruses as the gene source of Alphacoronavirus and Betacoronavirus and Avian coronaviruses as the gene source of Gammacoronavirus and Deltacoronavi. *J Virol.* (2012) 86:3995–4008. doi: 10.1128/JVI.06540-11

17. Wang L, Byrum B, Zhang Y. Detection and genetic characterization of deltacoronavirus in pigs, Ohio, USA, 2014. *Emerg Infect Dis.* (2014) 20:1227–30. doi: 10.3201/eid2007.140296

18. Gong L, Li J, Zhou Q, Xu Z, Chen L, Zhang Y, et al. A new bat-HKU2-like coronavirus in swine, China, 2017. *Emerg Infect Dis.* (2017) 23:1607–9. doi: 10.3201/eid2309.170915

19. Xu Z, Zhang Y, Gong L, Huang L, Lin Y, Qin J, et al. Isolation and characterization of a highly pathogenic strain of Porcine enteric alphacoronavirus causing watery diarrhoea and high mortality in newborn piglets. *Transbound Emerg Dis.* (2018) 66:119–30. doi: 10.1111/tbed.12992

20. Fu X, Fang B, Liu Y, Cai M, Jun J, Ma J, et al. Newly emerged porcine enteric alphacoronavirus in southern China: identification, origin and evolutionary history analysis. *Infect Genet Evol.* (2018) 62:179–87. doi: 10.1016/j.meegid.2018.04.031

21. Zhou P, Fan H, Lan T, Yang X-L, Shi WF, Zhang W, et al. Fatal swine acute diarrhoea syndrome caused by an HKU2-related coronavirus of bat origin. *Nature.* (2018) 556:255–9. doi: 10.1038/s41586-018-0010-9

22. Pan Y, Tian X, Qin P, Wang B, Zhao P, Yang Y-L, et al. Discovery of a novel swine enteric alphacoronavirus (SeACoV) in southern China. *Vet Microbiol.* (2017) 211:15–21. doi: 10.1016/j.vetmic.2017.09.020

23. Kim O, Choi C, Kim B, Chae C. Detection and differentiation of porcine epidemic diarrhoea virus and transmissible gastroenteritis virus in clinical samples by multiplex RT-PCR. *Vet Rec.* (2000) 146:637–43. doi: 10.1136/vr.146.22.637

24. Kim S, Song D, Park B. Differential detection of transmissible gastroenteritis virus and porcine epidemic diarrhea virus by duplex RT-PCR. *J Vet Diagnostic Investig.* (2001) 13:516–20. doi: 10.1177/104063870101300611

25. Ding G, Fu Y, Li B, Chen J, Wang J, Yin B, et al. Development of a multiplex RT-PCR for the detection of major diarrhoeal viruses in pig herds in China. *Transbound Emerg Dis.* (2019) 67:678–85. doi: 10.1111/tbed.13385

26. Huang YW, Dickerman AW, Piñeyro P, Li L, Fang L, Kiehne R, et al. Origin, evolution, and genotyping of emergent porcine epidemic diarrhea virus strains in the united states. *MBio.* (2013) 4:1–8. doi: 10.1128/mBio.00737-13

27. Chen Q, Li G, Stasko J, Thomas J, Stensland W, Pillatzki A, et al. Isolation and characterization of porcine epidemic diarrhea viruses associated with the 2013 disease outbreak among swine in the United States. *J Clin Microbiol.* (2014) 52:234–43. doi: 10.1128/JCM.02820-13

28. Kumar S, Stecher G, Li M, Knyaz C, Tamura K. MEGA X: molecular evolutionary genetics analysis across computing platforms. *Mol Biol Evol.* (2018) 35:1547–9. doi: 10.1093/molbev/msy096

29. Valkó A, Biksi I, Cságola A, Tuboly T, Kiss K, Ursu K, et al. Porcine epidemic diarrhoea virus with a recombinant S gene detected in Hungary, 2016. *Acta Vet Hung.* (2017) 65:253–61. doi: 10.1556/004.2017.025

30. Valkó A, Albert E, Cságola A, Varga T, Kiss K, Farkas R, et al. Isolation and characterisation of porcine epidemic diarrhoea virus in Hungary – short communication. *Acta Vet Hung.* (2019) 67:307–13. doi: 10.1556/004.2019.031

31. Choudhury B, Dastjerdi A, Doyle N, Frossard J-P, Steinbach F. From the field to the lab — an European view on the global spread of PEDV. *Virus Res.* (2016) 226:40–9. doi: 10.1016/j.virusres.2016.09.003

32. Dortmans JCFM, Li W, van der Wolf PJ, Buter GJ, Franssen PJM, van Schaik G, et al. Porcine epidemic diarrhea virus (PEDV) introduction into a naive Dutch pig population in 2014. *Vet Microbiol.* (2018) 221:13–8. doi: 10.1016/j.vetmic.2018.05.014

33. Zhang J. Porcine deltacoronavirus: overview of infection dynamics, diagnostic methods, prevalence and genetic evolution. *Virus Res.* (2016) 226:71–84. doi: 10.1016/j.virusres.2016.05.028

34. Alvarez J, Sarradell J, Morrison R, Perez A. Impact of porcine epidemic diarrhea on performance of growing pigs. *PLoS ONE.* (2015) 10:e0120532. doi: 10.1371/journal.pone.0120532

35. Boniotti MB, Papetti A, Bertasio C, Giacomini E, Lazzaro M, Cerioli M, et al. Porcine epidemic diarrhoea virus in Italy: disease spread and the role of transportation. *Transbound Emerg Dis.* (2018) 65:1935–42. doi: 10.1111/tbed.12974

36. Li C, Li W, Lucio de Esesarte E, Guo H, van den Elzen P, Aarts E, et al. Cell attachment domains of the porcine epidemic diarrhea virus spike protein are key targets of neutralizing antibodies. *J Virol.* (2017) 91:1–16. doi: 10.1128/JVI.00273-17

18

High Co-Infection Status of Novel Porcine Parvovirus 7 with Porcine Circovirus 3 in Sows that Experienced Reproductive Failure

Jinhui Mai[†], Dongliang Wang[†], Yawen Zou, Sujiao Zhang, Chenguang Meng, Aibing Wang and Naidong Wang*

Hunan Provincial Key Laboratory of Protein Engineering in Animal Vaccines, Laboratory of Functional Proteomics (LFP), Research Center of Reverse Vaccinology (RCRV), College of Veterinary Medicine, Hunan Agricultural University, Changsha, China

*Correspondence:
Naidong Wang
naidongwang@hunau.edu.cn

[†] These authors have contributed equally to this work

Porcine parvoviruses (PPVs) and porcine circoviruses (PCVs) infect pigs worldwide, with PPV1–7 and PCV2 infections common in pigs. Although PPV7 was only identified in 2016, co-infection of PPV7 and PCV2 is already common, and PPV7 may stimulate PCV2 replication. PCV3, a novel type of circovirus, is prevalent in pig populations worldwide and considered to cause reproductive disorders and dermatitis nephrotic syndrome. In recent studies, pigs were commonly infected with both PCV3 and PPV7. Our objective was to investigate the co-infections between PPV7 and PCV3 in samples from swine on farms in Hunan, China, and assess the potential impacts of PPV7 on PCV3 viremia. A total of 209 samples, known to be positive (105) or negative (104) for PCV3, were randomly selected from serum samples that were collected from commercial swine herds in seven regions from 2016 to 2018 in our previous studies; these samples were subjected to real-time PCR to detect PPV7. Of these samples, 23% (48/209) were positive for PPV7. Furthermore, the PPV7 positive rate was significantly higher in PCV3 positive serum (31.4%, 33/105) than in PCV3 negative serum (14.4%, 15/104). Another 62 PCV3 positive sow serum samples and 20 PCV3 positive aborted fetuses were selected from 2015 to 2016 in our other previous study. These samples were designated as being from farms with or without long-standing histories of reproductive failure (RF or non-RF), respectively, and they were also subjected to real-time PCR to detect PPV7 and to determine whether PPV7 affected PCV3 viremia. Among the 62 serum samples (39 PCV3 positive RF-serum and 23 PCV3 positive non-RF-serum), 45.1% (28/62) were positive for PPV7 and PCV3, and the PPV7 positive rate was significantly higher in PCV3 positive RF-serum (51.2%, 20/39) than in PCV3 positive non-RF-serum (34.8%, 8/23). In addition, there was a higher positive rate of PPV7 (55%, 11/20) in PCV3 positive aborted fetus samples. In addition, the copy number of PCV3 in PPV7 positive samples was significantly higher than that in PPV7 negative serum samples. Based on these findings, we concluded that PPV7 may stimulate PCV3 replication.

Keywords: porcine parvovirus 7, porcine circovirus type 3, co-infections, viremia, RT-PCR

INTRODUCTION

Porcine parvoviruses (PPVs) have been prevalent in pigs globally, and PPV1 is considered as one of the main pathogens causing reproductive failure in pigs around the world (1). However, genotypes PPV2–PPV6 with pathogenic potential were also detected, e.g., by genome sequencing. Porcine parvovirus 7 (PPV7) was initially identified in 2016 by metagenomics sequencing of rectal swabs from healthy adult pigs in the United States and subsequently from pigs in Brazil, China, South Korea, Poland, and Sweden. In China, PPV7 is already prevalent in Guangxi, Hunan, Anhui, Fujian, Shandong, and Northeast China (2, 3), although the detailed information of its pathogenicity in pigs remains unavailable. Regarding novel PPVs, PPV4, PPV6, and PPV7 were detected in aborted fetuses, which implied that these viruses may cause reproductive failure (4–6). Moreover, detection of PPV7 in semen implies that this virus may cause reproductive dysfunction through vertical transmission (7).

PPV7 is a single-stranded DNA (ssDNA, ~4 kb), non-enveloped virus, with low homology with PPV1-6 (~30%). It belongs to the family *Parvovirinae* and is an emerging species of the genus *Chapparvovirus*. PPV7 can be isolated from healthy and sick pigs of all ages and was present in various tissues (liver, lung, lymph node, kidney, and spleen). Nucleotide mutation rates of *NS1* and *cap* genes of PPV7 were higher than those of PPV1-4 (8), perhaps enabling PPV7 to adapt to various environmental conditions and posing a major threat to health security of pig herds.

PPV1-7 and porcine circovirus 2 (PCV2) co-infections are common in pigs. In recent studies, the level of PCV2 viremia was greater in serum samples that were positive for PPV1 and PPV7 than in those that were negative for PPVs (9, 10). Furthermore, there was a correlation between the Ct values of PPV7 and PCV2 (11). As a consequence, we inferred that, in addition to PPV1, PPV7 may potentially act as a co-factor infection by stimulating the replication of PCV2. PCV3, a novel type of circovirus discovered in 2016, is prevalent in many countries around the world and is regarded as causing reproductive disorders and dermatitis nephrotic syndrome, although the pathogenesis is not well established. It was reported that PCV3 positive samples have a high co-infection rate with PPV7 (12), although nothing is known about the impact of PPV7 on PCV3 viremia. In this study, we investigated co-infections between PPV7 and PCV3 in samples from swine on farms in Hunan, China, and assessed potential impacts of PPV7 on PCV3 viremia.

MATERIALS AND METHODS

Serum and Aborted Fetuses

We previously detected PCV3 IgG antibodies in sow sera from commercial swine herds ($n = 1038$) in seven regions of Hunan Province, China using capsid protein-based indirect ELISA (13). Among them, a total of 209 serum samples (105 PCV3 positive and 104 PCV3 negative serum samples, **Table 1**), based on PCV3 detection by quantitative PCR (qPCR), as described (13, 14), were randomly selected and used to determine PPV7 prevalence in

TABLE 1 | Presence of PPV7 in PCV3 positive and negative serum samples.

Region	PCV3 positive	PPV7 positive	PCV3 negative	PPV7 negative
Chenzhou	15	2	15	2
Hengyang	15	9	15	3
Shaoyang	15	7	15	4
Yueyang	15	4	14	1
Changde	15	4	15	2
Yiyang	15	5	15	3
Loudi	15	2	15	0
Total	105	33	104	15

the present study. In other studies, we reported identification of PCV3 (using qPCR and ELISA, respectively) in sow sera ($n = 190$), which were selected from the farms (A–E) with or without reproductive failure (RF) in various regions in Hunan, China (14). In more detail (**Table 2**), 85 samples (with 39 PCV3 positive) were from sows that had aborted or had a history of reproductive failure (+RF), whereas the remaining 105 (with 23 PCV3 positive) were from healthy sows (from herds with no history of reproductive failure, −RF), among which copy numbers of PCV3 genome based on qPCR were determined and reported (13, 14). It was noteworthy that the PCV3 positive rate was significantly higher in sows with reproductive failure [+RF, 45.9% (39/85)] than in healthy sows [−RF, 21.9% (23/105)] (14). In addition, 60.6% (20/33) of aborted fetuses from Farms C and E were positive for PCV3 (13), based on qPCR assays (**Table 2**).

As these important samples have already been tested for PCV3 and its viral load, they can also be used to detect co-infection with PPV7, facilitating an in-depth study of the co-infection of PCV3 and PPV7 and the interaction by co-infection to enhance or stimulate virus replication.

Real-Time PCR Assay for PCV3 and PPV7

qPCR for copy numbers of PCV3 genomic DNA with primers (QP3-F: YAGTGCTCCCCATTGAACGG and QP3-R: GCTCCAAGACGACCCTTATGC) in our previous report (13) was used to determine the copy number of PCV3 in the samples. In addition, a SYBR Green real-time PCR assay with primers (F1: GCGACCAGTCGAAAGTCTTC and R1: TTGGTGTTGCCCATTCTGTA) targeting a 165-bp region of PPV7, the conserved capsid gene for PPV7 detection, was done, as described (15). Based on results of real-time PCR, samples were deemed negative or positive for PCV3 and for PPV7.

In brief, we used a 20-µl reaction mixture containing 10 µl of AceQ qPCR SYBR Green Master Mix (Vazyme Biotech Co., Piscataway, NJ, USA), 0.4 µl PCV3 primer pairs or 0.6 µl PPV7 primer pairs (10 µM), 0.4 µl of 50 × ROX Reference Dye 1, 2 µl of DNA template, and 6.8 µl of RNase-free ddH$_2$O. In addition, a pSP72 plasmid clone containing the full-length *cap* gene of PCV3 (pSP72-PCV3; GenBank accession number KY484769) or the full-length *VP2* gene of PPV7 (pSP72-PPV7; GenBank accession number KU563733) and ddH$_2$O were used as positive and negative controls, respectively. Copy numbers of

TABLE 2 | Presence of PCV3 and PPV7 co-infections in serum of sows, with and without reproductive failure (RF), and in aborted fetuses.

Farm	No.	PCV3 positive				Co-infection with PPV7			
		Sow serum		Aborted fetus		Sow serum		Aborted fetus	
		+RF	−RF			+RF	−RF		
A	23	3/8	2/15	–	–	3/3	1/2	–	–
B	24	3/9	2/15	–	–	2/3	1/2	–	–
C	41	11/26	6/15	17	11/17	5/11	1/6	11	6/11
D	22	2/7	3/15	–	–	2/2	2/3	–	–
E	35	13/20	7/15	16	9/16	5/13	2/7	9	5/9
F	20	3/5	2/15	–	–	1/3	0/2	–	–
G	25	4/10	1/15	–	–	2/4	0/1	–	–
Total	190	39/85(45.9%)	23/105 (21.9%)	33	20/33 (60.6%)	20/39(51.2%)	8/23 (34.8%)	20	11/20 (55%)

viral genomic DNA extracted from samples were calculated based on a standard curve.

Statistical Analyses

All statistical analyses were performed using SPSS 21.0 software (SPSS Inc., Chicago, IL, USA) and GraphPad Prism version 8.0.0 for Windows (GraphPad Software, San Diego, CA, USA; www.graphpad.com). PCV3 and PPV7 serum categories were investigated using Fisher's exact test by pairwise comparisons. The one-way ANOVA was used for statistical comparison between PCV3 and PPV7 serum categories expressed as copy numbers. Pearson's correlations of copy numbers in PCV3 and PPV7 positive samples were determined. Statistical significance was set at $p < 0.05$, and confidence intervals were calculated.

RESULTS

PPV7 Infections Occur Frequently in Pigs Affected With PCV3

The 209 samples (105 PCV3 positive and 104 PCV3 negative serum samples), derived from our previous study (13), were randomly selected from each region in Hunan, China, from 2016 to 2018. Among these 209 serum samples, 23% (48/209) were positive for PPV7. Of these, 31.4% (33/105) were positive for PPV7 in PCV3 positive serum samples (**Table 1**), whereas PPV7 was detected in 14.4% (15/104) of the randomly selected PCV3 negative samples (**Table 1**). The PPV7 positive rate was significantly higher (2.2 times) in PCV3 positive serum samples (31.4%) than in PCV3 negative serum samples (14.4%).

In this study, we also used sow sera and aborted fetuses that had been collected between 2015 and 2016 from seven sow farms with histories of long-standing reproductive problems (14). Among the 190 serum samples, there were 62 PCV3 positive and 128 PCV3 negative (14), whereas 24.7% (47/190) were positive for PPV7 (**Table 2**). The PPV7 positive rate was significantly higher (3.0 times) in PCV3 positive serum samples (28/62, 45.1%) than in PCV3 negative serum samples (19/128, 14.8%).

The PPV7 detection rates in PCV3 positive serum samples with RF (+RF) were 51.2% (20/39), whereas they were only 34.8%

(8/23) in PCV3 positive sera without RF (−RF). Furthermore, among 33 aborted fetuses from Farms C and E that had 20 PCV3 positive fetuses (14), 55% (11/20) were positive for both PPV7 and PCV3 (**Table 2**). In summary, the PPV7 positive rate was 1.5 times higher in PCV3 positive serum from sows with RF (+RF) vs. without RF (−RF); furthermore, there was a higher PPV7 prevalence (55%) in aborted fetus samples.

PCV3 Viremia Is Higher in PPV7 Positive Pigs

To evaluate impacts of PCV3 and PPV7 co-infections on their viremia, 190 sow serum samples (+RF and −RF) used in a previous report (14) were divided into the following groups: PCV3–PPV7 positive ($n = 28$), PCV3 positive–PPV7 negative ($n = 34$), and PCV3 negative–PPV7 positive ($n = 19$).

The copy number of PPV7 in PCV3 positive and negative serum samples was detected by real-time PCR; there was no significant difference in PPV7 between PCV3 positive ($n = 28$) and negative ($n = 19$) samples (**Figure 1A**). However, the copy number of PCV3 in PPV7 positive samples ($n = 28$, PCV3–PPV7 positive groups) was higher ($p < 0.001$) than that in PPV7 negative serum samples ($n = 27$, selected from 34 samples of PCV3 positive–PPV7 negative groups) (**Figure 1B**), and there was a very high correlation ($p = 0.0002$) in copy number between PCV3 and PPV7 from PCV3–PPV7 positive group samples (**Figure 2**). The linear correlation coefficient (r) between PPV7 and PCV3 copy numbers was 0.651. As the square of correlation (r^2) score was 0.424, 42.4% of PCV3 copy number could be accounted for by PPV7 copy number.

DISCUSSION

PPV1 co-infects with PCV2 and PCV3, porcine reproductive and respiratory syndrome virus (PRRSV), pseudorabies virus (PRV), and classical swine fever virus (CSFV). The prevalence of PPV1–PCV2 co-infections is high, and PPV1 may trigger PCV2 associated disease (PCVAD) by supporting PCV2 replication, and increase PCVAD severity (e.g., pathological lesions in lymphoid tissues) (16). In addition, there are co-infections between novel

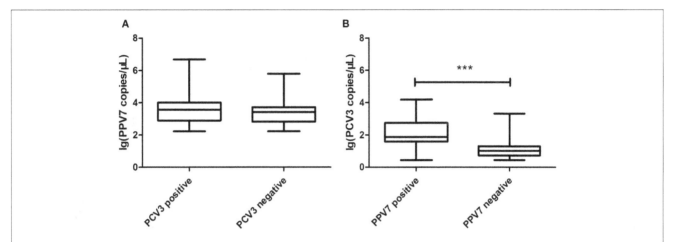

FIGURE 1 | Boxplot comparison of real-time PCR copy number of PPV7 and PCV3. **(A)** Boxplot comparison of real-time PCR copy number of PPV7 in PCV3 positive ($n = 28$) and PCV3 negative ($n = 19$) serum samples. **(B)** Boxplot comparison of real-time PCR copy number of PCV3 in PPV7 positive ($n = 28$) and PPV7 negative ($n = 27$) serum samples. *** $p < 0.001$.

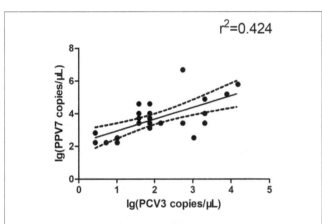

FIGURE 2 | Scatterplots with trends for real-time PCR copy number for PPV7 and PCV3 positive samples ($n = 28$, $p = 0.0002$).

PPVs and other well-known pathogens (e.g., PPVs, PCV2, PCV3, PRRSV, and TTSU) (3). Infections with PPV7 may become chronic, and PPV7 may contribute to virus persistence, with continuous excretion of virus in feces (17). In addition, fattening pigs without clinical symptoms had a high viral load ($Ct < 25$), for PPV7 in their feces; therefore, variations in PPV7 viral loads may indicate various effects of PPV7 infection in pigs (17), or perhaps other conditions (e.g., co-infection) that made PPV7 pathogenic in pigs.

The prevalence of PPV7 ranged from 8.6 to 61.5% (2, 9, 11, 17–20). In our study of pigs from Hunan, China, the prevalence of PPV7 for both PCV3 negative and positive serum samples combined was 23% (48/209), and the prevalence in sow serum samples with or without RF was 24.7% (47/190). There was no basis to conclude that PPV7 contributed to all observed pathologic changes, as not all pathogens were consistently detected in diseased pigs and the prevalence of PPV7 in serum samples was higher than that in other tissues (18). Furthermore,

none of the diseased pigs was only infected with PPV7. Therefore, it remains to be determined whether infection with PPV7 *per se* induces disease in pigs. It was also reported that the positive rate of PPV7 in PCV2 positive pig farms was significantly higher than that in negative farms (65.5 vs. 5.7%, respectively) (18). Moreover, the co-infection rate of PPV7 and PCV2 was high (17.4–59.5%) composed of 17.4% (67/385) and 59.5% (147/247) in Guangxi, 18.2% (29/159) in Poland, and 17.5% (21/120) in Anhui, respectively (9, 11, 19, 21). Therefore, it was speculated that PPV7 was an important cofactor of PCVAD (9). Although clinical symptoms and pathology of PPV7 remain unclear, it may act as a co-factor of disease caused by other porcine pathogens, or it may trigger disease development.

The co-infection rate of PCV3 and PPV7 was 9.1% (11/120) in samples from commercial farms with various clinical symptoms, including respiratory and gastrointestinal (19). In another report, in PCV3 positive samples, PCV3 had a high co-infection rate with both PPV6 (60.0%, 21/35) and PPV7 (74.3%, 26/35) (12). Based on these data, we inferred that there is a possible association between PCV3 and PPV7 infections. In our study, PCV3 also had a high co-infection rate with PPV7 [45.1% (28/62), 55% (11/20)]. Since both circovirus and parvovirus are ssDNA viruses, active proliferation of target cells is required for efficient viral replication. Virus-induced lymphocyte proliferation or immunosuppression can enhance the susceptibility to other virus replication and infection (22–25). For PCV2, its infection directly targets immune cells and causes immunosuppression (26–28), which leads to secondary or mixed infections with other pathogens. Furthermore, evidence that PPV-induced immune dysfunction could promote PCV2 replication (29) supports our notion that a co-infection of PPV7 and PCV3 could enhance the pathogenicity of the latter virus.

In this study, the PPV7 positive rate was statistically significantly higher in PCV3 positive versus PCV3 negative samples, suggesting that PCV3 may also cause immunosuppression, similar to PCV2, leading to secondary infection. Interestingly, co-infection with PPV7 and PCV3 in sow serum with RF (+RF) was significantly higher than that in sow serum without RF (–RF), and we also noted a higher PPV7 prevalence in aborted fetus samples. Furthermore, there were higher PCV3 viral loads in samples that were PPV7 positive compared with PPV7 negative. It has been suggested that PPV7 may stimulate the replication of PCV2 (11, 30). We speculated that PPV7 stimulated the replication of PCV3, thereby enhancing PCV3 viremia. Based on the present results and previous studies, we concluded that PPV7 may be an important co-factor triggering PCV2 and PCV3-associated diseases. Regardless, the pathogenesis of PPV7 infections, with or without PCV3 co-infection, needs to be further confirmed. More frequent multifactorial co-infection in clinical conditions contributes to a range of disease syndromes and is one of the most difficult problems in swine production, where next-generation sequencing (NGS) will gain a new insight into how co-factor infections interact to cause syndromes.

ETHICS STATEMENT

We confirm that the ethical policies of the journal, as noted on the journal's author guidelines page, have been adhered to. This study was approved by the Animal Ethics Committee of Hunan Agricultural University, Hunan, China.

AUTHOR CONTRIBUTIONS

NW and JM conceived and designed the experiments. JM, DW, and YZ designed and carried out the PCV3 and PPV7 RT-PCR detection. JM, SZ, and CM conducted statistical analysis on the data. JM, AW, and NW contributed to writing and revision of the manuscript. All authors read and approved the final manuscript.

REFERENCES

1. Mengeling WL, Lager KM, Vorwald AC. The effect of porcine parvovirus and porcine reproductive and respiratory syndrome virus on porcine reproductive performance. *Anim Reprod Sci.* (2000) 60:199–210. doi: 10.1016/S0378-4320(00)00135-4
2. Palinski RM, Mitra N, Hause BM. Discovery of a novel Parvovirinae virus, porcine parvovirus 7, by metagenomic sequencing of porcine rectal swabs. *Virus Genes.* (2016) 52:564–7. doi: 10.1007/s11262-016-1322-1
3. Mai JH, Wang DL, Tan L, Wang ND. Advances in porcine parvovirus 7. *Chin Vet Sci.* (2021) 51:361–7. doi: 10.16656/j.issn.1673-4696.2021.0054
4. Cságola A, Lorincz M, Cadar D, Tombácz K, Biksi I, Tuboly, T. Detection, prevalence and analysis of emerging porcine parvovirus infections. *Arch Virol.* (2012) 157:1003–10. doi: 10.1007/s00705-012-1257-3
5. Ni J, Qiao C, Han X, Han T, Kang W, Zi Z, et al. Identification and genomic characterization of a novel porcine parvovirus (PPV6) in China. *Virol J.* (2014) 11:203. doi: 10.1186/s12985-014-0203-2
6. Ouh IO, Park S, Lee JY, Song JY, Cho IS, Kim HR, et al. First detection and genetic characterization of porcine parvovirus 7 from Korean domestic pig farms. *J Vet Sci.* (2018) 19:855–7. doi: 10.4142/jvs.2018.19.6.855
7. Chung HC, Nguyen VG, Park YH, Park KT, Park BK.. PCR-based detection and genetic characterization of porcine parvoviruses in South Korea in 2018. *BMC Vet Res.* (2020) 16:113. doi: 10.1186/s12917-020-02329-z
8. Wang D, Mai J, Yang Y, Wang ND. Porcine parvovirus 7: evolutionary dynamics and identification of epitopes toward vaccine design. *Viruses-Basel.* (2020) 8:359. doi: 10.3390/vaccines8030359
9. Wang W, Cao L, Sun W, Xin J, Zheng M, Tian M, et al. Sequence and phylogenetic analysis of novel porcine parvovirus 7 isolates from pigs in Guangxi, China. *PLoS ONE.* (2019) 14:e0219560. doi: 10.1371/journal.pone.0219560
10. Opriessnig T, Xiao CT, Gerber PF, Halbur PG. Identification of recently described porcine parvoviruses in archived North American samples from 1996 and association with porcine circovirus associated disease. *Vet Microbiol.* (2014) 173:9–16. doi: 10.1016/j.vetmic.2014.06.024
11. Miłek D, Wozniak A, Podgórska K, Stadejek T. Do porcine parvoviruses 1 through 7 (PPV1-PPV7) have an impact on porcine circovirus type 2 (PCV2) viremia in pigs? *Vet Microbiol.* (2020) 242:108613. doi: 10.1016/j.vetmic.2020.108613
12. Ha Z, Xie CZ, Li JF, Wen SB, Zhang KL, Nan FL, et al. Molecular detection and genomic characterization of porcine circovirus 3 in pigs from Northeast China. *BMC Vet Res.* (2018) 14:321. doi: 10.1186/s12917-018-1634-6
13. Zhang S, Wang D, Jiang Y, Li Z, Zou Y, Li M, et al. Development and application of a baculovirus-expressed capsid protein-based indirect ELISA for detection of porcine circovirus 3 IgG antibodies. *BMC Vet Res.* (2019) 15:79. doi: 10.1186/s12917-019-1810-3
14. Zou Y, Zhang N, Zhang J, Zhang S, Jiang Y, Wang D, et al. Molecular detection and sequence analysis of porcine circovirus type 3 in sow sera from farms with prolonged histories of reproductive problems in Hunan, China. *Arch Virol.* (2018) 163:2841–7. doi: 10.1007/s00705-018-3914-7
15. Li YD, Yu ZD, Bai CX, Zhang D, Sun P, Peng ML, et al. Development of a SYBR Green I real-time PCR assay for detection of novel porcine parvovirus 7. *Pol J Vet Sci.* (2021) 24:43–9.
16. Opriessnig T, Fenaux M, Yu S, Evans RB, Cavanaugh D, Gallup JM, et al. Effect of porcine parvovirus vaccination on the development of PMWS in segregated early weaned pigs coinfected with type 2 porcine circovirus and porcine parvovirus. *Vet Microbiol.* (2004) 98:209–20. doi: 10.1016/j.vetmic.2003.11.006
17. Miłek D, Wozniak A, Podgórska K, Stadejek T. The detection and genetic diversity of novel porcine parvovirus 7 (PPV7) on Polish pig farms. *Research in Vet Sci.* (2018) 120:28–32. doi: 10.1016/j.rvsc.2018.08.004
18. Xing X, Zhou H, Tong L, Chen Y, Sun Y, Wang H, et al. First identification of porcine parvovirus 7 in China. *Arch Virol.* (2018) 163:209–13. doi: 10.1007/s00705-017-3585-9
19. Wang Y, Yang KK, Wang J, Wang XP, Zhao L, Sun P, et al. Detection and molecular characterization of novel porcine parvovirus 7 in Anhui province from Central-Eastern China. *Infect Genet Evol.* (2019) 71:31–5. doi: 10.1016/j.meegid.2019.03.004
20. Da Silva MS, Budaszewski RF, Weber MN, Cibulski SP, Paim WP, Mósena ACS, et al. Liver virome of healthy pigs reveals diverse small ssDNA viral genomes. *Infect Genet Evol.* (2020) 81:104203. doi: 10.1016/j.meegid.2020.104203
21. Cao L, Sun WC, Wang W, Tian MY, Guo DD, Liu YX, et al. Sequence and phylogenetic analysis of porcine parvovirus 7 isolates from pigs in Guangxi Province, China. *Chin J Vet Sci.* (2020) 40:457–62.
22. Saekhow P, Kishizuka S, Sano N, Mitsui H, Akasaki H, Mawatari T, et al. Coincidental detection of genomes of porcine parvoviruses and porcine circovirus type 2 infecting pigs in Japan. *J Vet Med Sci.* (2016) 77:1581–6. doi: 10.1292/jvms.15-0167
23. Saekhow P, Mawatari T, Ikeda H. Coexistence of multiple strains of porcine parvovirus 2 in pig farms. *Microbiol Immunol.* (2014) 58:382–7. doi: 10.1111/1348-0421.12159
24. Ellis J, Clark E, Haines D, West K, Krakowka S, Kennedy S, et al. Porcine circovirus-2 and concurrent infections in the field. *Vet Microbiol.* (2004) 98:159–63. doi: 10.1016/j.vetmic.2003.10.008
25. Darwich L, Mateu E. Immunology of porcine circovirus type 2 (PCV2). *Adv Virus Res.* (2012) 164:61–67. doi: 10.1016/j.virusres.2011.12.003

26. Darwich L, Segalés J, Mateu E. Pathogenesis of postweaning multisystemic wasting syndrome caused by Porcine circovirus 2: an immune riddle. *Arch Virol.* (2004) 149:857–74. doi: 10.1007/s00705-003-0280-9

27. Meng XJ. Porcine circovirus type 2 (PCV2): pathogenesis and interaction with the immune system. *Annu Rev Anim Biosci.* (2013) 1:43–64. doi: 10.1146/annurev-animal-031412-103720

28. Segalés J, Rosell C, Domingo M. Pathological findings associated with naturally acquired porcine circovirus type 2 associated disease. *Vet Microbiol.* (2004) 98:137–49. doi: 10.1016/j.vetmic.2003.10.006

29. Cadar D, Cságola A, Kiss T, Tuboly T. Capsid protein evolution and comparative phylogeny of novel porcine parvoviruses. *Mol Phylogenet Evol.* (2013) 66:243–53. doi: 10.1016/j.ympev.2012.09.030

30. Allan GM, Kennedy S, McNeilly F, Foster JC, Ellis JA, Krakowka SJ, et al. Experimental reproduction of severe wasting disease by co-infection of pigs with porcine circovirus and porcine parvovirus. *J Comp Pathol.* (1999) 121:1–11. doi: 10.1053/jcpa.1998.0295

19

Current Status of Loop-Mediated Isothermal Amplification Technologies for the Detection of Honey Bee Pathogens

Timothy C. Cameron [1,2], Danielle Wiles [1,2] and Travis Beddoe [1,2]*

[1] Department of Animal, Plant and Soil Science, Centre for AgriBioscience, La Trobe University, Melbourne, VIC, Australia,
[2] Centre for Livestock Interactions With Pathogens, La Trobe University, Melbourne, VIC, Australia

*Correspondence:
Travis Beddoe
t.beddoe@latrobe.edu.au

Approximately one-third of the typical human Western diet depends upon pollination for production, and honey bees (*Apis mellifera*) are the primary pollinators of numerous food crops, including fruits, nuts, vegetables, and oilseeds. Regional large scale losses of managed honey bee populations have increased significantly during the last decade. In particular, asymptomatic infection of honey bees with viruses and bacterial pathogens are quite common, and co-pathogenic interaction with other pathogens have led to more severe and frequent colony losses. Other multiple environmental stress factors, including agrochemical exposure, lack of quality forage, and reduced habitat, have all contributed to the considerable negative impact upon bee health. The ability to accurately diagnose diseases early could likely lead to better management and treatment strategies. While many molecular diagnostic tests such as real-time PCR and MALDI-TOF mass spectrometry have been developed to detect honey bee pathogens, they are not field-deployable and thus cannot support local apiary husbandry decision-making for disease control. Here we review the field-deployable technology termed loop-mediated isothermal amplification (LAMP) and its application to diagnose honey bee infections.

Keywords: honey bee, pathogens, diagnostics, LAMP, in-field, viruses, bacteria

INTRODUCTION

The European honey bee, *Apis mellifera,* is a significant component of agricultural systems worldwide. The honey bee is classified as a livestock species due to being a food-producing animal specifically related to honey production (1). Honey bees also produce wax, pollen, royal jelly, and propolis which are all commercial products of the apiary industry. However, honey bees' most significant ecological impact is that they are a critical contributor to food production via pollination (2, 3). The majority of crop species depend on pollination, with some crops such as almonds, onions, sunflowers and avocados being 100% reliant on honey bees for pollination (2, 3). Despite the importance of honey bees to agricultural systems, there have been reports of large scale losses in managed honey bee populations in different parts of the world. These mass losses have been due to various environmental stressors such as pathogens, agrochemical exposure, lack of quality forage, climate change and reduced habitat (4–8).

The prevailing view is that the increasing prevalence of pathogens and parasites are a significant driver in honey bee colony losses. Honey bees are infected by a variety of pathogen and pests such as bacteria (*Paenibacillus larvae*, *Melissococcus plutonius*) (9), fungi (*Nosema* spp., *Ascosphaerea apis*) (10, 11), mites (*Varroa destructor*, *Acarapis woodi*, *Tropilaelaps* spp.) (12) and insect pests such as the greater wax moth (*Galleria melonella*) and the small hive beetle (*Aethina tumidae*) (13). In particular, honey bees are known to be infected by several viruses; most of these are positive-strand RNA viruses belonging to the order of Picornavirales (14). They include several important viruses, such as the Israeli acute bee paralysis virus (IAPV) and the black queen cell virus (BQCV), which belong to the Dicistroviridae family. In contrast, the Iflaviridae family contains the deformed wing virus (DWV) and sacbrood virus (SBV). These viral infections result in deformities, paralysis and/or death; however, most of these viral infections remain asymptomatic until external stress is applied (7, 15). Due to honey bees being predominantly asymptomatic when these virus species are present, molecular-based diagnostic techniques are critical for the accurate diagnosis of infection and making informed management decisions.

CURRENT MOLECULAR DETECTION OF HONEY BEE PESTS AND PATHOGENS

The majority of molecular techniques utilize the ability to detect specific pathogen or pest nucleic acids. The most common technique for detecting honey bee pests and pathogens is by quantitative PCR (qPCR), and in the case of a virus, this requires the use of reverse transcriptase to amplify the RNA, which is termed RT-qPCR. There are many individual qPCR assays to detect specific pathogens, such as *P. larvae* (16), *M. plutonis* (17), *A. woodi* (18), *Nosema* spp. (19). Furthermore, a range of viruses [described within (19)] with many of these qPCR tests being multiplexed to perform rapid detection of several pathogens within a single PCR run (20, 21). In recent years, the use of matrix-assisted laser desorption/ionization time-of-flight (MALDI-TOF) mass spectrometry (MS) has emerged as a clinical diagnostic method for the identification of bacterial species (22), and this technology has been applied to honey bee pathogen diagnostics in the identification of different strains of *P. larvae* (23). Despite these techniques' power to identify infected honey bees and hives, they still require specialized labs and trained personnel. The early identification of pests and pathogens in managed honey bees is crucial for the decision-making process regarding disease control, prevention, the strategy of treatment and, therefore, mitigation of the impact of a particular disease. This has been highlighted recently where an integrated management strategy was used to prevent outbreaks and eliminate American foulbrood (*P. larvae*) in a commercial beekeeping operation (24). Several field-based diagnostic technologies that can amplify nucleic acids have emerged in recent years, such as loop-mediated isothermal amplification (LAMP) and recombinase polymerase amplification (25, 26). These technologies have the potential to revolutionize disease management in livestock industries, including honey bees. Currently, the only field-based diagnostic technologies applied for the detection of honey bee pests and pathogens is LAMP. Here we review the current status of field-based nucleic acid amplification

techniques, with a particular focus on LAMP, to detect various honey bee pathogens and discuss the implications with which these new diagnostic techniques can impact and inform apiary management practices.

PRINCIPLES OF LAMP

Loop-mediated isothermal amplification (LAMP) is a novel nucleic acid amplification technology that rapidly amplifies nucleic acids under isothermal conditions (27). LAMP utilizes *Bst* or *Bsm* DNA polymerase with a strong strand displacing ability and functions at isothermal conditions between 60 and 65°C, thereby eliminating the need for thermal cycling. LAMP does not require an additional reverse transcription step for the amplification of RNA viral gene products and amplifies DNA with high specificity, sensitivity, and speed (27). Additionally, the LAMP amplification is very robust, which is ideal when using a crude DNA extract purified from a range of environmental sources (25). This allows the use of non-invasive sampling techniques to be implemented, such as swabbing hive entrances rather than sampling honey bees themselves, minimizing stress applied to the hive due to excessive human handling. However, to avoid false-positive (due to contamination) and -negative results, in-hive samples/bees should be recommended. These characteristics allow LAMP assays to be performed in field-based settings with cheap and portable equipment (28). It has been proven to be a suitable molecular diagnostic method for field detection of a range of pathogens (29–31).

LAMP reactions are highly specific, involving four primary primers designed to target six distinct sequences on the target DNA (27) (**Supplementary Figure 1**). These primers are termed the forward and backward inner primer (FIP and BIP) as well as the forward (F3) and backward outer (B3) primer (**Supplementary Figure 1**). Both the FIP and BIP primers contain complementary regions that bind to form loop structures, providing more sites for primers to bind, initiating further amplification. Optional loop forward (LF) and loop backward (LB) primers can also be added to increase reaction speed by hybridizing to the loop structure to provide additional amplification initiation sites (32). Overall, LAMP is an ideal method for providing cheap (≈AU$ 5–7 per sample), rapid and robust detection of pathogens in-field with high sensitivity and specificity using minimal, simple equipment.

APPLICATION OF LAMP FOR THE DETECTION OF FUNGAL PATHOGENS OF HONEY BEES

Nosemosis is a worldwide distributed infectious disease and constitutes a severe problem in both managed European (*A. mellifera*) and Asian honey bee (*A. cerana*) populations as well as wild bumble bees (11, 33, 34). There are three causative agents of nosemosis; *Nosema ceranae* and *N. apis*, which infect both *A. mellifera* and *A. cerana*, while *N. bombi* is a major pathogen of wild bumble bees (34). *Nosema* spp. belongs to a spore-forming fungal family termed microsporidia. They are obligatory unicellular parasites that infect a range of agricultural

TABLE 1 | LAMP assays developed for the detection of pathogens and pests of honey bees.

Pathogen	Target gene	Specimen	Detection limit	Loop primers	Field samples[a]	References
Fungal						
Nosema ceranae	16S rRNA	Adult bees[a]	0.3 ng	No	Yes	(42)
	16S rRNA	Adult bee[c]	100 fg	Yes	No	(43)
	Polar tube protein 3 (PTP3)	Adult bees[b], Spores	1 pg	Yes	Yes	(44)
N. apis	16S rRNA	Adult bee[c]	100 fg	Yes	Yes	(43)
N. bombi	SSU rRNA	Adult bees[b]	4.57×10^1 spores/μl	Yes	No	(45)
Aspergillus flavus	18S rRNA	Adult bees[b]	N.D.[4]	No	Yes	(46)
	18S rRNA	Adult bees[b]	10^5 copies/reaction	No	Yes	(47)
Viral						
Sacbrood virus	SBV-pol gene	Adult bees[b]	10 copies/reaction	Yes	No	(48)
	SBV-pol gene	*cerana indica* Larvae, Pre pupae	N.D	Yes	Yes	(49)
Korean *Sacbrood virus*	VP1 gene	Adult bees[b], Larvae	1,000 copies/reaction	No	Yes	(50)
Chinese *Sacbrood virus*	VP1 gene	Larvae	1 pg	No	Yes	(51)
Bacterial						
Melissococcus plutonius	DNA gyrase subunit B	Adult bee[c], Larvae	2 fg	No	No	(52)
Insect pests						
Aethina tumida (Small hive beetle)	28S rRNA	*tumida* Adults, Pupae, Eggs	12 pg	yes	No	(53)
Vespa velutina nigrithorax (yellow-legged Asian hornet)	COX1 (cytochrome oxidase subunit 1)	*V. velutina nigrithorax* Adults, I Larva, Egg, Nest material	5 pg	yes	Yes	(54)

[a] *Samples collected from the field.*
[b] *Pool of adult honey bees were used for extraction of nucleic acid for LAMP assay.*
[c] *Individual adult honey bee was used for extraction of nucleic acid for LAMP assay.*
[d] *N.D., not determined.*

important livestock (35, 36). In particular, *N. ceranae* is the major pathogen of *A. mellifera* that results in a range of symptoms such as suppressed immune function, lipid synthesis, pheromone and hormone production (37–39). If an infection is severe, it can lead to death and the resulting colonies' collapse (40, 41). Transmission of *N. ceranae* between hives can occur via honey, pollen, nectar and bee fecal matter. It can be controlled by treatment with fumagillin if the infection has been diagnosed in the field. The application of antibiotics has several problems, such as the potential to lead to resistant strains and honey's residue contamination. In many parts of the world, such as the European Union, antibiotics for Nosemosis treatment are banned. There have been three separate LAMP assays developed to detect *N. ceranae* and one for the detection of *N. apis* (**Table 1**) (42–44). Also, one has been developed for *N. bombi* infection within wild bumble bee populations (45). All three of the *N. ceranae* LAMP assays are extremely sensitive for the detection of infection; however, the LAMP assay developed by Lannutti et al. (44) uses

primers targeting the polar tube protein 3 (PTP3) gene, a highly specific and conserved gene of *N. ceranae*. Targeting the *PTP3* gene overcomes non-specific amplification that can occur due to polymorphisms in the 16S rRNA gene, which is the other two assays' target gene (55). Furthermore, only the PTP3-LAMP assay has been successfully evaluated using a panel of field samples (44).

Two brood diseases, stonebrood and chalkbrood, are caused by the fungal species *Aspergillus flavus* and *Ascophaera apis*, respectively. Diagnosis based on visual symptoms is difficult as both diseases have very similar clinical symptoms (56). Two LAMP assays have been developed to amplify different regions of the 18S rRNA gene to allow detection of an infected hive (46, 47). In laboratory testing, both assays were shown to be highly specific for the target species only, detecting *A. flavus* with no amplification of *A. apis* and *N. ceranae* DNA. To date, neither test has been optimized for field sampling and detection, with in-field validation of these tests required.

APPLICATION OF LAMP FOR THE DETECTION OF VIRAL PATHOGENS OF HONEY BEES

Honey bees can be infected with a range of RNA viruses. However, most of the time, the bees are asymptomatic until external stress is applied, which results in severe loss of honey bees and reduced hive functionality (57). For example, the deformed wing virus (DWV) is often present in low levels in *A. mellifera* with no impacts on hive health; however, the *Varroa destructor* mite's introduction causes the virus to become more virulent, which results in massive mortality (58, 59). Current detection for honey bee viruses has mainly focused on molecular techniques in specialized laboratories (19, 20). Currently, LAMP tests have been developed only for the sacbrood virus (SBV) for country-specific outbreaks (**Table 1**). SBV causes the larvae to die shortly after capping; however, the disease incidence is higher after stress events such as a shortage of nectar or pollen (60). The assays either amplify the SBV polymerase gene or viral protein gene with a range of sensitivities from 1 pg to 1,000 copies per reaction (**Table 1**). The range of sensitivity of detection is most likely due to sampling processing. Apart from SBV, there is significant scope for developing LAMP assays to detect a range of viruses that affect honey bees, particularly DWV. Currently, Australia is free of DWV (as well as the Varroa mite), thus has not suffered large colony loss due to these pathogens. It would be advantageous to have an assay to detect this virus in honey bees imported into the country to maintain Australia's DWV free status (61).

APPLICATION OF LAMP FOR THE DETECTION OF BACTERIAL PATHOGENS OF HONEY BEES

Of the several pathogenic bacteria species that cause disease of managed honey bees, there are only two economically relevant pathogens, *Paenibacillus larvae* and *Melissococcus plutonius*, the causative agents of American Foulbrood (AFB) and European Foulbrood (EFB), respectively (9). *P. larvae* and *M. plutonius* are listed by OIE (World Organisation for Animal Health) as category B organisms, which are defined as disease-causing agents considered to be of socio-economic and/or public health importance within countries. There are limited control options against theses pathogens; antibiotics such as Terramycin are effective against *M. plutonius* though in many parts of the world such European Union antibiotic treatments are strictly prohibited while there are no effective treatment options for *P. larvae* as antibiotics will not kill the infective spore stage thus burning of infected hives are required to minimize the spread of the pathogen (62). Prevention is better than the cure, and to this aim, there are commercial lateral flow devices that detect AFB and EFB infections; however, they all work only on larval samples. However, there is a demand for highly sensitive field tests from environmental samples to aid in disease control, prevention, monitoring and treatment strategies for bacterial diseases of honey bees. The predominant method utilized to distinguish the two diseases is visual inspection, which requires subjective expertise. Given the differences in treatment of AFB and EFB, more precise diagnostic methods are urgently required for use in the field. Currently, there is only a LAMP test for *M. plutonius*, which is extremely sensitive (detection limit of 2 fg) on laboratory prepared samples; however, this test has not been used in the field. Future work should be directed toward developing and validating LAMP assays for the causative agents of AFB and EFB in the field. A multiplex assay for the differentiation of these two species would be ideal.

APPLICATION OF LAMP FOR THE DETECTION OF INSECT PESTS AND MITES OF HONEY BEES

Several species of insect pests and mites of *A. mellifera* can cause significant problems in commercial apiaries worldwide. The *Varroa destructor* mite is the primary biotic cause of colony collapse syndrome and is found in nearly every continent except Australia (63, 64). Other exotic pests such as the small hive beetle (SHB, *Aethina tumida*) and various species of hornets that have been introduced into a range of non-native countries can have a devastating effect on honey bees (65, 66). The ability to rapidly and reliably identify invasive species at all life stages, and within the nest and hive debris is crucial in mounting an effective control response. As LAMP technology is well suited to aid biosecurity, there have been two reported LAMP assays for insect pests of honey bees (**Table 1**). The small hive beetle LAMP assay targets the 28S ribosomal gene and is able to detect the presence of SHB DNA down to 12 pg within 20 min (53). True hornets belong to the *Vespa* family and are naturally found only in Asia, Europe and Africa. They all prey on other insects, including honey bees; thus, introductions into non-native areas can have severe consequences for honey bee populations in these areas. Only one of the 20 species of true hornets have had a LAMP assay developed for their identification (**Table 1**). The yellow-legged Asian hornet (*Vespa velutina nigrithorax*) has been rapidly spreading throughout Europe after being accidentally introduced into France from China (67). The LAMP assay can reliably identify all life stages of *V. v. nigrithorax* as well as from nest material as low as 5 pg in 10 min. Both assays allow rapid unequivocal identification of insect pests which are normally identified via manual inspection of morphological features. An additional benefit of using LAMP is it can provide identification on decomposing or incomplete insect samples; thus, these assays will be useful in control programs to limit the damage caused by these pests. In the future, an entire suite of LAMP assays should be developed for the rapid identification of insect pests of honey bees to aid effective biosecurity control measures.

APPLICATION OF LAMP FOR IN-FIELD DETECTION OF PESTS AND PATHOGENS OF HONEY BEES

Several LAMP assays have been developed to detect pests and pathogens of honey bees; however, none have been applied in the field. The current sampling methods for detecting pathogens require the use of specialized equipment in a laboratory setting. Further research is required to establish methods for lysing honey bees in the field such as the use of ball bearing and small capped tubes which have been used previously for plant and insect samples (68). The majority of LAMP assays are performed in an 8-strip tube, thus providing a negative and positive control and six tubes for testing. The six sample tubes could contain a single or duplex reaction and have the ability to analyze six different samples or you can have six different individual assays and the ability to use a single sample. What configuration the field-based LAMP test kits are will be determined mainly by consumer demand.

CONCLUSIONS

The increasing awareness about the important roles honey bees play in food production and security has led to many advances in understanding honey bees' health and well-being. Honey bees are under threat from a range of environmental

stress and infection from a large variety of pathogens. The ability to identify specifically and rapidly infection at the hive-site will allow for improved management and treatment strategies. LAMP assays in the last few years have become an important tool to aid in the detection of both exotic and endemic pathogens in the livestock industry. Several LAMP assays have been developed for honey bee pathogens, with a number of these still requiring in-field validation to confirm its use as an on-site diagnostic tool. It is important that researchers continue to develop assays against other honey bee pathogen and promote them for use in the field, with consideration given to non-invasive sampling methods to maximize the benefit from LAMP assays and reduce stress on honey bee hives introduced by humans.

AUTHOR CONTRIBUTIONS

TC, DW, and TB conceived, designed, and wrote the manuscript. All authors contributed to the article and approved the submitted version.

REFERENCES

1. Geldmann J, Gonzalez-Varo JP. Conserving honey bees does not help wildlife. *Science*. (2018) 359:392–3. doi: 10.1126/science.aar2269
2. Aizen MA, Garibaldi LA, Cunningham SA, Klein AM. Long-term global trends in crop yield and production reveal no current pollination shortage but increasing pollinator dependency. *Curr Biol*. (2008) 18:1572–5. doi: 10.1016/j.cub.2008.08.066
3. Aizen MA, Harder LD. The global stock of domesticated honey bees is growing slower than agricultural demand for pollination. *Curr Biol*. (2009) 19:915–8. doi: 10.1016/j.cub.2009.03.071
4. Cox-Foster DL, Conlan S, Holmes EC, Palacios G, Evans JD, Moran NA, et al. A metagenomic survey of microbes in honey bee colony collapse disorder. *Science*. (2007) 318:283–7. doi: 10.1126/science.1146498
5. Cornman RS, Tarpy DR, Chen Y, Jeffreys L, Lopez D, Pettis JS, et al. Pathogen webs in collapsing honey bee colonies. *PLoS ONE*. (2012) 7:e43562. doi: 10.1371/journal.pone.0043562
6. Gonzalez-Varo JP, Biesmeijer JC, Bommarco R, Potts SG, Schweiger O, Smith HG, et al. Combined effects of global change pressures on animal-mediated pollination. *Trends Ecol Evol*. (2013) 28:524–30. doi: 10.1016/j.tree.2013.05.008
7. Goulson D, Nicholls E, Botias C, Rotheray EL. Bee declines driven by combined stress from parasites, pesticides, and lack of flowers. *Science*. (2015) 347:1255957. doi: 10.1126/science.1255957
8. Hoppe PP, Safer A, Amaral-Rogers V, Bonmatin JM, Goulson D, Menzel R, et al. Effects of a neonicotinoid pesticide on honey bee colonies: a response to the field study by Pilling et al. (2013). *Environ Sci Eur*. (2015) 27:28. doi: 10.1186/s12302-015-0060-7
9. Fünfhaus A, Ebeling J, Genersch E. Bacterial pathogens of bees. *Curr Opin Insect Sci*. (2018) 26:89–96. doi: 10.1016/j.cois.2018.02.008
10. Evison SEF, Jensen AB. The biology and prevalence of fungal diseases in managed and wild bees. *Curr Opin Insect Sci*. (2018) 26:105–13. doi: 10.1016/j.cois.2018.02.010
11. Burnham AJ. Scientific advances in controlling *Nosema ceranae* (Microsporidia) infections in honey bees (*Apis mellifera*). *Front Vet Sci*. (2019) 6:79. doi: 10.3389/fvets.2019.00079
12. Sammataro D, Gerson U, Needham G. Parasitic mites of honey bees: life history, implications, and impact. *Annu Rev Entomol*. (2000) 45:519–48. doi: 10.1146/annurev.ento.45.1.519
13. Kwadha CA, Ong'amo GO, Ndegwa PN, Raina SK, Fombong AT. The biology and control of the greater wax moth, *Galleria mellonella*. *Insects*. (2017) 8:61. doi: 10.3390/insects8020061

14. Grozinger CM, Flenniken ML. Bee viruses: ecology, pathogenicity, and impacts. *Ann Rev Entomol*. (2019) 64:205–26. doi: 10.1146/annurev-ento-011118-111942
15. O'Neal ST, Anderson TD, Wu-Smart JY. Interactions between pesticides and pathogen susceptibility in honey bees. *Curr Opin Insect Sci*. (2018) 26:57–62. doi: 10.1016/j.cois.2018.01.006
16. Martínez J, Simon V, Gonzalez B, Conget P. A real-time PCR-based strategy for the detection of *Paenibacillus larvae* vegetative cells and spores to improve the diagnosis and the screening of American foulbrood. *Lett Appl Microbiol*. (2010) 50:603–10. doi: 10.1111/j.1472-765X.2010.02840.x
17. Budge GE, Barrett B, Jones B, Pietravalle S, Marris G, Chantawannakul P, et al. The occurrence of *Melissococcus plutonius* in healthy colonies of *Apis mellifera* and the efficacy of European foulbrood control measures. *J Invertebr Pathol*. (2010) 105:164–70. doi: 10.1016/j.jip.2010.06.004
18. Cepero A, Martin-Hernandez R, Prieto L, Gomez-Moracho T, Martinez-Salvador A, Bartolome C, et al. Is *Acarapis woodi* a single species? A new PCR protocol to evaluate its prevalence. *Parasitol Res*. (2015) 114:651–8. doi: 10.1007/s00436-014-4229-6
19. D'Alvise P, Seeburger V, Gihring K, Kieboom M, Hasselmann M. Seasonal dynamics and co-occurrence patterns of honey bee pathogens revealed by high-throughput RT-qPCR analysis. *Ecol Evol*. (2019) 9:10241–52. doi: 10.1002/ece3.5544
20. Meeus I, Smagghe G, Siede R, Jans K, de Graaf DC. Multiplex RT-PCR with broad-range primers and an exogenous internal amplification control for the detection of honey bee viruses in bumble bees. *J Invertebr Pathol*. (2010) 105:200–3. doi: 10.1016/j.jip.2010.06.012
21. De Smet L, Ravoet J, de Miranda JR, Wenseleers T, Mueller MY, Moritz RF, et al. BeeDoctor, a versatile MLPA-based diagnostic tool for screening bee viruses. *PLoS ONE*. (2012) 7:e47953. doi: 10.1371/journal.pone.0047953
22. Clark AE, Kaleta EJ, Arora A, Wolk DM. Matrix-assisted laser desorption ionization-time of flight mass spectrometry: a fundamental shift in the routine practice of clinical microbiology. *Clin Microbiol Rev*. (2013) 26:547–603. doi: 10.1128/CMR.00072-12
23. Schäfer MO, Genersch E, Fünfhaus A, Poppinga L, Formella N, Bettin B, et al. Rapid identification of differentially virulent genotypes of *Paenibacillus larvae*, the causative organism of American foulbrood of honey bees, by whole cell MALDI-TOF mass spectrometry. *Vet Microbiol*. (2014) 170:291–7. doi: 10.1016/j.vetmic.2014.02.006
24. Locke B, Low M, Forsgren E. An integrated management strategy to prevent outbreaks and eliminate infection pressure of American foulbrood disease in a commercial beekeeping operation. *Prev Vet Med*. (2019) 167:48–52. doi: 10.1016/j.prevetmed.2019.03.023

25. Francois P, Tangomo M, Hibbs J, Bonetti EJ, Boehme CC, Notomi T, et al. Robustness of a loop-mediated isothermal amplification reaction for diagnostic applications. *FEMS Immunol Med Microbiol.* (2011) 62:41–8. doi: 10.1111/j.1574-695X.2011.00785.x

26. James A, Macdonald J. Recombinase polymerase amplification: emergence as a critical molecular technology for rapid, low-resource diagnostics. *Expert Rev Mol Diagn.* (2015) 15:1475–89. doi: 10.1586/14737159.2015.1090877

27. Notomi T, Okayama H, Masubuchi H, Yonekawa T, Watanabe K, Amino N, et al. Loop-mediated isothermal amplification of DNA. *Nucleic Acids Res.* (2000) 28:E63. doi: 10.1093/nar/28.12.e63

28. Lee PL. DNA amplification in the field: move over PCR, here comes LAMP. *Mol Ecol Resour.* (2017) 17:138–41. doi: 10.1111/1755-0998.12548

29. Tao ZY, Zhou HY, Xia H, Xu S, Zhu HW, Culleton RL, et al. Adaptation of a visualized loop-mediated isothermal amplification technique for field detection of *Plasmodium vivax* infection. *Parasit Vectors.* (2011) 4:115. doi: 10.1186/1756-3305-4-115

30. Nkouawa A, Sako Y, Li T, Chen X, Nakao M, Yanagida T, et al. A loop-mediated isothermal amplification method for a differential identification of *Taenia* tapeworms from human: application to a field survey. *Parasitol Int.* (2012) 61:723–5. doi: 10.1016/j.parint.2012.06.001

31. Best N, Rawlin G, Suter R, Rodoni B, Beddoe T. Optimization of a loop mediated isothermal amplification (LAMP) assay for in-field detection of *Dichelobacter nodosus* with aprV2 (VDN LAMP) in Victorian Sheep Flocks. *Front Vet Sci.* (2019) 6:67. doi: 10.3389/fvets.2019.00067

32. Nagamine K, Hase T, Notomi T. Accelerated reaction by loop-mediated isothermal amplification using loop primers. *Mol Cell Probes.* (2002) 16:223–9. doi: 10.1006/mcpr.2002.0415

33. Fries I, Feng F, Silva A, Slemenda SB, Pieniazek NJ. *Nosema ceranae* n. sp. (Microspora, Nosematidae), morphological and molecular characterization of a microsporidian parasite of the Asian honey bee *Apis cerana* (Hymenoptera, Apidae). *Eur J Protistol.* (1996) 32:356–65. doi: 10.1016/S0932-4739(96)80059-9

34. Brown, M.J.F. Microsporidia: an emerging threat to bumble bees? *Trends Parasitol.* (2017) 33:754–62. doi: 10.1016/j.pt.2017.06.001

35. James TY, Kauff F, Schoch CL, Matheny PB, Hofstetter V, Cox CJ, et al. Reconstructing the early evolution of Fungi using a six-gene phylogeny. *Nature.* (2006) 443:818–22. doi: 10.1038/nature05110

36. Stentiford GD, Becnel J, Weiss LM, Keeling PJ, Didier ES, Williams BP, et al. Microsporidia - emergent pathogens in the global food chain. *Trends Parasitol.* (2016) 32:336–48. doi: 10.1016/j.pt.2015.12.004

37. Antunez K, Martin-Hernandez R, Prieto L, Meana A, Zunino P, Higes M. Immune suppression in the honey bee (*Apis mellifera*) following infection by *Nosema ceranae* (Microsporidia). *Environ Microbiol.* (2009) 11:2284–90. doi: 10.1111/j.1462-2920.2009.01953.x

38. Mayack C, Natsopoulou ME, McMahon DP. *Nosema ceranae* alters a highly conserved hormonal stress pathway in honey bees. *Insect Mol Biol.* (2015) 24:662–70. doi: 10.1111/imb.12190

39. Li W, Chen Y, Cook SC. Chronic *Nosema ceranae* infection inflicts comprehensive and persistent immunosuppression and accelerated lipid loss in host *Apis mellifera* honey bees. *Int J Parasitol.* (2018) 48:433–44. doi: 10.1016/j.ijpara.2017.11.004

40. Higes M, Martin-Hernandez R, Garrido-Bailon E, Gonzalez-Porto AV, Garcia-Palencia P, Meana A, et al. Honey bee colony collapse due to *Nosema ceranae* in professional apiaries. *Environ Microbiol Rep.* (2009) 1:110–3. doi: 10.1111/j.1758-2229.2009.00014.x

41. Bromenshenk JJ, Henderson CB, Wick CH, Stanford MF, Zulich AW, Jabbour RE, et al. Iridovirus and microsporidian linked to honey bee colony decline. *PLoS ONE.* (2010) 5:e13181. doi: 10.1371/journal.pone.0013181

42. Chupia V, Patchanee P, Krutmuang P, Pikulkaew S. Development and evaluation of loop-mediated isothermal amplification for rapid detection of *Nosema ceranae* in honey bee. *Asian Pac J Trop Dis.* (2016) 6:952–6. doi: 10.1016/S2222-1808(16)61163-5

43. Ptaszyńska AA, Borsuk G, Wozniakowski G, Gnat S, Małek W. Loop-mediated isothermal amplification (LAMP) assays for rapid detection and differentiation of *Nosema apis* and *N. ceranae* in honey bees. *FEMS Microbiol Lett.* (2014) 357:40–8. doi: 10.1111/1574-6968.12521

44. Lannutti L, Mira A, Basualdo M, Rodriguez G, Erler S, Silva V, et al. Development of a loop-mediated isothermal amplification (LAMP) and a direct LAMP for the specific detection of *Nosema ceranae*, a parasite of honey bees. *Parasitol Res.* (2020) 119:3947–56. doi: 10.1007/s00436-020-06915-w

45. Kato Y, Yanagisawa T, Nakai M, Komatsu K, Inoue MN. Direct and sensitive detection of a microsporidian parasite of bumble bees using loop-mediated isothermal amplification (LAMP). *Sci Rep.* (2020) 10:1118. doi: 10.1038/s41598-020-57909-8

46. Lee JS, Yong SJ, Lim HY, Yoon BS. A simple and sensitive gene-based diagnosis of *Aspergillus flavus* by loop-mediated isothermal amplification in honey bee. *J Apicult.* (2015) 30:53. doi: 10.17519/apiculture.2015.04.30.1.53

47. Lee JS, Luong GT, Yoon BS. Development of in-field-diagnosis of *Aspergillus flavus* by loop-mediated isothermal amplification in honey bee. *J Apicult.* (2016) 31:25. doi: 10.17519/apiculture.2016.04.31.1.25

48. Jin-Long Y, Rui Y, Ke-Fei S, Xiang-Wei P, Tao X, Zuo-Hua L. Rapid detection of sacbrood virus (SBV) by one-step reverse transcription loop-mediated isothermal amplification assay. *Virol J.* (2012) 9:1–4. doi: 10.1186/1743-422X-9-47

49. Tamilnayagan T, Srinivasan MR, Selvarajan R, Subramanian S, Saravanan PA, Muthuswami M, et al. Designing of rt-lamp primers and detection of sac brood virus from Indian honey bee *Apis cerana indica* (F.). *Ind J Entomol.* (2020) 82:162–6. doi: 10.5958/0974-8172.2020.00037.1

50. Yoo MS, Noh JH, Yoon BS, Reddy KE, Kweon CH, Jung SC, et al. Reverse transcription loop-mediated isothermal amplification for sensitive and rapid detection of Korean sacbrood virus. *J Virol Methods.* (2012) 186:147–51. doi: 10.1016/j.jviromet.2012.08.009

51. Ma M, Ma C, Li M, Wang S, Yang S, Wang S. Loop-mediated isothermal amplification for rapid detection of Chinese sacbrood virus. *J Virol Methods.* (2011) 176:115–9. doi: 10.1016/j.jviromet.2011.05.028

52. Van Nguyen P, Lee B, Yoo MS, Yoon BS. Development and clinical validation of a DNA gyrase subunit B gene based loop-mediated isothermal amplification method for detection of *Melissococcus plutonius*. *J Apicult.* (2012) 27:51–8.

53. Ponting S, Tomkies V, Stainton K. Rapid identification of the invasive small hive beetle (*Aethina tumida*) using LAMP. *Pest Manag Sci.* (2021) 77:1476–81. doi: 10.1002/ps.6168

54. Stainton K, Hall J, Budge GE, Boonham N, Hodgetts J. Rapid molecular methods for in-field and laboratory identification of the yellow-legged Asian hornet (*Vespa velutina nigrithorax*). *J Appl Entomol.* (2018) 142:610–6. doi: 10.1111/jen.12506

55. Sagastume S, Martin-Hernandez R, Higes M, Henriques-Gil N. Ribosomal gene polymorphism in small genomes: analysis of different 16S rRNA sequences expressed in the honey bee parasite *Nosema ceranae* (Microsporidia). *J Eukaryot Microbiol.* (2014) 61:42–50. doi: 10.1111/jeu.12084

56. Jensen AB, Aronstein K, Flores JM, Vojvodic S, Palacio MA, Spivak M. Standard methods for fungal brood disease research. *J Apic Res.* (2013) 52:1–20. doi: 10.3896/IBRA.1.52.1.13

57. McMenamin AJ, Flenniken ML. Recently identified bee viruses and their impact on bee pollinators. *Curr Opin Insect Sci.* (2018) 26:120–29. doi: 10.1016/j.cois.2018.02.009

58. Martin SJ, Highfield AC, Brettell L, Villalobos EM, Budge GE, Powell M, et al. Global honey bee viral landscape altered by a parasitic mite. *Science.* (2012) 336:1304–6. doi: 10.1126/science.1220941

59. Wilfert L, Long G, Leggett HC, Schmid-Hempel P, Butlin R, Martin SJ, et al. Deformed wing virus is a recent global epidemic in honeybees driven by Varroa mites. *Science.* (2016) 351:594–7. doi: 10.1126/science.aac9976

60. Grabensteiner E, Ritter W, Carter MJ, Davison S, Pechhacker H, Kolodziejek J, et al. Sacbrood virus of the honey bee (*Apis mellifera*): rapid identification and phylogenetic analysis using reverse transcription-PCR. *Clin Diagn Lab Immunol.* (2001) 8:93–104. doi: 10.1128/CDLI.8.1.93-104.2001

61. Roberts JMK, Anderson DL, Durr PA. Absence of deformed wing virus and *Varroa destructor* in Australia provides unique perspectives on honey bee viral landscapes and colony losses. *Sci Rep.* (2017) 7:6925. doi: 10.1038/s41598-017-07290-w

62. Genersch E. American Foulbrood in honeybees and its causative agent, *Paenibacillus larvae*. *J Invertebrate Pathol*. (2010) 103:S10–9. doi: 10.1016/j.jip.2009.06.015

63. Noel A, Le Conte Y, Mondet F. *Varroa destructor*: how does it harm *Apis mellifera* honey bees and what can be done about it? *Emerg Top Life Sci*. (2020) 4:45–57. doi: 10.1042/ETLS20190125

64. Traynor KS, Mondet F, de Miranda JR, Techer M, Kowallik V, Oddie MAY, et al. *Varroa destructor*: a complex parasite, crippling honey bees worldwide. *Trends Parasitol*. (2020) 36:592–606. doi: 10.1016/j.pt.2020.04.004

65. Neumanna P, Elzenc PJ. The biology of the small hive beetle (*Aethina tumida*, Coleoptera: Nitidulidae): gaps in our knowledge of an invasive species. *Apidologie*. (2004) 35:229–47. doi: 10.1051/apido:2004010

66. Budge GE, Hodgetts J, Jones EP, Ostoja-Starzewski JC, Hall J, Tomkies V, et al. The invasion, provenance and diversity of *Vespa velutina Lepeletier* (Hymenoptera: Vespidae) in Great Britain. *PLoS ONE*. (2017) 12:e0185172. doi: 10.1371/journal.pone.0185172

67. Arca M, Mougel F, Guillemaud T, Dupas S, Rome Q, Perrard A, et al. Reconstructing the invasion and the demographic history of the yellow-legged hornet, *Vespa velutina*, in Europe. *Biol Invasions*. (2015) 17:2357–71. doi: 10.1007/s10530-015-0880-9

68. Colosi JC, Schaal BA. Tissue grinding with ball bearings and vortex mixer for DNA extraction. *Nucleic Acids Res*. (1993) 21:1051–2. doi: 10.1093/nar/21.4.1051

20

Serum Metabolomic Profiles of Paratuberculosis Infected and Infectious Dairy Cattle by Ambient Mass Spectrometry

Alessandra Tata[1], Ivana Pallante[1], Andrea Massaro[1], Brunella Miano[1], Massimo Bottazzari[1], Paola Fiorini[1], Mauro Dal Prà[1], Laura Paganini[1], Annalisa Stefani[1], Jeroen De Buck[2], Roberto Piro[1] and Nicola Pozzato[1]*

[1] *Istituto Zooprofilattico delle Venezie (IZSVe), Legnaro, Italy,* [2] *Department of Production Animal Health, University of Calgary, Calgary, AB, Canada*

*Correspondence:
Nicola Pozzato
npozzato@izsvenezie.it

Mycobacterium avium subsp. paratuberculosis (MAP) is the causative agent of paratuberculosis [Johne's disease (JD)], a chronic disease that causes substantial economic losses in the dairy cattle industry. The long incubation period means clinical signs are visible in animals only after years, and some cases remain undetected because of the subclinical manifestation of the disease. Considering the complexity of JD pathogenesis, animals can be classified as infected, infectious, or affected. The major limitation of currently available diagnostic tests is their failure in detecting infected non-infectious animals. The present study aimed to identify metabolic markers associated with infected and infectious stages of JD. Direct analysis in real time coupled with high resolution mass spectrometry (DART-HRMS) was, hence, applied in a prospective study where cohorts of heifers and cows were followed up annually for 2–4 years. The animals' infectious status was assigned based on a positive result of both serum ELISA and fecal PCR, or culture. The same animals were retrospectively assigned to the status of infected at the previous sampling for which all JD tests were negative. Stored sera from 10 infected animals and 17 infectious animals were compared with sera from 20 negative animals from the same herds. Two extraction protocols and two (-/+) ionization modes were tested. The three most informative datasets out of the four were merged by a mid-level data fusion approach and submitted to partial least squares discriminant analysis (PLS-DA). Compared to the MAP negative subjects, metabolomic analysis revealed the m/z signals of isobutyrate, dimethylethanolamine, palmitic acid, and rhamnitol were more intense in infected animals. Both infected and infectious animals showed higher relative intensities of tryptamine and creatine/creatinine as well as lower relative abundances of urea, glutamic acid and/or pyroglutamic acid. These metabolic differences could indicate altered fat metabolism and reduced energy intake in both infected and infectious cattle. In conclusion, DART-HRMS coupled to a mid-level data fusion approach allowed the molecular features that identified preclinical stages of JD to be teased out.

Keywords: metabolomic, paratuberculosis, biomarker, cattle, DART-MS, Jonhe's disease, *mycobacterium avium subsp paratubercolosis*

INTRODUCTION

Bovine paratuberculosis, known as Johne's disease (JD), is a chronic infectious disease of ruminants resulting in diarrhea, wasting, weight loss, emaciation, and eventual death (1–3). The etiologic agent of JD is *Mycobacterium avium* subsp. *paratuberculosis* (MAP), a slow growing, obligate intracellular pathogen (4).

JD is widespread worldwide, causes great economic losses, and is mainly transmitted through the fecal-oral route (2, 5, 6). The susceptibility is age-dependent, with young calves highly sensitive to infection. The susceptibility decreases in heifers, with adult cows being infected only in the case of high infectious doses or long exposure time (2, 5, 7). In JD, animals can be classified into three groups: infected when MAP is present intracellularly in the animal, infectious when the animal is shedding MAP via feces and affected when clinical signs are visible (8). Common diagnostic tests, such as fecal Polymerase Chain Reaction (PCR) and enzyme-linked immunosorbent assay (ELISA) lack of sensitivity in earlier stages of infection, characterized by intermittent MAP shedding and absence of specific Th-2 response (9). The biology of MAP infection, the long incubation period, the pathogenesis, and the difficulties in detecting infected animals in the absence of accurate diagnostic tests entail delayed diagnosis of JD, so disease control in infected herds is a challenge (10).

Over recent years, genomics, transcriptomics and proteomics were introduced to overcome the lack of efficient diagnostic methods in the preclinical stages of the disease (11–16); the aim was to identify specific pathways related to disease progression through the study of the expression of genes and proteins. In this way, biomarkers related to MAP infection can be determined (11, 14–16). In addition, metabolomics has emerged as a means to identify altered metabolic pathways in infected animals, by characterizing the metabolic profiles of cattle experimentally infected with MAP (13). Serum lipidomics of control and MAP infected cattle were also explored, utilizing high-resolution mass spectrometry, with the data showing that altered availability of choline-containing lipids occurs late in the disease process, and it is most likely a result of malnutrition and altered biosynthetic capacities of the liver and the gastrointestinal tract (17). Volatile organic signatures of breath were defined by gas-chromatography to differentiate healthy cattle from MAP infected cattle (18). In human medicine, the metabolomic approach was used to differentiate latent infection caused by *Mycobacterium tuberculosis* from active tuberculosis. The identification of mycobacterial biomarkers of infection could contribute to faster and more accurate diagnosis than the tuberculin skin or interferon gamma tests (19).

In the field of metabolomics, direct analysis in real time coupled to high resolution mass spectrometry (DART-HRMS) is considered an innovative, ambient mass spectrometric approach, successfully applied in clinical screening, microbiology, food safety, and toxicology (20–30). DART-HRMS requires minimal sample preparation and it has already demonstrated its accuracy, intra-sample repeatability and rapidity, with the aim of reducing the burden of chemical laboratories. In addition, DART-HRMS allows screening the metabolic profile without any prior knowledge of the identity of the metabolic features or their physicochemical characteristics (31). In parallel with genomic and transcriptomic analysis (11, 14–16, 32), this non-targeted approach produces a large amount of information within a very short time by the application of different extraction procedures and instrumental modalities. Statistical strategies called data fusion can then be applied to adequately integrate the data into a unique global dataset that can be submitted to multivariate analysis (33, 34).

In the present study, sera collected from MAP infected, infectious and negative animals were submitted to polar and non-polar extraction, then analyzed by DART-HRMS in positive and negative ion modes. Latent variables extracted from partial least squares discriminant analysis (PLS-DA) of single datasets were merged and submitted to a fused-PLS-DA with the aim of teasing out the characteristic molecular markers of the MAP infected, infectious and negative status.

MATERIALS AND METHODS

Animal Selection and Time Course of the Study

Holstein cattle were selected from four dairy farms with known paratuberculosis initial seroprevalences of >10% and were divided into age-cohorts by reproduction cycle: heifers, primiparous, and pluriparous cows. A total of 356 animals were monitored up to 4 lactations, with blood and fecal sample collections at 30 ± 15 days before the expected calving date to minimize individual metabolic variations except for young heifers that were recruited at 13–15 months of age. During the pre-calving period, cows do not produce milk and the metabolic-hormonal changes that prepare the animal for calving are not established yet. MAP affected animals and cattle in bad health condition were excluded from the study. Blood sample collection was performed under authorization n. 506/2015 of the Italian Ministry of Health for the use of animals for experimental purposes.

Sample Collection and Testing for JD

Blood samples were collected from the jugular vein in an anticoagulant free vacutainer tube, left to coagulate at room temperature for 2–4 h and centrifuged at 2,500 rpm for 5 min. Aliquots from the sera obtained were used for detecting serum antibodies against MAP using a commercial enzyme-linked immunosorbent assay (ELISA) (IDEXX Paratuberculosis Screening Ab, IDEXX Laboratories, Inc.) and applying the manufacturer's instructions for analysis. Two other aliquots of each serum were stored at $-80°C$ for metabolomic analyses and for possible future analyses. Suspect and positive sera were submitted to an ELISA biphasic confirmation test (IDEXX Paratuberculosis Verification Ab, IDEXX Laboratories, Inc.).

Individual fecal samples were collected from the rectal ampulla and analyzed applying microbiological and molecular diagnostic methods for MAP identification. One fecal aliquot from each animal was stored at $-80°C$ for possible future analyses.

All samples were processed for testing by direct real-time PCR (qPCR) and culture on modified Middlebrook 7H9 liquid media (7H9+). In brief, 2 g of feces were resuspended in 10 ml of water; mixtures were rocked on a horizontal shaker for 30 min and left to sediment for an additional 30 min. At the end of this step, an aliquot of 300 μl of supernatant was collected for PCR testing and 5 ml were processed for culture following a modified double-decontamination and centrifugation method (35). In brief, the supernatant was resuspended in 10 ml of 0.75% hexadecylpyridinium, incubated overnight at 37°C, centrifuged, resuspended in PANTA antimicrobial mixture and reincubated overnight at 37°C. The next day, 200 μl were inoculated into two 7H9+ tubes and incubated at 37°C for 6 weeks. At the end of the period, the 7H9+ cultures were examined by Ziehl-Nielsen staining and the broth cultures were confirmed by real-time PCR.

The same PCR protocol was used for both confirmatory test and direct analysis. In brief, 300 μl of supernatant or culture medium was subjected to a bead-beating step in order to enhance MAP DNA recovery as previously described (36). DNA extraction was performed manually with the High Pure PCR preparation kit (Roche Diagnostic, Mannheim, Germany) or by the automated MagMAX™ 96 Viral Isolation Kit (Ambion, Austin, USA) using the Microlab Starlet automated extraction platform (Hamilton Robotics, Bonaduz, Switzerland) or the KingFisher Flex instrument (ThermoFisher Scientific Inc., Worcester, MA, USA). In all cases, DNA extraction was performed according to the manufacturer's instructions. Real-time amplification was performed in a 7300 Real-Time PCR System (Applied Biosystems, Nieuwerkerk a/d IJssel, The Netherlands) or a CFX96 Touch Deep Well real-time PCR system (Bio-Rad Laboratories, Segrate, Italy). The amplification mixture contained 900 nM of each primer, 200 nM of probe, and 1X 1× Taq GOLD PCR Master Mix (Applied Biosystems) in a volume of 25 μl. The primers (Map668F-5'-GGCTGAT CGGACCCG-3', Map791R-5'-TGGTAGCCAGTAAGCAG GATCA-3') and probe (Map718 5'-FAM-ATACTTTCGG CGCTGGAACGCGC-TAMRA) were designed on a MAP-specific portion of IS900. The real-time PCR program was 2 min at 50°C followed by 10 min at 95°C, 40 cycles at 95°C for 15 s and 60°C for 1 min. A cut-off value of 38 cycles was set according to the laboratory's validation procedure (35).

JD Health Status Assignment and Sample Selection for DART-HRMS Analysis

Out of 356 animals, a total of 854 samples were collected during the study period resulting in a mean value of 2.40 samplings per cattle (range 1–5). Regarding JD testing, the frequency of positive animals along the study period resulted to be 6.23% by serology and 11.05% by fecal PCR/culture. At the end of the prospective study, the infectious status was assigned to a serum sample based on a seroconversion for MAP by ELISA accompanied by a positive result to fecal PCR or culture. The infected status was retrospectively assigned to the previous sampling of the animals classified as infectious, in which all JD tests (ELISA, PCR and culture) produced negative results.

The negative status was eventually assigned to exposed cohort animals selected from the same infected herds with the presence of at least one subsequent JD negative result after the selected sampling. These control animals were matched to cases according to sampling date and age category (heifers, primiparous cows, and pluriparous cows) in order to minimize the variability due to dietary and management conditions. The average number of samplings for these animals was 2.84 (range 2–4).

From the collection of sera stored at −80°C, 17 sera of infectious animals, 10 sera of infected animals and 20 sera of negative animals were selected and then analyzed by "DART-HRMS." The age of the selected animals averaged 51.4 months (range 13–119 months).

DART-HRMS Analysis
Sample Extraction

Frozen aliquots of sera were thawed and submitted to two different extraction procedures. In the first protocol, 200 μL of serum were diluted in 800 μL of water and methanol (H_2O:MeOH; 20:80 v/v) solution (MilliQ water and methanol HPLC-grade with 99.9% purity, from VWR International, Radnor, USA), vortexed for 30 s, sonicated for 15 min, and centrifuged for 5 min at 12,000 rpm. In the second extraction procedure, 200 μL of serum were diluted in 800 μL of pure ethyl acetate (EtAc) (99.9% purity, Carlo Erba Reagents, Cornaredo, Italy), vortexed for 30 s, sonicated for 15 min, and centrifuged for 5 min at 12,000 rpm.

DART-HRMS

The instrumental analyses were carried out using a DART SVP 100 ion source (IonSense, Saugus, USA) coupled with an Exactive Orbitrap (Thermo Fisher Scientific, Waltham, USA). The DART source was coupled with a Dip-it[R] sampler (IonSense, Saugus, MA, USA). A Vapur interface (IonSense, Saugus, USA) facilitated the passage of the ions from the DART source to the mass spectrometer. The distance between the DART gun and the ceramic transfer tube of the Vapur interface was 12 mm. The optimized DART settings were as follows: grid voltage 250 V, temperature 300°C, sample speed 0.3 mm/s, and a single time analysis of 0.66 min. The system parameter settings for the mass spectrometer were as follows: 55 S-lens RF level, capillary temperature 300°C, and maximum injection time 10 ms. The resolution was set to 70.000 FWHM and the mass range was 50–1,000 Da in both positive and negative ion modes. In positive ion mode, a vial with an aqueous solution of 25% ammonia was positioned below the DART gun exit, working as a dopant to facilitate and stabilize the formation of $[M+NH_4]^+$ ions.

All DART-MS analyses were run with an automated gain control target setting of 3×10^6. Homemade Dip-it tips (IonSense, Saugus, USA) were inserted into a holder of the autosampler, and then 5 μL of each extract were spotted onto each Dip-it tip. Subsequently, the Dip-it tips automatically moved at a constant speed of 0.3 mm/s throughout the DART gun exit and ceramic tube of the Vapur interface. The duration of desorption from the surface of each tip was about 20 s.

The samples were analyzed in triplicate and XCalibur QualBrowser software (Thermo Fisher Scientific, Waltham,

USA) was used to visualize the entire spectra in raw format. These were converted to mzML files using Proteowizard and then opened with mMass software (http://www.mmass.org/), which allowed interpretation of the mass spectrometry data and assignment of ions using the online METLIN (https://metlin.scripps.edu) and HUMAN METABOLOME DATABASE (www.hmdb.ca) libraries. Prior to statistical analysis, the spectra of the four datasets (two extraction solvents *per* two ion modes) were converted into.csv files with Rstudio 3.6.1 software (RStudio Team, 2016; RStudio Integrated Development for R; RStudio, Inc., Boston, USA).

Data Processing and Statistical Analysis

The DART-HRMS spectral data, acquired in triplicate and not averaged, were statistically analyzed using MetaboAnalyst 4.0 web platform (www.metaboanalyst.ca) and Rstudio 3.6.1 software (37). The three replicates were used independently as done previously in several chemometric studies (38, 39). The signals of the four datasets were loaded onto MetaboAnalyst 4.0 web platform and aligned with a tolerance of 0.008 Da. We removed the ion signals with more than 75% of missing values (no detected ion intensity) over all the samples. The ions with <75% of missing values had them replaced with 1/5 of the recorded lowest intensity (40). Isotopes were removed. Normalization by sum was applied to the signals, whereby each feature was normalized by Pareto scaling. First, supervised partial least squared discriminant analysis (PLS-DA) was performed on the four separate datasets (2 extraction solvents × 2 instrumental ion modes) to evaluate the possible improved discrimination achieved by mid-level data fusion (**Supplementary Figures 1–4**).

A low level data fusion was also tested and described in the **Supplementary Material (Supplementary Figure 5)**.

Mid-Level Data Fusion

Using Rstudio 3.6.1 software, the first five PLS-DA score components of each dataset were fused (concatenated) and submitted to a new PLS-DA with the aim at discriminating the three groups of samples (30). Evaluating the R^2, Q^2, and accuracy of each separate PLS-DA, (−)DART-HRMS spectra of polar extraction were excluded because they provided poor information. Mid-level data fusion of the three most informative datasets was performed and the merged data submitted to fused-PLS-DA clustering (41). Ten-fold cross-validation was performed on the entire dataset to evaluate the performance of the fused-PLS-DA and to select the best number of components within the loading tables of each separate PLS-DA. As recommended by Borràs et al. (41), to extract the PLS-DA features, the best number of components (5) was chosen when the classification error obtained by cross-validation was minimized.

Finally, only the ions whose loadings had an absolute value higher than 0.3 were retained from the first five components of the three separate PLS-DA (**Figure 1**, blue boxes). A table with the samples in the rows and the selected significant ions in the columns was built (**Figure 1**, pink box). The obtained table was used to calculate Pearson's distance and Ward linkage to

determine the correlation of the selected ions among the three JD health status groups.

RESULTS

In this study, a dual mode DART-HRMS analysis was performed on sera extracted using polar and non-polar solvents with the aim of finding the changes in metabolites' level in MAP-infected and infectious cattle as compared to those negative. Four DART-HRMS spectral datasets were thus acquired. Once pre-processed, each dataset was submitted to PLS-DA.

To overcome the difficulty of handling high dimensional datasets, a data reduction was conducted to fade out the most significant variables capable of discriminating the three MAP status groups. To this aim, a mid-level data fusion strategy was attempted by operating at the level of features and thus capturing only the relevant differences in the four datasets (33, 41, 42). In this case, good separation was obtained within the PC1 vs. PC2 score space (**Supplementary Figure 6**), explaining 32.9 and 10.6% of the total variance of the model. Although we obtained a good separation, we removed the less informative dataset.

To further improve the discrimination, we evaluated the R^2, Q^2, and accuracy of each separate PLS-DA (data not shown) and realized that (−)DART-HRMS of polar extractions provided no informative data for the discrimination of the groups. Hence, we merged the scores of the three most informative datasets and performed a PLS-DA. The score plot showed an improvement in clustering (**Figure 2**), with most samples from the MAP negative group correctly assigned to their 0.95-ellipsis confidence interval, and some samples that overlapped between the infected and infectious groups. In this case, PC1 vs. PC2 explained 37.3 and 11.9% of the total variance of the model.

The 12 most informative m/z values were extrapolated by selecting the loadings with absolute value higher than 0.3. They were then fused in a single dataset and submitted to Pearson's distance and Ward linkage calculation. In this way, correlation between ions and MAP status groups was obtained. **Table 1** reports the m/z values that codified each MAP status group in terms of the most abundant molecular features. Representative DART-HRMS spectra showing the most informative m/z values are reported in the **Supplementary Material (Supplementary Figures 8–10)**.

Figure 3 shows box plots with the relative intensities of the observed biomarkers. Sera of infected cattle presented higher relative abundances (compared to the other MAP groups studied) of dimethylethanolamine (m/z 72.0815 in positive ion mode), isobutyric acid (m/z 106.0867 in positive ion mode), creatine a/o creatinine (m/z 114.0665 in positive ion mode), rhamnitol (m/z 167.0917 in positive ion mode), tryptamine (m/z 178.1339 in positive ion mode), palmitic acid (m/z 255.2333 in positive ion mode), and the unassigned ion, m/z 90.0919. The serum profiles of infected cattle were also characterized by lower relative intensity of urea (the dimer of m/z 121.0722 in positive ion mode). In addition, the molecular signature of sera from infectious cattle showed higher relative abundance of dimethylethanolamine (m/z 72.0815 in positive ion mode),

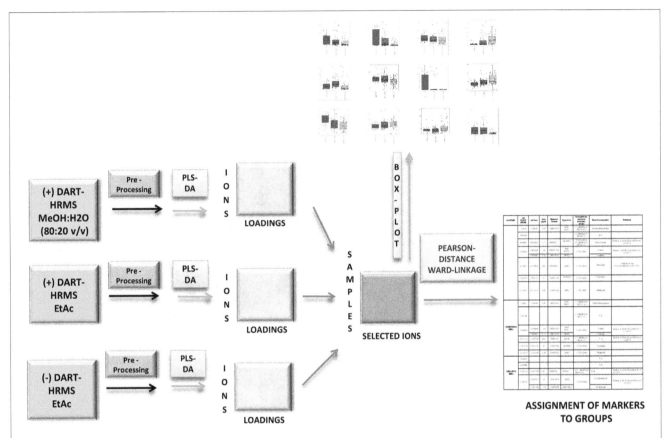

FIGURE 1 | Flow chart of the mid-level data fusion and consequent statistical analysis of the three most informative (+/−) direct analysis in real time high resolution mass spectrometry (DART-HRMS) datasets with the aim selecting the most discriminative variables. After DART-HRMS data pre-processing (gray boxes), three exploratory partial least squares discriminant analysis were carried out (green boxes) and their most discriminative loadings (threshold value higher than 0.3) were selected and merged (red box). Box plots that denote differences in normalized ion abundance of biomarker ions were extrapolated from pre-processed data (orange box). A hierarchical cluster analysis (HCA) by the Pearson's distance criterion and Ward linkage allowed markers to be correlated to groups.

isobutyric acid (m/z 106.0867 in positive ion mode), creatine a/o creatinine (m/z 114.0665 in positive ion mode), tryptamine (m/z 178.1339 in positive ion mode), and the unassigned ions, m/z 76.0764 and m/z 90.0919.

Compared to sera of infected and infectious animals, negative cattle showed higher levels of pyroglutamic acid a/o glutamic acid (observed in negative ion mode at m/z 128.0353), urea (m/z 121.0722), and the unassigned ions of m/z 61.0404 and 59.9855.

To further investigate the discriminatory capacity of the selected biomarkers, internal cross-validation was performed on the PLS-DA of the three most informative DART-HRMS datasets after fusion. The outcomes of the cross-validation, expressed as accuracy (0.91), $Q^2 = 0.57$, and $R^2 = 0.48$, are summarized in **Supplementary Figure 7**. The accuracy, with a maximum theoretical value of 1, is the capability of the model to correctly classify the samples. While the R^2 parameter indicates how well the PLS-DA model explains the current dataset, Q^2 provides a qualitative measure of consistency between the predicted and actual data (43). The parameters Q^2 and R^2 each have a theoretical maximum of 1 and acceptable values of ≥0.4 for a biological model (44). Note that in metabolomics, the values of these parameters strongly depend on the individuals that

constitute the validation subsets. Since cross-validation requires systematic deletion of large portions of the dataset during training, non-trustable values of Q^2 can be produced (44, 45). Since no large difference between R^2 and Q^2 values was observed in the present study, overfitting can be excluded (46).

DISCUSSION

In metabolomics, the selection of the most appropriate statistical analysis method allows extrapolation of significant features that can characterize each group in terms of its metabolic content. In a non-targeted approach, statistical analysis is often employed in two modes: (i) "model building," for the purpose of unravel important molecular markers that describe each group of samples, and; (ii) "classification," for the purpose of sample assignment through matching its spectrum to a previously built model.

In the present study, characterized by small sized and slightly unbalanced groups, we focused on model building aiming to tease out and identifying informative m/z values capable of describing each group (i.e., the infected, infectious and negative animals in infected herds.

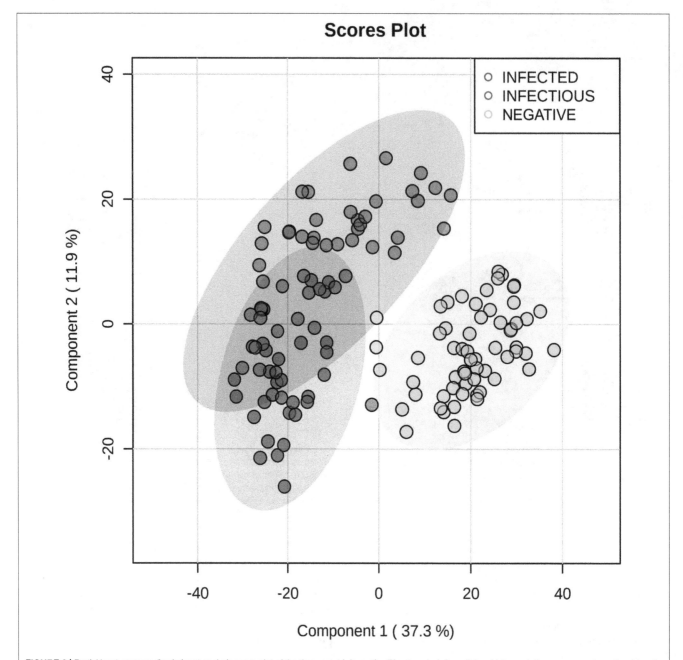

FIGURE 2 | Partial least squares discriminant analysis score plot of the three most informative Direct analysis in real-time high-resolution mass spectrometry datasets merged by mid-level data fusion. MAP infected (blue) and infectious (red) cattle are successfully discriminated from negative (green) cattle. A slight overlap can be seen between infected and infectious groups. Three repetitions for each sample were used.

We applied multimodality DART-HRMS that allows more comprehensive information to be obtained, although with the counterpart of its over-dispersion in the case of big dimensional data. To overcome this issue, we exploited a mid-level data fusion strategy, which demonstrated good discriminatory power. We confirmed that this technique can catch the existent variability among groups and that compression of the high dimensional data was imperative to fade out the existent correlations between markers (33, 34). DART-HRMS coupled

to statistical analysis demonstrated its capability to discriminate the negative group from infected and infectious cattle. On the other hand, this approach provided a tendency to discrimination between MAP infected and infectious animals due to a partial superposition of their metabolic profiles (**Figure 2** and **Supplementary Figures 8–10**).

MAP infected and infectious cattle had higher serum levels of creatine/creatinine, palmitic acid, dimethylethanolamine and tryptamine than did negative cattle.

TABLE 1 | List of discriminant (+/−) direct analysis in real time high resolution mass spectrometry metabolites observed in sera from groups of MAP infected, infectious and negative cattle.

Samples	m/z DART-HRMS	m/z theor	error (ppm)	Elemental formula	Type of ion	Instrument ion mode and extraction solvent	Tentative assignment
INFECTED SERA	72.0815	72.0814	−1.39	$C_4H_{11}N_O$	$[M+H-H_2O]^+$	(+) Pure EtAc	Dimethylethanolamine
	90.0919					(+) MeOH:H_2O (80:20 v/v)	N/A
	106.0867	106.0863	−3.77	$C_4H_8O_2$	$[M+NH_4]^+$	(+) Pure EtAc	Isobutyric acid[+]
						(+) MeOH:H_2O (80:20 v/v)	
	114.0665	114.0668	−2.6	$C_4H_9N_3O_2$	$[M+H-H_2O]^+$	(+) MeOH:H_2O (80:20 v/v)	Creatine[+]
		114.0663	1.75	$C_4H_7N_3O$	$[M+H]^+$		Creatinine[+]
	167.0917	167.0914	1.80	$C_6H_{14}O_5$	$[M-H]^+$	(+) Pure EtAc	Rhamnitol
	178.1339	178.1339	0	$C_{10}H_{12}N_2$	$[M+NH_4]^+$	(+) MeOH:H_2O (80:20 v/v)	Tryptamine
	255.2333	255.2330	1.18	$C_{16}H_{32}O_2$	$[M-H]^-$	(-) Pure EtAc	Palmitic acid (16:0)
INFECTIOUS SERA	72.0815	72.0814	1.39	$C_4H_{11}NO$	$[M+H-H_2O]^+$	(+) MeOH:H_2O (80:20 v/v)	Dimethylethanolamine
	76.0764					(+) MeOH:H_2O (80:20 v/v)	N/A
	114.0665	114.0668	−2.6	$C_4H_9N_3O_2$	$[M+H-H_2O]^+$	(+) Pure EtAc	Creatine[+]
		114.0663	1.75	$C_4H_7N_3O$	$[M+H]^+$		Creatinine[+]
	121.0722	121.0720	1.65	CH_4N_2O	$[2M+H]^+$	(+) MeOH:H_2O (80:20 v/v)	Urea dimer[+]
	178.1339	178.1339	0	$C_{10}H_{12}N_2$	$[M+NH_4]^+$	(+) Pure EtAc	Tryptamine
	255.2333	255.2330	1.18	$C_{16}H_{32}O_2$	$[M-H]-$	(−) Pure EtAc	Palmitic acid (16:0)
NEGATIVE SERA	59.9855					(−) Pure EtAc	N/A
	61.0404					(+) MeOH:H_2O (80:20 v/v)	N/A
	121.0722	121.0720	1.65	CH_4N_2O	$[2M+H]^+$	(+) MeOH:H_2O (80:20 v/v)	Urea dimer[+]
	128.0353	128.0353	0	$C_5H_7NO_3$	$[M-H]^-$	(−) Pure EtAc	Pyroglutamic acid[+]
		128.0348	−3.9	$C_5H_9NO_4$	$[M-H-H_2O]^-$		Glutamic acid[+]

The m/z values, theoretical mass, error (ppm), elemental formula, type of ion, ion mode and extraction procedure, tentative assignment, and literature references are reported.
[+] *(13).*

The high creatine/creatinine abundances, already reported in experimental MAP infection (13), could be associated with muscle wasting due to the protein catabolism determined by the disease progression the led to a reduced energetic intake (47). In addition, we observed a higher abundance of palmitic acid in both MAP infected and infectious cattle than in negative animals. Alterations in the synthesis and absorption of phospholipids and sphingolipids presumably contribute to the circulation of high levels of the free fatty acid. In this context, Wood et al. found significant decrease in circulating levels of phospholipids and sphingolipids probably due to the dysfunction of the gastrointestinal (GI) epithelium and the liver (17). Furthermore, Thirunavukkarasu *et al* demonstrated the altered expression of genes associated with cholesterol and lipid metabolism (48). In parallel, in patients with active *Mycobacterium tuberculosis* infection, phosphatidylglycerol (PG 16:0_18:1), the structural components of which are oleic acid and palmitic acid, was one of the molecules significantly elevated in the plasma (49). In the present study, the hydrolysis of phospholipids could have occurred during the extraction procedure or DART ionization.

In the same vein, high relative abundances of dimethylethanolamine were found in sera of both infected and infectious cattle. Dimethylethanolamine is a structural analogue of choline that is involved in the metabolism of phospholipids, absorption of which can be altered by gastrointestinal microbiome alteration (50). High levels of tryptamine (involved in tryptophan metabolism), observed in both infected and infectious animals, can be explained by important changes in protein turnover or deficiencies in MAP infected cattle (13). Interestingly, higher levels of isobutyric acid were measured in infected animals than in negative animals (**Table 1** and **Figure 3**). Higher relative intensities of isobutyric acid in infected than in negative sera could be related to inflammation of the gut due to MAP infection.

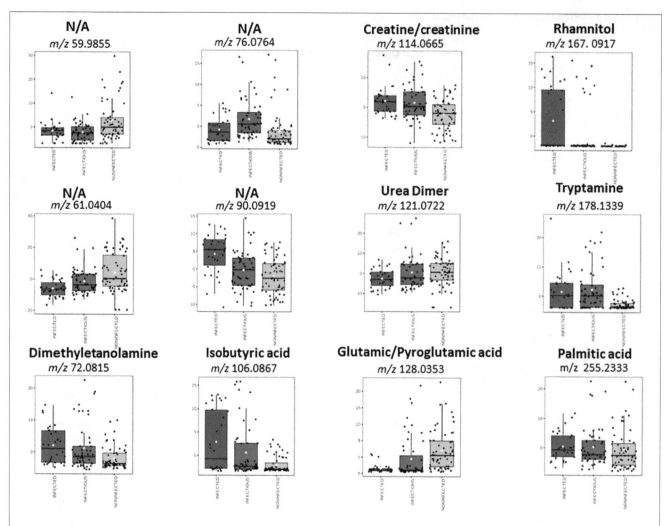

FIGURE 3 | Box plots that denote differences in normalized ion abundances for markers that contributed to the statistical discrimination between MAP infected, infectious and negative animals. The box plot diagrams were retrieved from Metaboanalyst web portal and used without further modification. The bottom and top of the boxes represent the 25th and 75th percentiles, the line in the middle indicates the 50th percentile or the median. The black circles represent the entire data range, including the extreme value outliers not taken into consideration. Three repetitions for each sample were used.

The lower urea level in MAP-infected cattle has already been reported by De Buck et al. (13), who interpreted this phenomenon as being due to increased muscle turnover, likely altering amino acid metabolism and reducing energy intake.

Interestingly, while De Buck et al. (13) observed increased glutamic acid in both MAP infected and control groups, due to the influence of developmental and diet changes of the life of the calves, we observed higher glutamic/pyroglutamic acid levels only in sera of negative animals. Glutamic acid is involved in energy metabolism, immunity and GI function. Its scarcity in infected and infectious animals could be explained by a low immune response when cattle are in the advanced JD stages and by the damage of GI system. Since glutamic acid is also produced by muscles, low serum levels could also be associated with muscle wasting.

Finally, pyroglutamic acid and glutamic acid are involved in glutathione (GSH) metabolism. Pyroglutamic acid is a downstream metabolite of GSH metabolism, and glutamic acid is involved in the synthesis of GSH. GSH is an important antioxidant that protects cells from oxidative stress. Both were lower in the sera of infected and infectious cattle than in that of negative cattle, suggesting that MAP alters GSH metabolism.

In conclusion potential caveats of this prospective field study on natural MAP infection in dairy cattle must be taken into account. Considering the long MAP incubation period, we do not exclude that negative animals could have changed their status after the latest sampling carried out at least 1 year after the selected time-point.

Note that we made any possible effort to reduce metabolic variability due to season, feeding and management, by: (i) testing all animals (except young heifers) during the pre-calving period and (ii) matching negative animals to cases by sampling date and age category. Finally, individual differences could have affected the results because of the small sized groups.

CONCLUSION

The main goal of mid-level data fusion is to optimize high dimensional information, exploit the synergies of information provided by different analytical strategies, and fade out the existent correlations between markers and groups. The construction of this model using DART-HRMS data revealed the characteristic serum metabolites of MAP infected, infectious, and negative cattle. The model, built by fusing the three most informative DART-HRMS datasets, produced a reasonably high degree of accuracy, suggesting the markers are capable of discriminating the health status of cattle with regard to MAP infection. In the future, the model will be populated with results from more animals in order to improve its robustness and performance. Proper validation of the model will be performed to evaluate its discriminative capacity and verify its potential

for diagnostic purposes. Prospectively producing an earlier diagnosis, it will then be easier to manage infected cattle, prevent the diffusion of the pathogen and, thus, control JD on dairy farms.

ETHICS STATEMENT

The animal study was reviewed and approved by authorization n. 506/2015 of the Italian Ministry of Health. Written informed consent was obtained from the owners for the participation of their animals in this study.

AUTHOR CONTRIBUTIONS

NP, RP, LP, and JD designed the research. BM, MB, PF, MD, and AS performed the experiments. LP contributed to sampling. AM performed the statistical analyses. AT, IP, and AM interpreted the data and wrote the manuscript. NP, RP, and JD interpreted the results and edited the manuscript. All contributed to the editing the manuscript.

REFERENCES

1. Chacon O, Bermudez LE, Barletta RG. Johne's disease, inflammatory bowel disease, and *Mycobacterium paratuberculosis*. *Annu Rev Microbiol.* (2004) 58:329–63. doi: 10.1146/annurev.micro.58.030603.123726
2. Clarke CJ. The pathology and pathogenesis of paratuberculosis in ruminants and other species. *J Comp Pathol.* (1997) 116:217–61. doi: 10.1016/S0021-9975(97)80001-1
3. Whitlock RH, Buergelt C. Preclinical and clinical manifestations of paratuberculosis (including pathology). *Vet Clin North Am Food Anim Pract.* (1996) 12:345–56. doi: 10.1016/S0749-0720(15)30410-2
4. Lambrecht RS, Collins MT. Mycobacterium paratuberculosis. Factors that influence mycobactin dependence. *Diagn Microbiol Infect Dis.* (1992) 15:239–46. doi: 10.1016/0732-8893(92)90119-E
5. Sweeney RW. Transmission of paratuberculosis. *Vet Clin North Am Food Anim Pract.* (1996) 12:305–12. doi: 10.1016/S0749-0720(15)30408-4
6. Whittington R, Donat K, Weber MF, Kelton D, Nielsen SS, Eisenberg S, et al. Control of paratuberculosis: who, why and how. A review of 48 countries. *BMC Vet Res.* (2019) 15:198. doi: 10.1186/s12917-019-1943-4
7. Rankin JD. The experimental infection of cattle with mycobacterium johnei: IV. Adult cattle maintained in an infectious environment. *J Comp Pathol.* (1962) 72:113–7. doi: 10.1016/S0368-1742(62)80013-7
8. Nielsen SS, Toft N. Ante mortem diagnosis of paratuberculosis: a review of accuracies of ELISA, interferon-γ assay and faecal culture techniques. *Vet Microbiol.* (2008) 129:217–35. doi: 10.1016/j.vetmic.2007.12.011
9. Whitlock RH, Wells SJ, Sweeney RW, Van Tiem J. ELISA and fecal culture for paratuberculosis (Johne's disease): sensitivity and specificity of each method. *Vet Microbiol.* (2000) 77:387–98. doi: 10.1016/S0378-1135(00)00324-2
10. Arsenault RJ, Maattanen P, Daigle J, Potter A, Griebel P, Napper S. From mouth to macrophage: mechanisms of innate immune subversion by *Mycobacterium avium* subsp. paratuberculosis *Vet Res.* (2014) 45:54. doi: 10.1186/1297-9716-45-54
11. Casey JL, Sanalla AM, Tamvakis D, Thalmann C, Carroll EL, Parisi K, et al. Peptides specific for *Mycobacterium avium* subspecies paratuberculosis infection: diagnostic potential. *Protein Eng Des Sel.* (2011) 24:589–96. doi: 10.1093/protein/gzr026
12. David J, Barkema HW, Mortier R, Ghosh S, De Buck J. Gene expression profiling and putative biomarkers of calves 3 months after infection

with *Mycobacterium avium* subspecies paratuberculosis. *Vet Immunol Immunopathol.* (2014) 160:107–17. doi: 10.1016/j.vetimm.2014.04.006
13. De Buck J, Shaykhutdinov R, Barkema HW, Vogel HJ. Metabolomic profiling in cattle experimentally infected with *Mycobacterium avium* subsp. Paratuberculosis. *PLoS One.* (2014) 9:e111872. doi: 10.1371/journal.pone.0111872
14. Seth M, Lamont EA, Janagama HK, Widdel A, Vulchanova L, Stabel JR, et al. Biomarker discovery in subclinical mycobacterial infections of cattle. *PLoS One.* (2009) 4:e5478. doi: 10.1371/journal.pone.0005478
15. Skovgaard K, Grell SN, Heegaard PM, Jungersen G, Pudrith CB, Coussens PM. Differential expression of genes encoding CD30L and P-selectin in cattle with Johne's disease: progress toward a diagnostic gene expression signature. *Vet Immunol Immunopathol.* (2006) 112:210–24. doi: 10.1016/j.vetimm.2006.02.006
16. Zhong L, Taylor D, Begg DJ, Whittington RJ. Biomarker discovery for ovine paratuberculosis (Johne's disease) by proteomic serum profiling. *Comp Immunol Microbiol Infect Dis.* (2011) 34:315–26. doi: 10.1016/j.cimid.2011.03.001
17. Wood PL, Erol E, Hoffsis GF, Steinman M, DeBuck J. Serum lipidomics of bovine paratuberculosis: disruption of choline-containing glycerophospholipids and sphingolipids. *SAGE Open Med.* (2018) 6:2050312118775302. doi: 10.1177/2050312118775302
18. Bergmann A, Trefz P, Fischer S, Klepik K, Walter G, Steffens M, et al. *In vivo* volatile organic compound signatures of *Mycobacterium avium* subsp. Paratuberculosis. *PLoS One.* (2015) 10:e0123980. doi: 10.1371/journal.pone.0123980
19. Mehaffy C, Kruh-Garcia NA, Graham B, Jarlsberg LG, Willyerd CE, Borisov A, et al. Identification of *Mycobacterium tuberculosis* peptides in serum extracellular vesicles from persons with latent tuberculosis infection. *J Clin Microbiol.* (2020) 58:e00393-20. doi: 10.1128/JCM.00393-20
20. Cody RB, McAlpin CR, Cox CR, Jensen KR, Voorhees KJ. Identification of bacteria by fatty acid profiling with direct analysis in real time mass spectrometry. *Rapid Commun Mass Spectrom.* (2015) 29:2007–12. doi: 10.1002/rcm.7309
21. Gu H, Pan Z, Xi B, Asiago V, Musselman B, Raftery D. Principal component directed partial least squares analysis for combining nuclear magnetic resonance and mass spectrometry data in metabolomics: application to the detection of breast cancer. *Anal Chim Acta.* (2011) 686:57–63. doi: 10.1016/j.aca.2010.11.040

188   Handbook of Veterinary Microbiology and Disease

22. Guo T, Yong W, Jin Y, Zhang L, Liu J, Wang S, et al. Applications of DART-MS for food quality and safety assurance in food supply chain. *Mass Spectrom Rev.* (2017) 36:161–87. doi: 10.1002/mas.21466

23. Halouzka R, Zeljković SC, Klejdus B, Tarkowski P. Analytical methods in strigolactone research. *Plant Methods.* (2020) 16:1–13. doi: 10.1186/s13007-020-00616-2

24. Li Y. Application of DART-MS in clinical and pharmacological analysis. *Direct Anal Real Time Mass Spectrom.* (2018) 223–40. doi: 10.1002/9783527803705.ch9

25. Miano, B., Righetti, L., Piro, R., Dall'Asta, C., Folloni, S., Galaverna, G., et al. (2018). Direct analysis real-time-high-resolution mass spectrometry for *Triticum* species authentication. *Food Addit Contam A* 35:2291–7. doi: 10.1080/19440049.2018.1520398

26. Pavlovich MJ, Musselman B, Hall AB. Direct analysis in real time-Mass spectrometry (DART-MS) in forensic and security applications. *Mass Spectrom Rev.* (2018) 37:171–87. doi: 10.1002/mas.21509

27. Pozzato N, Piva E, Pallante I, Bombana D, Stella R, Zanardello C, et al. Rapid detection of asperphenamate in a hay batch associated with constipation and deaths in dairy cattle. The application of DART-HRMS to veterinary forensic toxicology. *Toxicon.* (2020) 187:122–8. doi: 10.1016/j.toxicon.2020.08.022

28. Song, Y.-,q., Liao, J., Zha, C., Wang, B., and Liu, C. C. (2015). A novel approach to determine the tyrosine concentration in human plasma by DART-MS/MS. *Anal Methods.* 7:1600–5. doi: 10.1039/C4AY02566K

29. Wang C, Zhu H, Cai Z, Song F, Liu Z, Liu S. Newborn screening of phenylketonuria using direct analysis in real time (DART) mass spectrometry. *Anal Bioanal Chem.* (2013) 405:3159–64. doi: 10.1007/s00216-013-6713-8

30. Riuzzi G, Tata A, Massaro A, Bisutti V, Lanza I, Contiero B, et al. Authentication of forage-based milk by mid-level data fusion of (+/−) DART-HRMS signatures. *Int Dairy J.* (2021) 112:104859. doi: 10.1016/j.idairyj.2020.104859

31. Aszyk J, Kubica P, Wozniak MK, Namieśnik J, Wasik A, Kot-Wasik A. Evaluation of flavour profiles in e-cigarette refill solutions using gas chromatography-tandem mass spectrometry. *J Chromatogr A.* (2018) 1547:86–98. doi: 10.1016/j.chroma.2018.03.009

32. You Q, Verschoor CP, Pant SD, Macri J, Kirby GM, Karrow NA. Proteomic analysis of plasma from Holstein cows testing positive for *Mycobacterium avium* subsp. paratuberculosis (MAP). *Vet Immunol Immunopathol.* (2012) 148:243–51. doi: 10.1016/j.vetimm.2012.05.002

33. Biancolillo A, Bucci R, Magrì AL, Magrì AD, Marini F. Data-fusion for multiplatform characterization of an Italian craft beer aimed at its authentication. *Anal Chim Acta.* (2014) 820:23–31. doi: 10.1016/j.aca.2014.02.024

34. Pirro V, Oliveri P, Ferreira CR, González-Serrano AF, Machaty Z, Cooks RG. Lipid characterization of individual porcine oocytes by dual mode DESI-MS and data fusion. *Anal Chim Acta.* (2014) 848:51–60. doi: 10.1016/j.aca.2014.08.001

35. Pozzato N, Gwozdz J, Gastaldelli M, Capello K, Dal Ben C, Stefani E. Evaluation of a rapid and inexpensive liquid culture system for the detection of *Mycobacterium avium* subsp. paratuberculosis in bovine faeces. *J. Microbiol. Methods.* (2011) 84:413–7. doi: 10.1016/j.mimet.2011.01.019

36. Pozzato N, Stefani E, Capello K, Muliari R, Vicenzoni G. *Mycobacterium avium* subsp. paratuberculosis as a template in the evaluation of automated kits for DNA extraction from bovine organs. *World J Microbiol Biotechnol.* (2011) 27:31–7. doi: 10.1007/s11274-010-0423-6

37. Chong, J., Soufan, O., Li, C., Caraus, I., Li, S., Bourque, G., et al. (2018). MetaboAnalyst 4.0: towards more transparent and integrative metabolomics analysis. *Nucleic Acids Res.* 46:W486–W94. doi: 10.1093/nar/gky310

38. Alves JO, Botelho BG, Sena MM, Augusti R. Electrospray ionization mass spectrometry and partial least squares discriminant analysis applied to the quality control of olive oil. *J Mass Spectrom.* (2013) 48:1109–15. doi: 10.1002/jms.3256

39. Woolman M, Ferry I, Kuzan-Fischer CM, Wu M, Zou J, Kiyota T, et al. Rapid determination of medulloblastoma subgroup affiliation with mass spectrometry using a handheld picosecond infrared laser desorption probe. *Chem Sci.* (2017) 8:6508–19. doi: 10.1039/C7SC01974B

40. Chong J, Wishart DS, Xia J. Using MetaboAnalyst 4.0 for comprehensive and integrative metabolomics data analysis. *Curr Protoc Bioinfor.* (2019) 68:e86. doi: 10.1002/cpbi.86

41. Borràs, E., Ferré, J., Boqué, R., Mestres, M., Aceña, L., Calvo, A., et al. Olive oil sensory defects classification with data fusion of instrumental techniques and multivariate analysis (PLS-DA). *Food Chem.* (2016) 203:314–22. doi: 10.1016/j.foodchem.2016.02.038

42. Borràs E, Ferré J, Boqué R, Mestres M, Aceña L, Busto O. Data fusion methodologies for food and beverage authentication and quality assessment - a review. *Anal Chim Acta.* (2015) 891:1–14. doi: 10.1016/j.aca.2015.04.042

43. Blasco H, Błaszczyński J, Billaut J-C, Nadal-Desbarats L, Pradat P-F, Devos D, et al. Comparative analysis of targeted metabolomics: dominance-based rough set approach versus orthogonal partial least square-discriminant analysis. *J Biomed Inform.* (2015) 53:291–9. doi: 10.1016/j.jbi.2014.12.001

44. Worley B, Powers R. Multivariate analysis in metabolomics. *Curr Metab.* (2013) 1:92–107. doi: 10.2174/2213235X130108

45. Triba MN, Le Moyec L, Amathieu R, Goossens C, Bouchemal N, Nahon P, et al. PLS/OPLS models in metabolomics: the impact of permutation of dataset rows on the K-fold cross-validation quality parameters. *Mol BioSyst.* (2015) 11:13–9. doi: 10.1039/C4MB00414K

46. Kiralj R, Ferreira M. Basic validation procedures for regression models in QSAR and QSPR studies: theory and application. *J Braz Chem Soc.* (2009) 20:770–87. doi: 10.1590/S0103-50532009000400021

47. Roy GL, De Buck J, Wolf R, Mortier RAR, Orsel K, Barkema HW. Experimental infection with *Mycobacterium avium* subspecies paratuberculosis resulting in decreased body weight in Holstein-Friesian calves. *Can Vet J.* (2017) 58:296–8.

48. Thirunavukkarasu S, Plain KM, de Silva K, Begg D, Whittington RJ, Purdie AC. Expression of genes associated with cholesterol and lipid metabolism identified as a novel pathway in the early pathogenesis of Mycobacterium avium subspecies paratuberculosis-infection in cattle. *Vet Immunol Immunopathol.* (2014) 160:147–57. doi: 10.1016/j.vetimm.2014.04.002

49. Collins JM, Walker DI, Jones DP, Tukvadze N, Liu KH, Tran VT, et al. High-resolution plasma metabolomics analysis to detect *Mycobacterium tuberculosis*-associated metabolites that distinguish active pulmonary tuberculosis in humans. *PLoS One.* (2018) 13:e0205398. doi: 10.1371/journal.pone.0205398

50. Shipkowski KA, Sanders JM, McDonald JD, Garner CE, Doyle-Eisele M, Wegerski CJ, et al. Comparative disposition of dimethylaminoethanol and choline in rats and mice following oral or intravenous administration. *Toxicol Appl Pharmacol.* (2019) 378:114592. doi: 10.1016/j.taap.2019.05.011

21

A Virulent *Trueperella pyogenes* Isolate, which Causes Severe Bronchoconstriction in Porcine Precision-Cut Lung Slices

Lei Qin [1,2†], Fandan Meng [1†], Haijuan He [3], Yong-Bo Yang [1], Gang Wang [1], Yan-Dong Tang [1], Mingxia Sun [1], Wenlong Zhang [2], Xuehui Cai [1*] and Shujie Wang [1*]

[1] National Key Laboratory of Veterinary Biotechnology, Harbin Veterinary Research Institute, Chinese Academy of Agricultural Sciences, Harbin, China, [2] College of Veterinary Medicine, Northeast Agricultural University, Harbin, China, [3] Institute of Animal Husbandry, Heilongjiang Academy of Agriculture Sciences, Harbin, China

*Correspondence:
Xuehui Cai
caixuehui@caas.cn
Shujie Wang
wangshujie@caas.cn

† These authors have contributed equally to this work

Trueperella pyogenes causes disease in cattle, sheep, goats and swine, and is involved occasionally in human disease worldwide. Most reports implicating *T. pyogenes* have been associated with clinical cases, whereas no report has focused on pathogenicity of *T. pyogenes* in mouse models or precision-cut lung slice (PCLS) cultures from swine. Here, we isolated and identified a virulent, β-hemolytic, multidrug-resistant *T. pyogenes* strain named 20121, which harbors the virulence marker genes *fimA*, *fimE*, *nanH*, *nanP* and *plo*. It was found to be highly resistant to erythromycin, azithromycin and medemycin. Strain 20121 was pathogenic in mouse infection models, displaying pulmonary congestion and inflammatory cell infiltration, partial degeneration in epithelial cells of the tracheal and bronchiolar mucosa, a small amount of inflammatory cell infiltration in the submucosa, and bacteria ($>10^4$ CFU/g) in the lung. Importantly, we used *T. pyogenes* 20121 to infect porcine precision-cut lung slices (PCLS) cultures for the first time, where it caused severe bronchoconstriction. Furthermore, dexamethasone showed its ability to relieve bronchoconstriction in PCLS caused by *T. pyogenes* 20121, highlighting dexamethasone may assist antibiotic treatment for clinical *T. pyogenes* infection. This is the first report of *T. pyogenes* used to infect and cause bronchoconstriction in porcine PCLS. Our results suggest that porcine PCLS cultures as a valuable 3D organ model for the study of *T. pyogenes* infection and treatment *in vitro*.

Keywords: *Trueperella pyogenes*, porcine precision-cut lung slices, virulent, bronchoconstriction, infection

INTRODUCTION

Trueperella pyogenes is a Gram-positive, non-motile, non-spore-forming, short, rod- to coccobacillus-shaped bacterium that occurs singly, in pairs or in clusters. *T. pyogenes* was previously called *Corynebacterium pyogenes*, *Actinomyces pyogenes* and *Arcanobacterium pyogenes*, in chronological order (1, 2). In 2011, according to Yassin et al., *Arcanobacterium pyogenes* was renamed as *T. pyogenes* based on phylogenetic and chemotaxonomic observations (2).

T. pyogenes expresses several established and putative virulence factors. To date, known virulence factors mainly include exotoxin pyolysin (PLO), and others promote adhesion factors such as fimbriae (Fim), neuraminidase (NanH, NanP) and collagen-binding protein (CbpA) (3, 4). The cytolysin PLO is considered to be a major virulence factor, associated with cell damage induced by *T. pyogenes* infection (5). Adhesion factors may be associated with mucosal adherence and colonization of host tissues, thereby contributing to the pathogenicity of *T. pyogenes* (3).

The use of precision-cut lung slices (PCLS) in three-dimensional (3D) organ models is becoming an area of intensive research due to its close similarity to the host environment (6, 7). There are many advantages in the use of PCLS, including isolated tracheal rings and bronchial rings, and the contraction of airway (7). PCLS have been commonly used in the study of viral infections (8), but there have been few studies on bacterial pathogens (9). Porcine PCLS have been reported for the study of *Streptococcus suis* (10, 11), but never for *T. pyogenes*.

Here, we used a porcine PCLS model to study a *T. pyogenes* isolate, showing that infection of lung tissues by strain 20121 (isolated and characterized from lung tissues of clinically diseased pigs) resulted in severe bronchoconstriction. This study demonstrates that porcine PCLS is a suitable 3D organ model for the study of pathogenicity of *T. pyogenes* in vitro.

MATERIALS AND METHODS

Ethics Statement

All animal experiments were conducted in accordance with the Guide for the Care and Use of Laboratory Animals of the Ministry of Science and Technology of the People's Republic of China. Mouse infection experiments (approval number 210119-02) were carried out in the animal biosafety level 2 facilities under the supervision of the Committee on the Ethics of Animal Experiments of the Harbin Veterinary Research Institute of the Chinese Academy of Agricultural Sciences (CAAS) and the Animal Ethics Committee of Heilongjiang Province, China.

Bacterial Strains

The novel *T. pyogenes* strain 20121 was isolated from the lungs of two sick nursery pigs with pneumonia and severe abdominal effusion from a pig farm in Heilongjiang Province of China in 2020. The lung samples were cultured on Columbia-based blood agar media (ThermoFisher Scientific, Beijing, China) for 36 h at 37 °C. The isolated colonies were cultured for 36–48 h in tryptic soy agar (TSA, Difco, Loveton Circle Sparks, MD, USA) plates supplemented with 5% fetal bovine serum (FBS, CLARK, USA) at 37 °C and inoculated in tryptic soy broth (TSB, Difco, Loveton Circle Sparks, MD, USA) supplemented with 5% FBS for extraction of genomic DNA.

The isolate 20121 in TSB was observed after rapid Gram stain (AOBOX, Beijing, China) following standard procedure using an optical microscope (Primo Star, ZEISS). Furthermore, the isolate was prepared with standard electron microscopy procedures and the morphological structure was observed using a Hitachi H-7650 transmission electron microscope.

TABLE 1 | 16S RNA and the virulence factor genes used in this study.

Target gene	Primers (5′-3′)	Size of target amplicon (bp)
16S rRNA	5′-AGAGTTTGATCCTGGCTCAG-3′	1,465
	5′-TACGGCTACCTTGTTACGACTT-3′	
cbpA	5′-GCAGGGTTGGTGAAAGAGTTTACT-3′	124
	5′-GCTTGATATAACCTTCAGAATTTGCA-3′	
fimA	5′-CACTACGCTCACCATTCACAAG-3′	605
	5′-GCTGTAATCCGCTTTGTCTGTG-3′	
fimC	5′-TGTCGAAGGTGACGTTCTTCG-3′	843
	5′-CAAGGTCACCGAGACTGCTGG-3′	
fimE	5′-GCCCAGGACCGAGAGCGAGGGC-3′	775
	5′-GCCTTCACAAATAACAGCAACC-3′	
fimG	5′-ACGCTTCAGAAGGTCACCAGG-3′	929
	5′-ATCTTGATCTGCCCCCATGCG-3′	
nan-H	5′-CGCTAGTGCTGTAGCGTTGTTAAGT-3′	781
	5′-CCGAGGAGTTTTGACTGACTTTGT-3′	
nan-P[1]	5′-ATGATGAGCGCCCGCGTGGGCGGGGGTA-3′	2,275
	5′-TAACCGAGTTCGCCGCAAGCGCTAGTTT-3′	
plo	5′-GGCCCGAATGTCACCGC-3′	270
	5′-AACTCCGCCTCTAGCGC-3′	

1, Designed for use in current study.

PCR Detection

Genomic DNA of *T. pyogenes* 20121 was extracted by a Bacterial DNA Extraction Kit (Tiangen, Beiing, China) following the manufacturer's instructions. *T. pyogenes* was positively identified by detecting the 16S rRNA (12) products through PCR. The virulence factors of *T. pyogenes* 20121 were detected by PCR (13), including hemolysin (pyolysin, PLO), collagen-binding protein (CbpA), neuraminidase (NanH and NanP), and fimbriae (FimA, FimC, FimE and FimG). The primer sequences and reaction conditions are listed in **Table 1**. PCR products were subsequently analyzed by loading to 1% agarose gels with 2000 bp marker (Tiangen, Beiing, China) and purified with a Gel Extraction Kit (OMEGA, New York, USA). Then, the PCR products were cloned into a pMD18-T vector (Takara, Dalian, China) and positive clones were sequenced by Comate Bioscience Company Ltd.

Antibiotic Susceptibility Test

The susceptibility of *T. pyogenes* 20121 to different antibiotics was determined by the drug sensitive paper disc diffusion method, according to the Clinical and Laboratory Standards Institute (CLSI) guidelines (2016). The following antimicrobials were used: cefazolin, nitrofurantoin, erythromycin, chloramphenicol, kanamycin, ampicillin, ceftazidime, clarithromycin, meropenem, azithromycin, trimethoprim, medemycin, spiramycin, fosfomycin, ceftriaxone, cefoxitin, streptomycin, tetracycline, ciprofloxacin and vancomycin (Tianhe, Hangzhou, China). The quality control strain *Streptococcus pneumoniae* (ATCC49619) was stored in our lab (12).

TABLE 2 | *Trueperella pyogenes 16S rRNA* genes referenced in this study.

Strain	Isolation source	Host	Country	Accession no.
NIAH 13535	Abscess in leg of swine	Sus scrofa	Japan	LC500012
NIAH 13534	The lung of diseased swine	Sus scrofa	Japan	LC500011
24398	Vaginal discharge	Okapia johnstoni	Germany	MN946520
HC-H 13-2	Uterine secretions	Cattle	China, Liaoning	EU268191
TP6375	Uterus with metritis	Dairy cow	USA	CP007519
DAT1453	Ileum	Sus scrofa	Japan	LC500013
Bu8-2B2	Abortion material	Bubalus bubalis	India	MG461533
H9	Intrauterine fluid	Buffalo	China, Guangxi	KC894522
DTK434	Abscess in the brain of goat	Capra hircus	Japan	LC500006
DTK435	The lung of diseased sheep	Ovis aries	Japan	LC500004
G	Lung	Calf	China, Hebei	KP159746
S 1276/1/18	Lung	Lynx	Germany	MN135984
171003246	Kidney	Python regius	Germany	MN712476
141010414	Brain abscess	Capreolus capreolus	Germany	KX815984
TP8	Pus	forest musk deer	China, Sichuan	CP007003
TP2	Knee joint	Bovine	China, Jilin	CP033903
XJXBMY-11-4NF	Lung with pneumonia	Bos Taurus	China, Xinjiang	JQ975936
M29	Pus samples	Forest musk deer	China, Sichuan	JN578115
scnu001	Pus	Goat	South Korea	MT775813
11-07-D-03394	Facial abscess	gray slender lorises	Germany	HG530069
TP3	Lung	Swine	China, Jilin	CP033904
Truep25	Pus	Swine	Brazil	KJ930040
AUVF-TRU_19	Vaginal swab	Cattle	Turkey	MN907639
FL-1	Pus	Goat	China, Chongqing	KX462008
XJALT-127-2YF1	Lung	Goat	China, Xinjiang	JX975440
HJ-4	Pus	Dairy cattle	China, Hei Longjiang	GU372928
TP-2849	Lung	Swine	China, Jilin	CP029004
2012CQ-ZSH	Goat lung tissue	Capra aegagrus	China, Chongqing	CP012649
15A0121	Abortion (placenta)	Bos taurus	Switzerland	CP063213
19OD0592	Lung	Sus scrofa	Switzerland	CP063212
SCDR 1	Patient	Homo sapiens	Saudi Arabia	CP034038
jx18	Lung	Swine	China, Jiangxi	CP050810
TP4	Lung	Swine	China, Jilin	CP033905
TP1	Lung	Bovine	China, Jilin	CP033902
Arash114	Uterine secretions	Water Buffalo	Iran: Tehran	CP028833
FC3480	Patient	Homo sapiens	China	MK611773
nck254a04c1	Skin, antecubital fossa	Homo sapiens	USA	KF098604
S350	Cord blood unit	Bovine	Portugal	KR232876
P504064-19-1	Abortion material	Pig	United Kingdom	MW332266
IMMIB L-1653	Abortus	Sus scrofa	Germany	HE575404
JCM 14813	Sow placenta after abortion	Sow	Japan	LC500014
Murakami	Placenta of an aborted sow	Sow	Japan: Chiba	NR 041607

Phylogenetic Analysis

The similarities between the nucleotide sequences recovered from isolate 20121 and the reference *T. pyogenes* sequence published in GenBank were aligned using BLAST online search tool (http://blast.ncbi.nlm.nih.gov). Phylogenetic trees of genes *16S rRNA* and *plo* sequences were constructed with MEGA V 7.0 using the neighbor-joining method and a bootstrap validation with 1,000 replications. Branches corresponding to partitions reproduced in <50% bootstrap replicates were collapsed and shown above the branches. Data from the *T. pyogenes 16S rRNA* and *plo* genes used for phylogenetic trees are listed in **Tables 2, 3**.

Experimental Mouse Infection

To investigate the virulence of *T. pyogenes* 20121, a mouse survival experiment was carried out. Briefly, 35 six-week-old

TABLE 3 | *Trueperella pyogenes pyolysin* genes referenced in this study.

Strain	Isolation source	Host	Country	Accession no.
24398	Vaginal discharge	Okapia johnstoni	Germany	MN956806
S 1276/1/18	Lung	Lynx	Germany	MN163264
171003246	Kidney	Python regius	Germany	MN741110
DTK435	The lung of diseased sheep	Ovis aries	Japan	LC500001
DTK434	Abscess in the brain of goat	Capra hircus	Japan	LC500002
FMV13	Uterus	Bovine	Portugal	KJ150328
HJ-3	Pus	Dairy cattle	China, Helongjiang	HQ637573
TP2	Knee joint	Bovine	China, Jilin	CP033903
jx18	Lung	Swine	China, Jiangxi	CP050810
NIAH 13534	The lung of diseased swine	Sus scrofa	Japan	LC500003
2012CQ-ZSH	Goat lung tissue	Capra aegagrus hircus	China, Chongqing	CP012649
TP6375	Uterus with metritis	Dairy cow	USA	CP007519
Arash114	Uterine secretions	Water Buffalo	Iran: Tehran	CP028833
TP8	Pus	Forest musk deer	China, Sichuan	CP007003

(18–20 g) female C57BL/6 mice (Changsheng Biotechnology, Liaoning, China) were randomly divided into 5 groups including a non-infection control. The mice were challenged intraperitoneally (i.p.) with 0.2 ml bacterial suspension containing strain 20121 (2×10^6, 2×10^7, 2×10^8 and 2×10^9 CFU) or sterile TSB. Each group contained 6 mice except for the group receiving 2×10^6 CFU, which had 11 mice. Clinical symptoms and mortality were recorded for 14 days, during which any mice exhibiting extreme lethargy were considered moribund and were humanely euthanized. Samples of blood and organs (lung, trachea, heart, liver, ileum, duodenum, spleen and thymus) of infected mice were collected and observed for gross pathological changes. Organ/body weight (g/g) × 100% was calculated and organ samples were fixed immediately in 3.7% formaldehyde (Amresco, Fountain Parkway, USA) for histopathological examination. 5 µl of anticoagulated blood and lung samples were serially diluted in PBS, and plated on blood agar medium for 36 h, and the bacteria in blood and lung samples were quantified by colony counting. 60 µl of anticoagulated blood was tested by a ProCyte Dx automatic blood cell analyzer (IDEXX, USA), determining white blood cell count (WBC), reticulocyte (RET), platelet (PLT), neutrophilic granulocyte percentage (NEUT%), lymphatic number percentage (LYMP%), monocyte percentage (MONO%), eosinophil percentage (EO%) and hematocrit percentage (HCT%).

T. pyogenes 20121 Infection of Porcine PCLS

Fresh lung tissue was obtained after euthanasia from three 3-month-old SPF pigs from Harbin Veterinary Research Institute. The cranial, middle, and intermediate lobes were filled with low-melting agarose (Promega, Madison WI, USA) along the bronchus gently as described previously (14). The filling tissue were covered by ice until the agarose became solidified, then the tissue was stamped out as cylindrical portions with 8-mm tissue coring tool and precision slices were further prepared by a

Krumdieck tissue slicer (model MD6000-01; TSE Systems). The PCLS were carefully picked up into 24-well plat (one slice/well) maintained with 1ml fresh medium for additional cultivation for 24 h. Then the airway epithelial cells with 100% ciliary activity were divided randomly into three groups. PCLS were washed 3 times with PBS, then inoculated with *T. pyogenes* 20121 (8×10^4 CFU or 8×10^5 CFU per slice) in a humidified atmosphere containing 5% CO_2 at 37 °C, mock-infected slices were used as control. Infected slices were washed three times with PBS to remove non-attached bacteria at 4 h post-inoculation (hpi), and 1 ml fresh medium (1640, Gibco, Beijing, China) was added for further cultivation.

T. pyogenes 20121-induced bronchoconstriction was detected by imaging and measurement of bronchial cavity area. Initial bronchial cavity area was calculated for each PCLS by imaging at 0 hpi by inverted light microscope (EVOS FL Auto, ThermoFisher Scientific). To quantify the relative bronchoconstriction of the lung tissue, bronchial cavity positions in each infected and mock-infected PCLS were imaged at 4 and 24 hpi. Bronchial cavity areas were measured and calculated using ImageJ/Fiji and the results were presented as bronchial contraction percentage (BCP) using the formula, BCP = [reduced bronchial cavity area / initial bronchial cavity area] × 100%. Treatments were carried out in triplicate and experiments were repeated at least three times.

In order to evaluate the drug intervention effect on bronchoconstriction induced by *T. pyogenes* 20121, several bronchodilators were selected and applied in this study. Dexamethasone (785 µg/ml in final concentration), atropine (300 µg/ml in final concentration), aminophylline (420.43 µg/ml in final concentration), α-Terpineol (168 µg/ml in final concentration) or salbutamol (250 µg/ml in final concentration) were added at the time of inoculation with strain 20121 (8×10^5 CFU), and then non-attached bacteria were removed at 4 hpi followed by adding fresh medium containing the appropriate drugs.

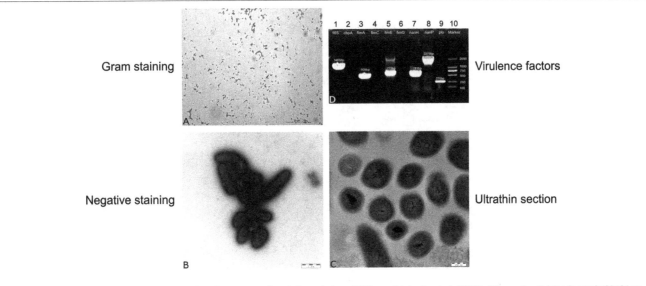

FIGURE 1 | Morphological evaluation and screening of genes encoding virulence factors. **(A)** Gram staining for strain 20121, **(B)** negative staining for strain 20121 on transmission electron microscope **(C)** ultrathin section for strain 20121 on transmission electron microscope, **(D)** PCR analysis of virulence factors genes, 1: *16S-rRNA*, 2: *cbpA*, 3: *fimA*, 4: *fimC*, 5: *fimE*, 6: *fimG*, 7: *nan-H*, 8: *nan-P*, 9: *plo*, 10: Marker.

Statistical Analyses

Numerical data were expressed as the mean ± standard deviation (SD). Statistical analysis of the results was performed with one- or two-way ANOVA using GraphPad Prism version 9.00 (GraphPad, San Diego, CA, USA). Statistical significance was evaluated based on Bonferroni post-tests, and $p < 0.05$ was considered statistically significant.

RESULTS

Morphological Evaluation and Virulence Factors of *T. pyogenes* 20121

Strain 20121 was isolated from two lungs of two sick pigs from Heilongjiang Province of China in December 2020. The isolate shows a narrow zone of β-hemolysis with 0.1-mm hemolytic rings and formed small, white, wet, smooth, and glossy colonies on Columbia blood agar media after culturing for 48 h. It is a Gram-positive coccobacilli or short coryneform occuring in single or pairs (**Figure 1A**). Electron micrographs of negative staining showed that the isolate were corynebacteria (**Figure 1B**). Electron micrographs of ultrathin sections showed the strain was most likely encapsulated with 10–25 nm cell wall thickness (**Figure 1C**). *16S rRNA* sequencing indicated that the isolate was *T. pyogenes*, which harbored virulence factor genes *plo*, *fimA*, *fimE*, *nanH* and *nanP*.

Sequence Comparison and Phylogenetic Analysis of Strain 20121

Genes *16S rRNA, plo, fimA, fimE, nanH, nanP* of strain 20121 were sequenced and compared to *T. pyogenes* strains in NCBI GenBank. *16S rRNA* sequence of strain 20121 shared >94% nucleotide identity with sequences in GenBank (**Figure 1D**). In addition, the virulence factors *plo* (accession MZ189360), *fimA* (accession MZ189359), *fimE* (accession MZ579543) and *nanP*

(accession MZ579545) were highly similar, sharing >96, >98, >96, and >97% nucleotide identity, respectively, with sequences in GenBank. The *nanH* sequence (accession MZ579544) from strain 20121 was less similar, with only 81–89% nucleotide identity with homologous sequences from *T. pyogenes* strains in GenBank.

To analyze the evolutionary relationship between strain 20121 and other *T. pyogenes* strains, we constructed phylogenetic trees based on the *16S rRNA* **Figure 2A** and *plo* **Figure 2B**. As shown in **Figure 2**, strain 20121 is located within lineage 1 of the trees based on the *16S rRNA* and *plo* genes, in the same lineage as most Chinese and other Asian isolates, and some European ones. The sequences within lineage 1 shared >99 and >98% nucleotide identity, respectively.

Antimicrobial Susceptibility Profiles of Strain 20121

In order to determine the drug resistance profile and thus the best way to potentially treat sick animals, we tested strain 20121 for susceptibility to cefazolin, nitrofurantoin, erythromycin, chloramphenicol, kanamycin, ampicillin, ceftazidime, clarithromycin, meropenem, azithromycin, trimethoprim, medemycin, spiramycin, fosfomycin, ceftriaxone, cefoxitin, streptomycin, tetracycline, ciprofloxacin and vancomycin. The test strain was highly resistant to erythromycin, azithromycin and medemycin, with growth exclusion diameters of 6 mm, 10 mm, and 8 mm, respectively, while it was sensitive to the other antibiotics.

Virulence Evaluation of 20121 Isolate in Mice

To evaluate the virulence of strain 20121 *in vivo*, we injected six-week-old C57BL/6 mice and tracked their survival and clinical signs. The mice infected with 20121 exhibited depression,

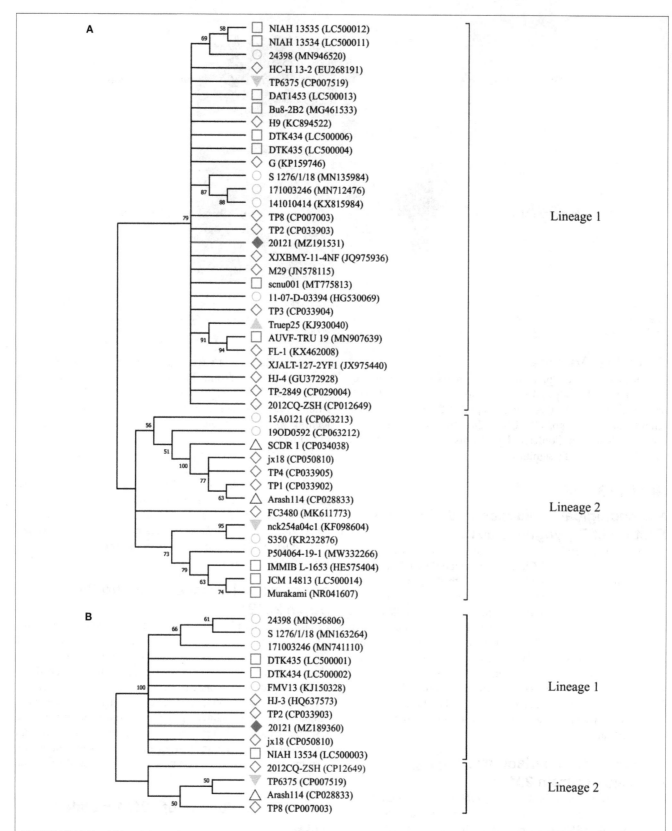

FIGURE 2 | Neighbor-joining phylogenetic trees for *16S RNA* and *plo* genes. **A**: the phylogenetic trees for 16S RNA gene; **B**: the phylogenetic trees for plo genes. Branches corresponding to partitions reproduced in <50% bootstrap replicates are collapsed. The percentage of replicate trees in which the associated taxa clustered together in the bootstrap test (1,000 replicates) are shown above the branches. ♦ denotes the genes sequenced in this study; ◇ indicates the reference sequences isolated from China; while □ indicates sequences isolated from the rest of Asia; ○ are sequences isolated from European countries; △ indicates isolated reports from the Middle Eastern countries, ▲ was from a South American country and ▼ denotes isolates from North American countries.

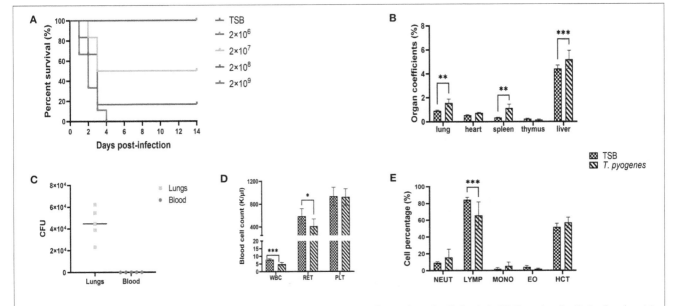

FIGURE 3 | Virulence of *T. pyogenes* strain 20121 in a mouse model. Mice were challenged intraperitoneally with the strain 20121, as described in the Experimental Procedure. **(A)** Survival percentage of mice inoculated with strain 20121 or tryptic soy broth (TSB; control). **(B)** Organ coefficients after 20121 infection at 2 dpi. **(C)** Bacterial loads in lung (CFU/g of tissue) and blood (CFU/ml). **(D)** White blood cell (WBC), reticulocyte (RET) and platelet (PLT) count after *T. pyogenes* infection. **(E)** Percentage of neutrophilic granulocyte (NEUT), lymphatic number (LYMP), monocyte (MONO), eosinophil (EO), hematocrit (HCT) after *T. pyogenes* infection. Results are expressed as means ± S.D., and significance was determined using two-way ANOVA and the Sidak multiple-comparison test. *$p < 0.05$; **$p < 0.01$; ***$p < 0.001$.

trembling, exuberant periocular secretion and fecal adhesions at the anus after injecting 20121, and the clinical signs were bacteria dose-dependent. In the higher dose groups, all of the mice receiving 2×10^9 CFU and most (5/6) of the mice who received 2×10^8 CFU died. The survival percentage of the 2×10^7 CFU and 2×10^6 CFU groups were 50% and 100%, respectively (**Figure 3A**).

On 2 dpi, five mice in the 2×10^6 CFU group and three control mice were sacrificed, and the main gross lesions in various organs were visualized. Organ-body weight ratios for lung, heart, spleen, thymus and liver were calculated. As shown in **Figure 3B**, all coefficients of the lungs, spleen and liver were significantly increased ($p < 0.01$). In addition, bacteria were detected in the lungs of infected mice, revealing higher levels (>10^4 CFU/g tissue) on 2 dpi (**Figure 3C**). No bacteremia was observed at 2 dpi as determined by colony count after plating 5 μl blood on blood agar media (**Figure 3C**).

T. pyogenes 20121 Infection Induces Abnormal Hematological Parameters

We used an automatic blood cell analyzer to detect WBC, RET, PLT, NEUT%, LYMP%, MONO%, EO% and HCT% at 2 dpi. *T. pyogenes* 20121 infection altered the expression of hematological parameters which can influence immunity. As shown in **Figure 3D**, the blood levels of WBC decreased significantly ($p < 0.001$) and RET decreased slightly ($p < 0.05$) at 2 dpi, and no significant differences in the levels of blood of PLT. Meanwhile, LYMP% in blood of infected mice had a significant decrease ($p < 0.001$), with 18.8% less than control mice at 2 dpi,

but no significant differences in NEUT, MONO, EO, and HCT% in blood (**Figure 3E**).

T. pyogenes 20121 Causes Histopathological Lesions in a Mouse Model

Histopathological lesions were determined in mice that were euthanized on 2 dpi (**Figure 4A**). In 20121-infected mice, the main histopathological lesions observed in the lungs were pulmonary congestion and inflammatory cell infiltration, moderately broadened alveolar diaphragm, partial degeneration in the epithelial cells of the tracheal and bronchial mucosa, and a small amount of inflammatory cell infiltration in the submucosa. In infected livers, extensive degeneration of hepatocytes, partial necrosis, and small focal clusters of Kupffer cells could be seen locally. Extensive necrosis and nuclear pyknosis of thymocytes and infiltration of inflammatory cells into the lamina propria of the chorionic mucosa were seen, along with massive necrosis of lymphocytes in the submucosal lymphatic tissue of the duodenum. A small amount of mucosal epithelial cells degenerated, necrosed and fell off, and Paneth cell degeneration was observed in the ileum (**Figure 4B**). The main histopathological lesions observed in the spleen were white pulp atrophy and lymphopenia. However, there was no significant changes in the infected heart tissue.

T. pyogenes 20121 Induces Severe Bronchoconstriction in PCLS Cultures

It has been reported that bacterial infection in the respiratory tract may contribute to development of bronchospasm and

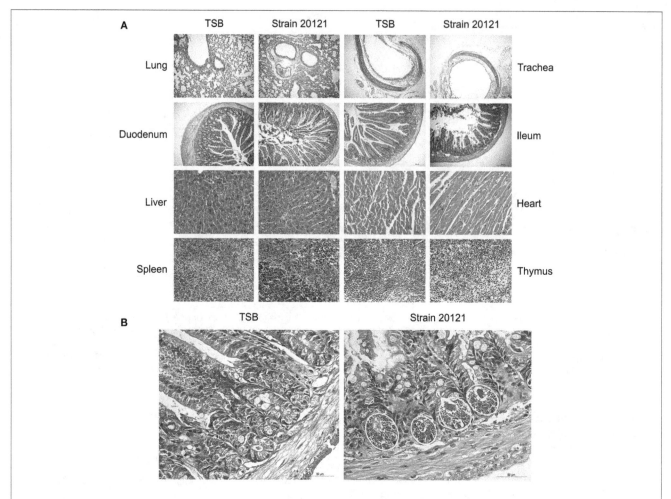

FIGURE 4 | Organ histopathology in mice infected with *T. pyogenes*. **(A)** Mice were infected with 2×10^6 CFU of *T. pyogenes* strain 20121 or inoculated with tryptic soy broth (TSB) as control. Lung, trachea, duodenum, ileum (scale bars = 200 μm), liver, heart, spleen and thymus (scale bars = 50 μm) were collected on 2 dpi for observation of histopathological lesions. **(B)** Ileum at 2 dpi, showing degeneration of mucosal epithelial cells, necrosis and sloughing, and Paneth cell degeneration (yellow oval); scale bars = 50 μm.

the progression of chronic obstructive pulmonary disease (COPD) (15). To further evaluate the damage to pig lungs induced by *T. pyogenes* 20121, we prepared the porcine PCLS and the preparation process was showed in **Figure 5A**. Then different doses were used to inoculate PCLS for 4 or 24 h. Interestingly, we found that *T. pyogenes* infection was able to cause obvious bronchoconstriction on PCLS (**Figure 5B**). A slightly constriction can be observed in bronchus of infected PCLS at 2 hpi. The bronchial cavities of infected PCLS showed obvious reduction in area relative to control PCLS at 4 hpi; the BCP of the 8×10^4 CFU group and 8×10^5 CFU group were nearly 77.11 and 82.44% (**Figure 5C**), respectively. At 24 hpi, the bronchial cavity area remained nearly 14% (BCP: 86.31%) in the 8×10^4 CFU group, and the area of bronchial cavity almost disappeared completely in 8×10^5 CFU group (BCP: 99.53%) comparing with controls (**Figure 5**). The observed airway closure was persistent and could not be relieved by the replacement of fresh medium. The high dose infectious group induced a faster bronchoconstriction response,

which indicates a dose-dependent capability of strain 20121 to trigger bronchoconstriction.

Dexamethasone Relieves the Bronchoconstriction Caused by Strain 20121

Bronchodilating drugs can dilate the bronchi and bronchioles to improve lung ventilation and relieve wheezing. Five common bronchodilators (dexamethasone, atropine, aminophylline, α-Terpineol and salbutamol) were selected and applied to the PCLS infection model in order to improve bronchospasm and relieve bronchoconstriction caused by *T. pyogenes* infection. Among the five, our results showed that only dexamethasone relieved the bronchoconstriction caused by *T. pyogenes* 20121 at 4 hpi and 24 hpi, keeping 14.70 and 19.17% of bronchiole luminal area open, respectively, compared to the no-drug group (**Figure 6**). Thus, our results indicated that dexamethasone is a candidate for relief of bronchospasm in the treatment of *T. pyogenes* infection resulting in wheezing.

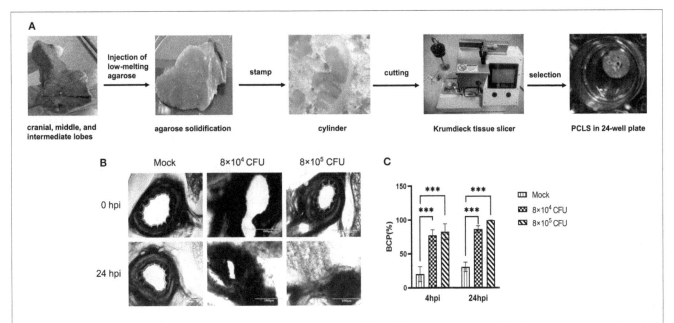

FIGURE 5 | *T. pyogenes* 20121 induced bronchoconstriction in porcine PCLS cultures. **(A)** The PCLS preparation process; **(B)** Light microscope imaging of bronchial cavities in infected (8×10^4 or 8×10^5 CFU) and mock PCLS cultures at 4 and 24 hpi; **(C)** Bronchial cavity area was measured and calculated as bronchial contraction percentage (BCP). Results are expressed as means ± S.D., and significance was determined using two-way ANOVA and the Tukey multiple-comparison test. ***$p < 0.001$.

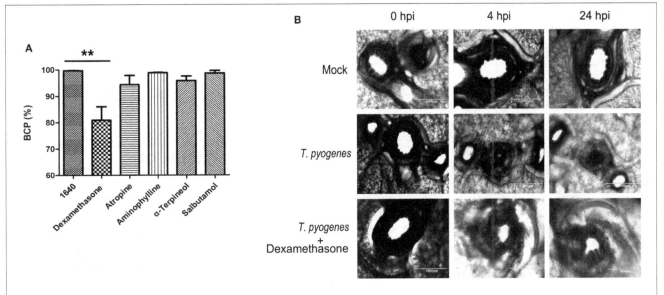

FIGURE 6 | Therapeutic effect of bronchodilators on bronchoconstriction in infected PCLS cultures. **(A)** The BCP after five common bronchodilators were used to treat bronchoconstriction resulting from *T. pyogenes* infection. Results are expressed as means ± S.D., and significance was determined using one-way ANOVA and the Tukey multiple-comparison test. **$p < 0.01$. **(B)** Therapeutic effect of dexamethasone on bronchoconstriction in PCLS cultures infected with *T. pyogenes*.

DISCUSSION

Although *T. pyogenes* has been especially linked to bovine mastitis, it is a well-known causative agent of diverse clinical presentations among domestic ruminants, pigs, companion animals and gray slender lorises (16). In domestic animals, there have been more bacterial species isolated from cattle and sheep than pigs over the last 10 years (17, 18). However, *T. pyogenes*

infections in pigs have become an increasingly serious clinical problem on large-scale farms (19, 20). *T. pyogenes* had a high isolation rate in bacterial swine pneumonia in Jilin Province (21). Pneumonia in pigs is caused mainly by viruses and bacteria. In this study, we firstly detected common viruses on the lungs of sick pigs, and the results were all negative. Furthermore, we isolated bacteria and most of clones on the blood plate are *T. pyogenes*. In order to know the best way to potentially treat the sick animals, we conducted a drug sensitivity experiment and made recommendations to the affected pig farm that resulted in effective control of the disease.

Strain 20121 showed a β-hemolytic phenotype, implying that it could produce a hemolysin that dissolves red blood cells completely. This finding was further confirmed by detecting the virulence factor PLO in the strain. The genotype of virulence factors in strain 20121 was *plo/fimA/fimE/nanH/nanP*, genes which have also been identified in bovine mastitis, pneumonia and abscesses, as well as encephalitis in goats (22). This is the first report of the genotype *plo/fimA/fimE/nanH/nanP* identified in swine pneumonia. The sequences of *plo*, *fimA*, *fimE* and *nanP* were highly similar to sequences in GenBank, indicating that these genes are highly conserved in *T. pyogenes* species. However, the *nanH* sequence of strain 20121 was relatively less similar to other *nanH* sequences from GenBank, suggesting that it may be less conserved among *T. pyogenes* isolates.

This is the first report of *T. pyogenes* infection in a mouse model causing massive necrosis of lymphocytes in the submucosal lymphatic tissue of the duodenum. Intestinal Paneth cells are the "gatekeepers" of intestinal innate immunity, thus impacts to Paneth cells can cause intestinal inflammation and inflammatory bowel disease. Therefore, our results suggest that *T. pyogenes* infection of mice induces abnormal mucosal immune response, thereby downregulating the immune response. Also, the levels of WBC and LYMP% in blood decreased significantly at 2 dpi, indicating that *T. pyogenes* infection reduced the immune function in mice. What's more, there was extensive necrosis in thymocytes, suggesting that the central immune organ thymus was destroyed after *T. pyogenes* infection in mice. Altogether, we provided evidence to show that *T. pyogenes* decreases immune function in the early stages of infection, though much remains undetermined and warrants further investigation.

For the first time in swine PCLS cultures, we showed that infection of *T. pyogenes* induced severe bronchoconstriction and led to a narrowing of the luminal area of bronchioles, suggesting PCLS are a suitable 3D model for the study *T. pyogenes* infection. Narrowing of bronchioles would affect lung ventilation and cause severe airflow limitations, which may aggravate damage to the lungs and cause the host to die suddenly from asphyxiation. We speculate that an inflammatory response may responsible for contraction of airway smooth muscle induced by *T. pyogenes* infection. However, the mechanisms by which *T. pyogenes* causes bronchoconstriction remain unclear and warrants further study in the future.

PCLS cultures have been reported to preserve lung functions for around 10 days (23), during which the bronchioles can maintain reversible constriction after methacholine treatment (24). Thus, as a good model for analyzing the effect of drugs on lung tissue, PCLS cultures have been applied for toxicological and functional studies (25, 26). In the current study, we found that dexamethasone dilated airways and kept the bronchioles open, showing a protective effect for bronchoconstriction caused by *T. pyogenes* infection in porcine PCLS. Dexamethasone is a long-acting glucocorticoid that is widely used due to its anti-inflammatory and immunosuppressive properties (27). High-dose glucocorticoid intervention is used for the treatment of mild or severe asthma with sudden onset in human to improve alveolar ventilation while treating the underlying illness (28). With respect to treatment of *T. pyogenes* infection, we suggest that a combination therapy of dexamethasone and antibiotics should be taken into account in swine clinical practice. Moreover, PCLS can be used in the hunt for more effective therapeutic drugs for *T. pyogenes* infection.

In conclusion, we isolated and identified a multidrug-resistant *T. pyogenes* strain from the lungs of sick pigs. It was virulent in a mouse infection model and also led to heavy bronchoconstriction in porcine PCLS cultures. What's more, bronchodilators showed their ability to antagonize bronchoconstriction in the same cultures. In summary, our results highlight porcine PCLS cultures as a valuable 3D organ model for the study of *T. pyogenes* infection and treatment in *vitro*.

CONCLUSION

A virulent, multidrug-resistant *T. pyogenes* strain induced severe bronchoconstriction in porcine PCLS, highlighting a valuable 3D organ model for the study of *T. pyogenes* infection *in vitro*.

AUTHOR CONTRIBUTIONS

SW, FM, and XC conceived the study and designed the experimental procedures. LQ, FM, and SW performed the experiments. LQ, FM, HH, MS, WZ, and SW analyzed the data. HH, Y-BY, Y-DT, GW, MS, WZ, and XC contributed reagents and materials. LQ, FM, and SW wrote the manuscript. All authors contributed to the article and approved the submitted version.

REFERENCES

1. Collins MD, Jones D, Kroppenstedt RM, Schleifer KH. Chemical studies as a guide to the classification of *Corynebacterium pyogenes* and "*Corynebacterium haemolyticum*". *J Gen Microbiol.* (1982) 128:335–41. doi: 10.1099/00221287-128-2-335
2. Yassin AF, Hupfer H, Siering C, Schumann P. Comparative chemotaxonomic and phylogenetic studies on the genus *Arcanobacterium* 1 emend. Lehnen et al. 2006: proposal for Trueperella gen nov and emended description of the genus Arcanobacterium. *Int J Syst Evol Microbiol.* (2011) 61:1265–74. doi: 10.1099/ijs.0.020032-0
3. Jost BH, Billington SJ. *Arcanobacterium pyogenes*: molecular pathogenesis of an animal opportunist. *Antonie Van Leeuwenhoek.* (2005) 88:87–102. doi: 10.1007/s10482-005-2316-5
4. Yang L, Liang H, Wang B, Ma B, Wang J, Zhang W. Evaluation of the potency of two pyolysin-derived recombinant proteins as vaccine candidates of *Trueperella Pyogenes* in a mouse model: pyolysin oligomerization and structural change affect the efficacy of pyolysin-based vaccines. *Vaccines (Basel).* (2020) 8. doi: 10.3390/vaccines8010079
5. Rudnick ST, Jost BH, Billington SJ. Transcriptional regulation of pyolysin production in the animal pathogen, *Arcanobacterium pyogenes*. *Vet Microbiol.* (2008) 132:96–104. doi: 10.1016/j.vetmic.2008.04.025

6. Henjakovic M, Martin C, Hoymann HG, Sewald K, Ressmeyer AR, Dassow C, et al. Ex vivo lung function measurements in precision-cut lung slices (PCLS) from chemical allergen-sensitized mice represent a suitable alternative to in vivo studies. *Toxicol Sci.* (2008) 106:444–53. doi: 10.1093/toxsci/kfn178

7. Weldearegay YB, Müller S, Hänske J, Schulze A, Kostka A, Rüger N, et al. Host-Pathogen Interactions of *Mycoplasma mycoides* in Caprine and Bovine Precision-Cut Lung Slices (PCLS) Models. *Pathogens.* (2019) 8. doi: 10.3390/pathogens8020082

8. Dobrescu I, Levast B, Lai K, Delgado-Ortega M, Walker S, Banman S, et al. In vitro and ex vivo analyses of co-infections with swine influenza and porcine reproductive and respiratory syndrome viruses. *Vet Microbiol.* (2014) 169:18–32. doi: 10.1016/j.vetmic.2013.11.037

9. Ebsen M, Mogilevski G, Anhenn O, Maiworm V, Theegarten D, Schwarze J, et al. Infection of murine precision cut lung slices (PCLS) with respiratory syncytial virus (RSV) and chlamydophila pneumoniae using the Krumdieck technique. *Pathol Res Pract.* (2002) 198:747–53. doi: 10.1078/0344-0338-00331

10. Meng F, Wu NH, Nerlich A, Herrler G, Valentin-Weigand P, Seitz M. Dynamic virus-bacterium interactions in a porcine precision-cut lung slice coinfection model: swine influenza virus paves the way for *Streptococcus suis* Infection in a two-step process. *Infect Immun.* (2015) 83:2806–15. doi: 10.1128/IAI.00171-15

11. Dresen M, Schenk J, Berhanu Weldearegay Y, Vötsch D, Baumgärtner W, Valentin-Weigand P, et al. *Streptococcus suis* Induces Expression of Cyclooxygenase-2 in Porcine Lung Tissue. *Microorganisms.* (2021) 9. doi: 10.3390/microorganisms9020366

12. Wang S, Zhang D, Jiang C, He H, Cui C, Duan W, et al. Strain characterization of *Streptococcus suis* serotypes 28 and 31, which harbor the resistance genes optrA and ant(6)-Ia. *Pathogens.* (2021) 10. doi: 10.3390/pathogens10020213

13. Zastempowska E, Lassa H. Genotypic characterization and evaluation of an antibiotic resistance of Trueperella pyogenes (Arcanobacterium pyogenes) isolated from milk of dairy cows with clinical mastitis. *Vet Microbiol.* (2012) 161:153–8.

14. Barton KT, Conklin DR, Ranabhat RS, Harper M, Holmes-Cobb LM, Martinez Soto MH, et al. Methacholine induced airway contraction in porcine precision cut lung slices from indoor and outdoor reared pigs. *Am J Transl Res.* (2020) 12:2805–13.

15. Cazzola M, Matera MG, Rossi F. Bronchial hyperresponsiveness and bacterial respiratory infections. *Clin Ther.* (1991) 13:157–71.

16. Ribeiro MG, Risseti RM, Bolaños CA, Caffaro KA, De Morais AC, Lara GH, et al. *Trueperella pyogenes* multispecies infections in domestic animals: a retrospective study of 144 cases (2002 to 2012). *Vet Q.* (2015) 35:82–7. doi: 10.1080/01652176.2015.1022667

17. Nagib S, Rau J, Sammra O, Lämmler C, Schlez K, Zschöck M, et al. Identification of *Trueperella pyogenes* isolated from bovine mastitis by Fourier transform infrared spectroscopy. *PLoS ONE.* (2014) 9:e104654. doi: 10.1371/journal.pone.0104654

18. Jaureguiberry M, Madoz LV, Giuliodori MJ, Wagener K, Prunner I, Grunert T, et al. Identification of Escherichia coli and *Trueperella pyogenes* isolated from the uterus of dairy cows using routine bacteriological testing and Fourier transform infrared spectroscopy. *Acta Vet Scand.* (2016) 58:81. doi: 10.1186/s13028-016-0262-z

19. Galán-Relaño Á, Gómez-Gascón L, Luque I, Barrero-Domínguez B, Casamayor A, Cardoso-Toset F, et al. Antimicrobial susceptibility and genetic characterization of *Trueperella pyogenes* isolates from pigs reared under intensive and extensive farming practices. *Vet Microbiol.* (2019) 232:89–95. doi: 10.1016/j.vetmic.2019.04.011

20. Jarosz ŁS, Gradzki Z, Kalinowski M. *Trueperella pyogenes* infections in swine: clinical course and pathology. *Pol J Vet Sci.* (2014) 17:395–404. doi: 10.2478/pjvs-2014-0055

21. Dong WL, Liu L, Odah KA, Atiah LA, Gao YH, Kong LC, et al. Antimicrobial resistance and presence of virulence factor genes in *Trueperella pyogenes* isolated from pig lungs with pneumonia. *Trop Anim Health Prod.* (2019) 51:2099–103. doi: 10.1007/s11250-019-01916-z

22. Risseti RM, Zastempowska E, Twaruzek M, Lassa H, Pantoja JCF, De Vargas APC, et al. Virulence markers associated with *Trueperella pyogenes* infections in livestock and companion animals. *Lett Appl Microbiol.* (2017) 65:125–32. doi: 10.1111/lam.12757

23. Meng F, Punyadarsaniya D, Uhlenbruck S, Hennig-Pauka I, Schwegmann-Wessels C, Ren X, et al. Replication characteristics of swine influenza viruses in precision-cut lung slices reflect the virulence properties of the viruses. *Vet Res.* (2013) 44:110. doi: 10.1186/1297-9716-44-110

24. Punyadarsaniya D, Liang CH, Winter C, Petersen H, Rautenschlein S, Hennig-Pauka I, et al. Infection of differentiated porcine airway epithelial cells by influenza virus: differential susceptibility to infection by porcine and avian viruses. *PLoS ONE.* (2011) 6:e28429. doi: 10.1371/journal.pone.0028429

25. Ressmeyer AR, Larsson AK, Vollmer E, Dahlèn SE, Uhlig S, Martin C. Characterisation of guinea pig precision-cut lung slices: comparison with human tissues. *Eur Respir J.* (2006) 28:603–11. doi: 10.1183/09031936.06.00004206

26. Lavoie TL, Krishnan R, Siegel HR, Maston ED, Fredberg JJ, Solway J, et al. Dilatation of the constricted human airway by tidal expansion of lung parenchyma. *Am J Respir Crit Care Med.* (2012) 186:225–32. doi: 10.1164/rccm.201202-0368OC

27. Becker DE. Basic and clinical pharmacology of glucocorticosteroids. *Anesth Prog.* (2013) 60:25–31. doi: 10.2344/0003-3006-60.1.25

28. Fitzgibbons JP. Fluid, electrolyte, and acid-base management in the acutely traumatized patient. *Orthop Clin North Am.* (1978) 9:627–48. doi: 10.1016/S0030-5898(20)30597-6

22

Impact of Network Activity on the Spread of Infectious Diseases through the German Pig Trade Network

Karin Lebl[1]*, Hartmut H. K. Lentz[1], Beate Pinior[2] and Thomas Selhorst[3]

[1] Institute of Epidemiology, Friedrich-Loeffler-Institute, Greifswald, Insel Riems, Germany, [2] Institute for Veterinary Public Health, University of Veterinary Medicine Vienna, Vienna, Austria, [3] Unit Epidemiology, Statistics and Mathematical Modelling, Federal Institute for Risk Assessment, Berlin, Germany

Correspondence:
Karin Lebl
k.lebl@gmx.at

The trade of livestock is an important and growing economic sector, but it is also a major factor in the spread of diseases. The spreading of diseases in a trade network is likely to be influenced by how often existing trade connections are active. The activity α is defined as the mean frequency of occurrences of existing trade links, thus $0 < \alpha \leq 1$. The observed German pig trade network had an activity of $\alpha = 0.11$, thus each existing trade connection between two farms was, on average, active at about 10% of the time during the observation period 2008–2009. The aim of this study is to analyze how changes in the *activity* level of the German pig trade network influence the probability of disease outbreaks, size, and duration of epidemics for different disease transmission probabilities. Thus, we want to investigate the question, whether it makes a difference for a hypothetical spread of an animal disease to transport many animals at the same time or few animals at many times. A SIR model was used to simulate the spread of a disease within the German pig trade network. Our results show that for transmission probabilities <1, the outbreak probability increases in the case of a decreased frequency of animal transports, peaking range of α from 0.05 to 0.1. However, for the final outbreak size, we find that a threshold exists such that finite outbreaks occur only above a critical value of α, which is ~0.1, and therefore in proximity of the observed activity level. Thus, although the outbreak probability increased when decreasing α, these outbreaks affect only a small number of farms. The duration of the epidemic peaks at an activity level in the range of $\alpha = 0.2$–0.3. Additionally, the results of our simulations show that even small changes in the activity level of the German pig trade network would have dramatic effects on outbreak probability, outbreak size, and epidemic duration. Thus, we can conclude and recommend that the network activity is an important aspect, which should be taken into account when modeling the spread of diseases within trade networks.

Keywords: network analysis, disease spread, trade activities, temporal network, animal movements, epidemiology

INTRODUCTION

Live animal trade represents an important economic sector but is permanently subject to fluctuations. For instance, consignments of pigs increased to 48% within EU-27 member states between 2005 and 2009 (1). However, the financial crisis in the subsequent years might have lessened this effect. The importance of live animal trade on the economy is also demonstrated during animal disease outbreaks. Trade restrictions with movement bans cause enormous financial losses for the affected livestock holdings and countries. For example, the outbreak of classical swine fever (CSF) in the 1990s in Germany led to an economical loss of approximately €1 billion (2). Thus, as demonstrated during CSF outbreak in Germany, livestock trade between farms is one of the major routes for the spread of animal diseases, although other infection routes, like proximity to infected herds or contact with contaminated persons and vehicles, exist as well (2).

Scientific research has primarily focused on the influence of the trade structure of farms on disease dynamics (3, 4). Farms differ with respect to their trade activity, i.e., with respect to the number of trading partners, trade connections, trade volume, and time intervals (5). Within the trade network, farms with greater trade activities are the most important contributors to disease spread (6). Veterinary epidemiology assessments utilized social network analysis (SNA) tools, such as centrality measures, developed within the field of social sciences, to calculate the importance of farms for the spread of animal infections. Numerous centrality measures, such as in- and out-degree, betweenness, and closeness (7), were correlated with standard epidemiological parameters, such as size of an epidemic, duration of the epidemic, time to peak of the epidemic, and the basic reproduction number R_0 (4, 8–10).

Previous studies applying SNA on pig trade networks have already provided important insight for disease prevention and control. One aspect of this research was the identification of the structure of trade communities (11, 12). Another essential finding was that there is a large degree of heterogeneity associated with movements of pigs at the movement level and at the premise specific network level as well (13). As a result, pig trade has a right-skewed distribution of all centrality parameters, i.e., few holdings have high centrality, while most have a low centrality. Thus, strategic removal of the most central nodes would result in a decomposition of the network into fragments, which would interrupt infection chains and prevent further disease spread (14–16). It was also shown that the holding types differ in their centrality measures, which allow for a targeted removal of specific holding types in the case of a disease outbreak (16–18). Further, SNA has been utilized to simulate the spread of specific diseases to estimate the effects of an outbreak, e.g., the spread of Methicillin-resistant *Staphylococcus aureus* (MRSA) through the Danish pig trade network (19).

Although SNA provides useful insights into epidemic dynamics on trade systems, the methods used in SNA do not take into account the temporal ordering of trade links. Whenever a network is traversed using trade links, each traversal has to follow a causal sequence of connections. This constraint can have a significant impact on the spreading paths for pathogens in networks (20). For this reason, recent work has been focused on *temporal network analysis*, where each connection has a time stamp marking its occurrence time. The probability of contagion between two individuals is not constant in time and depends, beside the transmission rate and infectious period, also on the frequency and duration of the contact (21–24). Studies that considered the heterogeneity and duration of contacts and their importance for the epidemic showed the importance to elucidate the time dependency of activities in order to investigate disease dynamics (22, 24–26). Previously, it has been shown that the aggregation of trade links into static networks leads to an overestimation of the epidemic size (27–30), the outbreak probability (31), and the epidemic duration. Thus, scientific research in the veterinary field has increasingly focused on time-dependent networks. Methods have been adapted and extended from static analyses to time-dependent analyses (20, 27, 31–37).

A temporal network view on livestock trade networks includes the frequency of trade links. For the whole system, this frequency can be considered as the pace of trading. This raises the question, whether it makes a difference for a potential spread of an animal disease to transport many animals at the same time (low frequency) or few animals at many times (high frequency). From the economic point of view, it is appropriate to choose a low trade frequency and transport many animals at the same time.

In this work, we analyze the impact of the overall trade frequency on the spread of infectious disease. Hereby, we keep the total trade volume of the network constant and systematically investigate the impact of a changing frequency of traded animals. We define the *activity* of a network by averaging the frequency of all existing trade connections between node pairs and analyze how changes in the activity influence the probability of a disease outbreak, the final outbreak size, and the duration of an epidemic. A discrete stochastic SIR model is used to simulate the spread of a hypothetical disease through the trade network of the German pig production chain.

MATERIALS AND METHODS

In order to analyze the influence of network activity on the course of an epidemic, an outbreak model predicting the course of a hypothetical animal disease on a contact network between holdings belonging to the German pig production chain was set up. Besides the outbreak model, we propose a method how to systematically adjust the activity of the network.

Data and Network Setup

According to the EU directive EC/2000/15 (38), EU member states are obliged to collect and record livestock movement data in a national database. Pursuant to the German Animal Movement Directive (Viehverkehrsverordnung), each holding in the pig production chain (including piglet production, breeding, raising, fattening, slaughtering, and trading) is obliged to notify the movement of pigs within 7 days. All data are stored in a database, "Herkunftssicherungs- und Informationssystem für Tiere" (HI-Tier). In Germany, movement data for pigs are collected on a daily basis. In general, movement data of livestock comprise information about the source and target farms (unique identifiers), the date of movement, and the number of animals moved (batch size).

For this study, pig movement data from the federal states of Bavaria and Baden-Württemberg between the years 2008 and 2009 were used. It has previously been shown that a period of 2 years is suitable to cover all characteristic properties of the German pig trade network (31). In our data set in most cases (90%), only one movement per week took place between a supplier and buyer. Consequently, we decided to use a weekly timescale for our analysis. In the case of two movements per week, those were merged into one occasion.

To describe the pattern of trade activity over time, a temporal network was constructed. By implementing a temporal network, it is possible to take into account causality for network transversal. In other words, consecutive trade connections have to be temporally ordered in order to make up a valid indirect connection between farms (**Figure 1**). The network comprised nodes and edges, where each edge connected a node pair. Farms were represented by nodes, and movements of animals between farms at a certain point in time were represented by directed edges. A temporal network is defined as $\mathcal{G}(V, \mathcal{E}, T)$, where V is the set of nodes within the network, $\mathcal{E}$ is the set of directed edges, and T represents the length of the observation period, as we considered weekly time steps, $T = 104$ weeks. An edge $(u, v, t, w) \in \mathcal{E}$ describes the movement of w pigs from farm u to farm v at time $t \leq T$. This network comprises $|V| = 45,065$ and $|\mathcal{E}| = 1,237,753$ edges (i.e., overall number of transports during the observation period). Further, the static representation of the network was constructed by summing all observations in the temporal network over the study period, such as the static network is the time-aggregated network of $\mathcal{G}$. In the static representation of the network $G(V, E)$, V represents the set of nodes and E the set of directed edges ($|E| = 112,826$). A directed edge between two nodes exists in the static network if a certain animal movement has taken place at least once during the observation period.

The aim of this analysis was to investigate the influence of the network activity on the outbreak size of an epidemic. However, this outbreak size would be strongly influenced by differences in the reachability of the nodes, i.e., nodes form distinct reachability

classes where a significant number of nodes may only cause trivial outbreak (11, 12). To reduce this bias, the data were first tailored to include only nodes, which are, in the static representation of the network, reachable from each other. We used the static network to identify the *largest strongly connected component* (LSCC; in a strongly connected component, each node is reachable by any other node in the component). The further analysis was limited to this LSCC, which we denote as G. Thus, the static representation of the network enables the disease to reach all nodes in finite time, no matter which node is the source of infection. All nodes and edges, which were not elements of the LSCC in the static network, were removed, as well as the corresponding elements from the temporal network. We hereby implicitly assumed that the concept of connectivity (35, 36) is preserved for the temporal network. In the resulting network, pigs moved between $|V| = 7,455$ farms (number of nodes in the LSCC) and $|E| = 27,149$ transport routes (number of edges in the LSCC) were recorded during the observational period, corresponding to $|\mathcal{E}| = 315,481$ transports in the temporal network.

Setting the Network Activity α

Starting from the network generated as described above, we changed the activity systematically. The *activity of a single edge* in a temporal network $\mathcal{G}$ can be described by its frequency, i.e., how often a certain edge was active during the study period divided by the length of the study period. The *network activity* α was defined as the mean edge frequency of a network, with $0 < \alpha \leq 1$. The network activity α of a temporal network $\mathcal{G}(V, \mathcal{E}, T)$ and its according static representation $G(V, E)$ can be calculated as follows.

$$\alpha = \frac{|\mathcal{E}|}{|E| \times T}, \quad (1)$$

where $|\mathcal{E}|$ is the number of edges in the temporal network, $|E|$ is the number of edges in the aggregated network, and T is the observation period.

In order to investigate the influence of α on disease dynamics, we propose a method to systematically change the network activity. Since the results for a network with shifted α should be comparable to the original network, following constraints had to be considered: (i) the aggregated network G remained the same for all α, (ii) the total trade volume remained constant for all α, (iii) the temporal sequence of existing trade routes had to be preserved (see details below), and (iv) the observation period T was preserved.

In order to highlight the activity of a temporal network, we computed the activity according to Eq. 1 and denoted a temporal network with a certain network activity as $\mathcal{G}_\alpha$. For our observed network, we found α = 0.11, and we denote the observed network as $\mathcal{G}_{\alpha=0.11} \equiv \mathcal{G}$.

In order to create networks with a reduced α, randomly chosen edges from $\mathcal{G}(V, \mathcal{E}, T)$ were removed. According to constraint (i), edges were removed in a way such that each edge of the aggregated network appeared at least once in the newly generated temporal network.

In order to increase α, we first considered our temporal network as a sequence of static network snapshots. In other

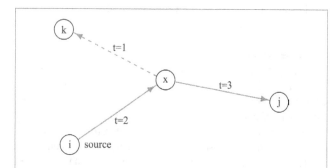

FIGURE 1 | Disease spread in a temporal network. If the source node i is infectious at time $t = 0$, the disease can spread *via* node x to node j. Node k cannot become infected, as the edge between node x and k is active at $t = 1$, thus before the disease has reached node x at $t = 2$.

words, a temporal network consists of an ordered sequence $\mathcal{G}_\alpha(V, \mathcal{E}, T) = G_1, G_2, \ldots, G_T$, where each $G_t \in \mathcal{G}$ is a static snapshot of the temporal network at time t. In order to increase α, each snapshot was first duplicated (once or multiple times) and time-shifted by a certain value chosen at random. Second, these snapshots were merged into a new temporal network. In the case of overlapping edges occurring between the same node pairs (i.e., multiple occurrences of directed edges active at the same time; regardless of their edge weights), the edge weights w (i.e., number of transported pigs) were averaged. Using this approach, the existing trade routes remain preserved as required by constraint (iii).

In order to satisfy constraint (iv), we used periodic boundary conditions, i.e., for each edge $(u, v, t, w) = (u, v, t + T, w)$. In other words, if the new times exceeded the observation period T, the times were shifted by subtracting T.

The procedures described above would already be sufficient to change the activity α of the observed network $\mathcal{G}_*$. Nevertheless, both procedures would violate constraint (ii), as the overall sum of edge weights changes as well. Therefore, the new edge weights had to be adjusted. During the observation period, a total of $W = 24,995,162$ transported pigs were recorded. The new edge weights for $\mathcal{G}_\alpha$ were normalized, so that the sum of the new edge weights equaled the total of the observed edge weights W. Finally,

edge weights for the generated network were rounded to a whole number, with the minimum number of pigs per transport set to one [constraint (i)].

For example, in a first step, we duplicated the graph $\mathcal{G}_*$ once and conducted a 52-week shift (i.e., a shift of 1 year in the duplicate). Thus, an edge active in the original graph at weeks 2, 40, 63, and 92 would be active in a 52-week-shifted graph at weeks 54, 92, 11, and 40. Merging the original with the time-shifted graph would thus result in a graph where this certain edge is active at weeks 2, 11, 40, 54, 63, and 92 (see **Figure 2** for a more detailed example).

Overall, 22 different networks were generated with different activity values, including the original network $\mathcal{G}_* = \mathcal{G}_{0.11}$. The considered values for α were approximately evenly distributed in the interval (0; 1].

Disease Dynamics
SIR Model
In order to analyze the influence of network activity α on the course of an epidemic, we simulated the spread of a disease on different temporal networks $\mathcal{G}_\alpha$ with parameter α. Disease dynamics were modeled by applying a stochastic discrete-time SIR model (29). Farms were treated as epidemiological units that are assigned to one of the three epidemiological states: susceptible (S), infected (I), and recovered (R). The infection spread along an

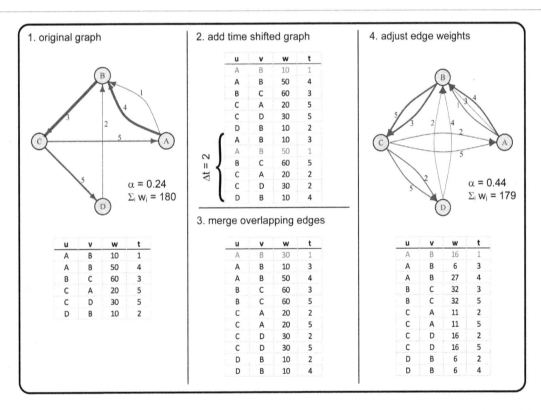

FIGURE 2 | Example for creating a graph with an increased α using a time shift of two time steps. In this example, the original graph has $|V| = 4$ nodes (A, B, C, D) and $|\mathcal{E}| = 6$ directed edges (with u as the starting node and v as the receiving node), corresponding to $|E| = 5$ in the time-aggregated network. The edges are active at times $t \in \{1, 2, \ldots, 5\}$ (numbers next to the drawn edges), thus $T = 5$. The line widths of the edges correspond to the edge weights w. Overlapping edges (i.e., edges with the same u, v, t) are marked in red. The newly generated graph has the same number of nodes, but an increased number of edges ($|\mathcal{E}| = 11$). Note that, due to rounding errors, the sum of edge weights in the original and the new graph are only approximately equal.

edge (u, v, t, w), if at time t the supplying node u was in state I, and the receiving node v in state S. Thus, a receiving farm could only became infected, if a transport took place from the supplying farm to the receiving farm during the time period in which the supplying farm was in the I state. Infectious nodes stayed in the I state for μ time steps, thereafter they passed to the R state. Nodes in the R state remained in this state until the end of a simulation run. Infectious farms infect susceptible farms with probability p_e.

Due to the fact that certain information was not available, the following model assumptions were made. (I) farms representing the nodes within the network were all treated identically (8, 29, 31, 39). Thus, in this model, the number of animals on the farm, breed, farm type, or farm practices did not have an effect on the transmission dynamics. (II) the epidemiological status does not alter the trade contact structure. The latter is a strong assumption, but it allowed an examination of the influence of network topology on unmanaged disease dynamics (29).

Model Parameters

In order to compute the transmission probability p_e for each edge, we first considered the risk of infection for each transported animal. For every transport from an infected to a susceptible farm, each transported animal has a probability p to infect the receiving node. In this work, the probabilities $p = \{0.25, 0.5, 0.75, 1\}$ were considered. The receiving node became infected, when at least one transported animal spread the disease. The probability p_e can be described with a binomial function $B(w, p)$, whereas the function depends on the parameters edge weight w and an animals' transmission probability p.

$$p_e = P(X > 0) \sim B(w, p) = 1 - (1 - p)^w. \quad (2)$$

A transmission probability of $p = 1$ corresponds to a highly infectious disease: the supplied farm always became infected, independent of the batch size w. This corresponds to a worst-case scenario and is therefore often used in studies investigating the spread of diseases within the trade networks (6, 8, 31).

Nodes remain in the I state for the *infectious period* μ and then pass to the R state. Nodes in the R state remained in this state. In this paper, we considered a constant infectious period of $\mu = 4$ weeks [as estimated for cases, such as CSF, African swine fever, foot-and-mouth disease; Ref. (40)].

Initial Conditions

In the analysis presented here, the model predicted the disease dynamics for discrete intervals of 1 week. Initially, all farms were in the susceptible state (S). At a randomly chosen time, the state of one randomly selected farm was set to infected (I).

The disease dynamics were simulated on a temporal network $\mathcal{G}_\alpha$. All possible start times and initially infected nodes (index nodes) had the same selection probability. The start times were selected from the interval $[1; T - 40]$ to avoid that the durations of the epidemics exceed the observation period of 104 weeks. We chose 40 weeks arbitrarily, as the first test runs showed that the duration of the epidemic only rarely exceeded this time period. However, in some cases, the duration of the epidemic still exceeded the study period – those cases were excluded from

the further analysis. The simulation stopped when the number of infectious nodes reached 0.

Summary of Parameters

For each value of the activity parameter coming from one of the 22 investigated $\mathcal{G}_\alpha$, each with the 4 transmission probabilities as described above, the simulation was repeated 2,000 times, as test runs showed that this number of iterations provided robust results. Thus, 176,000 simulation experiments were run in total (**Table 1**). In 175,877 of those simulations, the duration of the infection did not exceed the observation period and were used for further analysis.

Analysis

We wanted to determine the probability that a disease outbreak occurs for a certain level of α. The *outbreak probability* was estimated as the proportion of the 2,000 simulation runs, in which the disease spread beyond the starting node. In those cases where the disease spread beyond the starting node, the *outbreak size* was calculated as the total number of infected nodes. In addition, the *outbreak duration* was defined as the number of weeks in which infected nodes occurred. The distribution of the latter two measures was skewed to the right, and thus we give the median and the first and third quartiles (Q1, Q3).

All analyses were conducted using the open-source software R version 3.2.1 (41). The package *igraph* (42) was used to generate and analyze the network.

RESULTS

Descriptors of G.

For this static representation G., we found an average shortest length of 6.33; the path length between the two most distant nodes (diameter) was 17. The median in-degree, measuring the number of trade partners delivering animals to a certain node was only one, while the median for the number of trade partners a certain holding delivers to (out-degree) was two (**Table 2**). The values for the median ingoing and outgoing closeness centrality were rather similar (**Table 2**), indicating that the number of steps required to reach a certain node equals the number of steps required to reach

TABLE 1 | Description and value bound of the used parameters.

	Parameter	Description	Value
Network	α	Network activity	22 values in the interval (0; 1]
Infection parameters	p	Infection probability per transported animal	{0.25, 0.5, 0.75, 1}
	p_e	Infection probability per edge, depending on batch size	calculated according to Eq. 2
	μ	Infectious period	4 weeks (constant)
Initial conditions	u	Starting node	2,000 random samples from V
	t	Starting time	2,000 random samples from $[1; T - 40]$
Total runs			176,000

any other node from a certain node. The number of shortest paths going through a certain node (betweenness centrality, **Table 2**) showed a high variation, ranging from 0 to 15,166,160.

Outbreak Probability

We observed that the outbreak probability is finite, independent of the particular values of transmission probability p and network activity α (**Figure 3**). Even for the smallest considered activity values ($\alpha = 0.01$), the outbreak probabilities was in the region of 5% for all considered transmission probabilities.

TABLE 2 | Minimum, 25% quartile, median, 75% quartile and maximum of the calculated centrality parameters for G·, the static representation of the observed network.

	Min	Q1	Median	Q3	Max
In-degree	1	1	1	2	665
Out-degree	1	1	2	3	358
Ingoing closeness centrality	0.000011	0.000018	0.000023	0.000026	0.000041
Outgoing closeness centrality	0.000012	0.000019	0.000022	0.000024	0.000037
Betweenness centrality	0.0	1.0	316.2	7,490.2	15,166,160.0

We now focus on the outbreak probability for a transmission probability of $p = 1$, i.e., the worst-case scenario, in which transports of any size spread the infection. In this scenario, a monotonous increase of the outbreak probability with increasing activity was observed. The outbreak probability saturated for larger values of α. More precisely, the outbreak probability was greater than 99% for all $\alpha > 0.80$. For small and intermediate values of α, it can be observed that even relatively small changes in α had a strong effect on the outbreak probability. Our observed network ($\alpha = 0.11$) lies in this region. Consequently, small changes in the real system would result in large changes in the outbreak probability.

We now focus on transmission probabilities of $p < 1$. For all considered $p < 1$, a qualitatively similar behavior could be observed. Contrary to the worst-case scenario ($p = 1$), the outbreak probabilities for $p < 1$ did not increase monotonously, but rather showed a maximum. The location of these maxima was shifted to the right for increasing values of p. It should be noted that the location of these maxima was relatively close to the activity of the observed network G·.

Final Outbreak Size

We now consider the cases where the infection spread beyond the starting node and the corresponding outbreak sizes for different values for α and p (**Figure 4**). For the worst-case scenario $p = 1$, the outbreak size increased monotonously with increasing α. The

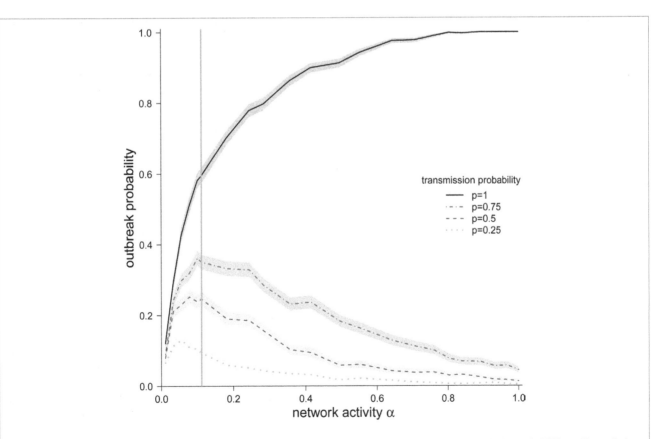

FIGURE 3 | Outbreak probability (±95% CI) depending on the network activity level α for different disease transmission probabilities p. The vertical orange line represents α for the observed pig trade network G·.

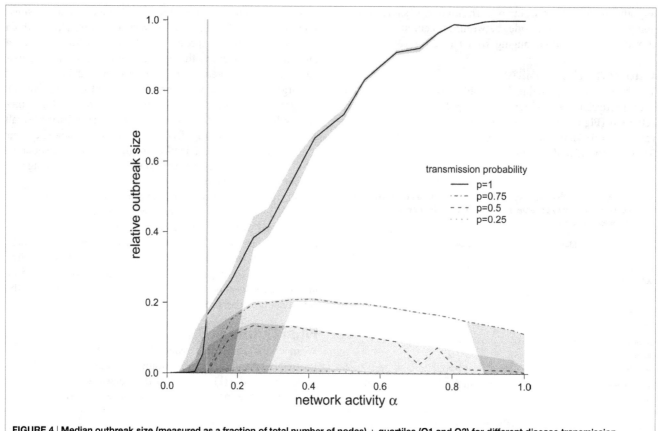

FIGURE 4 | Median outbreak size (measured as a fraction of total number of nodes) ± quartiles (Q1 and Q3) for different disease transmission probabilities _p_ (in the case the disease spread beyond the starting node). The vertical orange line represents α for the observed pig trade network $\mathcal{G}_\cdot$.

possibility that all nodes in the network became infected was only found at this scenario ($p = 1$), but only for very high network activities. For the observed network ($\alpha = 0.11$), ~15% of the nodes would become infected in the worst-case scenario.

For smaller transmission probabilities ($p < 1$), we observed that outbreak sizes are significantly smaller than in the worst-case scenario. In contrast to the worst-case scenario, the outbreak sizes showed a maximum at approximately $\alpha = 0.3$.

The authors would like to stress the fact that the outbreak size showed a critical threshold regarding the network activity. This means that there was a _critical activity_ α_{crit}, such that finite outbreaks occurred only if $\alpha > \alpha_{crit}$. To estimate α_{crit}, we calculated the central point between the last value of α below and the first value above the threshold. For transmission probability $p = 1$, we found $\alpha_{crit} = 0.1$, and for transmission probabilities of 0.75, 0.5, 0.25, we found $\alpha_{crit} = 0.15$. Interestingly, the activity of the observed network was close to the critical region. For $p = 1$, the activity of the observed network $\mathcal{G}_\cdot$ was only slightly above the critical threshold, whereas for transmission probabilities $p < 1$, the observed network was subcritical. As it is typical for such critical regimes, small changes in the activity result in large changes in the outbreak size (**Figure 4**).

Outbreak Duration

Although the shapes of the outbreak durations were similar for different transmission probabilities, we found that the outbreak

duration increased with higher transmission probabilities (**Figure 5**). However, for all transmission probabilities, a maximum in the outbreak probability at approximately $\alpha = 0.2$ could be found, with the exception of $p = 0.25$, where the maximum was at approximately $\alpha = 0.3$. The reason for these maxima is the existence of two dueling effects. (i) For small α, the outbreak duration correlates with the outbreak size. Outbreaks were typically small here, and increasing α increased the possible number of paths to other nodes. Topological and temporal shortcuts played a minor role here. (ii) For large values of α, the network was likely to form a number of shortcuts, accelerating the spread of a disease.

DISCUSSION

In this study, we investigated how the spreading of hypothetical infectious diseases through a trade network is influenced by the networks activity level. For the observed German pig trade network $\alpha = 0.11$, thus each existing trade connection between two farms was on average active at about 10% of the time during the observation period (using weekly time steps). At this observed low network activity, the chances for a disease to spread beyond the starting node were relatively low, especially for low transmission probabilities (e.g., 10% at $p = 0.25$). Even in the case that an infection spread, the total number of infected farms was for all but the worst-case scenario only about 0.2% of the nodes within the network. Previously, the size of the largest connected component

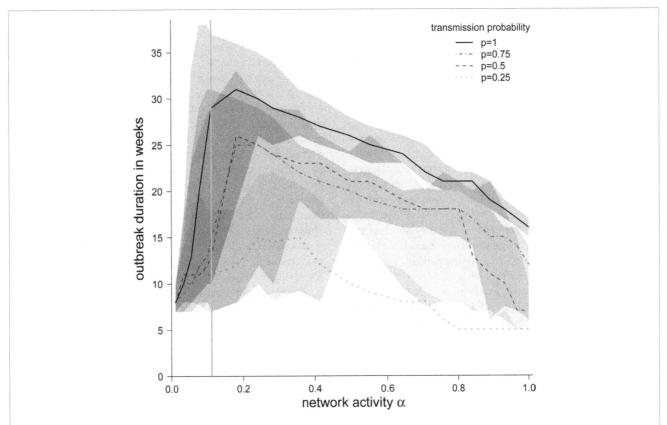

FIGURE 5 | Median duration of the epidemic in weeks (in the case the disease spread beyond the starting node) ± quartiles (Q1 and Q3) depending on the network activity level α for different disease transmission probabilities *p*. The vertical orange line represents α for the observed pig trade network 𝒢.

has often been used as an estimate for the potential final size of an epidemic spreading through a network (43). However, even at the applied worst-case scenario ($p = 1$), the size of the epidemic in our simulation was only a fraction (around 16%) of the total number of nodes for the observed trade data. Using the LSCC would therefore have considerably overestimated the final size of the epidemic. Thus, our results indicate that, at the observed level of the network activity, the threat of large epidemics spreading through the German pig trade network is relatively low, especially for diseases with low transmission rates. However, as we focused in our study on the spread of diseases through the trade network, the actual number of infected farms could be higher due to additional spreading *via* other infection routes (2).

For our analysis, we limited the trade network to the LSCC in order to avoid bias in the results caused by differences in the reachability of the nodes. The observed network activity of the untailored network ($α = 0.105$) was very similar to the activity in the LSCC ($α = 0.112$), indicating that changes from the observed network activity would have the same effect on the outbreak probability, -size, and -duration. However, due to the differences in the reachability of the nodes, a much higher variation in the results is to be expected (20).

Interestingly, the German pig trade network seems to be at a rather unstable state, as even small changes in the networks activity level would have a large impact on the spreading of

diseases. The main factor that could change the network activity of the German pig trade network is likely to be the farm size. In the last years, the pig production in Germany and other EU countries increased, resulting in larger farm sizes and increased number of traded pigs (1, 44). This would also result in increasing animal transports, which could by archived either by increasing the animals per transport (i.e., edge weights) or by a higher frequency of transports (i.e., higher activity level), whereby the latter would likely have a higher impact on disease dynamics. If an increase in the network activity is to be expected in the long term, the probability for an outbreak and outbreak size are likely to increase, as shown in this study. Considering all three investigated measurements (outbreak probability, final outbreak size, and duration of epidemic), it becomes apparent that an increase in the network activity should be avoided. Further, in order to confine disease spreads, a decrease in the activity of the German pig trade network would be conducive, even if this reduction would only be minor. In our model, a decrease of the activity is realized by random deletion of edges. We assume that a targeted deletion of edges might even have a larger effect (45). From a practical point of view, a reduction in the network activity would mean that animal transports from one farm to another would have to be concentrated to fewer occasions. This also implies that a matching pig production schedule would be necessary, favoring "all-in-all-out" production systems.

The final outbreak size for different network activities shows, as depicted in **Figure 4**, strong similarities to the threshold behavior known from epidemic SIR-type models (46). This epidemic threshold describes a condition above which an epidemic becomes global, while below this threshold only a limited number of nodes become infected (46, 47). To estimate the epidemic threshold in a given network is thus important as it allows predicting the possibility that an infection spreads on a large scale. Hence, it is essential for the planning control and intervention strategies. Different methods exist to identify the epidemic thresholds, with the performance of those methods depending on the topology of the network (48, 49). The results of our study show not only the existence of a threshold but also that its position varies with the transmission probability. Read and colleagues (22) demonstrated for a small-scale human contact network that the encounter rate had a strong effect on the outbreak size at high transmission rates but could find no significant effect at low transmission rates. This concurs with our results, where the effects of the network activity on the outbreak size were most produced at high transmission rates. Again, it seems that the actual activity of the investigated system is close to this threshold value, as even a small increase in the activity level has a large impact on the outbreak size of an epidemic.

The outbreak probability peaked in a region below this threshold for a global epidemic. As the total number of transported animals was kept constant for all network activities, the batch sizes per transport increased, while the frequency of transports decreased at low network activities. Thus, as the edge infection probability p_e depends on the batch size, the chance to transmit a disease beyond the starting node is rather high at low network activity levels, given the case that a transport occurs. As the number of transports is low at low levels of α, the epidemics are restricted to only a few livestock holdings. On the other hand, a decrease in the observed outbreak probabilities for large values of α can be observed, which can be explained by the fact that the batch sizes are small in this regime. Thus, disease spread was dominated by strong fluctuations in edge infection probability p_e. These described effects only apply to transmission probabilities <1, as in the case of $p = 1$, the spreading of diseases is independent of the batch size.

As the necessary information was not available to us, we had to made several simplifications for our analysis. Especially, the farm type has already been shown to be an important factor in the spreading of the disease in animal trade networks (15). The farm type defines how long animals remain at a certain node. It is likely, that if the network activity would change due to an overall increase or decrease in the German pig production, the change in the activity of the individual trade connections would be irregular and vary according to the type of the source and the receiving node. This would be an important point to consider in further studies, as heterogeneous waiting times have been shown to influence the spread of diseases in networks (50, 51). For our simulation, we neglected within-herd transmission dynamics as well. Within-herd transmission depends not only on the specifics of a disease but is also influenced by several external factors that were not available to us (e.g., farm size or biosecurity measures on the farm level). The numbers of infected animals within a

farm vary over time (52), and it is unlikely that all animals are simultaneously infected over a certain time period, as assumed in our simulation. Consequently, the presented results could overestimate the probability of a disease outbreak and the size of the epidemic. For our model, we assumed that the epidemiological status of the farms does not alter the trade contact structure. This applies to rather harmless diseases, like porcine reproductive and respiratory syndrome (PRRS), porcine circovirus type 2 (PCV2), or MRSA. However, depending on the severity of a disease, trade connections with an infected farm could cease. The withdrawal of trade connections would not be instantaneous but depend on various factors like incubation period or the occurring of clinical symptoms, resulting in a high variation between the time of infection of a farm and the potential termination of trade connections. Thus, the more likely a disease results in trade restrictions and the faster those restrictions are applied, the more our model is prone to overestimate the size of an epidemic. In case of an outbreak of a severe disease, trade connections could change due to the targeted implementation of trade restrictions by veterinary authorities. However, the extent of trade restrictions often differs between countries. For instance, during the bluetongue virus outbreak in Europe starting in 2006, trade restrictions in France were directed to specific areas (53), while in Germany, as well as in Austria and Swiss, the whole country was declared a single restriction zone at an early stage of the epidemic (54–56). Thus, if the whole country is declared a single restriction zone, the within-country trade network would likely show only marginal changes. The effect of lowering the contact rate on outbreak probability, -size, and -duration is shown in this analysis, but the implementation of trade restrictions directed to specific areas could lead to different dynamics.

In our study, we presented the *network activity* as a new indicator value for networks. With this parameter, it is possible to investigate how changes in the mean frequency in the activation of existing trade connections can affect the spread of diseases. By setting the total trade volume constant, as we did in this study, it was possible to differentiate between effects of trade frequency and trade volume. There are two specific characteristics of α: first, it is designed to be a characteristic of a temporal network. It has been shown that several network parameters drawn from a static network correlate with standard epidemiological parameters. Especially in networks with a right-skewed degree distribution, as we found for the pig trade network, nodes with a high degree can play an important role in the spreading of diseases (8, 14, 16). However, the frequency of trade links cannot be represented by a static network; static networks generated from different levels of α would be identical and thus network measurements (like centrality measurements) would be identical as well. As static networks do not take the temporal causality of the paths into account, results drawn from such static representations can be problematic. For example, it has been shown that compared to a temporal network, its static representation overestimates the size of a disease outbreak (20). Thus, in the last years, measurements for temporal networks have been developed (20, 57), and their relation to disease spread, however, remains to be investigated. In comparison with most of those measurements, the calculation of the *network activity* is simple, as it is obtained from the total number of edges in the static and the temporal network. Second, the *network activity* is a measurement for the state of the whole network and not for single nodes. It can be used as a measurement of how well a temporal network is described by its static representation. An $\alpha = 1$ would be equal to network, where each existing trade link is active at all time steps, thus the static representation would be true at any time. The more closely the network activity is to one, the more accurate is its static representation. Still, for now, we would like to suggest carefulness in applying the results to other networks. While the general pattern is likely to stay the same, the exact location of the maxima/threshold of the investigated parameters could vary. Further, when comparing the *network activity* of different networks, care must be taken to use the same time period and time steps, as α changes with those two values.

In this study, we could demonstrate that the network activity α is an important factor in evaluating the effects of a disease spread in the German pig trade network. We would like to propose applying this indicator number to other networks used to demonstrate the spread of disease or other malicious agents as well, as the networks' activity is likely to have a strong impact on the spreading.

AUTHOR CONTRIBUTIONS

This work was designed by TS, KL, and HL. BP, HL, and KL processed the raw data, and KL performed the data analysis. The results of the analysis were interpreted by KL, HL, and TS. KL, BP, and HL drafted and wrote the manuscript. All authors revised the manuscript and approved to the final version.

ACKNOWLEDGMENTS

We thank A. Fröhlich and C. Firth for their comments, which substantially helped to improve the manuscript.

REFERENCES

1. Baltussen W, Gebrensbet G, deRoest K. *Study on the Impact of Regulation (EC) No 1/2005 on the Protection of Animals during Transport.* (2011). Final Report. Specific Contract N SANCO/2010/D5/S12.574298.
2. Fritzemeier J, Teuffert J, Greiser-Wilke I, Staubach C, Schlüter H, Moennig V. Epidemiology of classical swine fever in Germany in the 1990s. *Vet Microbiol* (2000) 77:29–41. doi:10.1016/S0378-1135(00)00254-6
3. Christley RM, Pinchbeck GL, Bowers RG, Clancy D, French N, Bennett J, et al. Infection in social networks: using network analysis to identify high-risk individuals. *Am J Epidemiol* (2005) 162:1024–31. doi:10.1093/aje/kwi308
4. Keeling M, Eames K. Networks and epidemic models. *J R Soc Interface* (2005) 2:295–307. doi:10.1098/rsif.2005.0051
5. Pinior B, Platz U, Ahrens U, Petersen B, Conraths F, Selhorst T. The German Milky Way: trade structure of the milk industry and possible consequences of a food crisis. *J Chain Netw Sci* (2012) 12:25–39. doi:10.3920/JCNS2012.x001
6. Pinior B, Konschake M, Platz U, Thiele H, Petersen B, Conraths F, et al. The trade network in the dairy industry and its implication for the spread of contamination. *J Dairy Sci* (2012) 95:6351–61. doi:10.3168/jds.2012-5809
7. Wasserman S, Faust K. *Social Network Analysis – Methods and Applications.* Cambridge: Cambridge University Press (1994).
8. Natale F, Giovannini A, Savini L, Palma D, Possenti L, Fiore G, et al. Network analysis of Italian cattle trade patterns and evaluation of risks for potential disease spread. *Prev Vet Med* (2009) 92:341–50. doi:10.1016/j.prevetmed.2009.08.026
9. Bajardi P, Barrat A, Savini L, Colizza V. Optimizing surveillance for livestock disease spreading through animal movements. *J R Soc Interface* (2012) 9:2814–25. doi:10.1098/rsif.2012.0289
10. Lentz HHK, Selhorst T, Sokolov I. Spread of infectious diseases in directed and modular metapopulation networks. *Phys Rev E Stat Nonlin Soft Matter Phys* (2012) 85:066111. doi:10.1103/PhysRevE.85.066111
11. Lentz HHK, Konschake M, Teske K, Kasper M, Rother B, Carmanns R, et al. Trade communities and their spatial patterns in the German pork production network. *Prev Vet Med* (2011) 98(2–3):176–81. doi:10.1016/j.prevetmed.2010.10.011
12. Lichoti JK, Davies J, Kitala PM, Githigia SM, Okoth E, Maru Y, et al. Social network analysis provides insights into African swine fever epidemiology. *Prev Vet Med* (2016) 126:1–10. doi:10.1016/j.prevetmed.2016.01.019
13. Bigras-Poulin M, Barfod K, Mortensen S, Greiner M. Relationship of trade patterns of the Danish swine industry animal movements network to potential disease spread. *Prev Vet Med* (2007) 80:143–65. doi:10.1016/j.prevetmed.2007.02.004

14. Nöremark M, Håkansson N, Lewerin SS, Lindberg A, Jonsson A. Network analysis of cattle and pig movements in Sweden: measures relevant for disease control and risk based surveillance. *Prev Vet Med* (2011) 99(2–4):78–90. doi:10.1016/j.prevetmed.2010.12.009
15. Büttner K, Krieter J, Traulsen A, Traulsen I. Efficient interruption of infection chains by targeted removal of central holdings in an animal trade network. *PLoS One* (2013) 8(9):e74292. doi:10.1371/journal.pone.0074292
16. Büttner K, Krieter J, Traulsen A, Traulsen I. Static network analysis of a pork supply chain in Northern Germany – characterisation of the potential spread of infectious diseases via animal movements. *Prev Vet Med* (2013) 110(3–4):418–28. doi:10.1016/j.prevetmed.2013.01.008
17. Dorjee S, Revie CW, Poljak Z, McNab WB, Sanchez J. Network analysis of swine shipments in Ontario, Canada, to support disease spread modelling and risk-based disease management. *Prev Vet Med* (2013) 112(1–2):118–27. doi:10.1016/j.prevetmed.2013.06.008
18. Rautureau S, Dufour B, Durand B. Structural vulnerability of the French swine industry trade network to the spread of infectious diseases. *Animal* (2012) 6(7):1152–62. doi:10.1017/S1751731111002631
19. Ciccolini M, Dahl J, Chase-Topping ME, Woolhouse ME. Disease transmission on fragmented contact networks: livestock-associated Methicillin-resistant *Staphylococcus aureus* in the Danish pig-industry. *Epidemics* (2012) 4(4):171–8. doi:10.1016/j.epidem.2012.09.001
20. Lentz HHK, Koher A, Hövel P, Gethmann J, Sauter-Louis C, Selhorst T, et al. Disease spread through animal movements: a static and temporal network analysis of pig trade in Germany. *PLoS One* (2016) 11(5):e0155196. doi:10.1371/journal.pone.0155196
21. Holme P. Epidemiologically optimal static networks from temporal network data. *PLoS Comput Biol* (2013) 9(7):e1003142. doi:10.1371/journal.pcbi.1003142
22. Read JM, Eames KTD, Edmunds WJ. Dynamic social networks and the implications for the spread of infectious disease. *J R Soc Interface* (2008) 5(26):1001–7. doi:10.1098/rsif.2008.0013
23. Stehlé J, Voirin N, Barrat A, Cattuto C, Colizza V, Isella L, et al. Simulation of an SEIR infectious disease model on the dynamic contact network of conference attendees. *BMC Med* (2011) 9:87. doi:10.1186/1741-7015-9-87
24. Smieszek T. A mechanistic model of infection: why duration and intensity of contacts should be included in models of disease spread. *Theor Biol Med Model* (2009) 6:25. doi:10.1186/1742-4682-6-25
25. Colizza V, Barrat A, Barthélemy M, Vespignani A. The role of the airline transportation network in the prediction and predictability of global epidemics. *Proc Natl Acad Sci U S A* (2006) 103(7):2015–20. doi:10.1073/pnas.0510525103

26. Chen S, White BJ, Sanderson MW, Amrine DE, Illany A, Lanzas C. Highly dynamic animal contact network and implications on disease transmission. *Sci Rep* (2014) 4:4472. doi:10.1038/srep04472

27. Lentz HH, Selhorst T, Sokolov I. Unfolding accessibility provides a macroscopic approach to temporal networks. *Phys Rev Lett* (2013) 110:118701. doi:10.1103/PhysRevLett.110.118701

28. Dubé C, Ribble C, Kelton D, McNab B. Comparing network analysis measures to determine potential epidemic size of highly contagious exotic diseases in fragmented monthly networks of dairy cattle movements in Ontario, Canada. *Transbound Emerg Dis* (2008) 55:382–92. doi:10.1111/j.1865-1682.2008.01053.x

29. Vernon M, Keeling M. Representing the UKs cattle herd as static and dynamic networks. *Proc R Soc B* (2009) 276:469–76. doi:10.1098/rspb.2008.1009

30. Karsai M, Kivelä M, Pan R, Kaski K, Kertész J, Barabási AL, et al. Small but slow world: how network topology and burstiness slow down spreading. *Phys Rev E Stat Nonlin Soft Matter Phys* (2011) 83:025102. doi:10.1103/PhysRevE.83.025102

31. Konschake M, Lentz H, Conraths F, Hövel P, Selhorst T. On the robustness of in- and out-components in a temporal network. *PLoS One* (2013) 8:e55223. doi:10.1371/journal.pone.0055223

32. Kao R, Green D, Johnson J, Kiss I. Disease dynamics over very different time-scales: foot-and-mouth disease and scrapie on the network of livestock movements in the UK. *J R Soc Interface* (2007) 4:907–16. doi:10.1098/rsif.2007.1129

33. Casteigts A, Flocchini P, Quattrociocchi W, Santoro N. Time-varying graphs and dynamic networks. *Int J Parallel Emergent Distrib Syst* (2012) 27:387–408. doi:10.1080/17445760.2012.668546

34. Holme P, Saramäki J. Temporal networks. *Phys Rep* (2012) 519:97–125. doi:10.1016/j.physrep.2012.03.001

35. Kiss I, Berthouze L, Taylor TJ, Simon P. Modelling approaches for simple dynamic networks and applications to disease transmission models. *Proc Roy Soc A* (2012) 468:1332–55. doi:10.1098/rspa.2011.0349

36. Nicosia V, Tang J, Musolesi M, Russo G, Mascolo C, Latora V. Components in time-varying graphs. *Chaos* (2012) 22:023101. doi:10.1063/1.3697996

37. Liu S-Y, Baronchelli A, Perra N. Contagion dynamics in time-varying metapopulation networks. *Phys Rev E Stat Nonlin Soft Matter Phys* (2013) 87:032805. doi:10.1103/PhysRevE.87.032805

38. EUR-Lex. Directive 2000/15/EC of the European Parliament and the Council of 10 April 2000 amending Council Directive 64/432/EEC on health problems affecting intra-community trade in bovine animals and swine. *Off J Eur Commun* (2000) 43:34–5.

39. Pinior B, Conraths F, Petersen B, Selhorst T. Decision support for risks managers in the case of deliberate food contamination: the dairy industry as an example. *Omega Int J Manage S* (2015) 53:41–8. doi:10.1016/j.omega.2014.09.011

40. Fernandeź PJ, White WR. *Atlas of Transboundary Animal Diseases*. Paris: OIE (World Organisation for Animal Health) (2010). 277 p.

41. Core Team R. *R: A Language and Environment for Statistical Computing.* Vienna: R Foundation for Statistical Computing (2015). Available from: http://www.R-project.org

42. Csardi G, Nepusz T. The igraph software package for complex network research. *Int J Complex Syst* (2006) 1695 Available from: http://igraph.org

43. Kao R, Danon L, Green D, Kiss I. Demographic structure and pathogen dynamics on the network of livestock movements in Great Britain. *Proc R Soc B* (2006) 273:1999–2007. doi:10.1098/rspb.2006.3505

44. Roguet C, Rieu M. The German pork industry responds to societal demands: from private labels to sectoral initiative. *Cahiers de l'IFIP* (2014) 1(1):1–12.

45. Borgatti S. Identifying sets of key players in a social network. *Comput Math Organ Theory* (2006) 12:21–34. doi:10.1007/s10588-006-7084-x

46. Pastor-Satorras R, Castellano C, Van Mieghem P, Vespignani A. Epidemic processes in complex networks. *Rev Mod Phys* (2015) 87:925. doi:10.1103/RevModPhys.87.925

47. Moreno Y, Pastor-Satorras R, Vespignani A. Epidemic outbreaks in complex heterogeneous networks. *Eur Phys J B* (2002) 26(4):521–9. doi:10.1140/epjb/e20020122

48. Shu P, Wang W, Tang M, Do Y. Numerical identification of epidemic thresholds for susceptible-infected-recovered model on finite-size networks. *Chaos* (2015) 25:063104. doi:10.1063/1.4922153

49. Wang W, Liu QH, Zhong LF, Tang M, Gao H, Stanley HE. Predicting the epidemic threshold of the susceptible-infected-recovered model. *Sci Rep* (2016) 6:24676. doi:10.1038/srep24676

50. Delvenne J-C, Lambiotte R, Rocha LEC. Diffusion on networked systems is a question of time or structure. *Nat Commun* (2015) 6:7366. doi:10.1038/ncomms8366

51. Yang GL, Yang X. Optimal epidemic spreading on complex networks with heterogeneous waiting time distribution. *Physica A* (2016) 447:386–91. doi:10.1016/j.physa.2015.12.033

52. Chis Ster I, Dodd PJ, Ferguson NM. Within-farm transmission dynamics of foot and mouth disease as revealed by the 2001 epidemic in Great Britain. *Epidemics* (2012) 4(3):158–69. doi:10.1016/j.epidem.2012.07.002

53. Tago D, Hammitt JK, Thomas A, Raboisson D. Cost assessment of the movement restriction policy in France during the 2006 bluetongue virus episode (BTV-8). *Prev Vet Med* (2014) 117(3–4):577–89. doi:10.1016/j.prevetmed.2014.10.010

54. Gethmann J, Hoffmann B, Probst C, Beer M, Conraths FJ, Mettenleiter TC. Drei Jahre Blauzungenkrankheit Serotyp 8 in Deutschland. *Tierärztl Umschau* (2010) 65:4–12.

55. Häsler B, Howe KS, Di Labio E, Schwermer H, Stärk KDC. Economic evaluation of the surveillance and intervention programme for bluetongue virus serotype 8 in Switzerland. *Prev Vet Med* (2012) 103(2):93–111. doi:10.1016/j.prevetmed.2011.09.013

56. Pinior B, Lebl K, Firth C, Rubel F, Fuchs R, Stockreiter S, et al. Cost analysis of Bluetongue virus serotype 8 (BTV-8) surveillance and vaccination programmes in Austria between 2005–2013. *Vet J* (2015) 206(2):154–60. doi:10.1016/j.tvjl.2015.07.032

57. Nicosia V, Tang J, Mascolo C, Musolesi M, Russo G, Latora V. Graph metrics for temporal networks. In: Holme P, Saramäki J, editors. *Temporal Networks*. Berlin, Heidelberg: Springer (2013). p. 15–40.

23

Rabies Virus Exploits Cytoskeleton Network to Cause Early Disease Progression and Cellular Dysfunction

Xilin Liu[1], Zeeshan Nawaz[2], Caixia Guo[1*], Sultan Ali[3], Muhammad Ahsan Naeem[4], Tariq Jamil[5], Waqas Ahmad[6*], Muhammad Usman Siddiq[7], Sarfraz Ahmed[4], Muhammad Asif Idrees[8] and Ali Ahmad[8]

[1] Department of Hand Surgery, Presidents' Office of China-Japan Union Hospital of Jilin University, Changchun, China, [2] Department of Microbiology, Government College University Faisalabad, Faisalabad, Pakistan, [3] Faculty of Veterinary Science, Institute of Microbiology, University of Agriculture, Faisalabad, Pakistan, [4] Department of Basic Sciences, University College of Veterinary and Animal Sciences, Narowal, Pakistan, [5] Department of Clinical Sciences, Section of Epidemiology and Public Health, College of Veterinary and Animal Sciences, Jhang, Pakistan, [6] Department of Clinical Sciences, University College of Veterinary and Animal Sciences, Narowal, Pakistan, [7] Institute of Microbiology, University of Veterinary and Animal Sciences, Lahore, Pakistan, [8] Department of Pathobiology, University College of Veterinary and Animal Sciences, Narowal, Pakistan

*Correspondence:
Caixia Guo
guocx@jlu.edu.cn
Waqas Ahmad
waqas.hussain@uvas.edu.pk

Rabies virus (RABV) is a cunning neurotropic pathogen and causes top priority neglected tropical diseases in the developing world. The genome of RABV consists of nucleoprotein (N), phosphoprotein (P), matrix protein (M), glycoprotein (G), and RNA polymerase L protein (L), respectively. The virus causes neuronal dysfunction instead of neuronal cell death by deregulating the polymerization of the actin and microtubule cytoskeleton and subverts the associated binding and motor proteins for efficient viral progression. These binding proteins mainly maintain neuronal structure, morphology, synaptic integrity, and complex neurophysiological pathways. However, much of the exact mechanism of the viral-cytoskeleton interaction is yet unclear because several binding proteins of the actin-microtubule cytoskeleton are involved in multifaceted pathways to influence the retrograde and anterograde axonal transport of RABV. In this review, all the available scientific results regarding cytoskeleton elements and their possible interactions with RABV have been collected through systematic methodology, and thereby interpreted to explain sneaky features of RABV. The aim is to envisage the pathogenesis of RABV to understand further steps of RABV progression inside the cells. RABV interacts in a number of ways with the cell cytoskeleton to produce degenerative changes in the biochemical and neuropathological trails of neurons and other cell types. Briefly, RABV changes the gene expression of essential cytoskeleton related proteins, depolymerizes actin and microtubules, coordinates the synthesis of inclusion bodies, manipulates microtubules and associated motors proteins, and uses actin for clathrin-mediated entry in different cells. Most importantly, the P is the most intricate protein of RABV that performs complex functions. It artfully operates the dynein motor protein along the tracks of microtubules to assist the replication, transcription, and transport of RABV until its egress from the cell. New remedial insights at subcellular levels are needed to counteract the destabilization of the cytoskeleton under RABV infection to stop its life cycle.

Keywords: Rabies virus, actin, microtubule, phosphoprotein, cytoskeleton, neuron, dynein, endocytosis

STRUCTURAL DYNAMICS OF CYTOSKELETON

Actin filaments, microtubules, and intermediate filaments are the 3 main components of the cell cytoskeleton. Actin filaments are composed of globular proteins that form small aggregates of actin monomers, and these actin monomers rapidly grow at the plus end of the actin filaments as compared to the minus end through a process called polymerization or nucleation (1, 2). There are 3 isoforms of globular actin, namely, α, β, and γ (2). The globular monomers are connected through weak forces to form long actin filaments. The actin cytoskeleton plays a vital role in viral endocytosis, cell motility, and membrane dynamics (3). The filamentous actin and the pool of globular actin are regulated and maintained by numerous actin-binding proteins (4, 5), while similar kinds of microtubule-binding proteins function to regulate the growth, polymerization, and depolymerization of microtubules (5). The microtubules are made up of α and β polar heterodimers which are arranged in a head-to-tail fashion, forming linear proto-filaments or tubular filaments, whereas 13 protofilaments combine to form microtubules (4, 5). Just like actin, the dynamic growing-end is denoted as the plus or barbed end (having GTP bound β subunit), facing the cell periphery. On the other hand, the depolymerizing or minus end (having α end) is attached to the microtubule organization center in the perinuclear area (4, 6, 7). Tubulins are abundantly present mainly in two pools, the free tubulin subunits and polymers (8, 9). The plus ends of the microtubules show a continuous dynamic state of growth and shrinkage with the intermittent pauses in dendrites, axons, and even in fully matured neurons (10). The microtubules have similar polarity in the axons, but mixed or heterogeneous polarity has been observed in dendrites (7, 11). The neuronal cytoskeleton is a set of complex proteins connected to strengthen the neurons in terms of guidance and growth in an early phase of neuronal development. The development of neuronal architecture, cell shape, homeostasis, and nerve plasticity are accomplished in the adult stage (1, 2, 4, 12). The cytoskeleton also provides support to transport molecular trafficking in the cytosol with the help of motor proteins. The bidirectional movement of molecular cargoes, cellular organelles, and viral genes within the environment of the cytoplasm is termed axonal transport (11). Microtubules extensively support the transport of the membrane-bounded vesicles either in retrograde (from axon to cell body) or anterograde (from cell body to axon) direction (4, 13, 14).

The actin and microtubule-binding proteins are the key elements that regulate the shape, structure, and polarity of actin and microtubule filaments, respectively (2, 4). For example, profilin is a noticeable actin-binding protein that is responsible for the binding of actin monomers to complete the cycle of polymerization by catalyzing the exchange of ATP in the actin filaments and thus helps in the growth and elongation of the actin filaments. The shorter nature of the β-thymosin peptides regulates the binding of the globular units (actin monomers) of the actin filaments. It also prevents the attachments of these monomers independently with the minus or plus end of the actin filaments. Cofilin is a vital actin slicing or severing protein that creates the dynamic instability among actin filaments by

providing free ends of the actin filaments from which the globular actin monomers can be dissociated or added. The capping proteins cap the plus or barbed ends of the actin filaments and prevent its further elongation by blocking the attachments of globular subunits at the polar ends of actin filaments. Contrary to the roles of capping proteins, the formins proteins normalize the actin dynamics by removing the capping proteins and elongating the actin filaments by exposing the corresponding end binding sites on these filaments to other actin-binding proteins (4, 14, 15). Similarly, the end binding proteins (EB family) of the microtubule are an important set of microtubule-binding proteins that regulate the dynamic nature of the microtubules. The carboxy-terminal tubulin tails (**Figure 1**) of the tubulin heterodimers coordinate the collective and individual assembly and growth rates of the microtubules. These terminal tails of the heterodimers also present the selective nature of the microtubules to the microtubule-binding proteins. Just like cofilin, stathmin is a microtubule depolymerizing protein (5, 14).

The various functions of these cytoskeleton binding proteins have been shown in **Figure 1** in which the dynamic turnover rates of both actin and microtubules have been summarized. This image describes the elongation (polymerization) and shrinkage (depolymerization) of actin and microtubule filaments with the help of these binding partners, and thus regulates the structure, integrity, and biochemical physiology of the nerve cell. Actin treadmilling is a phenomenon in which the actin monomers or individual units of the actin filaments are continuously released from the negative ends and join the positive ends. The profilin adds the ATP actin monomers to the plus ends, while formins uncap the negative ends. The hydrolysis of the ATP actin units occurs, and cofilin removes or slices the units of actin filaments. In this way, the detached actin monomers of the actin filaments present their hydrolyzed ADP in return to the ATP, and once again becomes eligible to perform another cycle of polymerization at the plus end of the actin filaments (15). In a similar fashion, the microtubule heterodimers (alpha and beta heterodimers) attach and detach to nucleate or polymerize the plus end of the microtubules, and hydrolysis of the beta bound GTP tubulin takes place, and similarly a slow rate of nucleation also takes place at the barbed end of the microtubule. The EB family proteins also aid in the process of nucleation. The catastrophic phenomena in the microtubules take place with the help of stathmin, just like the way cofilin does in the actin filaments (5). As a result, the pool of free alpha- and beta-tubulin heterodimers reduces and the length of the microtubule shrinks (**Figure 1**).

CELL BIOLOGY OF THE RABV

It is a bullet-shaped virus of around 180 nm long and 90 nm diameters. The virus is formed by an internal and an external unit linked together. The internal unit is composed of a nucleocapsid (NC) that includes the genomic RNA tied to the phosphoprotein (P), nucleoprotein (N), and viral polymerase (L). The external unit is formed by protruding spikes of the viral glycoprotein (G) and a bilayer lipid envelope acquired from the host cell

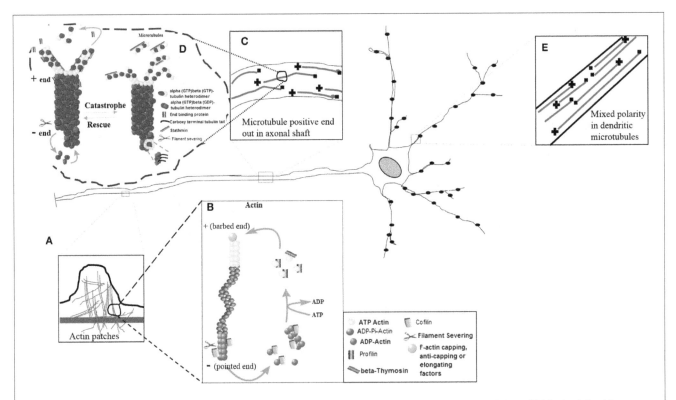

FIGURE 1 | The diagram of nerve cell showing different inset images of the active nature of the actin and microtubule cytoskeleton. **(E)** Mixed polarity of the microtubules exists in the dendrites of the neurons. **(C)** Positive ends are laid down in the axonal shaft for efficient bidirectional axonal transport. **(A)** The actin patches have been magnified in the inset image to show their presence in the axonal shaft. These actin patches act as a source to create further branches arising at different lengths of the axon. Further magnification of actin and microtubule images represent molecular structures showing the active phenomena of actin polymerization **(B)** and microtubule polymerization **(D)** or nucleation with the help of different binding proteins.

membrane. These two units are linked by the matrix protein (M) which interacts with the G protein and condenses the NC (16) (**Figure 2**).

Rabies virus (RABV) proteins (N, P, M, G, and L) are multifunctional. The N protein ensures the protection of the viral genome from RNAse and is the major component of the NC core. During transcription and replication, the N protein interacts with P and L proteins. The P protein participates in the replication and transcription process as a noncatalytic cofactor for the L protein and disrupts the host interferon-mediated antiviral response (16, 17). During N protein synthesis, the P protein regulates the positioning of the polymerase on the N-RNA template. It also prevents its binding to cellular RNA by acting as a chaperone. The M protein facilitates the budding, apoptosis, and intercellular membrane redistribution (16).

The life cycle of the RABV is dependent upon the clathrin-mediated endocytosis and acidic environment of the cytosol. RABV is coated with a spike-like G protein which is embedded in the lipid layer. The G protein of RABV is an essential indicator to induce pathogenesis inside host cells, and it also helps in the attachment of the RABV to the host cell surface. Moreover, it also assists in the long-distance transport of RABV from the neuromuscular junction to the central nervous system. After the attachment with the host cell receptors, various conformational changes occur in the G protein that uncoats the RABV genome

inside cytosol through an endocytic pathway (18). The negative-sense RNA genome is embedded in the N protein and acts as a template for transcription and replication. The ectodomain is the only external section of the G protein which provokes the synthesis of virus-neutralizing antibodies following the immune response mediated by cells. The role of replication and transcription are largely uptaken by the N and P proteins of RABV, while the M protein plays role in budding or viral exit (17–19).

MATERIALS AND METHODS

In this comprehensive critical review, a detailed analysis of different RABV proteins and their interactive features with the elements of the cytoskeleton have been discussed through a systematic strategy. All the relevant literature and published scientific research articles have been identified through various phrases and keywords with the help of boolean operators. These keywords and phrases included "Rabies virus and cytoskeleton," "RABV-Cytoskeleton," "Rabies virus and microtubule," "Rabies virus and actin," "Rabies virus with cytoskeleton binding proteins," "RABV-actin-microtubule," "Rabies pathogenesis in cytoskeleton," "Rabies-actin," "Rabies-microtubule," and "RABV depolymerizes cytoskeleton." In this regard, Google, PubMed, ScienceDirect, and Google Scholar were used as electronic

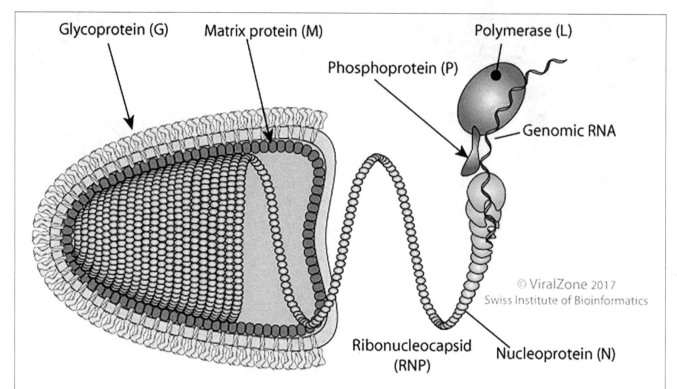

FIGURE 2 | Schematic diagram of bullet shape structure of RABV showing different proteins (original source of the image; Philippe Le Mercier, SIB Swiss Institute of Bioinformatics).

platforms to screen all the possible literature (20). All the materials that described the complete or partial association or interactive feature of RABV (or one of the related proteins of RABV) with the cytoskeleton elements (actin, microtubule, and binding proteins of cytoskeleton) were collected. Meaningful conclusions and interpretations have been made in the existing results to highlight the research findings of RABV pathogenesis and strategies to manipulate the host cytoskeleton using various models of *in vitro* and *in vivo* studies. These results have also been categorized in different subheadings to segregate similar findings under one subheading. Materials in a language other than English were excluded, while unindexed journals, websites, thesis reports, and magazine reports were also excluded (20).

RESULTS

Evasive Strategies of RABV With Cytoskeleton

Keeping in view the uniform integrity of the cytoskeleton in the neurons, it is believed that neurodegenerative diseases like rabies influence the dynamics, structure, and gene expression of the cytoskeleton and related proteins. Several studies support the fact that breach and discontinuity in the cytoskeleton network (microtubules and filamentous actin) develop neurodegenerative diseases, and rabies is one of the leading infectious diseases of the nervous system (14). RABV has many ways to manipulate the cell

cytoskeleton to induce pathological mechanisms that have been poorly understood so far. However, the followings are the most prevailing, but diversified sets of information that countercheck the host defense pathways using a variety of RABV-cytoskeleton interactions. These approaches also demonstrate that RABV sneakily exploits the actin and microtubule cytoskeleton for efficient viral replication, transcription, and intracellular transport.

RABV Alters the Gene Expression of Cytoskeleton-Related Proteins

Proteomic studies and real-time PCR assays quantify the viral proteins that aid molecular biologists and virologist to investigate the potential therapeutic agents, biomarkers, and foresee the generalized pathogenic pathways of the viruses (19). It has now been well established through *in vivo* and *in vitro* studies that RABV and related genotypes modulate the gene expression of cytoskeleton-related proteins in a variety of cell lines. Even humans nerve cells showed disturbances in the biological pathways of cytoskeleton organization or dynamics which control retrograde axonal transport, synaptic activity, and signaling events (4). The ingenuity pathways analysis shows that the RABV infected neurons in humans display abrupt alterations in the genetic expression of several key cytoskeleton-related proteins that regulate the intactness and structure of actin and microtubule cytoskeleton. Some of the notable genes increase the normal functioning of the cells which include calpastatin (CAST) and cyclin-dependent kinase inhibitor 1B (CDKN1B), while regulatory subunit 1 of the cyclin-dependent kinase (CDK5R1), clip associating protein 1 (CLASP1), and cAMP-responsive element-binding protein 1 (CREB1dec) decrease the cellular functions. Only doublecortin-like-kinase 1 (DCLK1) causes variable changes in the cellular functions. All of these genes are involved in the regulation and release of neurotransmitters, cell growth and differentiation, and stabilize microtubules (21). Another proteomic analysis shows the higher expression levels of tubulin, tropomyosin, and vimentin which are involved in the synthesis of elongated microtubules, development of axonal growth cones of filopodia (cytoplasmic projections larger than lamellipodia) or lamellipodia (thin membranous projections or protrusions of motile cells), and reinforce cytoskeleton to avoid external stress (22). The vimentin belongs to the intermediate filaments of the cytoskeleton, and preserves the cellular morphology by maintaining cytoskeleton shape, while tropomyosin also adjusts muscular contractions with the help of actin filaments (4, 14). Few studies of differential gene expression describe the abnormal neuronal structures due to the aberrations in the cytoplasmic proteins, and their corresponding pathways under RABV infections (22–24). Of these proteins, actin-related protein 2/3 complex subunit 3 and actin-related protein 2 showed higher gene expression, and the first one is meant for the actin polymerization, while the latter one maintains cellular polarity through the organization of the cytoskeleton in synaptosomes (24). However, neurofilament light polypeptide shows lower gene expression because it controls the axonal transport and aligns the assembly of axonal bundles (24). These are the salient proteins, and yet there are other actin-associated proteins (alpha-actinin-1 that anchors actin to various cellular structures, dynein light chain (DLC), capping proteins, and drebrin that generate stabilized actin filaments concentrated in the dendritic spines) and microtubule-associated proteins (microtubule-associated proteins-6) which are abundantly concentrated in the synaptosomes (5, 15, 24). The CVS strain of RABV also changes the 7 host proteins including the vimentin, stathmin, and capping proteins of the cytoskeletal in baby hamster kidney cell line (25). Interestingly, the protein-protein interactions discover that RABV transforms multiple neurochemical pathways related to synaptic plasticity, and nerve impulse transmission by renovating the organized proteins of the cytoskeleton (24, 26). A study also highlights the upregulation of the gene expression pattern of important microtubule-related proteins in cortical neurons of mouse brain tissue (27).

Microtubule-associated protein-2 (MAP-2) is a fundamental protein required to sustain neuronal shape and structure through the polymerization of dynamic microtubules. Most importantly, it also cross-links many biological pathways of neurotransmitters and maintains the assembly of other molecular trails involving different proteins of the cytoskeleton components (5, 28, 29). The downregulation pattern in the MAP-2 has already been observed under pathogenic infection of RABV (28, 30). In another study, RABV increases the genetic expression of NF-H (a protein that controls axonal growth) and MAP-2 which are integral proteins for the growing ends of tubulins as well (31), even though previously a proteomic approach reveal the similar findings in RABV infected human pyramidal nerve cells

(32). A CVS strain of RABV decreases the gene expression of more than 90% of the cytoskeleton-related genes while increasing the genetic expression of 39 important genes in mouse brain tissue (33). Keeping in view the importance of microtubule and actin-related proteins, end binding protein 3 (EB3) is one of the basic proteins that maintain microtubule-based signaling pathways, and also shapes the polar ends of the tubules, whereas p140cap protein controls actin dynamics and interacts with EB3 to optimize morphology of dendritic spines (29). Dendritic spines are the tiny protrusions at the end of dendrites that are abundant in other actin-binding proteins, namely, cortactin, drebrin, and CaMKIIβ. The cortactin performs actin polymerization and the rearrangement of actin filaments under the cell cortex, while CaMKIIβ controls neuronal growth and nerve plasticity with the help of the binding module of actin filaments (15, 34). Two different strains (the street and fixed RABVs) also downregulate the gene expression of EB3 and p140cap in cultured neuronal cells (29). These changes demonstrate that imbalance in the biochemical and neuronal homeostasis may lead to developing these degenerative changes in neuronal cells (14). The failure in the repair of the cytoskeleton network may lead to uncertainty in the maintenance of intact neuronal physiology which perhaps creates cellular dysfunctions (31, 35).

RABV Depolymerizes Microtubule and Actin

Rabies virus (RABV) causes depolymerization of microtubules by reducing the acetylated a-tubulin and this process facilitates the formation of RNA particles, while the M protein of RABV also up-regulates the gene expression of histone deacetylase 6 (HDAC6) which is a major structural protein to optimize actin and microtubule dynamics through the deacetylation of α-tubulin and cortactin. Moreover, the inhibition of HDAC6 also reduces the formation of RNA synthesis (36). The degenerative changes in the axons and dendritic tree are also caused by different strains of RABV. A recent study has shown that axonal degeneration occurs due to the depletion of nicotinamide adenine dinucleotide which is an energy producer molecule and accomplishes the proteolytic breakdown of MAP-2 and neurofilaments by calpain in extrinsic compartmental-nerve culture system (37).

In vivo and *in vitro* experiments show that street strain (MRV) of RABV causes dendritic injuries and depolymerization of actin filaments as dendritic spines are mostly enriched with filamentous actin (38). The decrease in the ratio between globular and filamentous actin in RABV-infected cells had also been calculated using western blot analysis (38). The alteration in neuronal actin was correlated with neuronal dysfunction. RABV depolymerizes the neuronal cytoskeleton by decreasing the actin bundle formation (39). Concisely, the N protein of RABV inhibited bundle formation of neuronal actin by inducing the dephospho-synapsin I which was an actin regulatory protein found in neurons. This was also experimentally demonstrated in confocal microscopy which showed the decreased intensity of immunofluorescence staining in the filamentous actin of neuroblastoma cells under RABV infection (40). A similar study was also conducted in different cell lines to observe the kinetics of focal adhesion kinase (FAK) and P protein of different RABV genomes. The FAK controlled the dynamic actin cytoskeleton through several actin-binding proteins. It also delimited the turnover rate of actin monomers in actin polymerization. Consequently, the decreased staining of filamentous actin was observed (41).

Clathrin-Mediated Endocytosis of RABV Requires Intact Actin

The G protein of RABV follows clathrin-mediated endocytosis for the receptor-mediated attachment and entry in the endothelial and vero cells with the help of actin filaments and associated proteins (35, 42–45). In vero cells, the internalized particles of RABV rely on microtubules for their motility as observed by the colocalization of SRV9 (an attenuated strain of RABV) with microtubules in immunofluorescence. Likewise, another study depicts similar results in which RABV is internalized in the peripheral neuronal cells (42). Vesicular stomatitis virus expressing recombinant G protein of RABV is experimentally internalized in the vero cell line using partially coated pits of clathrin-mediated endocytosis with the help of actin nucleation. The kinetics of G protein expressing viral particles is almost similar to vesicular stomatitis virus with respect to the time of attachment and association of pathogenic particles with the kidney cells (3). Similarly, different treatments of drugs that block or disrupt the clathrin-coated vesicles also inhibit the entry of RABV inside the cells. These drugs include sucrose, methyl-beta-cyclodextrin, and chlorpromazine, while the chlorpromazine also blocked the Australian bat lyssavirus G protein-mediated entry in HEK293T cells (3, 43). Latrunculin inhibits actin polymerization in the clathrin-coated pits. This drug also lessened the entry of Australian bat lyssavirus in HEK293T cells up to 62% (3). Similar types of drug tests verify that RABV does not follow the caveolar-dependent endocytosis (35, 43).

Nevertheless, experiments with HEP-2 and BHK-21 cells demonstrate that RABV might also employ additional passageways to enter the non-neuronal cell types (45, 46). For viruses, actin polymerization is an active process during receptor attachment and endocytosis. Therefore, further studies regarding drug experiments are needed to explore different cell types, interactions of RABV receptors, and the structure of the cytoskeleton elements so that a trajectory pathway can be envisaged (47). Cofilin is a well-known binding protein of actin and controls the remodeling and dynamic states of actin filaments. Remarkably, the M protein of RABV upregulates phosphorylated cofilin and promotes viral budding which is again dependent on the actin cytoskeleton (47). Hence, the internalization and budding of RABV require the assistance of actin and actin-based cytoskeleton (48). The trans-synaptic transmission of RABV has been shown in the diagram (**Figure 3**) where RABV is attached to the synaptic membrane *via* receptors, P75NTR and NCAM with the help of the G protein of RABV. The process of internalization is mediated by the clathrin protein, clathrin-coated pits, and actin proteins while the actin

has been densely populated beneath the cell membrane or in the synaptic terminal. The legend termed "invagination" shows that the RABV is coated within the clathrin-coated vesicle and formed with the surrounding actin filaments. As the clathrin protein uncoats, either the full genome is encapsulated within the endosome or the chelates of P/N protein are taken up by the dynein motor protein. The P and N proteins of RABV now interplay with the DLC to propagate the viral trafficking and transport it toward the cell body using the microtubule as tracks. All the process of retrograde transport has been diagrammed beneath the single microtubule. The RABV completes the transcription and replication within the nucleus (not shown), it then moves back to initiate its exit pathway once again using the stable tracks of microtubules. This reverse transport of the genome is designated as anterograde transport of the RABV which is accomplished by the kinesin motor proteins. These kinesin proteins harbor the fully replicated genome or the naked G protein of RABV and slide toward the cell periphery or the positive directed end of the microtubule to start the process of budding. The budding phenomena need the phosphorylated cofilin and M protein of RABV to exit and join the next cycle of infection.

RABV Requires Microtubules for Intracellular Trafficking

Viruses recruit motor proteins with the help of accessory proteins and employ the tracks of microtubules as pathways for the anterograde and retrograde transport of whole or partial viral parts for successful completion of the life cycle (12, 13). The intracellular transport of viruses is a complex system where the cytoplasmic environment is heavily crowded with various signaling and accessory proteins (7). In this situation, the microtubules act as polarized roads for the transport of viral cargoes to specific cellular destinations, while kinesins and dynein motor proteins act as energy vehicles to do the job of transportation of essential molecules from the plus or minus end of the microtubules to the other ends (49). Since cellular organelles are larger in size, therefore, energy is required to overcome the barriers of diffusion right after the internalization. Experiments conducted with the fluorescent-labeled G protein of RABV have shown long-range retrograde transport of virion using microtubules in neuroblastoma cells (6, 50, 51).

The mixed polarity of these microtubules in dendritic spines ensures the slow and fast axonal transport (adopted for RABV) inside the cells depending upon the availability of motor proteins in the absence of antiviral drugs, while plus ends are usually laid out in the axonal shaft as compared to the dendritic microtubules (12, 13). This fact has also been well established that RABV uses tracks of the microtubules for long-distance bidirectional transport with the help of motor proteins (7). In experiments in which the microtubule depolymerizing drugs such as vinblastine, nocodazole, and colchicine were used, the flow in the transport of various viruses (including RABV) was disrupted (6, 49).

Dynein deficient drosophila neurons produce transport defects leading to the misguided minus-end directed microtubules in axons (12). This suggests that the dynein

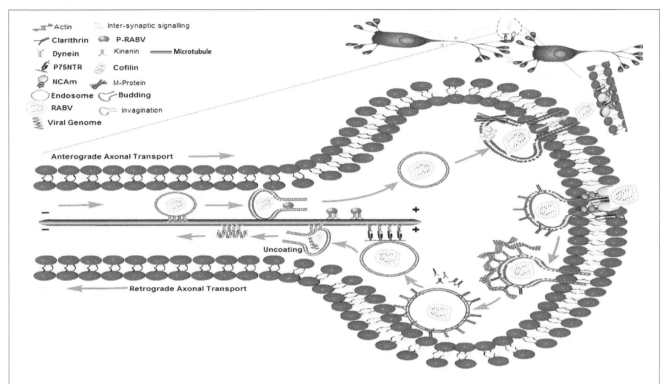

FIGURE 3 | The clathrin-mediated endocytosis and the transport (anterograde and retrograde) pathway of RABV within the nerve cell showing motor proteins, entry and exist paths of the RABV with the help of the cytoskeleton network.

motor is the most significant protein for retrograde axonal transport (6). The DLC is a microtubule minus-end-directed motor protein for retrograde transport of various molecular cargoes and organelles and also interacts with the actin in the early phase of RABV infection (11, 49). Modifications in the dynamics and spatial organization of microtubules play a critical role in the prognosis of infection. The P protein of RABV is a complex hub of protein with multiple binding sites that carries vital and multi-molecular interactive features in host-pathogen mechanisms including the cytoskeleton components. The structural or truncated forms of the P protein are p2, p3, p4, and p5 of which p3 has been extensively explored. The p3 interacts with the DLC in 2 different ways (52, 53). The p3 interacts with the DLC8 through the DLC association sequence that triggers the movement of the dynein motor proteins along the length of the microtubule, the second way is the formation of stable attachments with the microtubules with the help of microtubule-associated sequences (7).

Microtubules and Actin Are Required for RABV Inclusion Bodies

Nocodazole inhibited the dynamics and growth of microtubules. The RABV-infected BSR cells (cloned cells from the BHK-21 cell line) were treated with this drug that prevented the formation of "late" negri body-like inclusion bodies in the cells (40), while in another study, the same drug also diminished a few small size inclusion bodies. These negri bodies are viral replication

machinery and eject the RNP complex which is independent of the microtubule or actin network, but the transport of RNP is carried out with the help of microtubules. Moreover, the nearby movement of the RNP complex to negri bodies was restricted due to the inhibitory effect of the drug that ruptured or destabilized the tubulin filaments (43, 54). In the same way, the contribution of actin was also investigated by using cytochalasin D drug that depolymerizes actin dynamics. As a result, the inclusion bodies appeared smaller and scrappy in the cytoplasm (54).

Due to the overwhelming cellular stress, and overburdened viral replications, the misfolded viral aggregates are sequestered in the concentrated areas of the cytosol that give rise to ubiquitinated proteins which are known as aggresomes. These aggresomes structurally resembled some extent the negri bodies and are located at the microtubule organization center, but negri bodies are not covered externally with the microtubule protein vimentin. The negri bodies are also not connected to the microtubule organization center. These aggresomes are transferred to the inclusion bodies *via* microtubules using dynein-dependent transport. Microtubule inhibitory drug treatment increased the size and number of negri bodies per cell which further evidenced the fact that polymerization of microtubules coordinates the composition of negri bodies (55). The treatment of nocodazole also impaired the trajectories pathways, movement pattern, and velocities of viral particles which prove that microtubules are necessary for the intracellular transport of RABV (43).

The Interactions of N, P, and L Proteins of RABV With Cytoskeleton

Being a neurotropic virus, the intracellular transport of RABV depends on long-distance travel on axonal pathways. However, the approach by which RABV steals host cell transport machinery is equivocal. One strategy is the exploitation of host actin-microtubule cytoskeleton for invasion, and short or long-range trafficking at the cellular periphery even to reach the perinuclear region. The intracellular trafficking and transport of RABV rely on the stability of microtubule and actin filaments (56).

For example, microtubule and microtubule-associated proteins are involved in antiviral response by inducing interferon release that counters RABV intracellular replication. RABV handles this host cell strategy through its P protein by inhibiting the interferon production, and JAK/STAT signaling pathway which again depends upon the stability of the microtubules for intracellular trafficking of essential pathway building signaling proteins and molecular cues (8, 9, 52). Thus, in this way, the P protein is involved in the inhibition of IFN and promotes intracellular viral replication (9).

The P protein of RABV was also investigated using the FAK as an essential molecular ingredient in the yeast two-hybrid system. The dimerization domain of P protein was 106, while 131 was meant for the C-terminal domain of FAK. It has been well established that FAK interacts with the P protein of RABV to cause RABV infection in infected host cells. The P protein and FAK were experimentally colocalized and coimmunoprecipitated in negri bodies, and this experimental interaction between FAK and P protein was also reconfirmed through downregulation of FAK, which finally inhibited the expression of P protein of RABV. Hence, FAK is an imperative constituent for RABV pathogenesis and an important cellular partner of the P protein of RABV (41).

The P protein of all genotypes of RABV also interacts with the light chain of dynein motor protein (53, 57) and the RABV inclusion bodies are also closely in contact with the filamentous actin underneath the cell membrane or nearby the endocytic entry during the earlier events inside the cells. Thus, the light chain possesses a dual interactive role with the cytoskeleton components for the transport of the RNP complex in neuronal cells (53). DLC1 binding motif in L protein of RABV mediates microtubule binding with the help of dynein motors. As the motif was disrupted, the microtubule localization in the cell was disrupted. The L protein of RABV also regulates the post-translational modifications of the microtubule cytoskeleton. Hence, the microtubule is an essential structural element in controlling the intracellular transport (57).

The oligomeric state of P protein of RABV in the interactive process of more than one polypeptide chain of the protein gives rise to quaternary protein structure. The P protein has the unique ability to interact with the microtubules either through a microtubule-facilitated or inhibitory mechanism. Interestingly, the P protein can switch between these two states with the help of interferon-activated transcription factor STAT1 to regulate trafficking and motor-based bidirectional transport (9).

On the other hand, the N protein of RABV does not require the support of the cytoskeleton for its synthesis in the neuronal and non-neuronal cell cytoplasm of dorsal root ganglia (58), but the fluorescent-tagged L protein of RABV does interact with the microtubule cytoskeleton and facilitates the production of tubulin to enhance viral infection and transport. Further analysis also shows that the binding motif of DLC1 in the L protein of RABV can bind with the microtubules. As binding of P and L protein of RABV with DLC1 is valuable for transcription, both of these protein motifs regulate the gene expression of DLC1 inside the cells. The overexpression of DLC1 also enhances the tubulins' growth and maintenance to facilitate viral infections. The silencing or downregulation of the motif in the L destabilizes the microtubule and hence, the DLC1 is significantly associated with the L gene of RABV for smooth transport functions through the microtubule (59).

Two-dimensional far-western blotting confirmed that the M protein of RABV also interacts with six different proteins in rat brain stem including the actin cytoplasmic-1 that was verified in co-immunoprecipitation. All these proteins regulate vital cellular processes as described earlier and the findings were also verified in mouse neuro-N2a cells (60).

CONCLUSIONS

The review demonstrates a comprehensive analysis of various research studies to show that RABV attempt to dysfunction the axonal transport, structure of the neurons, and neurotransmitters in the synaptic terminal by modulating the cytoskeleton network. Subcellular transport is the best level of investigation to explore the individual lines of evidence used by the viruses. RABV sneakily exploits actin, microtubules, kinesin, and dynein motor proteins for its survival. However, the functional consequences and pathological outcomes are yet to be elucidated through experiments conducted through fluorescent-tagged proteins or cargoes in live cell imaging. The prospects of new research directions, identification of the existing gaps, and inconsistency in the development of new research insights were also identified. The review has highlighted that the host cytoskeleton provides tracks and assistance in each step from the entry of the RABV until its budding. This review will help scientists and virologists to further elucidate the pathogenesis of RABV and define new research questions to generate possible hypotheses. Further research is needed to address how RABV subverts the cellular motor proteins to complete a successful cycle of infection. Scientific reconsiderations of all the experimental studies and molecular approaches can provide helpful clues in determining the pathogenesis of RABV inside the host cell. It will also reveal the functional morphology of cytoskeleton elements that possibly aid RABV in disrupting the normal cellular physiology. The futuristic approaches are required to develop which should be based on the available findings and analysis of the reviews. Few helpful strategies include the development of therapeutic agents, biotechnological procedures, preventive drugs, and attenuated viruses for the production of efficient vaccines. The role of actin and microtubule-binding proteins, especially cofilin needs to be further explored in the pathogenesis and budding of RABV to verify whether RABV directly or indirectly interacts with actin.

AUTHOR CONTRIBUTIONS

XL and CG conceived the idea, designed the study plan, and managed funding. ZN and SAl collected the literature review and extracted meaningful contents. TJ, SAh, and WA wrote the manuscript. MAN and MUS drew the images. MAI and AA revised the manuscript, added further contents, and improved the language. All authors read and approved the final version of the manuscript.

REFERENCES

1. Kapitein Lukas C, Hoogenraad Casper C. Building the neuronal microtubule cytoskeleton. *Neuron.* (2015) 87:492–506. doi: 10.1016/j.neuron.2015.05.046
2. Pimm ML, Henty-Ridilla JL. New twists in actin–microtubule interactions. *Mol Biol Cell.* (2021) 32:211–7. doi: 10.1091/mbc.E19-09-0491
3. Weir DL, Laing ED, Smith IL, Wang LF, Broder CC. Host cell virus entry mediated by Australian bat lyssavirus G envelope glycoprotein occurs through a clathrin-mediated endocytic pathway that requires actin and Rab5. *Virol J.* (2014) 11:40. doi: 10.1186/1743-422X-11-40
4. Farhadi L, Ricketts SN, Rust MJ, Das M, Robertson-Anderson RM, Ross JL. Actin and microtubule crosslinkers tune mobility and control co-localization in a composite cytoskeletal network. *Soft Matter.* (2020) 16:7191–201. doi: 10.1039/C9SM02400J
5. Goodson HV, Jonasson EM. Microtubules and microtubule-associated proteins. *Cold Spring Harb Perspect Biol.* (2018) 10:a022608. doi: 10.1101/cshperspect.a022608
6. Dodding MP, Way M. Coupling viruses to dynein and kinesin-1. *EMBO J.* (2011) 30:3527–39. doi: 10.1038/emboj.2011.283
7. Brice A, Moseley GW. Viral interactions with microtubules: orchestrators of host cell biology? *Fut Virol.* (2013) 8:229–43. doi: 10.2217/fvl.12.137
8. Brice A, Whelan DR, Ito N, Shimizu K, Wiltzer-Bach L, Lo CY, et al. Quantitative analysis of the microtubule interaction of rabies virus P3 protein: roles in immune evasion and pathogenesis. *Sci Rep.* (2016) 6:33493. doi: 10.1038/srep33493
9. Moseley GW, Lahaye X, Roth DM, Oksayan S, Filmer RP, Rowe CL, et al. Dual modes of rabies P-protein association with microtubules: a novel strategy to suppress the antiviral response. *J Cell Sci.* (2009) 122:3652–62. doi: 10.1242/jcs.045542
10. Vitriol Eric A, McMillen Laura M, Kapustina M, Gomez Shawn M, Vavylonis D, Zheng James Q. Two functionally distinct sources of actin monomers supply the leading edge of lamellipodia. *Cell Rep.* (2015) 11:433–45. doi: 10.1016/j.celrep.2015.03.033
11. Richards A, Berth SH, Brady S, Morfini G. Engagement of neurotropic viruses in fast axonal transport: mechanisms, potential role of host kinases and implications for neuronal dysfunction. *Front Cell Neurosci.* (2021) 15:684762. doi: 10.3389/fncel.2021.684762
12. Zheng Y, Wildonger J, Ye B, Zhang Y, Kita A, Younger SH, et al. Dynein is required for polarized dendritic transport and uniform microtubule orientation in axons. *Nat Cell Biol.* (2008) 10:1172–80. doi: 10.1038/ncb1777
13. Arriagada G. Retroviruses and microtubule-associated motor proteins. *Cell Microbiol.* (2017) 19:e12759. doi: 10.1111/cmi.12759
14. Muñoz-Lasso DC, Romá-Mateo C, Pallardó FV, Gonzalez-Cabo P. Much more than a scaffold: cytoskeletal proteins in neurological disorders. *Cells.* (2020) 9:358. doi: 10.3390/cells9020358
15. Gupta CM, Ambaru B, Bajaj R. Emerging functions of actins and actin binding proteins in trypanosomatids. *Front Cell Dev Biol.* (2020) 8:587685. doi: 10.3389/fcell.2020.587685
16. Davis BM, Rall GF, Schnell MJ. Everything you always wanted to know about rabies virus (But Were Afraid to Ask). *Ann Rev Virol.* (2015) 2:451–71. doi: 10.1146/annurev-virology-100114-055157
17. Rieder M, Conzelmann KK. Interferon in rabies virus infection. *Adv Virus Res.* (2011) 79:91–114. doi: 10.1016/B978-0-12-387040-7.00006-8
18. Lafon M. Rabies virus receptors. *J NeuroVirol.* (2005) 11:82–7. doi: 10.1080/13550280590900427
19. Chienwichai P, Reamtong O. Application of multi-omics technologies to decipher rabies pathogenesis. *Thai J Vet Med.* (2020) 50:29–136. Available online at: https://he01.tci-thaijo.org/index.php/tjvm/article/view/243723
20. Lingard L. Writing an effective literature review. *Perspect Med Educ.* (2018) 7:133–5. doi: 10.1007/s40037-018-0407-z
21. Gomme EA, Wirblich C, Addya S, Rall GF, Schnell MJ. Immune clearance of attenuated rabies virus results in neuronal survival with altered gene expression. *PLoS Pathog.* (2012) 8:e1002971. doi: 10.1371/journal.ppat.1002971
22. Wang X, Zhang S, Sun C, Yuan ZG, Wu X, Wang D, et al. Proteomic profiles of mouse neuro N2a cells infected with variant virulence of rabies viruses. *J Microbiol Biotechnol.* (2011) 21:366–73. doi: 10.4014/jmb.1010.10003
23. Zandi F, Eslami N, Torkashvand F, Fayaz A, Khalaj V, Vaziri B. Expression changes of cytoskeletal associated proteins in proteomic profiling of neuroblastoma cells infected with different strains of rabies virus. *J Med Virol.* (2012) 85:336–47. doi: 10.1002/jmv.23458
24. Sun X, Shi N, Li Y, Dong C, Zhang M, Guan Z, et al. Quantitative proteome profiling of street rabies virus-infected mouse hippocampal synaptosomes. *Curr Microbiol.* (2016) 73:301–11. doi: 10.1007/s00284-016-1061-5
25. Zandi F, Eslami N, Soheili M, Fayaz A, Gholami A, Vaziri B. Proteomics analysis of BHK-21 cells infected with a fixed strain of rabies virus. *Proteomics.* (2009) 9:2399–407. doi: 10.1002/pmic.200701007
26. Farahtaj F, Zandi F, Khalaj V, Biglari P, Fayaz A, Vaziri B. Proteomics analysis of human brain tissue infected by street rabies virus. *Mol Biol Rep.* (2013) 40:6443–50. doi: 10.1007/s11033-013-2759-0
27. Ahmad W, Hussain FS, Ali A, Akram Q. Electron microscopy and differential gene expression of various neurotransmitters and cytoskeleton related proteins under rabies virus infection. *J Neurol Sci.* (2019) 405:14–6. doi: 10.1016/j.jns.2019.10.237
28. Hurtado AP, Rengifo AC, Torres-Fernández O. Immunohistochemical overexpression of MAP-2 in the cerebral cortex of rabies-infected mice. *Int J Morphol.* (2015) 33:465–70. doi: 10.4067/S0717-95022015000200010
29. Guo Y. *In vitro* infection of street and fixed rabies virus strains inhibit gene expression of actin-microtubule binding proteins EB3 and p140cap in Neurons. *Pak Vet J.* (2019) 39:359–64. doi: 10.29261/pakvetj/2019.007
30. Li XQ, Sarmento L, Fu ZF. Degeneration of neuronal processes after infection with pathogenic, but not attenuated, rabies viruses. *J Virol.* (2005) 79:10063–8. doi: 10.1128/JVI.79.15.10063-10068.2005
31. Monroy-Gómez J, Santamaría G, Torres-Fernández O. Overexpression of MAP2 and NF-H associated with dendritic pathology in the spinal cord of mice infected with rabies virus. *Viruses.* (2018) 10:112. doi: 10.3390/v10030112
32. Venugopal AK, Ghantasala SSK, Selvan LDN, Mahadevan A, Renuse S, Kumar P, et al. Quantitative proteomics for identifying biomarkers for Rabies. *Clin Proteomics.* (2013) 10:3. doi: 10.1186/1559-0275-10-3
33. Prosniak M, Hooper DC, Dietzschold B, Koprowski H. Effect of rabies virus infection on gene expression in mouse brain. *Proc Nat Acad Sci.* (2001) 98:2758–63. doi: 10.1073/pnas.051630298
34. McMahon HT, Boucrot E. Molecular mechanism and physiological functions of clathrin-mediated endocytosis. *Nat Rev Mol Cell Biol.* (2011) 12:517–33. doi: 10.1038/nrm3151

35. Guo Y, Duan M, Wang X, Gao J, Guan Z, Zhang M. Early events in rabies virus infection—attachment, entry, and intracellular trafficking. *Virus Res.* (2019) 263:217–25. doi: 10.1016/j.virusres.2019.02.006

36. Zan J, Liu S, Sun DN, Mo KK, Yan Y, Liu J, et al. Rabies virus infection induces microtubule depolymerization to facilitate viral RNA synthesis by upregulating HDAC6. *Front Cell Infect Microbiol.* (2017) 7:146. doi: 10.3389/fcimb.2017.00146

37. Sundaramoorthy V, Green D, Locke K, O'Brien CM, Dearnley M, Bingham J. Novel role of SARM1 mediated axonal degeneration in the pathogenesis of rabies. *PLoS Pathog.* (2020) 16:e1008343. doi: 10.1371/journal.ppat.1008343

38. Song Y, Hou J, Qiao B, Li Y, Xu Y, Duan M, et al. Street rabies virus causes dendritic injury and F-actin depolymerization in the hippocampus. *J Gen Virol.* (2013) 94:276–83. doi: 10.1099/vir.0.047480-0

39. Ceccaldi PE, Hellio R, Valtorta F, Tsiang H, Braud S. Alteration of the actin-based cytoskeleton by rabies virus. *J Gen Virol.* (1997) 78:2831–5. doi: 10.1099/0022-1317-78-11-2831

40. Lahaye X, Vidy A, Fouquet B, Blondel D. Hsp70 protein positively regulates rabies virus infection. *J Virol.* (2012) 86:4743–51. doi: 10.1128/JVI.06501-11

41. Fouquet B, Nikolic J, Larrous F, Bourhy H, Wirblich C, Lagaudrière-Gesbert C, et al. Focal adhesion kinase is involved in rabies virus infection through its interaction with viral phosphoprotein P. *J Virol.* (2015) 89:1640–51. doi: 10.1128/JVI.02602-14

42. Piccinotti S, Whelan SPJ. Rabies internalizes into primary peripheral neurons via clathrin coated pits and requires fusion at the cell body. *PLoS Pathog.* (2016) 12:e1005753. doi: 10.1371/journal.ppat.1005753

43. Xu H, Hao X, Wang S, Wang Z, Cai M, Jiang J, et al. Real-time imaging of rabies virus entry into living vero cells. *Sci Rep.* (2015) 5:11753. doi: 10.1038/srep11753

44. Wang C, Wang J, Shuai L, Ma X, Zhang H, Liu R, et al. The serine/threonine kinase AP2-Associated Kinase 1 plays an important role in rabies virus entry. *Viruses.* (2019) 12:45. doi: 10.3390/v12010045

45. Piccinotti S, Kirchhausen T, Whelan SPJ. Uptake of rabies virus into epithelial cells by clathrin-mediated endocytosis depends upon actin. *J Virol.* (2013) 87:11637–47. doi: 10.1128/JVI.01648-13

46. Hotta K, Bazartseren B, Kaku Y, Noguchi A, Okutani A, Inoue S, et al. Effect of cellular cholesterol depletion on rabies virus infection. *Virus Res.* (2009) 139:85–90. doi: 10.1016/j.virusres.2008.10.009

47. Zan J, An ST, Mo KK, Zhou JW, Liu J, Wang HL, et al. Rabies virus inactivates cofilin to facilitate viral budding and release. *Biochem Biophys Res Commun.* (2016) 477:1045–50. doi: 10.1016/j.bbrc.2016.07.030

48. Wang IH, Burckhardt C, Yakimovich A, Greber U. Imaging, tracking and computational analyses of virus entry and egress with the cytoskeleton. *Viruses.* (2018) 10:166. doi: 10.3390/v10040166

49. Leopold PL, Pfister KK. Viral strategies for intracellular trafficking: motors and microtubules. *Traffic.* (2006) 7:516–23. doi: 10.1111/j.1600-0854.2006.00408.x

50. Klingen Y, Conzelmann KK, Finke S. Double-labeled rabies virus: live tracking of enveloped virus transport. *J Virol.* (2008) 82:237–45. doi: 10.1128/JVI.01342-07

51. Gluska S, Zahavi EE, Chein M, Gradus T, Bauer A, Finke S, et al. Rabies virus hijacks and accelerates the p75NTR retrograde axonal transport machinery. *PLoS Pathog.* (2014) 10:e1004348. doi: 10.1371/journal.ppat.1004348

52. Leyrat C, Ribeiro EA, Gérard FC, Ivanov I, Ruigrok RW, Jamin M. Structure, interactions with host cell and functions of rhabdovirus phosphoprotein. *Fut Virol.* (2011) 6:465–81. doi: 10.2217/fvl.11.10

53. Jacob Y, Badrane H, Ceccaldi PE, TordoN. Cytoplasmic Dynein LC8 interacts with lyssavirus phosphoprotein. *J Virol.* (2000) 74:10217–22. doi: 10.1128/JVI.74.21.10217-10222.2000

54. Nikolic J, Le Bars R, Lama Z, Scrima N, Lagaudrière-Gesbert C, Gaudin Y, et al. Negri bodies are viral factories with properties of liquid organelles. *Nat Commun.* (2017) 8:58. doi: 10.1038/s41467-017-00102-9

55. Ménager P, Roux P, Mégret F, Bourgeois JP, Le Sourd AM, Danckaert A, et al. Toll-like receptor 3 (TLR3) Plays a major role in the formation of rabies virus negri bodies. *PLoS Pathog.* (2009) 5:e1000315. doi: 10.1371/journal.ppat.1000315

56. LoPachin RM. The changing view of acrylamide neurotoxicity. *Neurotoxicology.* (2004) 25:617–30. doi: 10.1016/j.neuro.2004.01.004

57. RauxH, Flamand A, Blondel D. Interaction of the rabies virus P protein with the LC8 dynein light Chain. *J Virol.* (2000) 74:10212–6. doi: 10.1128/JVI.74.21.10212-10216.2000

58. Hara Y, Hasebe R, Sunden Y, Ochiai K, Honda E, Sakoda Y, et al. Propagation of swine hemagglutinating encephalomyelitis virus and pseudorabies virus in dorsal root ganglia cells. *J Vet Med Sci.* (2009) 71:595–601. doi: 10.1292/jvms.71.595

59. Bauer A, Nolden T, Nemitz S, Perlson E, Finke S. A dynein light chain 1 binding motif in rabies virus polymerase L protein plays a role in microtubule reorganization and viral primary transcription. *J Virol.* (2015) 89:9591–600. doi: 10.1128/JVI.01298-15

60. Zandi F, Khalaj V, Goshadrou F, Meyfour A, Gholami A, Enayati S, et al. Rabies virus matrix protein targets host actin cytoskeleton: a protein–protein interaction analysis. *Pathog Dis.* (2020) 79:ftaa075. doi: 10.1093/femspd/ftaa075

24

Effect of Co-Infection of Low Pathogenic Avian Influenza H9N2 Virus and Avian Pathogenic *E. coli* on H9N2-Vaccinated Commercial Broiler Chickens

Sherif I. A. Mahmoud[1], Kamel A. Zyan[1], Mohamed M. Hamoud[2], Eman Khalifa[3], Shahin Dardir[4], Rabab Khalifa[4], Walid H. Kilany[5] and Wael K. Elfeil[6*]*

[1] Department of Avian and Rabbit Diseases, Faculty of Veterinary Medicine, Benha University, Benha, Egypt, [2] Department of Poultry and Rabbit Diseases, Faculty of Veterinary Medicine, Cairo University, Giza, Egypt, [3] Department Microbiology, Faculty of Veterinary Medicine, Matrouh University, Matrouh, Egypt, [4] Department Veterinary Care and Laboratories Department, Cairo Poultry Corporate, Giza, Egypt, [5] Reference Laboratory for Veterinary Quality Control on Poultry Production, Animal Health Research Institute, Agriculture Research Center, Ministry of Agriculture, Cairo, Egypt, [6] Department of Avian and Rabbit Department, Faculty of Veterinary Medicine, Suez Canal University, Ismailia, Egypt

Correspondence:
Wael K. Elfeil
elfeil@vet.suez.edu.eg
Mohamed M. Hamoud
Mohamed.hamoud@cu.edu.eg

In the last 40 years, low pathogenic avian influenza virus (LPAIV) subtype H9N2 has been endemic in most Middle Eastern countries and of course Egypt which is one of the biggest poultry producers in the middle east region. The major losses with the H9N2 virus infections come from complicated infections in commercial broiler chickens, especially *E. coli* infection. In this work, 2,36,345 Arbor acres broiler chickens from the same breeder flock were placed equally in four pens, where two pens were vaccinated against LPAIV of subtype H9N2 virus, and the other two pens served as non-vaccinated controls. All were placed on the same farm under the same management conditions. A total of twenty birds from each pen were moved to biosafety level–3 chicken isolators (BSL-3) on days 21 and 28 of life and challenged with LPAIV-H9N2 or *E. coli*. Seroconversion for H9N2 was evaluated before and after the challenge. The recorded results revealed a significant decrease in clinical manifestations and virus shedding in terms of titers of shedding virus and number of shedders in vaccinated compared to non-vaccinated chickens. In groups early infected with LPAIV-H9N2 virus either vaccinated or not vaccinated, there was no significant difference in clinical sickness or mortalities in both groups, but in late infection groups with H9N2 alone, non-vaccinated infected group showed significantly higher clinical sickness in comparison with infected vaccinated group but also without mortality. In groups co-infected with *E. coli* (I/M) and H9N2, it showed 100% mortalities either in vaccinated or non-vaccinated H9N2 groups and thus reflect the high pathogenicity of used *E. coli* isolates, whereas in groups co-infected with *E. coli* (per os to mimic the natural route of infection) and LPAIV-H9N2, mortality rates were significantly higher in non-vaccinated groups than those vaccinated with H9N2 vaccine (15 vs. 5%). In conclusion, the use of the LPAIV H9N2 vaccine has significantly impacted the health status, amount of virus shed, and mortality of challenged commercial broilers, as it can minimize the losses and risks after co-infection with *E. coli* (orally) and LPAIV-H9N2 virus under similar natural route of infection in commercial broilers.

Keywords: avian influenza, H9N2 AIV infection, *E. coli*, mixed infection, broiler - chicken, vaccine

INTRODUCTION

Low pathogenic avian influenza virus (LPAIV) subtype H9N2 virus infection is an endemic disease in nearly all Middle Eastern countries including Egypt, Iran, Israel, Saudi Arabia, Jordan, Kuwait, Lebanon, and the United Arab Emirates (1). LPAIV-H9N2 viruses found in the Middle East are mostly of the G1 "Western" sub-lineage, with occasional isolation of Y439 lineage viruses, possibly originating from wild birds (2). Whenever LPAIV of subtype H9N2 virus prevalence was investigated in developing countries, by surveys and sampling, the virus was found frequently, particularly in live bird markets "LBMs." LBMs are a major way of disease transmission and zoonotic infections (3). In Egypt, where LBMs are the main market for chicken consumers, the prevalence of LPAIV-H9N2 infections is about 10%. A degree of hyper-endemicity exists in all the previous countries, which is not the same for the other influenza virus subtypes such as H5N1 and H7 subtypes. This difference may be due to the nature of the LPAIV phenotype of the virus, allowing repeated re-infection of the same birds and the same flocks of layers and breeders chickens (with longer life span than broilers chickens). Silent spreading is frequently occurring between farms and backyards birds (2). Despite being detected by real-time reverse transcription polymerase chain reaction (RT-qPCR) in 2006, the first isolation of LPAIH9N2 in Egyptian birds' dates back to December 2010 (4). Serological surveillance done in February 2009 revealed the presence of antibodies against the LPAI H9N2 subtype in domestic poultry flocks (5). For the broiler industry In Egypt, the most common diseases that affect the flocks and causing severe economic losses are respiratory pathogens that act either singly or in combination with each other. Clinical signs caused by many poultry respiratory pathogens are similar and confusing (6). This includes avian influenza, Newcastle disease, and infectious bronchitis. All show a huge economic impact because of their ability to induce high mortality independently or in association with each other organisms (7, 8). Avian pathogenic *E. coli* (APEC) is the most common infectious pathogen of all poultry species, resulting in multiple diseases in commercial poultry flocks. The most common disease is colibacillosis, which results in severe economic losses (9). APEC virulence is related to the presence of multiple factors that help the pathogen in causing the disease. *E. coli* can cause significant necrosis to the host cells due to the various proteases, hydrogen peroxide, nitrous oxide, and the release of proinflammatory cytokines, inhibiting phagocytosis, and affecting the normal functions of B- and T-lymphocytes. The presence of *E. coli* may be a powerful predisposing factor for several viral and bacterial infections including LPAI H9N2 (10). No efficient vaccine has been declared for APEC and antibiotics have been used widely in poultry flocks for controlling this disease, leading to an extensive antimicrobial resistance (11). Infection of broiler chickens with *E.coli* before, after, or even during the infection with LPAI H9N2 induces severe clinical signs with high mortality; such two major pathogens can affect broiler chickens much more than each alone (12). Likewise, co-infections of LPAIV-H9N2 with other respiratory pathogens, such as infectious bronchitis virus (IBV),

Mycoplasma gallisepticum, Staphylococcus aureus, Escherichia coli, and Ornithobacterium rhinotracheale, can exacerbate H9N2 infection, resulting in high morbidity and mortality (13). The co-infection of H9N2 virus and avian pathogenic *E.coli* potentiates the pathological picture of each other as the replication of the AIV-H9N2 virus leads to significant upregulation of some essential proteins associated with avian pathogenic *E.coli* adhesion (transforming growth factor beta-1, E-cadherin, fibromodulin, and so on.), innate immunity associated protein (beta-2-microglobulin, alpha-1-acid glycoprotein, TAP-binding protein, and so on.), and cell proliferation, differentiation and apoptosis (apoptotic protease-activating factor 1, mitogen-activated protein kinase, transforming growth factor beta-1, and so on.), and the upregulation processes enhance the bacterial pathogenicity and pathological effect, as a result of the pathological effect of the bacterial, it increases the level of protease-like enzymes in the respiratory and digestive tract tissues, which enhance the cleavability of LPAIV-H9N2 and the immunosuppressive effect of *E.coli* infection decrease the birds response to the virus infection, so the virus replicates much higher and potentiates its pathological picture (14–18). Also, co-infection of avian pathogenic *E.coli* and AIV-H9N2 virus can elevate the inflammatory mediators (TNF-α and INF-γ), and the immunosuppressive effect of *E.coli* infection decreases the birds response to the virus infection and potentiates the losses from the co-infection process (10, 18–20). The objective of this study was to evaluate the benefit of vaccinating broiler chickens with LPAIV H9N2 and the role of combined infection with both avian pathogenic *E. coli* (APEC) and LPAIV H9N2.

MATERIALS AND METHODS
Ethical Approval
Animal studies were approved by the Animal Welfare and Research Ethics Committee of Benha University by approval no. BU2019421PX23, and all procedures were conducted strictly following the Guidelines for Care and Use of Laboratory Animals. Every effort was made to minimize animal suffering.

Birds and Vaccines
A total of 2,36,345 1-day-old Arbor Acres broiler chicks from vaccinated broiler breeders' flocks (1-day-old chicks with maternally derived immunity "MDA" against LPAIV-H9N2 virus) were obtained from the same breeder flock and placed in two closed broiler system farms in Elsaff, Giza Governorate. All were kept under commercial field conditions with proper biosecurity measures and received the same management standards. Farm A contained 117,170 birds and was vaccinated with MEFLUVAC H5+H9+ND7 combined vaccine "consist of H5N1 clade 2.2.1.2, H5N8 clade 2.3.4.4., NDV genotype-II, NDV-genotype-VII, and H9N2 inactivated vaccine seeds" (MEVAC Company, Egypt) at 10th day of age. Farm B was harbored 119,175 birds and vaccinated with MEFLUVAC H5+ND7 combined vaccine "containing H5N1 clade 2.2.1.2, H5N8 clade 2.3.4.4, NDV genotype-II and NDV-Genotype-VII inactivated vaccine seeds" (MEVAC Company, Egypt) at 10th day of age. The birds also received vaccines for IBD (Univax

BD "a live virus vaccine containing a mild strain (ST-12) of Infectious Bursal Disease," MSD company, USA on day one of life then Bursine plus "Live freeze-dried intermediate plus IBD virus, Lukert strain," Zoetis company, USA at day 13 of life), MEFLUVAC H5+ND7 combined vaccine (inactivated AIV-H5 vaccine (MEVAC Company, Egypt), and live bivalent ND-IB vaccine (Polimun ND Hitchner B1+IB H120, Biotest laboratory company at day one of life, Nobilis Clone 30+ IB Ma5 (MSD company at day 10 of life), Volvac LaSota (Boehringer-Ingelheim, Germany), Vaxsafe ND "ND V4 strain" (Bioproperties, Australia, at 16 day of life) as the part of routine vaccination program of commercial broilers in Egypt. All vaccines were used according to the manufacturer's recommendations.

Birds kept under field conditions underwent regular monitoring by RT-PCR on days 2, 4, 18, 21, 25, 27, and 31 of life for the detection of common circulating pathogens in the region, including AIV-H5, AIV-H9N2, NDV velogenic, IBV, IBD, avian nephritis virus, and chicken astrovirus using primer sets developed by Cairo Poultry Group diagnostic lab (house-made primers and probe, Unpublished data) and AgPath-ID™ One-Step RT-PCR Reagents Thermo Fisher Scientific Inc., Massachusetts, USA), according to the manufacturer's instructions (catalog number: 4387391, Thermo Fisher Scientific Inc., Massachusetts, USA) using Applied Biosystem 7500 RT-PCR engine, according to the manufacturer's instructions (Thermo Fisher Scientific Inc., Massachusetts, USA).

Experimental Design

The main objective of this work was to evaluate the effect of LPAIV-H9N2 vaccination (using inactivated vaccine) on the broiler chicks and response following challenge with LPAIV-H9N2 virus alone or combined with avian pathogenic E. coli under laboratory and commercial field conditions. The infection

was applied in two stages, an early challenge on 21 days of life, 120 birds moved to BSL-3 (early challenge) and grouped as G-1-3(a-b), and for late challenge applied on day 28 of life, another 120 birds moved to BSL-3 and grouped as G-3-5(a-b) (late challenge), birds in G3a/b were challenged on day 21 of life with E. coli per os and kept under monitoring for 7 days (till 28 day of life) and challenged on day 28 of life with LPAIV-H9N2 via IN route to evaluate the effect of infection of H9N2 following E. coli infection. All birds kept in commercial farms from 1 day of life and moved to the BSL-3, 48 h before the challenge date, and every 12 h, cloacal and tracheal swabs were collected and checked with RT-PCR for AIV-matrix gene, NDV velogenic virus, and IBV using specific primer for each disease, to ensure that it is free from any infection before conducting the experimental infection on BSL-3 according to the experimental design.

Challenge Groups Under Laboratory Conditions

On the 19th day of life, 60 birds from each of Farms A and B were moved to BSL-3 isolators at the animal house of Mevac laboratories to conduct the challenge at 21st day of age (groups 1–3a/b, 20 birds each group) as described in **Table 1** (challenge-1, early challenge). Group-1a from Farm A and G-1b from Farm B were challenged with H9N2 intranasally, and G-2a and G-2b were challenged with both H9N2 intranasally and E. coli intramuscularly. G-3a and G-3b were challenged with E. coli per the oropharyngeal route and then challenged 7 days later with H9N2 intranasally at 28th day of age.

On day 26th of life, 30 birds from each of Farms A and B were moved to BSL-3 isolators at the animal house of Mevac laboratories to conduct the challenge at 28th day of age as described in **Table 1** (challenge-2, late challenge). Birds were divided into 4 different experimental groups; Group-4a from Farm A and G-4b were challenged with H9N2 intranasally, and

TABLE 1 | Laboratory challenge groups, Groups:1a, 2a, 3, 4, 5a, and 6a (Challenge 1 at 21st day of life) and Groups 1b, 2b, 3, 4, 5b, and 6b (Challenge 2 at 28th day of life).

G-No.	Challenge time	Birds No.	Vaccine	Challenge	Evaluation parameters
G-1a	Early at 21st of life	20	H5H9ND	H9N2; IN	• Serum, swabs before Challenge.
G-1b	Early at 21st of life	20	H5ND	H9N2; IN	• Swabs for virus shedding at 3, 5, 7 DPC by RT-PCR
G-2a	Early at 21st of life	20	H5H9ND	H9N2; IN+ E-Coli; IM	• Develop clinical signs and mortalities
G-2b	Early at 21st of life	20	H5ND	H9N2; IN+ E-Coli; IM	• Serum samples at 10 DPC for challenge 2
G-3a	Early at 21st & late at 28th of life of life	20	H5H9ND	E. coli per os (at 21st day of life) then H9N2; IN 7 days later (at 28th day of life)	
G-3b	Early at 21st & late at 28th of life of life	20	H5ND	E. coli per os (at 21st day of life) then H9N2; IN 7 days later (at 28th day of life)	
G-4a	Late at 28th of life	15	H5H9ND	H9N2; IN	
G-4b	Late at 28th of life	15	H5ND	H9N2; IN	
G-5a	Late at 28th of life	15	H5H9ND	H9N2; IN+ E-Coli; IM	
G-5b	Late at 28th of life	15	H5ND	H9N2; IN+ E-Coli; IM	

No, number of birds; IN, intranasal; IM, intramuscular; Per Os., oropharyngeal; G, group; DPC, days post-challenge; RT-PCR, reverse transcription polymerase chain reaction.

G-5a and G-5b were challenged with H9N2 intranasally and *E. coli* intramuscularly. Birds in G-3a/b were previously challenged with *E. coli* per the oropharyngeal route in the first challenge "early challenge" (at 21st day of life) and kept under observation for 7 days and then challenged intranasally with LPAIV-H9N2 (at 28th day of life).

Hemagglutination Inhibition Test

Hemagglutination inhibition (HI) test was used to monitor the humoral immune response of each vaccine against the antigens of avian influenza H9N2, H5N1 (clade 2.2.1.1), H5N1 (clade 2.2.1.2), H5N8, and ND, which represents the circulating viruses in Egypt. HI test was performed according to the OIE manual (21, 22). Serial 2-fold serum dilutions in PBS were mixed with equal volumes (25 μl) of the virus-containing 4 hemagglutinating units (HAU), and then, 25 μl of washed chicken red blood cells was added. After incubation for 40 min at room temperature, HI titers were determined as reciprocals of the highest serum dilutions in which inhibition of hemagglutination was observed.

Challenge Virus

The LPAIV-H9N2 challenge was applied by the intranasal inoculation with 100 μl of allantoic fluid containing 6-$\log_{10}$ embryo infective dose 50 (EID^{50}) of previously isolated and identified LPAI-H9N2 virus (A/chicken/Egypt/Elfeil-26/2017(H9N2), with GenBank accession number: MF620130, kindly provided by Dr. Wael Elfeil, Suez Canal University, Egypt (23, 24).

Challenge Bacteria

Avian pathogenic *E. coli* "APEC" (Poly3:O157-H7) was applied either by oral or intramuscular route with 100 μl of 10^6 cfu/ml, this isolation previously evaluated its pathogenicity and showed 80% mortalities by IM injection in specific pathogen free chicks, and this bacterial isolate generously provided by Mevac bacteriology laboratory (25).

RT-QPCR for Virus Shedding

Tracheal and cloacal swabs were collected from the challenged birds for the detection of virus shedding by RT-PCR at 3, 5, and 7 days post-challenge, as per the OIE manual (22) using specific primers and probes as previously described (23); RT-qPCR titers were converted into $\log_{10}$ EID_{50}/ml as described previously (26). Briefly, a triplicate of six 10-fold dilutions of challenge AIV-H9N2 (AIV-H9N2; 10^6 EID_{50}/ml) was used to generate a standard curve using stock virus dilutions from 10^1 to 10^6. Since PCR cycle threshold "(CT.)" is defined as the point at which the curve crosses the horizontal threshold line, virus $\log_{10}$ titers of a specimen were plotted against the CT value, and the best fit line was constructed. The linear range of the assay was from 1 to 10^6 EID_{50}/ml, with a correlation coefficient of 0.99. System detection limit was 0.5 EID_{50}/ml as has been standardized and described previously (27). The AIV H9N2 titer in collected samples was derived by plotting the CT of an unknown against the standard curve and expressed in $\log_{10}$ EID_{50}/ml equivalents.

Statistical Analysis

Whenever necessary, data were analyzed by the Student's *t*-test or by ANOVA followed by the application of Duncan's new multiple range test to determine the significance of differences between individual treatments and corresponding control (28).

RESULTS

Serology Monitoring in Field Groups

AIV H9N2 Titers Monitoring in Field Groups and Pre-Challenge PCR Swabs

The findings from monitoring antibody titers in random serum samples collected from different farms at 4, 7, 14, 21, and 28 days of life for LPAIV-H9N2 are shown in **Table 2** and **Figure 1**. There was a significant seroconversion in titers of H9N2-vaccinated group (Farm A) at 21 days of life GMT 4.3 compared to the non-vaccinated group (Farm B) GMT 2.5, and at 28 days of life GMT 3.8 compared to GMT 2.3 in the non-vaccinated group.

All swabs were collected upon the arrival of the birds to the BSL-3 (3 successive cloacal and tracheal swabs each 12 h), and the RT-PCR showed its negative with AIV-H5, AIV-H9N2, and velogenic NDV primers, which declare that the birds did not expose to infection before moving from farms or during transportation process from farm to BSL-3 units either groups moved on day 21 or 28 of life.

Monitoring of Other Disease Titers in Field Groups

Random serum samples were collected from different farms at 4, 7, 14, 21, and 28 days of life for monitoring antibody titers for ND using LaSota, and ND Genotype VII antigens, AIV H5 antibodies against AIV (H5N1 clade 2.2.1.1), AIV (H5N1 clade 2.2.1.2), and AIV (H5N8 clade 2.3.4.4) antigens, and results did not show any significant difference between different field groups in titers for different antigens used compared to the significant difference observed in H9N2 titers as shown in **Figure 2**.

Laboratory Group Challenge Results

Experiment-1: Early Challenge Protection Results

The results of the early challenge in different laboratory groups on the 21st day indicated the presence of clinical signs,

TABLE 2 | AIV H9N2 HI GMT results for different field groups.

Antigen	Age (Days)	Farm A	Farm B
	0 (MDA)	7.5 ± 0.51	8.3 ± 0.73
AIV (H9N2)	4	7.3 ± 0.41	8.2 ± 0.33
	7	6.1 ± 0.27	7.8 ± 0.33
	14	3.8 ± 0.19	4.9 ± 0.20
	21	4.3 ± 0.12	2.5 ± 0.13
	28	3.8 ± 0.29	2.3 ± 0.15

MDA, maternal derived antibodies, GMT, geometric mean titer, HI, hemagglutination inhibition assay.

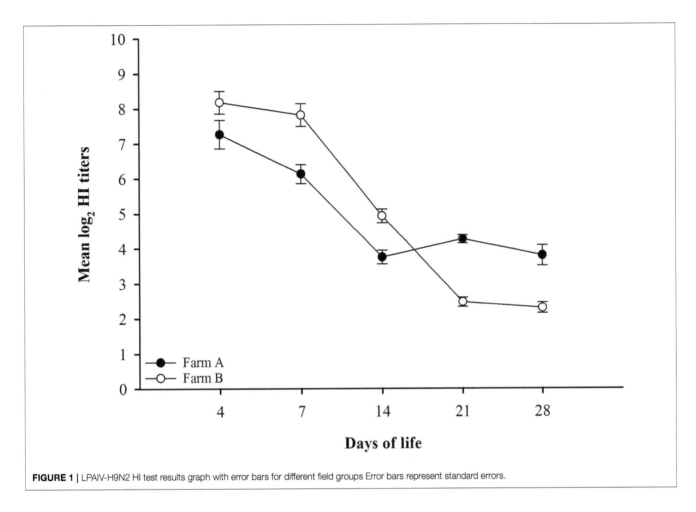

FIGURE 1 | LPAIV-H9N2 HI test results graph with error bars for different field groups Error bars represent standard errors.

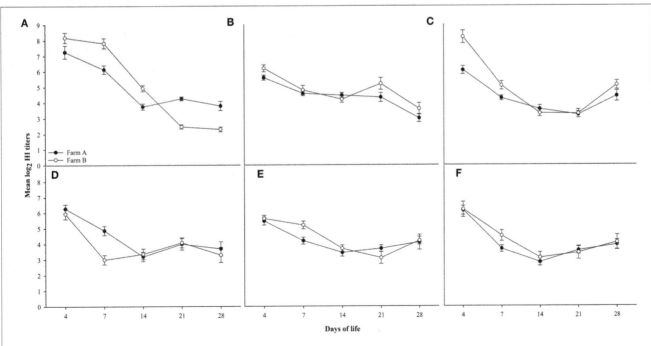

FIGURE 2 | shows HI titers for ages 4,7,14,21 and 28 days for farms A&B, **(A)**: AIV H9N2, **(B)**: ND Lasota, **(C)**: ND Genotype VII, **(D)**: H5N1 clade 2.2.1.1, **(E)**: H5N1 clade 2.2.1.2, **(F)**: H5N8 clade 2.3.4.4. Error bars represent standard errors.

TABLE 3 | Experiment 1 (early challenge) protection results.

Group	Clinical signs	Days post-challenge							Sick%	Clinical protection%	Mortality%	Protection%
		1	2	3	4	5	6	7	Sick/Total	Healthy/Total	Dead/Total	Alive/Total
Gr.1a	Normal	20	20	20	20	20	20	20	0.0% 0/20	100.0% 20/20	0.0% 0/20	100.0% 20/20
	Sick	0	0	0	0	0	0	0				
	Dead	0	0	0	0	0	0	0				
Gr.1b	Normal	20	20	20	20	20	20	20	0.0% 0/20	100.0% 20/20	0.0% 0/20	100.0% 20/20
	Sick	0	0	0	0	0	0	0				
	Dead	0	0	0	0	0	0	0				
Gr.2a	Normal	0	0	0	0	0	0	0	100.0% 20/20	0.0% 0/20	100.0% 20/20	0.0% 0/20
	Sick	14	3	3	0	0	0	0				
	Dead	6	11	3	0	0	0	0				
Gr.2b	Normal	0	0	0	0	0	0	0	100.0% 20/20	0.0% 0/20	100.0% 20/20	0.0% 0/20
	Sick	15	3	2	0	0	0	0				
	Dead	5	12	3	0	0	0	0				
Gr.3a (early challenge)	Normal	20	20	20	20	20	19	18	15.0% 03/20	85.0% 17/20	0.0% 0/20	100.0% 20/20
	Sick	0	0	0	0	0	1	2				
	Dead	0	0	0	0	0	0	0				
Gr.3b (early challenge)	Normal	20	20	20	20	20	19	18	15.0% 03/20	85.0% 17/20	0.0% 0/20	100.0% 20/20
	Sick	0	0	0	0	0	1	2				
	Dead	0	0	0	0	0	0	0				

Gr.1a, Group 1 (vaccinated + challenged with H9N2(IN)) No. = 20; Gr.1b, Group 5 (non-vaccinated + challenged with H9N2(IN)) No. = 20; Gr.2a, Group 2 (vaccinated + challenged with H9N2(IN) + E.coli(IM)) No. = 20; Gr.2b, Group 2b (non-vaccinated + challenged with H9N2(IN) + E.coli(IM)) No. = 20; Gr.3a, Group 3a (Vaccinated + challenged with E-Coli (Per Os.) then H9N2 7 days later(IN)) No. = 20; Gr.3b, Group 3b (non-vaccinated + challenged with E-Coli (Per Os.) then H9N2 7 days later(IN)) No. = 20. Sick birds mean birds showed lethargy, drop feather, nasal or ocular discharge and/ or respiratory manifestations. For birds in Gr3a/b the days post-challenge range 1–7 following to late challenge with H9N2 virus which equivalent to the first 7 out of17 days post-early challenge with APEC.

clinical protection, mortality, and total protection as shown in percentages in **Table 3**.

Experiment-2: Late Challenge Results

The results of the challenge on the 28th day of different laboratory groups indicated the presence of clinical signs, clinical protection percentage, mortality percentage, and total protection percentage as shown in **Table 4**.

Virus Shedding Following Experiment 1/2 of Challenge

Shedding was evaluated at 3, 5, and 7 days post-challenge for different groups in early and late challenge experiments (21st and 28th day of life, respectively.) as shown in **Table 5**.

Serology Monitoring Following Experiment 2 Challenge

Serum samples were collected from different groups at 10 days post-challenge for monitoring antibody titers for AIV H9N2, ND using LaSota antigen, AIV-H5 using AIV (H5N1 clade: 2.2.1.1), AIV (H5N1 clade: 2.2.1.2), and AIV (H5N8 clade: 2.3.4.4) antigens as shown in **Table 6**.

Bacterial Isolation Following Experiment 1/2 Challenge

E. coli was isolated from groups 2a and 2b following the challenge at 21 days of life, *E. coli* was isolated from groups 3a/b and 5a/b following challenge at 28 days of life as shown in **Table 7**.

DISCUSSION

This study aimed to evaluate the role of vaccinating broiler chickens with inactivated LPAIV-H9N2 and the results of protection either with single H9N2 infection or as co-infection of both avian pathogenic *E. coli* (APEC) and LPAIV-H9N2. Co-infection of LPAIV-H9N2 (intranasal) with E-coli O157 (intramuscular injection) either on days 21 or 28 of life showed 100% mortalities in both vaccinated and non-vaccinated groups (2a/b and 5a/b) due to a septicemic reaction following the parenteral infection of the avian pathogenic *E.coli* (APEC), which is supported by the previous findings of El-Sawah et al. (29) and by Elfeil et al. (30) for the same bacterial isolates which is associated with 100% mortalities following I/M infection and following per os infection mortalities started after 7 days post-infection (25, 29). Per os infection of birds with *E. coli* O157 (as a natural route

TABLE 4 | Experiment-2 (late challenge) protection results.

Group	Clinical signs	Days post-challenge										Sick%	Clinical protection%	Mortality%	Protection%
		1	2	3	4	5	6	7	8	9	10	Sick/Total	Healthy/Total	Dead/Total	Alive/Total
Gr.4a	Normal	15	15	15	15	14	15	15	15	15	15	6.7%	93.3%	0.0%	100.0%
	Sick	0	0	0	0	1	0	0	0	0	0	1/15*	14/15*	0/15	15/15
	Dead	0	0	0	0	0	0	0	0	0	0				
Gr.4b	Normal	15	10	9	9	12	15	15	15	15	15	40.0%	60.0%	0.0%	100.0%
	Sick	0	5	6	6	3	0	0	0	0	0	6/15*	9/15*	0/15	15/15
	Dead	0	0	0	0	0	0	0	0	0	0				
Gr.5a	Normal	0	0	0	0	0	0	0	0	0	0	100.0%	0%	100.0%	0.0%
	Sick	15	13	10	7	6	0	0	0	0	0	15/15	0/15	15/15	0/15
	Dead	0	2	3	3	1	6	0	0	0	0				
Gr.5b	Normal	0	0	0	0	0	0	0	0	0	0	100.0%	0.0%	100.0%	0.0%
	Sick	15	12	10	5	0	0	0	0	0	0	15/15	0/15	15/15	0/15
	Dead	0	3	2	5	5	0	0	0	0	0				
Gr.3a (late Challenge)	Normal	18	18	18	17	17	17	16	16	19	19	15.0%	85.0%	5.0%	95.0%
	Sick	2	2	2	3	3	3	3	3	0	0	3/20*	17/20*	1/20*	19/20*
	Dead	0	0	0	0	0	0	1	0	0	0				
Gr.3b (late challenge)	Normal	18	18	18	17	17	9	11	15	17	17	40.0%	60.0%	15.0%	85.0%
	Sick	2	2	2	3	3	8	6	2	0	0	8/20*	12/20*	3/20*	17/20*
	Dead	0	0	0	0	0	3	0	0	0	0				

Gr.4a, Group 4a (vaccinated + challenged with H9N2(IN)) No. = 15; Gr.5a, Group 5a (vaccinated + challenged with H9N2(IN)+ E. coli (IM)) No. = 15; Gr.3a, Group 3a (vaccinated + challenged with E-Coli (Per Os. At 21st day of age) then H9N2 (IN)at 28th day of age) No. =20; Gr.3b, Group 3b (non-vaccinated + challenged with E-Coli (Per Os. At 21st day of age) then H9N2 (IN)at 28th day of age) No. =20; Gr.4b, Group 4b (non-vaccinated + challenged with H9N2(IN)) No. = 15; Gr.5b, Group 5b (non-vaccinated + challenged with H9N2(IN)+ E. coli (IM)) No. = 15. Sick birds mean birds showed lethargy, drop feather, nasal or ocular discharge and/ or respiratory manifestations;. For birds in Gr3a/b the days post-challenge range 1–10 following to late challenge with H9N2 virus which equivalent to the second 10 out of 17 days post-early challenge with APEC. *: indicate significance difference between groups (p < 0.05).

of infection) followed by intranasal infection with LPAIV-H9N2 7 days later (allowing sufficient time to produce infection) resulted in significantly higher clinical protection in vaccinated birds (G3a) than non-vaccinated birds (G3b) (85 vs. 60%, respectively), thus agreeing with the previous report of Wang et al. (15), who recorded the exacerbation of clinical signs in a mouse model co-infected with both AIV-H9N2 and *E. coli* (15) and report by Ma et al. (14), who reported the synergistic effect of LPAIV-H9N2 infection with avian pathogenic *E.coli* as the replication of H9N2 virus upregulated some essential proteins associated with the APEC pathogenicity and invasion-like (14). Infection with H9N2 virus 7 days after per os administration of *E. coli* (O157) showed relatively higher mortality (15%, 3/20) in non-vaccinated birds (G3b) compared to the birds received H9N2-inactivated vaccine (G3a) (5%, 1/20), and this difference may be associated with the damage of internal tissues and accumulated protease enzymes after *E. coli* infection, in addition to increase in the level of invasion and adherence protein transcription rate following H9N2 replication in intestinal and respiratory tissues, which potentiate the replication and pathological picture of APEC and thus increase the level of trypsin-like enzyme in the respiratory and GIT tissues, which later support and exaggerate the cleavability of H9N2

virus and intern the replication rate and thus may reflect the significant higher effect of the co-infection of H9N2 with APEC in non-vaccinated birds over-vaccinated (10, 14, 15, 31–33). There was no humoral immune response against H9N2 virus in non-vaccinated chicken, rendering the ability of virus transmission higher than that of vaccinated birds, and thus can explain the significant higher clinical manifestation in non-vaccinated infected birds either with H9N2 alone or co-infected with H9N2 and APEC. The protective effect of the humoral immune response associated with the inactivated H9N2 vaccine will decrease the load of H9N2 infection and limited its replication out the respiratory and GIT tissues and thus decrease the lead of the virus inside the birds tissue and reduced the associated inflammatory mediators (TNF-α and INF-γ); the immunosuppressive effect of E.coli infection decreases the birds response to the virus infection and potentiates the losses from the co-infection process (10, 15, 18–20, 23, 31–33). There is a significant higher level of mortalities and clinical sickness rates between group infected with APEC O:157 *via* I/M route over per os route, respectively, and thus associate with the nature of the bacteria as applying the infection *via* the IM route to ensure the on spot onset of septicemic infection and developing the bacteremia directly and thus can associated

TABLE 5 | Virus shedding at 3, 5, and 7 days post-challenge, Experiment-1/2.

Group	Virus shedding EID_{50} 3 days post-challenge		Virus shedding EID_{50} 5 days post-challenge		Virus shedding EID_{50} 7 days post-challenge	
	Trachea	Cloaca	Trachea	Cloaca	Trachea	Cloaca
Gr.1a	3.5 ± 0.9	2.4 ± 1.2	3.5 ± 0.89	1.3 ± 0.94	1.07 ± 0.85	nd
Gr.1b	3.8 ± 0.17	0.7 ± 1.27	3.8 ± 0.31	1.7 ± 1.5	nd	1.7 ± 1.05
Gr.2a	4.2 ± 0.68	1.7 ± 1.66	nd	nd	nd	nd
Gr.2b	4.7 ± 0.81	2.6 ± 0.48	nd	nd	nd	nd
Gr.3a	2.3 ± 0.7	3.7 ± 0.48	1.04 ± 1.8	1.69 ± 0.69	nd	nd
Gr.3b	3.7 ± 0.15	2.5 ± 2.2	1.44 ± 1.25	1.88 ± 0.8	nd	nd
Gr.4a	2.4 ± 2.1	nd	nd		nd	nd
Gr.4b	1.68 ± 1.4	0.7 ± 1.27	nt	nd	nd	nd
Gr.5a	1.68 ± 1.4	0.7 ± 1.27	nd	nd	nd	nd
Gr.5b	2.9 ± 0.76	2.6 ± 0.48	nd	nd	nd	nd

EID_{50}, egg infectious dose50; No., Number of birds; IN, intranasal; IM, intramuscular; Per Os., oropharyngeal; Gr.1a, Group 1a (vaccinated + challenged with H9N2(IN)) No. = 20; Gr.1b, Group 1b (non-vaccinated + challenged with H9N2(IN)) No. = 20; Gr.2a, Group 2a (vaccinated + challenged with H9N2(IN) + E.coli(IM)) No. = 20; Gr.2b, Group 2b (non-vaccinated + challenged with H9N2(IN) + E.coli(IM)) No. = 20; Gr.3a, Group 3a (vaccinated + challenged with E-Coli (Per Os.) then H9N2 7 days later(IN)) No. =20; Gr.3b, Group 3b (non-vaccinated + challenged with E-Coli (Per Os.) then H9N2 7 days later(IN)) No. =20; Gr.4a, Group 4a (vaccinated + challenged with H9N2(IN)) No. = 15; Gr.4b, Group 4b (non-vaccinated + challenged with H9N2(IN)) No. = 15; Gr.5a, Group 5a (vaccinated + challenged with H9N2(IN) + E. coli (IM)) No. = 15; Gr.5b, Group 5b (non-vaccinated + challenged with H9N2(IN)

TABLE 6 | Serology results for different groups 10 days post-challenge, Experiment 2.

	GMT Log2 HI titer			
Antigen	Gr.3a No. = 8	Gr.3b No. = 8	Gr.4a No. = 8	Gr.4b No. = 8
AIV (H9N2)	10.13 ± 0.83	10 ± 0.76	10.8 ± 0.46	10 ± 0.93
ND (LaSota)	3 ± 0.93	4.13 ± 1.73	8.8 ± 0.71	3.13 ± 0.83
AIV (H5N1/a)	6.5 ± 0.53	4.88 ± 1.13	7.5 ± 0.53	6.5 ± 0.53
AIV (H5N1/b)	7.38 ± 0.52	6.38 ± 1.19	8.5 ± 0.53	6.75 ± 0.89
AIV (H5N8)	4.25 ± 1.04	3.75 ± 1.83	4.5 ± 0.76	4.25 ± 1.39

AIV (H5N1/b), Avian influenza H5N1 clade 2.2.1.1 antigen; AIV (H5N1/b): avian influenza H5N1 clade 2.2.1.2 antigen; Gr.3a, Group 3a (Vaccinated + challenged with E-Coli (Per Os. At 21st day of age) then H9N2 (IN)at 28th day of age); Gr.3b, Group 3b (non-vaccinated + challenged with E-Coli (Per Os. At 21st day of age) then H9N2 (IN)at 28th day of age); Gr.4a, Group 5a (non-vaccinated + challenged with H9N2(IN)); Gr.4b, Group 5b (non-vaccinated + challenged with H9N2(IN).

with 80–100% mortalities as previously described, while applying the vaccine *via* oral route needs more time to develop septicemia and may not develop it in all birds as we keeping commercial broilers and may exposed to *E.coli* during the first 21 day of live in the farm without clear clinical picture and developing systemic infection, and the 5% and 15% mortalities in H9N2-non-vaccinated and H9N2-vaccinated groups, respectively, agreed with the previous report by El-Sawah et al. (29), who reported that infection with APEC O:157 bacteria can associate with 5–25% mortalities in broiler chicks but needs 10–14 days following

infection to give sufficient time to bacteria to adhere, colonize, and develop the systemic infections status (29), but the co-infection of APEC O:157 with H9N2 and the synergistic effect between them lead to develop the losses from day 7 post-infection in H92-non-vaccinated groups and reached to 15%

TABLE 7 | Bacterial isolation post-challenge, Experiment-1/2.

Group	Time of isolation	Isolate
Gr.2a	18 h post-challenge	E. coli: O157-H7 (poly 3)
	1 DPC	E. coli: O157-H7 (poly 3)
	3 DPC	E. coli: O157-H7 (poly 3)
Gr.2b	1 DPC	E. coli: O157-H7 (poly 3)
	2 DPC	E. coli: O157-H7 (poly 3)
	3 DPC	E. coli: O157-H7 (poly 3)
Gr.3a	6 DPC	E. coli: O157-H7 (poly 3)
Gr.3b	6 DPC	E. coli: O157-H7 (poly 3)
Gr.5a	1 DPC	E. coli: O157-H7 (poly 3)
	3 DPC	E. coli: O157-H7 (poly 3)
Gr.5b	3 DPC	E. coli: O157-H7 (poly 3)
	3 DPC	E. coli: O157-H7 (poly 3)

Gr.2a, Group 2a (vaccinated + challenged with H9N2(IN)+ E. coli (IM)) on day 21 of life; Gr.2b, Group 2b (non-vaccinated + challenged with H9N2(IN) + E. coli (IM)) on day 21 of life; Gr.3a, Group 3a (vaccinated + challenged with E-Coli (Per Os. At 21st day of age) then H9N2 (IN)at 28th day of age); Gr.3b, Group 3b (non-vaccinated + challenged with E-Coli (Per Os. At 21st day of age) then H9N2 (IN)at 28th day of age); Gr.5a, Group 5a (vaccinated + challenged with H9N2(IN)) at day 28 of life; Gr.5b, Group 5b (non-vaccinated + challenged with H9N2(IN) + E. coli (IM)) at day 28 of life.

mortalities by day 14 post-infection and 40% clinical sickness vs. 5% mortalities and 15% clinical sickness in H9N2-vaccinated groups in birds kept at BSL3 with negative pressure and filtrated air flow, which can explain in partial the higher losses in commercial farms due to the extra effect of in proper ventilation, over-crowdedness, co-infection with other pathogen or vaccine seed replications as previously described by Elfeil et al. (34), who highlighted that the application the avian influenza and NDV vaccines in farms can associate with around 10–15% lower protection level in comparison with the laboratory conditions (30, 34, 35). The multidrug-resistant E. coli is a serious problem facing the poultry industry as previously reported (36–38). The results from this trial may explain in part the exaggerated effect of LPAIV-H9N2 infection in commercial broiler farms in the Middle East region as the co-infection of LPAIV-H9N2 with the APEC work in a synergism and exaggerate the pathological picture for both pathogen, and the LPAIV-H9N2 circulating in the Middle east region still low pathogenic virus and losses associated with its infection in poultry farms is not due to the increased pathogenicity of the LPAIV-H9N2 virus, but rather to the heavy infection with multidrug-resistant E. coli and other pathogen such as IB, NDV, and IBD viruses in commercial broiler flocks (35, 37, 39, 40). This kind of synergy between different pathogens in broilers results in exaggerated clinical pictures, loss of weight, and higher mortalities. Birds in all groups either vaccinated with H5H9ND7 (inactivated H9N2-"vaccinated birds") or H5ND7 (H9N2- "non-vaccinated birds") vaccines showed similar seroconversion for H5 and ND, and only birds in field group A (vaccinated group) showed seroconversion for AIV-H9N2 on days 21 and 28 of life. Birds in field group B (non-vaccinated) did not show seroconversion for AIV-H9N2 on 28 days of life, indicating that the combination of three different antigens in one inactivated vaccine (like the trivalent H5H9ND in MEFLUVAC H5+H9+ND7) provided an immune response similar to the bivalent vaccine (MEFLUVAC H5+ND7) and declare that there is no negative effect of any vaccine antigens on the protection and evaluation parameters associated with the H9N2 vaccination, which agreed with the previous report about the safety and efficacy of both used vaccines in commercial broiler chicks with maternal derived antibodies (41). Use of a vaccine containing H9N2 at day 10 of life developed seroconversion for AIV-H9N2 at 28 days of life, in agreement with previous reports, and thus highlighted delay of the inactivated H9N2 vaccination in commercial broiler chicks to the 2nd week of life better than the 1 day of life application, especially in commercial broiler with maternal derived antibodies "birds came from vaccinated breeders" (23). Data obtained from the early challenge by AIV-H9N2 virus on day 21 of life, either in vaccinated or non-vaccinated groups, revealed no mortalities in both groups (G1a/b), which confirms the previous findings of Elfeil et al. (24), who reported that the AIV-H9N2 virus is of low pathogenicity and did not show clinical manifestation as a single pathogen in birds in the presence of

humoral immune response (even remnants of maternally derived antibodies) (27) and thus may associated with the remnant of maternal derived immunity in the commercial broilers. On day 28 of life, the vaccinated group (G4a) showed significantly ($p < 0.05$) better clinical protection against chicken sickness and developing clinical manifestations (93.3%) after the challenge compared to the non-vaccinated group (G4b, 60% protection against chicken sickness and developing clinical manifestations); this is in agreement with the previous report of Talat et al. (23), who reported that using inactivated H9N2 vaccine on day 7 of life in commercial broilers chicks with MDA with homologs and high concentrated antigen can provide protection over 90% protection against infection with AIV-H9N2 virus (23). The LPAIV-H9N2-inactivated vaccine will not completely solve the problem but may significantly improve the vitality, performance, and survival rates following the infection of commercial boilers with LPAIV-H9N2, especially in complicated cases such as persistent co-infection of APEC, which is very common case in the commercial poultry farms.

CONCLUSIONS

Co-infection with LPAI-H9N2 and E. coli, especially the prolonged co-infection (over 7–14 days), may be the actual cause for the exaggerated losses associated with H9N2 infections in commercial broilers in endemic countries. The application of the LPAI-H9N2-inactivated vaccine strategy in commercial broilers may aid in controlling the complications associated with both LPAI-H9N2 and oral E. coli infections, by significant reduction the mortalities and clinical sickness. H9N2 vaccination should be associated with strict farm biosecurity measure to maintain superior clinical protection and minimize the bacterial co-infections especially with E. coli.

AUTHOR CONTRIBUTIONS

SM, KZ, and WE: conceptualization. SM, EK, KZ, MH, and WE: methodology. SM, MH, KZ, and WE: software. SM, MH, and WE: validation, writing—original draft preparation, writing—review and editing, visualization, supervision, project administration, and funding acquisition. SM, EK, and WE: formal analysis and investigation resources. SM, MH, SD, RK, and WE: resources. SM, MH, EK, SD, and WE: data curation. All authors contributed efficiently in this work. All authors have read and agreed to the published version of the manuscript.

ACKNOWLEDGMENTS

All authors acknowledge support provided by Dr. Mohamed Gamal, Dr. Mumtaz Wasify, Dr. Sara Salama, and Dr. Ahmed Sedeik for their technical support and providing the E. coli isolates.

REFERENCES

1. Nagy A, Mettenleiter TC, Abdelwhab EM, A. Brief summary of the epidemiology and genetic relatedness of avian influenza h9n2 virus in birds and mammals in the middle East and North Africa. *Epidemiol Infect.* (2017) 145:3320–33. doi: 10.1017/S0950268817002576

2. Peacock T, Reddy K, James J, Adamiak B, Barclay W, Shelton H, et al. Antigenic mapping of an H9n2 avian influenza virus reveals two discrete antigenic sites and a novel mechanism of immune escape. *Sci Rep.* (2016) 6:18745. doi: 10.1038/srep18745

3. Wan X-F, Dong L, Lan Y, Long L-P, Xu C, Zou S, et al. Indications that live poultry markets are a major source of human H5N1 influenza virus infection in China. *J Virol.* (2011) 85:13432–8. doi: 10.1128/JVI.05266-11

4. El-Zoghby EF, Arafa AS, Hassan MK, Aly MM, Selim A, Kilany WH, et al. Isolation of H9n2 avian influenza virus from bobwhite quail. (Colinus Virginianus) in Egypt. *Archives virology.* (2012) 157:1167–72. doi: 10.1007/s00705-012-1269-z

5. Afifi MAA, El-Kady MF, Zoelfakar SA, Abddel-Moneim AS. Serological surveillance reveals widespread influenza a H7 and H9 subtypes among chicken flocks in Egypt. *Trop Anim Health Prod.* (2013) 45:687–90. doi: 10.1007/s11250-012-0243-9

6. Taher M, Amer A, Arafa A, Saad F. Epidemiology of viral components causing respiratory problems in broilers in six egyptian governorates. *J Vet Med Res.* (2017) 24:308–20. doi: 10.21608/jvmr.2017.43266

7. Roussan D, Haddad R, Khawaldeh G. Molecular survey of avian respiratory pathogens in commercial broiler chicken flocks with respiratory diseases in Jordan. *Poult Sci.* (2008) 87:444–8. doi: 10.3382/ps.2007-00415

8. Haghighat-Jahromi M, Asasi K, Nili H, Dadras H, Shooshtari A. Coinfection of avian influenza virus. (H9n2 Subtype) with infectious bronchitis live vaccine. *Archives virology.* (2008) 153:651–5. doi: 10.1007/s00705-008-0033-x

9. Swayne DE, Boulianne M. *Diseases of Poultry.* Swayne DE, Boulianne M, Logue CM, McDougald LR, Nair V, Suarez DL, et al., editors. NJ, USA: John Wiley & Sons, Inc. (2020).

10. Jaleel S, Younus M, Idrees A, Arshad M, Khan AU. Ehtisham-ul-Haque S, et al. Pathological alterations in respiratory system during co-infection with low pathogenic avian influenza virus (H9N2) and escherichia coli in broiler chickens. *J veterinary research.* (2017) 61:253–8. doi: 10.1515/jvetres-2017-0035

11. Ammar AMAE-H, Elokshm AM. Studies on virulence genes of e. coli from different sources and their relation to antibiotic resistance pattern. *Zagazig Veterinary J.* (2014) 42:183–96. doi: 10.21608/zvjz.2014.59483

12. Mosleh N, Dadras H, Mohammadi A. Molecular quantitation of H9N2 avian influenza virus in various organs of broiler chickens using taqman real time pcr. *J Mol Genet Med.* (2009) 3:152–7. doi: 10.4172/1747-0862.1000027

13. Hassan KE, El-Kady MF, El-Sawah AAA, Luttermann C, Parvin R, Shany S, et al. Respiratory disease due to mixed viral infections in poultry flocks in egypt between 2017 and 2018: upsurge of highly pathogenic avian influenza virus subtype H5n8 since 2018. *Transbound Emerg Dis.* (2019). 68:21–36. doi: 10.1111/tbed.13281

14. Ma LL, Sun ZH, Xu YL, Wang SJ, Wang HN, Zhang H, et al. Screening host proteins required for bacterial adherence after H9N2 virus infection. *Vet Microbiol.* (2018) 213:5–14. doi: 10.1016/j.vetmic.2017.11.003

15. Wang S, Jiang N, Shi W, Yin H, Chi X, Xie Y, et al. Co-infection of h9n2 influenza a virus and escherichia coli in a Balb/C mouse model aggravates lung injury by synergistic effects. *Frontiers microbiology.* (2021) 12:670688. doi: 10.3389/fmicb.2021.670688

16. Mosleh N, Dadras H, Asasi K, Taebipour MJ, Tohidifar SS, Farjanikish G. Evaluation of the timing of the escherichia coli co-infection on pathogenecity of h9n2 avian influenza virus in broiler chickens. *Iranian j veterinary research.* (2017) 18:86.

17. Jiang X, Zhang M, Ding Y, Yao J, Chen H, Zhu D, et al. Escherichia coli prlc gene encodes a trypsin-like proteinase regulating the cell cycle. *J Biochem.* (1998) 124:980–5. doi: 10.1093/oxfordjournals.jbchem.a022216

18. Nakamura K, Imada Y, Maeda M. Lymphocytic depletion of bursa of fabricius and thymus in chickens inoculated with escherichia coli. *Vet Pathol.* (1986) 23:712–7. doi: 10.1177/030098588602300610

19. Dadras H, Nazifi S, Shakibainia M. Evaluation of the effect of simultaneous infection with e. coli O2 and H9N2 influenza virus on inflammatory factors in broiler chickens. *Veterinary Science Development.* (2014) 4:2. doi: 10.4081/vsd.2014.5416

20. Barbour EK, Mastori FA, Nour AA, Shaib HA, Jaber LS, Yaghi RH, et al. Standardisation of a new model of H9n2/escherichia coli challenge in broilers in the lebanon. *Vet Ital.* (2009) 45:317–22.

21. OIE. Newcastle Disease. In: 2012 VabtWaoDotOi, editor. *Oie Manual of Standers for Diagnosis Test and Vaccines.* France: OIE. (2012).

22. OIE. *Manual of Diagnostic Tests and Vaccines for Terrestrial Animals- Avian Influenza. Oie Terrestrial Manual 2015.* Rome, Italy: OIE. (2015).

23. Talat S, Abouelmaatti R, Almeer R, Abdel-Daim MM, Elfeil WK. Comparison of the effectiveness of two different vaccination regimes for avian influenza H9N2 in broiler chicken. *Animals.* (2020) 10:1–12. doi: 10.3390/ani10101875

24. Elfeil W, Abouelmaatti R, Diab M, Mandour M, Rady M. Experimental infection of chickens by avian influenza H9n2 virus: monitoring of tissue tropism and pathogenicity. *J Egypt Vet Med Assoc.* (2018) 78:369–83.

25. Elfeil W, Abu-Elala N, Rady M, Hamoud M, Wasfy M, Elsayed M. The Protective Role of Coli-Vac, a Heptavalent Vaccine against Extraintestinal Avian Pathogenic Escherichia Coli. (Apec) Infection. *American Assocaition of Avian Pthologist 2022-Meeting.* Philadelphia, PA,: The American Veterinary Medical Association. (AVMA). (2022).

26. Nolan T, Hands RE, Bustin SA. Quantification of mrna using real-time rt-pcr. *Nat Protoc.* (2006) 1:1559. doi: 10.1038/nprot.2006.236

27. Verma AK, Kumar M, Murugkar HV, Nagarajan S, Tosh C, Namdeo P, et al. Experimental infection and in-contact transmission of H9N2 avian influenza virus in crows. *Pathogens.* (2022) 11:304. doi: 10.3390/pathogens11030304

28. Steel RGD, Torrie JH. *Principles and Procedures of Statics* London: Mcgraw Hill Book Comp. Inc. (1960).

29. El-Sawah AA, Dahshan ALHM, El-Nahass E-S, El-Mawgoud AIA. Pathogenicity of escherichia coli O157 in commercial broiler chickens. *beni-suef university. J Basic Applied Sciences.* (2018) 7:620–5. doi: 10.1016/j.bjbas.2018.07.005

30. Elfeil W, Rady M, Kilany W, Sedeik A, Elkady M, Elsayed M. Evaluation protection of H5 vaccination regimes in commercail broilers with maternal immunity against early challenge with HPAI-H5N1. International Poultry Scientific Forum (IPSF); Georgia World Congress Center. *Atlanta, Georgia: Southern Poultry Science Society, USA.* (2022).

31. Awwad N, Elgendy E, Ibrahim M. The effect of some pathogenic bacterial proteases on avian influenza viruses H5N1 and H9N2. *European J Pharmaceutical Medical Research.* (2018) 5:50.

32. King M, Guentzel MN, Arulanandam B, Lupiani B, Chambers J. Proteolytic bacteria in the lower digestive tract of poultry may affect avian influenza virus pathogenicity. *Poult Sci.* (2009) 88:1388–93. doi: 10.3382/ps.2008-00549

33. Böttcher-Friebertshäuser E, Klenk H-D, Garten W. Activation of influenza viruses by proteases from host cells and bacteria in the human airway epithelium. *Pathog Dis.* (2013) 69:87–100. doi: 10.1111/2049-632X.12053

34. Elfeil W, Yousef H, Fawzy M, Ali A, Ibrahim H, Elsayed M. *Protective Efficacy of Mefluvac H9 in Turkey Poults in Both Lab and Field Condition. XXI- World Veterinary Poultry Association Congress.* Bangkok, Thailand: WVPA. (2019).

35. Sultan HA, Elfeil WK, Nour AA, Tantawy L, Kamel EG, Eed EM. et al. Efficacy of the newcastle disease virus genotype vii1-matched vaccines in commercial broilers. *Vaccines.* (2022) 10:29. doi: 10.3390/vaccines10010029

36. Eid HM, Algammal AM, Elfeil WK, Youssef FM, Harb SM, Abd-Allah EM. Prevalence, molecular typing, and antimicrobial resistance of bacterial pathogens isolated from ducks. *Veterinary World.* (2019) 12:677–83. doi: 10.14202/vetworld.2019.677-683

37. Eid HI, Algammal AM, Nasef SA, Elfeil WK, Mansour GH. Genetic variation among avian pathogenic e. coli strains isolated from broiler chickens Asian. *J Animal Veterinary Advances.* (2016) 11:350–6. doi: 10.3923/ajava.2016.350.356

38. Rady M, Ezz-El-Din N, Mohamed KF, Nasef S, Samir A, Elfeil WK. Correlation between Esβl salmonella serovars isolated from broilers and their virulence genes. *J Hellenic Veterinary Medical Society.* (2020) 71:2163–70. doi: 10.12681/jhvms.23645

39. Hassan KE, Ali A, Shany SAS, El-Kady MF. Experimental co-infection of infectious bronchitis and low pathogenic avian influenza H9N2

viruses in commercial broiler chickens. *Res Vet Sci.* (2017) 115:356–62. doi: 10.1016/j.rvsc.2017.06.024

40. Sedeik ME, Awad AM, Rashed H, Elfeil WK. Variations in pathogenicity and molecular characterization of infectious bursal disease virus. (IBDV) in Egypt. *AmJ Animal Veterinary Sciences.* (2018) 13:76–86. doi: 10.3844/ajavsp.2018.76.86

41. Elfeil W, Rady M, Kilany WE, Sedeik A, Elsayed M. *Evaluation Protection of H5 Vaccination Regimes Against Early Challenge with Hpai-H5N8 Clade 2.3.4.4.* Paris, France: *World Poultry Congress* (2022).

PERMISSIONS

LIST OF CONTRIBUTORS

Israel Barbosa Guedes, Gisele Oliveira de Souza, Juliana Fernandes de Paula Castro, Matheus Burilli Cavalini, Antônio Francisco de Souza Filho and Marcos Bryan Heinemann
Departamento de Medicina Veterinária Preventiva e Saúde Animal, Faculdade de Medicina Veterinária e Zootecnia, Universidade de São Paulo, São Paulo, Brazil

Murugan Subbiah, Nagaraja Thirumalapura, David Thompson and Deepanker Tewari
Pennsylvania Veterinary Laboratory, Harrisburg, PA, United States

Suresh V. Kuchipudi and Bhushan Jayarao
Animal Diagnostic Laboratory, Pennsylvania State University, University Park, PA, United States
Center for Infectious Disease Dynamics, Pennsylvania State University, University Park, PA, United States

Dehui Yin, Qiongqiong Bai, Xiling Wu, Jihong Shao and Jinpeng Zhang
Key Lab of Environment and Health, School of Public Health, Xuzhou Medical University, Xuzhou, China

Han Li
Department of Infection Control, The First Hospital of Jilin University, Changchun, China

Mingjun Sun
Laboratory of Zoonoses, China Animal Health and Epidemiology Center, Qingdao, China

Rui Jia, Gaiping Zhang, Jingming Zhou, Peiyang Ding and Aiping Wang
School of Life Sciences, Zhengzhou University, Zhengzhou, China

Hongliang Liu, Yankai Liu, Yanwei Wang and Weimin Zang
Henan Zhongze Biological Engineering Co. LTD, Zhengzhou, China

Yumei Chen
School of Life Sciences, Zhengzhou University, Zhengzhou, China
Henan Zhongze Biological Engineering Co. LTD, Zhengzhou, China

Elizabeth Ramirez-Medina, Sarah Pruitt, Nallely Espinoza, Douglas P. Gladue and Manuel V. Borca
Agricultural Research Service, United States Department of Agriculture, Plum Island Animal Disease Center, Greenport, NY, United States

Lauro Velazquez-Salinas
Agricultural Research Service, United States Department of Agriculture, Plum Island Animal Disease Center, Greenport, NY, United States
Department of Anatomy and Physiology, Kansas State University, Manhattan, KS, United States
Foreign Animal Disease Research Unit, Plum Island Animal Disease Center, United States Department of Agriculture-Agricultural Research Service, Greenport, NY, United States

Ayushi Rai
Agricultural Research Service, United States Department of Agriculture, Plum Island Animal Disease Center, Greenport, NY, United States
Oak Ridge Institute for Science and Education (ORISE), Oak Ridge, TN, United States

Elizabeth A. Vuono
Agricultural Research Service, United States Department of Agriculture, Plum Island Animal Disease Center, Greenport, NY, United States
Department of Pathobiology and Population Medicine, Mississippi State University, Mississippi, MS, United States

Kate Hole and Charles Nfon
National Centre for Foreign Animal Disease, Canadian Food Inspection Agency, Winnipeg, MB, Canada

Luis L. Rodriguez
Foreign Animal Disease Research Unit, Plum Island Animal Disease Center, United States Department of Agriculture-Agricultural Research Service, Greenport, NY, United States

Paola Dall'Ara, Stefania Lauzi, Joel Filipe and Roberta Caseri
Department of Veterinary Medicine, University of Milan, Lodi, Italy

Michela Beccaglia
Ambulatorio Veterinario Beccaglia, Lissone, Italy

Costantina Desario, Alessandra Cavalli, Giulio Guido Aiudi, Canio Buonavoglia and Nicola Decaro
Department of Veterinary Medicine, University of Bari, Bari, Italy

Xin Liu, Wenchao Zhang, Xinyue Zhu, Ying Chen, Kang Ouyang, Zuzhang Wei and Weijian Huang
College of Animal Science and Technology, Guangxi University, Nanning, China

Dongjing Wang
Institute of Animal Husbandry and Veterinary Medicine, Tibet Academy of Agriculture and Animal Husbandry Science, Lhasa, China

Huan Liu
Department of Scientific Research, The First Affiliated Hospital of Guangxi University of Chinese Medicine, Nanning, China

Virpi Sali
Department of Production Animal Medicine, University of Helsinki, Mäntsälä, Finland

Christina Veit and Janicke Nordgreen
Department of Paraclinical Sciences, Norwegian University of Life Sciences, Oslo, Norway

Mari Heinonen
Department of Production Animal Medicine, University of Helsinki, Mäntsälä, Finland
Department of Production Animal Medicine, Research Centre for Animal Welfare, University of Helsinki, Mäntsälä, Finland

Anna Valros
Department of Production Animal Medicine, Research Centre for Animal Welfare, University of Helsinki, Mäntsälä, Finland

Sami Junnikkala
Department of Veterinary Biosciences, Faculty of Veterinary Medicine, University of Helsinki, Helsinki, Finland

Xuexiang Yu, Xianjing Zhu, Xiaoyu Chen, Dongfan Li, Qian Xu, Lun Yao, Qi Sun and Qigai He
College of Veterinary Medicine, Huazhong Agricultural University, Wuhan, China
State Key Laboratory of Agricultural Microbiology, Wuhan, China
The Cooperative Innovation Center for Sustainable Pig Production, Wuhan, China

Shengxian Fan
College of Veterinary Medicine, Huazhong Agricultural University, Wuhan, China

Xugang Ku
College of Veterinary Medicine, Huazhong Agricultural University, Wuhan, China
The Cooperative Innovation Center for Sustainable Pig Production, Wuhan, China

Ahmed H. Ghonaim
College of Veterinary Medicine, Huazhong Agricultural University, Wuhan, China
The Cooperative Innovation Center for Sustainable Pig Production, Wuhan, China
Desert Research Center, Cairo, Egypt

Hanchun Yang
College of Veterinary Medicine, China Agricultural University, Beijing, China

Soyoun Hwang, Justin J. Greenlee and Eric M. Nicholson
Virus and Prion Research Unit, National Animal Disease Center, United States Department of Agriculture, Agricultural Research Service, Ames, IA, United States

Serenella Silvestri, Elisa Rampacci, Valentina Stefanetti, Chiara Brachelente and Fabrizio Passamonti
Department of Veterinary Medicine, University of Perugia, Perugia, Italy

Michele Trotta and Caterina Fani
CDVet Laboratorio Analisi Veterinarie, Rome, Italy

Lucia Levorato
Department of Medicine and Surgery, University of Perugia, Perugia, Italy

Richard Webby
Department of Infectious Diseases, St. Jude Children's Research Hospital, Memphis, TN, United States

Faten A. Okda
Veterinary Division, National Research Center, Cairo, Egypt
Department of Infectious Diseases, St. Jude Children's Research Hospital, Memphis, TN, United States

Elizabeth Griffith
Department of Chemical and Therapeutic, St. Jude Children's Research Hospital, Memphis, TN, United States

Ahmed Sakr
Department of Business Administration and Management, Dakota State University, Madison, SD, United States

Eric Nelson
Veterinary & Biomedical Sciences Department, Animal Disease Research and Diagnostic Laboratory, South Dakota State University, Brookings, SD, United States

Lars E. Larsen
Department of Veterinary and Animal Sciences, University of Copenhagen, Copenhagen, Denmark

Bodil H. Nielsen
Department of Animal Science, Aarhus University, Aarhus, Denmark

Mette B. Petersen
Department of Veterinary Clinical Sciences, University of Copenhagen, Copenhagen, Denmark

Alicia F. Klompmaker, Maria Brydensholt, Anne Marie Michelsen, Matthew J. Denwood, Carsten T. Kirkeby, Lars Erik Larsen, Nina D. Otten and Liza R. Nielsen
Department of Veterinary and Animal Sciences, Faculty of Health and Medical Sciences, University of Copenhagen, Copenhagen, Denmark

Nicole B. Goecke
Department of Veterinary and Animal Sciences, Faculty of Health and Medical Sciences, University of Copenhagen, Copenhagen, Denmark
Centre for Diagnostics, Technical University of Denmark, Kongens Lyngby, Denmark

Zhong Peng, Fei Wang, Xueying Wang, Lin Hua, Huanchun Chen and Bin Wu
State Key Laboratory of Agricultural Microbiology, The Cooperative Innovation Center for Sustainable Pig Production, College of Animal Science and Veterinary Medicine, Huazhong Agricultural University, Wuhan, China

Junyang Liu, Li Wang and Jia Wang
Hubei Key Laboratory of Agricultural Bioinformatics, College of Informatics, Huazhong Agricultural University, Wuhan, China

Wan Liang
State Key Laboratory of Agricultural Microbiology, The Cooperative Innovation Center for Sustainable Pig Production, College of Animal Science and Veterinary Medicine, Huazhong Agricultural University, Wuhan, China
Key Laboratory of Prevention and Control Agents for Animal Bacteriosis (Ministry of Agriculture and Rural Affairs), Animal Husbandry and Veterinary Institute, Hubei Academy of Agricultural Sciences, Wuhan, China

Brenda A. Wilson
Department of Microbiology, School of Molecular and Cellular Biology, University of Illinois at Urbana-Champaign, Urbana, IL, United States

Héctor Puente, Héctor Argüello, Óscar Mencía-Ares, Manuel Gómez-García, Pedro Rubio and Ana Carvajal
Department of Animal Health, Faculty of Veterinary Medicine, Universidad de León, León, Spain

Jinhui Mai, Dongliang Wang, Yawen Zou, Sujiao Zhang, Chenguang Meng, Aibing Wang and Naidong Wang
Hunan Provincial Key Laboratory of Protein Engineering in Animal Vaccines, Laboratory of Functional Proteomics (LFP), Research Center of Reverse Vaccinology (RCRV), College of Veterinary Medicine, Hunan Agricultural University, Changsha, China

Timothy C. Cameron, Danielle Wiles and Travis Beddoe
Department of Animal, Plant and Soil Science, Centre for Agri Bioscience, La Trobe University, Melbourne, VIC, Australia
Centre for Livestock Interactions With Pathogens, La Trobe University, Melbourne, VIC, Australia

Alessandra Tata, Ivana Pallante, Andrea Massaro, Brunella Miano, Massimo Bottazzari, Paola Fiorini, Mauro Dal Prà, Laura Paganini, Annalisa Stefani, Roberto Piro and Nicola Pozzato
Istituto Zooprofilattico delle Venezie (IZSVe), Legnaro, Italy

Jeroen De Buck
Department of Production Animal Health, University of Calgary, Calgary, AB, Canada

Lei Qin
National Key Laboratory of Veterinary Biotechnology, Harbin Veterinary Research Institute, Chinese Academy of Agricultural Sciences, Harbin, China
College of Veterinary Medicine, Northeast Agricultural University, Harbin, China

Fandan Meng, Yong-Bo Yang, Gang Wang, Yan-Dong Tang, Mingxia Sun, Xuehui Cai and Shujie Wang
National Key Laboratory of Veterinary Biotechnology, Harbin Veterinary Research Institute, Chinese Academy of Agricultural Sciences, Harbin, China

Wenlong Zhang
College of Veterinary Medicine, Northeast Agricultural University, Harbin, China

Haijuan He
Institute of Animal Husbandry, Heilongjiang Academy of Agriculture Sciences, Harbin, China

Karin Lebl and Hartmut H. K. Lentz
Institute of Epidemiology, Friedrich-Loeffler-Institute, Greifswald, Insel Riems, Germany

Beate Pinior
Institute for Veterinary Public Health, University of Veterinary Medicine Vienna, Vienna, Austria

Thomas Selhorst
Unit Epidemiology, Statistics and Mathematical Modelling, Federal Institute for Risk Assessment, Berlin, Germany

Xilin Liu and Caixia Guo
Department of Hand Surgery, Presidents' Office of China-Japan Union Hospital of Jilin University, Changchun, China

Zeeshan Nawaz
Department of Microbiology, Government College University Faisalabad, Faisalabad, Pakistan

Sultan Ali
Faculty of Veterinary Science, Institute of Microbiology, University of Agriculture, Faisalabad, Pakistan

Muhammad Ahsan Naeem and Sarfraz Ahmed
Department of Basic Sciences, University College of Veterinary and Animal Sciences, Narowal, Pakistan

Tariq Jamil
Department of Clinical Sciences, Section of Epidemiology and Public Health, College of Veterinary and Animal Sciences, Jhang, Pakistan

Waqas Ahmad
Department of Clinical Sciences, University College of Veterinary and Animal Sciences, Narowal, Pakistan

Muhammad Usman Siddiq
Institute of Microbiology, University of Veterinary and Animal Sciences, Lahore, Pakistan

Muhammad Asif Idrees and Ali Ahmad
Department of Pathobiology, University College of Veterinary and Animal Sciences, Narowal, Pakistan

Sherif I. A. Mahmoud and Kamel A. Zyan
Department of Avian and Rabbit Diseases, Faculty of Veterinary Medicine, Benha University, Benha, Egypt

Mohamed M. Hamoud
Department of Poultry and Rabbit Diseases, Faculty of Veterinary Medicine, Cairo University, Giza, Egypt

Eman Khalifa
Department Microbiology, Faculty of Veterinary Medicine, Matrouh University, Matrouh, Egypt

Shahin Dardir and Rabab Khalifa
Department Veterinary Care and Laboratories Department, Cairo Poultry Corporate, Giza, Egypt

Walid H. Kilany
Reference Laboratory for Veterinary Quality Control on Poultry Production, Animal Health Research Institute, Agriculture Research Center, Ministry of Agriculture, Cairo, Egypt

Wael K. Elfeil
Department of Avian and Rabbit Department, Faculty of Veterinary Medicine, Suez Canal University, Ismailia, Egypt

Index